Handbook of
INFECTIOUS DISEASES

Handbook of
INFECTIOUS DISEASES

Springhouse Corporation
Springhouse, Pennsylvania

STAFF

Senior Publisher
Donna O. Carpenter

Creative Director
Jake Smith

Design Director
John Hubbard

Executive Editor
H. Nancy Holmes

Clinical Project Managers
Patricia K. Fischer, RN, BSN; Joan M. Robinson, RN, MSN, CCRN

Clinical Editors
Kim Marie Falk, RN, MSN; Gloria McCartney, RN, BSN;
John Taylor, RN, BS; Kimberly A. Zalewski, RN, MSN, CEN

Editors
Naina D. Chohan, Jane V. Cray, Peter H. Johnson,
Jennifer P. Kowalak, Jacqueline Elizabeth Mills, Teresa Point

Designers
Arlene Putterman (associate design director),
BJ Crim (book design), Kathy Singel (design project
manager), Joseph John Clark, Mary Ludwicki,
Donna S. Morris, Jeffrey Sklarow

Copy Editors
Catherine B. Cramer, Carolyn Edlund, Joy Epstein,
Dolores P. Matthews, Celia McCoy, Barbara F. Ritter

Electronic Production Services
Diane Paluba (manager), Joyce Rossi Biletz (technician)

Manufacturing
Deborah Meiris (director), Patricia K. Dorshaw (manager),
Otto Mezei (book production manager)

Editorial and Design Assistants
Carol Caputo, Arlene Claffee, Tom Hasenmayer,
Elfriede Young

Indexer
Ellen S. Brennan

Cover Illustration
Electron micrograph of human cultured cells infected
with adenovirus, magnified 2,650 times;
© Dr. Gopal Murti/Phototake

The clinical procedures described and recommended in this publication are based on research and consultation with nursing, medical, and legal authorities. To the best of our knowledge, these procedures reflect currently accepted practice; nevertheless, they can't be considered absolute and universal recommendations. For individual application, all recommendations must be considered in light of the patient's clinical condition and, before administration of new or infrequently used drugs, in light of the latest package-insert information. The authors and the publisher disclaim responsibility for any adverse effects resulting directly or indirectly from the suggested procedures, from any undetected errors, or from the reader's misunderstanding of the text.

Printed in the United States of America.

HID-D N

03 02 01 00   10 9 8 7 6 5 4 3 2 1

Library of Congress Cataloging-in-Publication Data
Handbook of infectious diseases.
      p. ; cm.
   Includes bibliographical references and index.
   ISBN 1-58255-070-0 (flexible cover)
   1. Communicable diseases — Handbooks, manuals, etc.
   I. Springhouse Corporation.
   [DNLM: 1. Communicable Diseases — Handbooks.
   WC 39 H2361 2000]
RC112.H26 2000
616.9 — dc21   00-058807

Contents

Contributors
and consultants

Heather Boyd-Monk, SRN, BSN, CRNO
Assistant Director of Nursing for
  Ophthalmic Education Programs
Wills Eye Hospital
Philadelphia, Pa.

Janice T. Chussil, MSN, RNC, DNC, ANP
Nurse practitioner
Dermatology Associates
Portland, Ore.

Joann Coleman, RN, MS, ACNP, AOCN
Acute Care Nurse Practitioner,
  Gastrointestinal Surgery
Johns Hopkins Hospital
Baltimore, Md.

Diane Dixon, PA-C, M.A.E., MMSc
Assistant Professor
University of Southern Alabama
Mobile, Ala.

Clare Edelmayer, RN, MT(ASCP), MS, CIC
Infection Control Coordinator
Doylestown Hospital
Doylestown, Pa.

Mary Ellen Kelly, RN, BSN
Director of Staff Development/Infection
  Control
John L. Montgomery Care Center
Freehold, N.J.

Margaret M. Klein, RN, BSN
Staff Nurse, Surgicenter
Warminster Hospital
Warminster, Pa.

Elaine G. Lange, RN, MSN, CCRN, ANP-C
Adult Nurse Practitioner
Deerfield Valley Health Center
Wilmington, Vt.

David J. Lash, PA-C, MPAS
Department Head
Medical Annex, Camp H.M. Smith
U.S. Navy
Hawaii

Ernest H. Leber, MD
Resident
Medical College of Pennsylvania
Department of Emergency Medicine
Philadelphia, Pa.

Roger M. Morrell, MD, PhD, FACP, FAIC
Neurologist
Lathrup Village, Mich.

JoAnne Murphy, RN, MSN
Clinical Editor/Clinical Instructor
Virtua Homecare/Helene Fold School
  of Nursing
Camden, NJ/Blackwood, N.J.

Glenn Nordehn, DO
Assistant Professor
University of Minnesota
Duluth, Minn.

Kristine Anne Bludau Scordo, PhD, RN-C,
  ACNP
Director Acute Care Nurse Practitioner
Wright State University
Dayton, Ohio

Michael L. Silverman, MD
Attending Physician, Infectious Disease
Presbyterian Medical Center
University of Pennsylvania
Philadelphia, Pa.

David Toub, MD
Consultant
Lansdale, Pa

Jacqueline H. Zaremba, RN, BSN, CCRN
RN Clinical Analyst
The Medical Center at Princeton
Princeton, N.J.

Foreword

Medical historians will likely cite advances in the field of infectious diseases as among the most important accomplishments in medicine in the 20th century. These advances have included the discovery of many pathogens, the recognition of associated clinical syndromes, and advances in diagnosis and therapy. The 20th century witnessed the advent of antimicrobial chemotherapy, and with it, the hope and hubris that infectious diseases might become a thing of the past.

The hope engendered by advances in antimicrobial chemotherapy has been quickly tempered in more recent years by the sobering emergence of resistance in many organisms. The past 20 years have taught us that microbes are smarter than humans. In the new millennium, new and emerging infections — such as human immunodeficiency virus, cryptosporidiosis, and the *sin nombre* virus that causes hantavirus pulmonary syndrome — will remain daunting challenges. New pathogens will undoubtedly be discovered and old pathogens will likely resurface. Antimicrobial resistance is currently problematic among many bacterial, parasitic, fungal, and viral pathogens; this is unlikely to change in the foreseeable future. Increasing worldwide travel and the global economy will force clinicians to consider exotic infectious diseases in their patients in the coming years, as evidenced by the recent outbreaks of West Nile encephalitis and cryptosporidiosis in the United States. In the 21st century, infectious diseases will continue to represent a major cause of morbidity and mortality worldwide, and will pose an ongoing challenge in recognition, diagnosis, and therapy for health care professionals.

The *Handbook of Infectious Diseases* is designed for busy practitioners, such as nurses, physicians, physician assistants, nurse practitioners, and other health care professionals, who seek a broad-based yet concise and up-to-date reference. An introductory chapter discusses basic concepts of infection followed by more than 200 infectious diseases, arranged alphabetically for ease of reference. Each disease entry includes a concise discussion of its importance, common causes, associated signs and symptoms, methods of diagnosis, treatment, and special considerations.

Following the section on specific infections is a treatment guide to more than 150 anti-infective drugs, organized by therapeutic category. Each drug entry covers the drug's generic and brand names, pregnancy risk category, forms, actions, indications, contraindications, and dosage.

Also covered are possible adverse reactions, interactions, and effect on diagnostic tests. Special considerations discuss such information as patient age concerns, dosage timing, administration, and patient care and counseling.

The book is user friendly, with liberal use of bulleted information, charts, and highlighted take-home messages. The appendices discuss current immunization recommendations, national guidelines for standard and transmission-based precautions, infectious diseases that must be reported, alternative therapies for selected infections, and an overview of more than 75 rare infectious diseases.

Not meant to be an exhaustive textbook of infectious diseases, the *Handbook of Infectious Diseases* is nevertheless an extremely practical and useful source that the busy health care professional can use to retrieve clinically relevant information regarding the major infectious diseases encountered in clinical practice.

David L. Longworth, MD
Chairman,
Department of Infectious Diseases
The Cleveland Clinic Foundation
Cleveland, Ohio

UNDERSTANDING
INFECTION

Despite improved methods for treating and preventing infection — potent antibiotics, complex immunizations, and modern sanitation — infection remains the most common cause of human disease. Even in countries with advanced medical care, infections are a major cause of death.

Produced by such pathogens as bacteria, viruses, and fungi, infections may range from relatively mild illnesses (the common cold, for instance) to debilitating conditions such as chronic hepatitis to fatal diseases such as acquired immunodeficiency syndrome (AIDS).

Although large epidemics are rare in the United States, influenza still sweeps through parts of the country. In underdeveloped nations, cholera and malaria claim millions of lives every year. In addition, emerging new diseases threaten to trigger deadly worldwide epidemics, as AIDS has done.

Infections can have devastating effects in the health care setting, where a combination of circumstances leaves patients especially vulnerable. Hospitalized patients are commonly exposed to a wide range of microbes at a time when they're least able to fight them. Already under the stress brought on by illness and hospitalization, their defense mechanisms may be further taxed by surgery, drug treatment, or invasive procedures, which compromise skin integrity and may allow microbes to enter the body. Thus, many patients who don't have infections when admitted to a health care facility are at risk of developing them during their stay.

WHAT IS INFECTION?

Infection is the invasion and multiplication of microbes in or on body tissues, resulting in signs and symptoms as well as an immunologic response. Microbial reproduction injures the patient either by competing with host metabolism or by causing cellular damage from toxins produced by the microbe or from intracellular multiplication. The patient's own immune response may compound the tissue damage; such damage may be localized (as in an infected pressure ulcer) or systemic. The severity of the infection varies with the disease-producing ability and number of the invading microbes, the strength of host defenses, and various other factors.

Communicable and contagious diseases

A communicable disease is transmitted from one person to another. Childhood diseases such as chickenpox, measles, and mumps are considered communicable.

A contagious disease is a communicable disease that is easily transmitted from one person to another. Influenza and Norwegian scabies are examples.

Why outbreaks occur

Many infectious diseases are now preventable or treatable with antibiotics and other effective therapies. Yet infection remains a problem in all societies. There are many complex reasons why the microbes that cause infectious diseases are so difficult to overcome.

▶ Some bacteria develop a resistance to antibiotics — a growing problem. (See *When microbes grow resistant.*)
▶ Some microbes such as influenza virus have so many different strains that a single vaccine can't protect against them all.
▶ Most viruses resist antiviral drugs.
▶ New infectious agents, such as human immunodeficiency virus (HIV) and *Legionella*, occasionally arise.
▶ Some microbes localize in areas of the body that make treatment difficult, including bone and the central nervous system.
▶ Opportunistic microbes can cause infections in immunocompromised patients.
▶ Much of the world's ever-increasing population has not received immunizations.

WHEN MICROBES GROW RESISTANT

Over the last few decades, many microbes have developed resistant strains — those that won't succumb to the antibiotics normally used to combat them. Resistant strains pose serious problems for health care facilities and for the general population because the infections are increasingly difficult to treat.

REASONS FOR RESISTANT STRAINS

Practices by health care professionals, patients, and certain industries have contributed to the emergence of resistant bacterial strains. These practices include:
▶ unnecessary use of antibiotics
▶ inappropriate prescribing of antibiotics (such as prescribing a drug that doesn't specifically combat the infecting organism)
▶ patient failure to complete the full course of antibiotic treatment
▶ use of antibiotics in animal feed.

Contributing to the problem are easy access to over-the-counter antibiotics (in many countries) and symptomless carriers who harbor and spread resistant microbes.

FROM ADAPTATION TO RESISTANCE

A microbe develops resistance by continuously adapting to the changing environment in an effort to survive. Through adaptation, some microbes have developed the ability to enzymatically destroy an antibiotic, such as by inducing cellular or metabolic changes at target areas.

Some bacteria decrease cellular intake of a drug. Others have receptor sites on the bacteria that have less attraction for a drug.

New strains of gonococci emerging during the last 20 years are resistant to the antibiotics typically recommended for gonorrhea treatment. Penicillin was the drug of choice until a resistant strain developed in 1976;

tetracycline-resistant *Neisseria gonorrhoeae* emerged in 1986. Consequently, eradicating endemic antibiotic-resistant gonorrhea is now difficult.

HEREDITARY RESISTANCE

Hereditary drug resistance is commonly carried by extrachromosomal genetic elements with cell resistance (R) factors. These factors can be transferred among bacterial cells in a population and between different, but closely related, bacteria populations.

EFFECTS OF HOSPITALIZATION

Lengthy hospital stays and frequent hospitalization place some patients at special risk for drug-resistant infections. Most vulnerable are the very young, the very old, the seriously ill, or those using invasive equipment such as drains and ventilation equipment. Many of these patients already have weakened immune systems, making them all the more susceptible.

ANTIBIOTIC THERAPY

Persons already taking antibiotics are at an increased risk of infection by resistant microbes because the antibiotic kills off susceptible microbes, allowing resistant strains to take hold.

STRIKING BACK

When an outbreak of a resistant microbe occurs, researchers use molecular typing techniques to identify the microbe, track it to the source, and contain it. Medicine has managed to stay just ahead of resistant microbes, thanks to the development of new antibiotic drugs. But recently, some microbes have emerged that resist all antibiotics. Some experts even fear that most infections may eventually result from drug-resistant microbes.

SPORADIC, EPIDEMIC, OR ENDEMIC?

To determine if an infection problem exists in a particular health care facility or geographic area, investigators study the current incidence of the disease in that facility or area and compare it to past incidence rates.

SPORADIC DISEASES
If investigators find cases occurring occasionally and irregularly with no specific pattern, they classify the infection as sporadic. Examples of diseases that typically occur sporadically are tetanus and gas gangrene.

EPIDEMIC DISEASES
If a greater-than-expected number of cases of a given disease arises suddenly in a specific area over a specific period, investigators label it an epidemic. A highly publicized epidemic occurred during an American Legion convention in Philadelphia in 1976, resulting in the naming of a new illness, Legionnaire's disease.

A *pandemic* is an epidemic that affects several countries or continents. A current example is the ac-

quired immunodeficiency syndrome pandemic.

ENDEMIC DISEASES
Endemic diseases are those that are present in a population or community at all times. They usually involve relatively few people during a specified time. Hepatitis B, for example, is endemic in certain Asian cultures.

HERD IMMUNITY
When a high proportion of a population has developed immunity to a specific infectious agent, herd immunity exists. For example, thanks to the measles vaccine, the population of the United States has herd immunity to measles, and most Americans are able to resist it.

▶ Increased air travel by the world's population can speed a virulent microbe to a heavily populated urban area within hours.
▶ The use of biological warfare and bioterrorism with organisms such as anthrax, plague, and smallpox is an increasing threat to public health and safety throughout the world.
▶ The expanded use of immunosuppressive drugs and invasive procedures increase the risk of infection for many.

HOW INFECTION IS STUDIED

The study of infection involves three major disciplines: microbiology, epidemiology, and immunology. Microbiologists study infectious microbes and their effects on the body. Epidemiologists investigate the factors that influence the frequency

and distribution of diseases and their causes in a defined population, with the goal of establishing programs to prevent and control their development and spread. Immunologists study the body's responses to antigenic challenges, specifically those involving the immune mechanisms.

Determining morbidity
Morbidity rates indicate the frequency of an illness within a given population. For infections, the most useful types of morbidity rates are incidence and prevalence. Incidence is an expression of the rate of new cases of a disease in a given population over a specified period. (See S*poradic, epidemic, or endemic?*) When used in hospital infection surveillance programs, incidence reflects the number of new cases of a particular disease in the hospital population during a given time period.

Prevalence is the number of cases—both old and new—of a given disease occurring in a certain population over a specified period.

NORMAL MICROBIAL FLORA

Large numbers of microbes exist in the air we breathe, on the surfaces we touch, and on and within our bodies. Microbes naturally found on and within the body are called normal flora; they concentrate in certain body regions, such as the skin, mouth, and GI tract. (See *Where normal flora live.*) The skin harbors more than 10,000 microbes/cm^2; scrapings from the surface of the teeth or gums may show millions of organisms per mg of tissue.

The human body and its normal flora live together in a sort of ecosystem whose equilibrium is essential to health. Under normal circumstances, these microbes are nonpathogenic and harmless. In fact, they may aid the body by competing for nutrients with disease-producing microbes or by performing special tasks; in the lumen of the bowel, for instance, resident microbes carry out many chemical functions. Moreover, disruption of the normal ecology of the microbial flora can pose substantial risks to the host. (See *How microbes interact with the body,* page 6.)

Only relatively few of the many species of microbes living in the environment become adapted to the environments of various body tissues. Thus, to a certain degree, the flora of a given species—even of specific body tissues—is predictable.

HOW INFECTION OCCURS

Whether or not an infection develops hinges on variables relating to three crucial factors:
▶ an infectious organism (pathogen)
▶ a host (any organism that can support the nutritional and physical growth of another organism)

WHERE NORMAL FLORA LIVE

Normal microbial flora occur in the regions of the body identified here. At any given time, certain species of microbes may dwell in these regions.

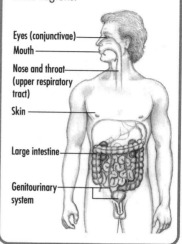

Eyes (conjunctivae)
Mouth
Nose and throat (upper respiratory tract)
Skin
Large intestine
Genitourinary system

▶ a favorable environment.

As long as all three factors are in balance, infection does not occur. However, if an imbalance develops—for example, if a patient's immune system is suppressed and can't fight off pathogens—the potential for infection increases.

Infection starts when a microbe invades body tissues. Once the microbe breaches the patient's immune defenses and enters the body, it multiplies and causes harmful effects. The severity of the infection depends on such factors as microbial characteristics, the number of microbes present, and the way in which the microbes enter the body and spread.

The inflammatory response

The body reacts to microbial invasion by producing an inflammatory response. The five classic signs and symptoms of inflammation are pain, heat, redness,

HOW MICROBES INTERACT WITH THE BODY

Microbes may interact with their host in various ways. For instance, some species of the normal human flora interact with the body in a mutually beneficial way. *Escherichia coli* bacteria, common in the normal intestinal flora, obtain nutrients from the human host; in return they secrete vitamin K, which the body needs for blood clotting.

Other normal body microbes live as commensals — while only they gain a benefit from the relationship, they do not harm the body.

PARASITIC INTERACTION

Some pathogenic organisms, such as helminths (worms), are parasites. They derive benefit from their interaction with the body but cause harm to it as well. For instance, the *Trichinella* worm severely damages the muscle tissues in which it lives.

---

swelling, and disordered function. Other manifestations include fever, malaise, nausea, vomiting, and purulent discharge from wounds.

Not all infections are apparent or symptomatic. With subclinical, or asymptomatic, infection, the infectious microbe is present and an immune system response is initiated, but the person shows no signs or symptoms of the disease. (See *Types of infection*.)

Endogenous and exogenous microbes

Microbes may be endogenous or exogenous. Endogenous microbes are found on the skin and in such body substances as saliva, feces, and sputum. They can cause disease in a susceptible individual.

Exogenous microbes originate from sources outside the body. Usually, humans and exogenous microbes live together in harmony. However, if something disrupts this harmonious relationship, the microbes may cause infection.

Invasion and colonization

The presence of microbes in or on an individual is called colonization. Colonized microbes grow and multiply but may not invade tissue and thus don't produce cellular injury. In these cases colonization results in positive results on tissue cultures, but the patient lacks evidence of infection.

However, some people who are colonized with bacteria do develop localized signs and symptoms of infection — tenderness, swelling, redness, and pus — because the bacteria has invaded the tissue, producing cellular injury. A culture of the pus typically elicits the microbe. Colonized bacteria may also cause systemic infection, producing fever, an elevated white blood cell count and possibly shock.

Pathogenicity

Pathogenicity refers to a microbe's ability to cause pathogenic changes, or disease. An example of a highly pathogenic microbe is the rabies virus; it always causes clinical disease in the host. In contrast, alpha-hemolytic streptococci have low pathogenicity; although they commonly colonize humans, they rarely produce clinical disease. Poliomyelitis and tuberculosis also have low pathogenicity.

Factors affecting pathogenicity include the microbe's mode of action, virulence, dose, invasiveness, toxigenicity, specificity, and antigenicity.

Mode of action

The means by which a microbe produces disease is called its mode of action. Viruses, for example, cause infection by invading host cells and interfering with cell metabolism. Other modes of microbial action include:

▶ evasion or destruction of host defenses by preventing host phagocytes (scavenger cells) from engulfing and digesting them (used by *Klebsiella pneumoniae*)

▶ secretion of enzymes or toxins, which allows the microbe to penetrate and spread through host tissues (used by the measles virus)

▶ production of toxins that interfere with intercellular responses (used by tetanus bacilli)

▶ stimulation of a pathologic immune response (used by group A beta-hemolytic streptococci)

▶ destruction of T-helper lymphocytes (used by HIV).

Virulence

Virulence refers to the degree of a microbe's pathogenicity. Virulence can vary with the condition of the body's defenses. For instance, *Mycobacterium avium-intracellulare* (MAI), a bacteria commonly found in water and soil, can cause severe pulmonary and systemic disease in AIDS patients. Virulence can be enhanced by several factors:

▶ toxins produced by bacteria such as Streptococci and *Clostridium*

▶ the ability of microorganisms to elude host defenses (*Pneumococcus* with its polysaccharide capsule)

▶ persistence in the environment (spores and cysts)

▶ genetic variation (influenza).

Dose

A microbe must be present in a sufficient dose to cause human disease. The size of the pathogenic dose varies from one microbe to the next and from person to person and may be affected by the mode of transmission. The patient's immune system also plays an important role in the pathogenic dose requirement.

TYPES OF INFECTION

A laboratory-verified infection that causes no signs and symptoms is called a *subclinical, silent, or asymptomatic infection*. A multiplication of microbes that produces no signs, symptoms, or immune response is called a *colonization*. A person with a subclinical infection or colonization may be a carrier and transmit infection to others.

A *latent infection* occurs after a microorganism has been dormant in the host, sometimes for years. An *exogenous infection* results from environmental pathogens; an *endogenous infection*, from the host's normal flora (for instance, *Escherichia coli* displaced from the colon may cause urinary tract infection).

Generally, the infective dose of hepatitis B virus is approximately 100,000 viral particles. The infective dose of *Salmonella* required to cause typhoid fever is 1,000 bacterial particles. The infective dose of hepatitis B viral particles is much smaller than that required to cause HIV infection. A lower infective dose does not necessarily imply that the organism causes more severe immediate disease.

Invasiveness

Invasiveness (sometimes called infectivity) refers to the ability of a microbe to invade tissues. Some microbes can enter the human body through intact skin; others can penetrate only through a break in the skin or mucous membranes. *Leptospira interrogans* usually enters the body through a minor skin abrasion; *Clostridium tetani*, through a deep puncture wound. The invasiveness of some microbes is increased by the enzymes they produce.

Toxigenicity

Toxigenicity, which is related to virulence, refers to a microbe's potential to damage host tissues by producing and releasing toxins. Some bacteria, such as diphtheria and tetanus, release exotoxins that are quickly disseminated in the blood, causing systemic and neurologic manifestations. Other bacteria, such as *Shigella*, release endotoxins that can cause diarrhea and shock.

Specificity

Specificity refers to the attraction of a microbe to a specific host or range of hosts. For example, the flavivirus that causes St. Louis encephalitis has a number of hosts including birds and humans; whereas rubeola, the virus that causes measles, is only carried by humans.

Viability

Viability refers to the ability of a microbe to survive outside the body. Microbes can live and multiply in a reservoir, which provides what the microbes need to survive. The microbes can then be transmitted from the reservoir to another person.

Antigenicity

Antigenicity, the degree to which a microbe can induce a specific immune response, varies among microbes. Those that invade and localize in tissue initially stimulate a cellular response, while those that disseminate more quickly generate an antibody response.

Bacterial resistance

Certain gram-positive microbes have become resistant to many of the antimicrobial drugs previously used to treat them. (See *Mechanisms of resistance.*) Resistant microbial strains that pose a serious challenge to health care facilities (especially acute-care hospitals and long-term care facilities) include methicillin-resistant *Staphylococcus aureus* (MRSA), resistant *Streptococcus pneumoniae,* and vancomycin-resistant *Enterococcus.* These strains, which are rapidly becoming part of the flora in many health care facilities, must be controlled to prevent hospital-acquired (nosocomial) infections.

Resistant Staphylococcus aureus infections

Staphylococcus aureus commonly occurs on the skin without producing any disease, but it can produce a variety of signs and symptoms ranging from a skin pustule to bloodstream infections and death. It's also a frequent cause of pneumonia, septicemia, and surgical site infections in hospitalized patients. Disease can also be caused by community-acquired infections.

Methicillin is an antibiotic commonly used to treat staph infections. Although methicillin is very effective in treating most staph infections, some staph bacteria have developed resistance to methicillin and can no longer be killed by this antibiotic. These methicillin-resistant *Staphylococcus aureus* (MRSA) infections account for approximately 40% of *S. aureus*-linked hospital infections.

The antibiotic used to treat MRSA infections is vancomycin. However, in 1996, an infection caused by a strain of *S. aureus* with reduced susceptibility to vancomycin was diagnosed in a patient in Japan. This strain of *S. aureus* was referred to as vancomycin intermediate resistant *S. aureus* or VISA. Since then several more infections with VISA have been identified.

A great concern among infectious disease experts is the emergence of a strain of *S. aureus* with full resistance to vancomycin. This could leave doctors with no antibiotics for the treatment of *S. aureus* infections.

Some persons are asymptomatic carriers of resistant *S. aureus,* with colonies in the nose and on the skin. The infection spreads from patient to patient, mainly on the hands of health care providers as they become contaminated during patient care.

Appropriate control measures to prevent the spread of MRSA and VISA include strict handwashing, barrier protection (gloves, gowns, and masks) and contact precautions.

Resistant Streptococcus pneumoniae infections

Streptococcus pneumoniae is the most common cause of bacterial pneumonia in the United States and is a major cause of ear infections, bloodstream infections, and meningitis. Each year, the microbe causes approximately 500,000 cases of pneumonia, 7 million ear infections, 50,000 bloodstream infections, and 3,000 cases of meningitis. Among older patients with S. pneumoniae–related bloodstream infections, roughly 40% die.

The emergence of drug-resistant S. pneumoniae has complicated the treatment of these infections. Authorities estimate that about 30% of S. pneumoniae microbes are now penicillin-resistant. Infections involving these microbes may eventually necessitate treatment with costly broad-spectrum antibiotics.

Resistant Enterococcal infections

Enterococci exist as part of the normal flora of the GI tract and female genital tract. Most enterococcal infections can be traced to endogenous sources. However, in the health care setting, patient-to-patient transmission of Enterococci can occur through direct contact with the hands of health care workers or indirectly through contaminated surfaces. This highlights the need for strict adherence to infection control measures such as handwashing and the use of gowns, gloves, and disinfectants.

Vancomycin-resistant Enterococcus infections

Vancomycin-resistant Enterococcus, a relatively new resistant organism, is causing great concern among infectious disease specialists. It's responsible for a rising

MECHANISMS OF RESISTANCE

Bacteria become resistant to antibiotics through several known mechanisms.

NATURAL RESISTANCE
Within a bacterial population, some microbes may have a natural resistance to a certain antibiotic. If so, the antibiotic will eliminate the sensitive microbe, leaving the resistant ones to proliferate. This is especially likely to occur in health care facilities.

MUTANT RESISTANCE
Within a population of bacteria, resistant mutants may arise spontaneously and then proliferate as described above.

GENETIC RESISTANCE
Drug resistance may be transferred from one microbe to another through the exchange of genes, called plasmids, that confer such resistance.

number of nosocomial infections over the past 5 years. Doctors lack effective antibiotics to treat vancomycin-resistant Enterococcus infections; most of these microbes also resist other drugs used against enterococcal infections. Also, there's a possibility that vancomycin-resistant genes present in the microbes may be transferred to other gram-positive microbes such as Staphylococcus aureus.

The risk of vancomycin-resistant Enterococcus colonization and infection is associated with the following conditions:
▶ previous vancomycin or multiple antimicrobial therapy, or both
▶ severe underlying disease
▶ immunosuppression
▶ intra-abdominal or cardiac surgery.

COMBATING RESISTANT ORGANISMS

In the past, medicine has been able to stay a step ahead of resistant strains thanks to the development of new drugs. Today, however, we may be losing the battle. This makes education — of both health care professionals and the public at large — the strongest weapon against the spread of resistant bacteria. Teaching efforts should center on proper antibiotic use and on hand washing and other measures that reduce the risk of transmission.

Using antibiotics properly

Not all bacterial infections warrant antibiotics. Doctors and other professionals with prescribing power must prescribe antibiotics only when warranted. Also, whenever possible, an exact bacteriological or antigenic diagnosis should be made before antibiotic treatment begins to avoid inappropriate drug therapy, which promotes drug resistance.

Promoting patient compliance

If your patient has been prescribed antibiotics, emphasize the importance of completing the entire course of therapy exactly as prescribed, even if the patient feels better. Caution against storing antibiotics in medicine cabinets, where they could deteriorate from heat, and warn patients never to take antibiotics that have been prescribed for another person.

Reducing the transmission risk

Keep in mind that MRSA is usually carried on the hands. Enterococci species are present in the bowel, and vancomycin-resistant *Enterococcus* lives on bed rails and equipment. Because these organisms can be spread to patients from your hands, wash your hands thoroughly and frequently — not just between patients but also between care activities involving the same patient.

Barrier precautions

Besides hand washing, precautions that reduce the risk of transmission include use of protective gear when appropriate. Gloves provide a physical barrier between the hands and the patient's skin and mucous membranes.

To avoid transferring an organism from one site to another on the same patient, always use a clean pair of gloves for each patient care activity. To protect yourself, be sure to wash your hands after removing gloves.

Gowns and aprons protect your clothing while providing a barrier against organisms. Masks and protective eyewear guard your face against anticipated splashes of blood and body fluids.

UNDERSTANDING THE CHAIN OF INFECTION

Knowing how infection occurs can help you prevent or control its spread. To better understand infection transmission, visualize it as a chain with the following six vital links:

- causative agent
- reservoir of infection
- portal of exit from the reservoir
- mode of transmission
- portal of entry into the body
- susceptible individual (host).

Each link must be present for the infection to proceed. Therefore, breaking any of the links can prevent the infection. (See *The fragile chain of infection*.)

Causative agent

The causative agent for infection is any microbe capable of producing disease. Forms of microbes responsible for infectious diseases include bacteria, viruses, rickettsiae, chlamydiae, fungi (yeasts and molds), protozoa, and parasites. Larger

THE FRAGILE CHAIN OF INFECTION

An infection can occur only if the six components described here are present. Removing any one link prevents the infection.

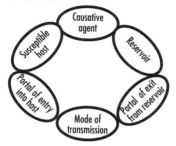

CAUSATIVE AGENT
A causative agent for infection is any microbe capable of producing disease.

RESERVOIR
The reservoir is the environment or object in or on which a microbe can survive and, in some cases, multiply. Inanimate objects, human beings, and other animals can all serve as reservoirs, providing the essential requirements for a microbe to survive at specific stages in its life cycle.

PORTAL OF EXIT
The portal of exit is the path by which an infectious agent leaves its reservoir. Usually, this portal is the site where the organism grows. Common portals of exit associated with human reservoirs include the respiratory, genitourinary, and GI tracts; the skin and mucous membranes; and the placenta (in transplacental disease transmission from other to fetus). Blood, sputum, emesis, stool, urine, wound drainage, and genital secretions also serve as portals of exit. The portal of exit varies from one infectious agent to the next.

MODE OF TRANSMISSION
The mode of transmission is the means by which the infectious agent passes from the portal of exit in the reservoir to the susceptible host. Infections can be transmitted through one of four modes: contact, airborne, vehicle, and vector-borne. Some organisms use more than one transmission mode to get from the reservoir to a new host. As with portals of exit, the transmission mode varies with the specific microbe.

Contact transmission is subdivided into direct contact, *indirect contact,* and droplet spread (contact with droplets that enter the environment). *Direct contact* refers to person-to-person spread of organisms through actual physical contact. *Indirect contact* occurs when a susceptible person comes in contact with a contaminated object. *Droplet transmission* results from contact with contaminated respiratory secretions. Droplet transmission differs from airborne transmission in that the droplets don't remain suspended in the air but settle to surfaces.

Airborne transmission occurs when fine microbial particles containing pathogens remain suspended in the air for a prolonged period, and then are spread widely by air currents and inhaled.

A *vehicle* is a substance that maintains the life of the microbe until it's ingested or inoculated into the susceptible host. The vehicle isn't harmful in itself but may harbor pathogenic microbes and thus serve as an agent of disease transmission. Examples of vehicles are water, blood, serum, plasma, medications, food, and feces.

Vector-borne transmission occurs when an intermediate carrier, or vector, such as a flea or a mosquito,

THE FRAGILE CHAIN OF INFECTION (continued)

transfers a microbe to another living organism. Vector-borne transmission is of most concern in tropical areas, where insects commonly transmit disease.

PORTAL OF ENTRY

Portal of entry refers to the path by which an infectious agent invades a susceptible host. Usually, this path is the same as the portal of exit.

SUSCEPTIBLE HOST

A susceptible host is also required for the transmission of infection. The human body has many defense mechanisms for resisting the entry and multiplication of pathogens. When these mechanisms function normally, infection doesn't occur. However, in a weakened host, an infectious agent is more likely to invade the body and launch an infectious disease.

---

organisms such as helminths (worms) may also cause infection. Each of these agents has its own mode of survival.

Bacteria

Bacteria are simple, one-celled microbes with a double cell membrane that protects them from many of the body's defense mechanisms. Although they lack a nucleus, bacteria possess all the other mechanisms they need to survive and rapidly reproduce. In developing countries, where poor sanitation predisposes the population to infection, bacterial diseases are prevalent causes of death and disability. Even in industrialized countries, bacterial infections are the most common fatal infectious diseases.

Bacteria can be classified according to shape. Spherical bacterial cells are called *cocci;* rod-shaped bacteria, *bacilli;* and spiral-shaped bacteria, *spirillae.* Bacteria can also be classified according to their need for oxygen (aerobic or anaerobic); their response to staining (gram-positive, gram-negative, or acid-fast); their motility (motile or nonmotile); their tendency to capsulation (encapsulated or nonencapsulated); and their capacity to form spores (sporulating or nonsporulating).

Spirochetes

Spirochetes are bacteria with flexible, slender, undulating spiral rods that possess cells walls. Most spirochetes are anaerobic. Three forms of spirochetes that cause disease in humans include *Treponema, Leptospira,* and *Borrelia.*

Mycoplasma

Mycoplasma, a genus of bacteria-like organisms, is the smallest of the cellular microbes that can live outside a living cell. Lacking cell walls, it can assume various distinct shapes ranging from coccoid to filamentous. Absence of cell walls also gives it resistance to penicillin and other antibiotics that work by inhibiting cell wall synthesis.

Mycoplasma organisms may be free-living or parasitic and are capable of causing disease in many animals and some plants. In humans, they are responsible for primary atypical pneumonia as well as many secondary infections.

How bacteria produce disease

Bacteria damage body tissues by interfering with essential cell function or by releasing toxins that cause cell damage. (See *How bacteria damage tissue.*) Several types of bacterial toxins exist.

HOW BACTERIA DAMAGE TISSUE

The human body is constantly infected by bacteria and other infectious microbes. Some are beneficial, such as the intestinal bacteria that produce vitamins. Others are harmful, causing illnesses ranging from the common cold to life-threatening septic shock.

To infect the body, bacteria must first enter it. They do this either by adhering to the mucosal surface and directly invading the cell or by attaching to epithelial cells and producing toxins, which invade adjacent cells. The result is a disruption of normal cell function or cell death (see illustration below). For example, the diphtheria toxin damages heart muscle by inhibiting protein synthesis. In addition, as some microbes multiply, they extend into deeper tissue and eventually gain access to the bloodstream.

Some toxins cause blood to clot in small blood vessels. The tissues supplied by these vessels may be deprived of blood and damaged (see illustration below).

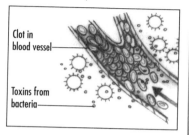

Other toxins can damage the cell walls of small blood vessels, causing leakage. This fluid loss results in decreased blood pressure, which in turn impairs the heart's ability to pump enough blood to vital organs (see illustration below).

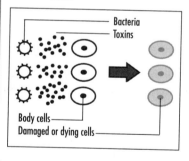

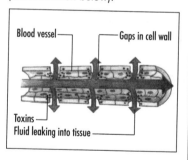

▶ *Exotoxins.* Most exotoxins are proteins released from bacterial cells into the surrounding medium. Diphtheria, botulism, and tetanus are examples of diseases caused by bacterial exotoxins.

▶ *Enterotoxins. Staphylococcus aureus, Vibrio cholerae, Shigella dysenteriae,* and other microbes that live in the GI tract secrete enterotoxins, which are exotoxins that affect the vomiting centers of the brain and cause gastroenteritis.

▶ *Endotoxins.* The cell walls of gram-negative bacteria contain endotoxins that cause disease when microbes are present in large numbers, typically inducing fever, vomiting, and diarrhea. Diseases associated with such endotoxins include septic shock, meningitis, and cholera.

Viruses
Perhaps the most common pathogens, viruses are subcellular microbes made up

only of a nucleus of deoxyribonucleic acid or ribonucleic acid surrounded by a protein coat. The smallest known microbes, they range from 0.02 mm to 0.3 mm — so tiny they're visible only through an electron microscope. Viruses can't replicate independently of host cells. Rather, they invade a host cell and stimulate it to participate in the formation of additional virus particles. Some viruses destroy surrounding tissue and release toxins. (See *Viral infection of a host cell*.)

Viruses lack the genes necessary for energy production. They depend on the ribosomes and nutrients of infected cells for protein production.

The estimated 400 viruses that infect humans are classified by size, shape (spherical, rod-shaped, or cubic), or means of transmission (respiratory, fecal, oral, or sexual).

Viral diseases
Viruses can produce a wide variety of illnesses. Clinical effects depend on the status of the host cell, the specific virus, and the environment. For instance, varicella zoster, a herpes virus, can cause chickenpox in the active stage or zoster (shingles) in the latent stage.

The immune system rapidly controls some viral invasions, producing permanent immunity to that particular virus. For example, a person who gets sick with the measles or receives measles immunization becomes permanently immune to the measles virus.

Other viruses, such as the Epstein-Barr virus (the virus that causes mononucleosis) and varicella zoster, remain in the body for months or years after the initial infection. Most of the time, the person's immune system controls the infection; however, during times of lowered resistance, the disease may reappear.

Most viruses enter the body through the respiratory, GI, or genital tract. A few, such as HIV, are transmitted in blood and body fluids.

Rickettsiae
Relatively uncommon in the United States, rickettsiae are small, gram-negative, bacteria-like microbes that can induce life-threatening infections. They may be round, rod-shaped, or irregularly shaped.

Like viruses, rickettsiae require a host cell for replication. Because of their leaky cell membranes, they must live inside another cell to retain all the necessary cellular substances.

Rickettsiae are transmitted through the bites of arthropod carriers, such as lice, fleas, and ticks, as well as through waste products. Three genera of rickettsiae include *Rickettsia, Coxiella,* and *Rochalimaea.*

Rickettsial diseases
Rickettsial infections that occur in the United States include Rocky Mountain spotted fever (*Rickettsia rickettsii*), typhus (*R. typhi*), and Q fever (*Coxiella burnetii*).

Chlamydiae
Chlamydiae are smaller than rickettsiae and bacteria but larger than viruses. They, too, depend on host cells for replication, but unlike viruses, they are susceptible to antibiotics.

Lacking the enzymes to perform many essential metabolic activities, Chlamydiae live off other organisms as intracellular parasites. After invading the host cell, they produce offspring, which are then released by cell rupture. The offspring, capable of living outside the cell, commonly serve as infectious particles.

Chlamydial infections
Chlamydiae are transmitted by direct contact such as occurs during sexual activity. They are a common cause of infections of the urethra, bladder, fallopian tubes, and prostate gland.

The most common type of chlamydial infection is the sexually transmitted disease caused by *Chlamydia trachomatis* (which also causes conjunctivitis and pneumonitis). In underdeveloped countries, *C. trachomatis* causes trachoma, a leading cause of blindness. Birds may transmit another species, *Chlamydia psittaci,* which can lead to an influenza-like disease called psittacosis.

Fungi

Fungi have rigid walls and nuclei that are enveloped by nuclear membranes. They occur as yeasts (single-celled, oval-shaped organisms) or molds (organisms with hyphae, or branching filaments). Depending on the environment, some fungi may occur in both forms.

Found almost everywhere on earth, fungi live on organic matter, in water and soil, on animals and plants, and on a wide variety of unlikely materials. For instance, fungi can cause deterioration of leather, plastics, and such foods as jam and pickles. They can also live inside and outside the human body.

Fungi are the vultures of the microbial world, obtaining nutrients from dead organic matter. They may be harmful or beneficial. Beneficial fungi are used in the production of cheeses, yogurt, beer, wine, and certain drugs (such as corticosteroids and penicillin).

One important function of fungi is breaking down plant matter. In fact, fungi are sometimes classified as plants because they have cell walls of cellulose or chitin. However, they lack chlorophyll, the green matter necessary for photosynthesis.

Fungal diseases

In humans, superficial fungal infections cause athlete's foot and vaginal infections. *Candida albicans,* part of the normal human flora, can cause yeast infection of the mouth, skin, vagina, GI tract, and virtually any other part of the body. *Histoplasma capsulatum* causes a systemic fungal infection carried by birds.

VIRAL INFECTION OF A HOST CELL

The virion becomes attached to receptors on the host cell's plasma membrane and releases enzymes that weaken the membrane, allowing the virion to penetrate the cell.

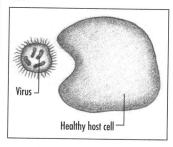

Virus

Healthy host cell

The virion uncoats itself and replicates within the host cell.

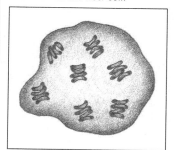

New virus particles mature within the cell and escape by budding from the plasma membrane. The viruses then infect other host cells.

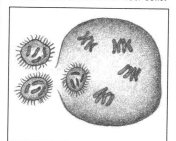

Patients at special risk for fungal infections include those receiving chemotherapy, steroid therapy, prolonged I.V. therapy, total parenteral nutrition, and other long term therapies. Patients receiving antibiotics are also at increased risk because these drugs suppress bacteria, which allows for an overgrowth of *Candida*.

Protozoa

Much larger than bacteria, protozoa are the simplest single-celled organisms of the animal kingdom. Although outwardly simple, protozoa show a high level of cellular specialization. Their cells have membranes rather than walls, and their nuclei are surrounded by nuclear membranes.

Protozoa are grouped according to their method of locomotion or the presence or absence of cilia and flagella. Most protozoa are free-living organisms found in soil and water. They lack chlorophyll and cannot make their own foods by photosynthesis. Some ingest algae, yeasts, bacteria, and smaller protozoans; others live on decaying organic matter. Parasitic protozoa absorb nutrients from the body of the host.

Although a few protozoa are pathogens, others cause no harm and a few are even beneficial to the host. For instance, protozoa that live in the intestines of termites digest the wood eaten by the termite, then return the nutrients to the termite.

Protozoal diseases

Worldwide, protozoa are important infectious agents, causing malaria and schistosomiasis. Giardiasis, caused by the protozoal species *Giardia lamblia*, has occurred in hikers after they drank untreated surface water and in children who attended certain day care centers. Trichomonas, a common sexually transmitted disease, is caused by *Trichomonas vaginalis*. Many AIDS patients and other immunocompromised persons develop serious infections from *Pneumocystis carinii*, *Cryptosporidium*, and *Toxoplasma gondii*.

Protozoal diseases are difficult to control because the microbes can evade the body's immune response and can adapt easily to different host environments. Many protozoa produce infection by depressing immune function, thereby limiting the body's ability to fight infection.

Parasites

Parasites are multicellular organisms that live on or within another organism and obtain nourishment from that organism. Parasites usually do not kill their hosts, but take only the nutrients they need.

Examples of parasites include helminths, such as pinworms and tapeworms, which infect the human GI tract, and arthropods, such as mites, fleas, and ticks, which commonly cause skin disease and systemic disease.

Parasitic diseases

In the United States, treatment of water and sewage keeps parasitic infections to a minimum. However, travelers to other countries and campers in areas with contaminated water may become ill with parasitic diseases such as schistosomiasis.

Infections caused by normal flora

Sometimes, microbes that are part of the normal flora of one body region can act as pathogens when transferred to another region. For instance, under the right conditions, *Neisseria meningitidis*, part of the normal respiratory tract flora, can cause meningitis if transferred to the spinal canal due to a wound or another infection. *Escherichia coli*, part of the normal GI tract flora, can cause infection if transferred to the bladder, such as by an indwelling urinary catheter.

RESERVOIR OF INFECTION

The second link in the chain of infection is the reservoir — the environment or object in or on which a microbe can survive and, in some cases, multiply. Inanimate objects, humans, and other animals can all serve as reservoirs, providing the essential requirements for a microbe to survive at specific stages in its life cycle.

Here are some examples of reservoirs for specific infectious agents:

▶ *Salmonella* survives and multiplies in milk.

▶ *Pseudomonas* survives and multiples in reservoir humidifiers.

▶ The hepatitis A virus survives but does not multiply in clams.

▶ The hepatitis B virus survives but does not multiply on the surfaces of hemodialysis machines.

Infectious reservoirs abound in health care settings, and may include everything from patients, visitors, and staff members to furniture, medical equipment, medications, food, water, and blood.

Cases and carriers

A human reservoir may be either a case or a carrier. A *case* is a patient with an acute clinical infection such as chickenpox. A *carrier* is a person colonized by a specific microbe but showing no signs or symptoms of infection. A carrier may have a subclinical or asymptomatic infection, such as in certain types of hepatitis. One of the most famous carriers in history, known as Typhoid Mary, transmitted the typhoid fever microbe (*Salmonella typhi*) to many people but wasn't ill with the disease herself.

Types of carriers

Carriers fall into four categories.

▶ An *incubatory carrier* — one who is incubating the illness — has acquired the infection but does not yet show symptoms. Incubation periods vary from one infectious organism to the next; a person may incubate chickenpox for 2 to 3 weeks.

▶ A *convalescent carrier* is in the recovery stage of an illness but continues to shed the pathogenic organism — perhaps for an indefinite period. A patient who has had a *Salmonella* infection commonly sheds the organism in feces even after symptoms disappear.

▶ An *intermittent carrier* occasionally sheds the pathogenic organism. Some people are intermittent carriers of *S. aureus*.

▶ A *chronic* or *sustained carrier* always has the infectious organism in his system. Some people are chronic carriers of hepatitis B; their blood harbors the hepatitis B surface antigen for years.

PORTAL OF EXIT

The portal of exit, the third link in the chain of infection, is the path by which an infectious agent leaves its reservoir. Usually, this portal is the site where the organism grows.

Common portals of exit associated with human reservoirs include the respiratory, genitourinary, and GI tracts; the skin and mucous membranes; and the placenta (in transplacental disease transmission from mother to fetus). Blood, sputum, emesis, stool, urine, wound drainage, and genital secretions also serve as portals of exit.

The portal of exit varies from one infectious agent to the next. The respiratory tract is the portal for the microbes that cause tuberculosis and the common cold; the GI tract, for those that produce typhoid fever.

MODE OF TRANSMISSION

The mode of transmission is the means by which the infectious agent passes from the portal of exit from the reservoir to the susceptible host. Of the six links in the chain of infection, the mode of transmission is the easiest link to break.

Infections can be transmitted through one of four modes: contact, airborne, vehicle, and vector-borne. Some microbes use more than one transmission mode to get from the reservoir to a new host.

As with portals of exit, the transmission mode varies with the specific microbe. For example, chickenpox and rubella are transmitted by contact; tuberculosis, by the airborne mode; cholera, by vehicle; and Lyme disease, by vector.

Contact transmission

Contact is the most common mode of infection transmission in health care settings. Contact transmission is subdivided into direct contact, indirect contact, and droplet spread (contact with droplets that occur from coughs and sneezes).

Direct contact

Direct contact refers to person-to-person spread of organisms through actual physical contact. Microbes with a direct mode of transmission can be transferred during such patient care activities as bathing, dressing changes, and insertion of invasive devices if the health care provider's hands or gloves are contaminated.

Diseases that spread by direct contact include herpes simplex (if direct contact with infected oral lesions or secretions occurs), and scabies.

Indirect contact

Indirect contact occurs when a susceptible person comes in contact with a contaminated object. In health care settings, virtually any item could be contaminated with microbes — thermometers, syringes, endoscopes, irrigating solutions, urinary and intravascular catheters, respiratory equipment, diapers, and toys.

Droplet spread

Transmission by droplet spread results from contact with contaminated respiratory secretions. A person with a droplet-spread infection coughs, sneezes, or talks, releasing infected secretions that spread through the air to the oral or nasal mucous membranes of a person nearby. Microbes carried in mucus droplets can travel up to about 3 feet (1 m).

Droplet transmission differs from airborne transmission in that the droplets don't remain suspended in the air but settle on surfaces. Examples of diseases spread by droplets include influenza, pneumonia, and whooping cough.

Airborne transmission

Airborne transmission occurs when fine microbial particles or dust particles containing microbes remain suspended in the air for a prolonged period and then are spread widely by air currents and inhaled.

When a person with pulmonary tuberculosis coughs or sneezes, for instance, particles containing *Mycobacterium tuberculosis* are expelled into the air. The tiny particles remain suspended in the air for several hours and may cause infection when a susceptible person inhales them and the tubercle bacillus travels to the lung.

Vehicle transmission

A vehicle is a substance that maintains the life of the microbe until it's ingested or inoculated into a susceptible person. The vehicle is not harmful in itself but may harbor pathogenic microbes and thus serve as an agent of disease transmission. Examples of vehicles are water, blood, serum, plasma, medications, food, and feces. Vehicle transmission usually occurs in the community and is uncommon in the hospital setting.

Examples of transmission by vehicle include food-borne diseases such as salmonellosis and hepatitis A. Unwashed fruit and vegetables are likely vehicles. For instance, salmonellosis may occur if the outer skin of a cantaloupe grown in a field contaminated with *Salmonella* is cut before it's washed and the knife transfers the bacteria into the cantaloupe. Enteric transmission is a type of vehicle transmission.

Vector-borne transmission

Vector-borne transmission occurs when an intermediate carrier, or vector, such as a flea, tick, or a mosquito, transfers a microbe to another living organism. Vector-borne transmission is of most concern in tropical areas, where insects commonly transmit disease.

In the United States, vector-borne transmission is responsible for Lyme disease. The deer tick, the vector for Lyme disease, carries the pathogenic spirochete *Borrelia burgdorferi* in its saliva. The tick injects spirochete-laden saliva into a person's bloodstream when it bites.

Preventive measures

Much can be done to prevent transmission of infectious diseases:
▶ comprehensive immunization (including the required immunization of travelers to or emigrants from endemic areas)
▶ drug prophylaxis
▶ improved nutrition, living conditions, and sanitation
▶ correction of environmental factors.

Immunization can now control many diseases, including diphtheria, tetanus, pertussis, measles, rubella, some forms of meningitis, poliovirus, hepatitis B, pneumococcal pneumonia, influenza, rabies, and tetanus. Smallpox (variola) — which killed or disfigured millions — is believed to have been successfully eradicated by a comprehensive World Health Organization program of surveillance and immunization.

Vaccines — which contain live but attenuated (weakened) or killed microbes — and toxoids — which contain modified bacterial exotoxins — induce active immunity against bacterial and viral diseases by stimulating antibody formation. Natural active immunity is produced as a patient who has the disease forms antibodies against it, thus preventing recurrence of disease.

Immune globulins contain previously formed antibodies from hyperimmunized donors or pooled plasma and provide temporary passive immunity. Generally, passive immunization is used when active immunization is perilous or impossible or when complete protection requires both active and passive immunization. Maternal passive immunity crosses the placental barrier from mother to fetus and is also provided to the infant by antibodies present in breast milk.

Although prophylactic antibiotic therapy may prevent certain diseases, the risk of superinfection and the emergence of drug-resistant strains may outweigh the benefits, so prophylactic antibiotics are usually reserved for patients at high risk for exposure to dangerous infections. Antibiotic-resistant bacteria are on the rise mainly because antibiotics are misused and overused. Some bacteria, such as enterococci, have developed mutant strains that do not respond to antibiotic therapy.

PORTAL OF ENTRY

The portal of entry, the fifth link in the chain of infection, refers to the path by which an infectious agent invades a susceptible person. Usually, this path is the same as the portal of exit.

Typical portals of entry for specific microbes include the following:
▶ The microbes that cause tuberculosis, common colds, diphtheria, influenza, and whooping cough enter through the respiratory tract.
▶ Hepatitis B virus and HIV enter through the bloodstream or body fluids.
▶ *Salmonella* enters through the GI tract.
▶ The microbes responsible for gonorrhea and syphilis enter through the mucous membranes (usually those of the genitourinary tract).

▶ The rabies virus and *Clostridium tetani* (the microbe that causes tetanus) enter the body through puncture wounds.

SUSCEPTIBLE INDIVIDUAL

The final link in the chain of infection is a susceptible individual, or host. The human body has many defenses against the entry and multiplication of microbes. When these defenses function normally, infection does not occur. However, in a weakened host, a microbe is more likely to invade the body and launch an infectious disease.

Defense mechanisms

The body's defense mechanisms fall into two general categories: first-line and second-line.

First-line defenses

External and mechanical barriers — such as the skin, other body organs, and secretions — serve as the body's first line of defense. Intact skin, mucous membranes, certain chemical substances, specialized structures such as cilia, and normal microbial flora can stop pathogens from establishing themselves in the body. The gag and cough reflexes and GI tract peristalsis work to remove pathogens before they can establish a foothold.

Chemical substances that help prevent infection or inhibit microbial growth include secretions such as saliva, perspiration, and GI and vaginal secretions as well as interferon (a naturally occurring glycoprotein with antiviral properties).

Normal flora control the growth of potential pathogens through a mechanism called microbial antagonism. In this mechanism, they use nutrients that pathogens need for growth, compete with pathogens for sites on tissue receptors, and secrete naturally occurring antibiotics to kill the pathogens. When microbial antagonism is disturbed, such as by prolonged antibiotic therapy, an infection may develop; for example, antibiotic therapy may destroy the normal flora of the mouth, leading to overgrowth of *Candida albicans* and the development of thrush.

Second-line defenses

If an organism gets past the first line of defense — say, by entering the body through a break in the skin — white blood cells and the inflammatory response come into play. Because these components respond to any type of injury, their response is termed nonspecific.

The main function of the inflammatory response is to bring phagocytic cells (neutrophils and monocytes) to the inflamed area to destroy the invading microbes and rid the tissue spaces of dead and dying cells so that tissue repair can begin. Inflammation produces four cardinal signs and symptoms: redness, swelling, pain, and heat. The first three result from local vasodilation, fluid leakage into extravascular spaces, and blockage of lymphatic drainage. Pain results from tissue space distention caused by swelling and pressure and from chemical irritation of nociceptors (pain receptors).

By raising the body's temperature, fever defends against infection by enabling host defenses to inhibit the growth of pathogens. Certain microbes, such as *Cryptococcus,* are unable to replicate at body temperatures above 100.4° F (38° C).

The acute phase of the inflammatory response typically lasts 2 weeks; the subacute phase (a less intense version of the acute phase) lasts another 2 weeks.

A pathogen that gets past the body's nonspecific defenses confronts specific immune responses in the form of cell-mediated immunity or humoral immunity.

Cell-mediated immunity involves T cells (a type of white blood cell). Some T cells synthesize and secrete lymphokines. Others become killer (cytotoxic) cells, setting out to track down infected body cells. Once the infection is under control, suppressor T cells bring the immune response to a close.

Humoral immunity, mediated by antibodies, involves the action of B lymphocytes in conjunction with helper T cells. Antibodies produced in response to the infectious agent help fight the infection. In response to the effects of suppressor T cell activity, antibody production then wanes.

When defenses are impaired

Impaired host defenses can open the door to infection. Conditions that may weaken a person's defenses include poor hygiene, malnutrition, extremes of age, climate, inadequate physical barriers, inherited and acquired immune deficiencies, emotional and physical stressors, chronic disease, medical and surgical treatments, and inadequate immunization.

Hygiene

Poor hygiene increases the risk of infection because untended skin is more likely to crack and break, allowing microbes to enter. Also, dirty skin harbors transient microbes, and microbial colonization of the skin increases.

Good hygiene promotes normal host defenses. Washing (with the addition of topical moisturizers if necessary) lubricates the skin and maintains the epidermis against breaks. Removing microbial accumulations on clothing through frequent laundering is another important step toward controlling infection.

Nutrition

The body produces antibodies from proteins, which are obtained through nutritional intake. With inadequate protein, a malnourished person lacks the energy to mount an adequate attack against invading organisms.

Age

The very young and the very old are at higher risk for infection. The immune system doesn't fully develop until about age 6 months; at the infant's first exposure to an infectious agent, the infection usually wins out — especially if it's an upper respiratory infection, the most common type among toddlers. Also, young children tend to put toys and other objects in their mouths, play in the dirt, or soil their clothes with urine and feces, bringing further exposure to microbes.

Exposure to communicable diseases continues throughout childhood. Preschoolers are exposed in day care facilities; school-age children, in school. Skin diseases, such as impetigo and lice (scabies), commonly pass from one child to the next. Childhood accidents, such as abrasions, lacerations, and fractures, may also allow microbes to enter the body.

Lack of immunization contributes to childhood infection. Measles, virtually eradicated by the measles vaccine several decades ago, resurfaced in community outbreaks in 1988 and 1989. Its revival has been linked to lax immunization efforts and primary vaccine failure, particularly in those vaccinated before 1980. Some people have simply become careless about getting their children vaccinated.

At the opposite end of the age spectrum, advancing age is associated with declining immune system function as well as with chronic diseases that weaken host defenses. What's more, the increase in long term care facilities such as nursing homes and personal care units have added to the risk of disease transmission among the elderly.

INFECTIONS IN HEALTH CARE FACILITIES

In health care facilities, patients of all ages stand a higher chance for developing an infection. Invasive procedures and devices, drugs that suppress the immune system, increased use of blood products, and inhalation therapy add to the potential threat. Heroic techniques such as massive radical surgery with prolonged anesthesia and organ transplants also place tremendous stress on the patient's immune system. Poor aseptic technique by health care providers also increase the risk of infection.

Infections among patients in health care facilities are classified as nosocomial, community acquired, or iatrogenic.

▶ A *nosocomial infection* develops during the patient's stay and was not present or incubating at the time of admission. Most nosocomial infections appear before the patient is discharged, although some (such as hepatitis B and surgical wound infections) typically are incubating at discharge and don't become apparent until later.

▶ A *community-acquired infection* is present or incubating at the time of admission in a patient who has no history of previous admission to the same facility.

▶ An *iatrogenic infection* is caused by the actions or treatments of a health care provider. Such an infection may also represent a secondary condition caused by treatment of a primary condition. Depending on when an iatrogenic infection develops, it may be nosocomial or community acquired.

Nosocomial infections

Approximately 5% to 10% of hospitalized patients in the United States (roughly 2 million persons) develop nosocomial infections every year. The 11th leading cause of death in this country, nosocomial in-

fections directly cause 19,000 deaths and contribute to another 58,000.

Nosocomial infections lengthen patients' hospital stays and increase their risk of death. Diagnosing and treating them costs billions of dollars annually. The longer a patient remains in the hospital, the greater his chance for developing a nosocomial infection.

The microbes that flourish in health care settings, along with patients' weakened defense mechanisms, help set the stage for nosocomial infections. The microbes responsible for nosocomial infections may be either endogenous (from normal flora) or exogenous (from external sources). (See *A dangerous combination.*)

Invasion sites

Nosocomial infections most commonly invade the body through the urinary tract. Other common portals of entry include surgical wounds, the respiratory tract, and the bloodstream.

Urinary tract infections

UTIs account for 40% of nosocomial infections. These infections may lengthen a patient's hospital stay by 3.8 days and cost nearly $2 billion yearly to treat.

Most nosocomial UTIs develop after urinary tract manipulation. Evidence of UTI arises in 20% to 25% of the hospitalized patients who have an indwelling urinary catheter.

Normal bowel flora are also implicated in UTIs. These microbes can gain access to the urinary tract through the use of contaminated equipment or irrigant solutions, through inadequate cleaning at the time of catheter insertion, or from the unwashed hands of health care providers.

Respiratory infections

Most respiratory nosocomial infections are linked to respiratory devices used to aid breathing or administer medications. Pneumonia, the second most common nosocomial infection in the United States, typically lengthens a patient's hospital stay by 4 to 9 days and adds an extra $1.3 billion to U.S. health care costs every year.

Nosocomial pneumonia most commonly stems from gram-negative bacteria, although it can also result from other bacteria, fungi, and viruses. Typically, the pathogen invades the lower respiratory tract by one of three routes:

▶ aspiration of oropharyngeal organisms
▶ inhalation of aerosols contaminated with bacteria
▶ spread by the bloodstream from another infection site.

Surgical wound infections

The third most common type of nosocomial infection, surgical wound infections account for approximately 25% of all nosocomial infections and occur in about 5% to 12% of surgical patients. Such infections lengthen hospital stays by about 6 days.

Surgical wound infections can occur in the incision as well as in the deep tissues of a wound. Most are thought to originate from bacteria that enter the wound during surgery.

Bloodstream infections

Called bacteremia, nosocomial infections of the bloodstream account for about 6% of nosocomial infections. Bacteria and fungi are common culprits.

Although local infections outside the bloodstream are sometimes the source of the infection, most bacteremias (more than 75% of those seen in hospitals) are related to intravascular devices such as IV catheters. The microbe can move from the patient's skin to the catheter tip and along the outer surface of the catheter, then enter the bloodstream.

With the growing use of intravascular devices, the incidence of bloodstream infections has climbed. Studies indicate that the risk of bacteremia increases for every hour that an invasive device remains in a

A DANGEROUS COMBINATION

This diagram shows how the coexistence of three major factors — compromised host, microbes that flourish in health care settings, and the chain of infection transmission — can combine to cause nosocomial infections.

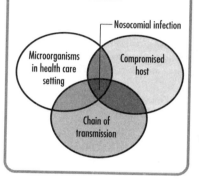

patient's body, rising significantly after 72 hours.

Also, the sicker a patient is, the more central and peripheral lines he is likely to have, bringing more opportunities for microbes to invade the bloodstream.

BREAKING THE WEAKEST LINK

The best way to control nosocomial infections is to break the weakest link in their chain of infection — usually, the mode of transmission. Many hospitals have developed strategies to prevent or control the transmission of infectious agents. These strategies fall into four general categories:

▶ control or elimination of infectious agents by appropriate sanitation, disinfection and sterilization
▶ control of transmission through proper handwashing, effective ventilation, and aseptic technique

❯ reservoir control. Interventions directed at controlling or destroying infectious reservoirs in health care settings include:
– using disposable equipment and supplies whenever possible
– disinfecting or sterilizing equipment as soon as possible after use
– using appropriate equipment for each patient
– handling and disposing of patient secretions, excretions, and exudates properly
– helping to identify and treat persons who are infection carriers. To help reduce the number of reservoirs in both the community and the health care setting, encourage patients to obtain active and passive immunizations, to practice positive health behaviors, to avoid high-risk behavior, and to maintain first-line defenses.

❯ isolating patients with infections, according to Centers for Disease Control and Prevention (CDC) recommendations, to limit the chance that they will transmit the infection.

PERFORMING ACCURATE ASSESSMENT

Accurate assessment helps identify infectious diseases and prevents avoidable complications. Complete assessment consists of patient history, physical examination, and laboratory data. The history should include the patient's sex, age, address, occupation, and place of work; known exposure to illness; and date of disease onset. Signs and symptoms, including their duration and whether they occurred suddenly or gradually; precipitating factors; relief measures; and weight loss or gain should also be included in the history. Detail information about recent hospitalization, blood transfusion, blood donation denial by Red Cross or other agencies, vaccination, travel or camping trips, and exposure to animals. If applicable, ask about possible exposure to sexually transmitted diseases or about drug abuse. Also, try to determine the patient's resistance to infectious disease. Ask about usual dietary patterns, unusual fatigue, and any conditions, such as neoplastic disease or alcoholism, that may predispose him to infection. Notice if the patient is listless or uneasy, lacks concentration, or has any obvious abnormality of mood or affect.

In suspected infection, a physical examination must assess the skin, mucous membranes, liver, spleen, and lymph nodes. Check for and note the type and location of drainage from skin lesions. Record skin color, temperature, and turgor; ask if the patient has pruritus. Take his temperature, using the same route consistently, and watch for a fever (the best indicator of many infections). Note and record the pattern of temperature change and the effect of antipyretics. Be aware that certain analgesics may contain antipyretics. In high fever, especially in children, watch for seizures.

Check the pulse rate. Infection commonly increases pulse rate, but some infections, notably typhoid fever and psittacosis, may decrease it. In severe infection or when complications are possible, watch for hypotension, hematuria, oliguria, hepatomegaly, jaundice, bleeding from gums or into joints, and altered level of consciousness. Obtain laboratory studies and appropriate cultures, as ordered. (See *How to collect culture specimens.*)

HOW TO COLLECT CULTURE SPECIMENS

Proper identification of the causative organism requires proper culture collection. Always try to obtain cultures before the first dose of antibiotics. If antibiotics are given before specimen collection, obtain the specimen as soon as possible. Label culture specimens with the date, time, patient's name, suspected diagnosis, and source of culture.

CULTURE SITE	SPECIMEN SOURCE	SPECIAL CONSIDERATIONS
Infected wound	▶ Aspiration of exudate with syringe	▶ Use only a sterile syringe. A pungent odor suggests the presence of anaerobes. Use oxygen-free collection tubes, if available.
	▶ Applicator swab	▶ Firmly but gently insert the swab deep into the wound, and saturate it with exudate from the infected site. If the surface is dry, moisten the swab with sterile saline solution first.
Skin lesions	▶ Excision or puncture	▶ Thoroughly clean the skin before excision or puncture, and follow the procedure for an infected wound.
Upper respiratory tract	▶ Nasopharyngeal swab (generally used to detect carriers of *Staphylococcus aureus* and viral infections)	▶ Gently pass the swab through the nose into the nasopharynx. Send the specimen to the laboratory for culture immediately.
	▶ Throat swab	▶ Under adequate light, swab the area of inflammation or exudation.
Lower respiratory tract	▶ Expectorated sputum	▶ Instruct the patient to cough deeply and to expectorate into a cup. Culture requires expectorated sputum, not just saliva. The best time to obtain a sputum specimen is first thing in the morning, before eating.
	▶ Induced sputum	▶ Use aerosol mist spray of saline solution or water to induce sputum production. Perform cupping and postural drainage, if needed.
	▶ Nasotracheal suction	▶ Measure the approximate distance from the patient's nose to his ear. Note the distance; then insert a sterile suction catheter this length, with a collection vial attached, into his nose. Maintain suction during catheter withdrawal.
	▶ Pleural tap	▶ Warn the patient that he may feel discomfort even though his skin will be anesthetized before this procedure. After the tap, check the site often for local swelling, and report dyspnea and other adverse reactions.

(continued)

HOW TO COLLECT CULTURE SPECIMENS (continued)

CULTURE SITE	SPECIMEN SOURCE	SPECIAL CONSIDERATIONS
Lower intestinal tract	▶ Rectal swab	▶ A lesion on the colon or rectal wall may require a colonoscopy or sigmoidoscopy to obtain the specimen. If so, explain the procedure. Help the patient to assume a left lateral decubitus or knee-chest position.
	▶ Stool specimen	▶ The specimen should contain any pus or blood present in the feces and a sampling of the first, middle, and last portion of stool. Urine with stool can invalidate results. Send the specimen to the laboratory at once in a clean, tightly covered container, especially stools being examined for ova and parasites.
Eye	▶ Cotton swab	▶ Carefully retract the lower lid, and gently swab the conjunctiva.
	▶ Corneal scrapings	▶ The doctor uses a swab loop to scrape the specimen from the site of corneal infection. Reassure the patient that the procedure is short and discomfort is minimal.
Genital tract	▶ Swab specimen	▶ A specimen from a male should contain urethral discharge or prostatic fluid; from a female, urethral or cervical specimens. Always collect specimens on two swabs simultaneously.
Urinary tract	▶ Midstream clean-catch urine (avoids specimen contamination with microbes commonly found in the lower urethra and perineum)	▶ A midstream clean-catch specimen in an infected person should contain fewer than 10,000 bacteria/ml. ▶ Teach the patient how to collect the specimen or supervise collection. In males, retract the foreskin and clean the glans penis; in females, clean and separate the labia so the urinary meatus is clearly visible; then clean the meatus. Tell the patient to void 25 to 30 ml first, then, without stopping the urine stream to collect the specimen. ▶ In infants, apply the collection bag carefully and check it frequently to avoid mechanical urethral obstruction. ▶ Send the urine specimen to the laboratory immediately, or refrigerate it to retard growth.
	▶ Indwelling urinary catheter specimen	▶ Clean the specimen port of the catheter with povidone-iodine, and aspirate urine with a sterile needle, or form a latex catheter, at a point distal to the "Y" branch.

HOW TO COLLECT CULTURE SPECIMENS *(continued)*

CULTURE SITE	SPECIMEN SOURCE	SPECIAL CONSIDERATIONS
Body fluids	▶ Needle aspiration	▶ Send peritoneal and synovial fluid and cerebrospinal fluid (CSF) to the laboratory at once. Don't retard the growth of the CSF organisms by refrigerating the specimen. After pericardial and pleural fluid aspiration, observe the patient carefully and check vital signs often. Watch for signs of pneumothorax or cardiac tamponade.
Blood	▶ Venous or arterial aspiration	▶ Prepare the skin according to your facility's policy. ▶ Using a sterile syringe, collect 12 to 15 ml of blood, changing needles before injecting blood into the aerobic and anaerobic collection bottles. Continue the procedure accordingly to your facility's policy. ▶ If the patient is receiving antibiotics, note this on the laboratory slip because the laboratory may add enzymes or resins to the culture to inactivate the drug.

MANAGING
INFECTIOUS DISEASES

A

ACQUIRED IMMUNODEFICIENCY SYNDROME

Currently one of the most widely publicized diseases, acquired immunodeficiency syndrome (AIDS) is marked by progressive failure of the immune system. Although it's characterized by gradual destruction of cell-mediated (T-cell) immunity, it also affects humoral immunity and even autoimmunity because of the central role of the CD4+ T lymphocyte in immune reactions. The resultant immunodeficiency makes the patient susceptible to opportunistic infections, unusual cancers, and other abnormalities that define AIDS.

This syndrome was first described by the Centers for Disease Control and Prevention (CDC) in 1981. Since then, the CDC has declared a case surveillance definition for AIDS and has modified it several times, most recently in 1993.

A retrovirus — the human immunodeficiency virus (HIV) Type I — is the primary etiologic agent. Transmission of HIV occurs by contact with infected blood or body fluids and is associated with identifiable high-risk behaviors. As a result, it's most common in homosexual and bisexual men, I.V. drug users, neonates of HIV-infected women, recipients of contaminated blood or blood products (dramatically decreased since mid-1985), and heterosexual partners of persons in the former groups. Because of similar routes of transmission, AIDS shares epidemiologic patterns with hepatitis B and sexually transmitted diseases (STDs).

The natural history of AIDS infection begins with infection by the HIV retrovirus, detectable only by laboratory tests, and ends with the severely immunocompromised, terminal stage of this disease. The course of the disease varies greatly in individuals but always progresses from acute HIV infection to the appearance of symptoms (mild to severe) to a diagnosis of AIDS and eventually to death. The average time between exposure to the virus and diagnosis of AIDS is 8 to 10 years, but shorter and longer incubation times are known.

However, current combination antiretroviral therapy (for example, with zidovudine, ritonavir, and others) and treatment and prophylaxis of common opportunistic infections can delay HIV's natural progression and prolong survival.

Causes

AIDS results from infection with HIV, which strikes cells bearing the CD4+ antigen; this antigen, normally a receptor for major histocompatibility complex molecules, serves as a receptor for the retrovirus and lets it enter the cell. HIV prefers to infect the CD4+ lymphocyte or macrophage, but may also infect other CD4+ antigen-bearing cells of the GI tract, uterine cervical cells, and neuroglial cells. The virus gains access by binding to the CD4+ molecule on the cell surface along with a coreceptor (thought to be the chemokine receptor CCR5). After invading a cell, HIV replicates, leading to cell death, or becomes latent. HIV infection leads to profound pathology, either directly, through destruction of CD4+ cells, other immune cells, and neuroglial cells, or indirectly, through the secondary effects of CD4+ T-cell dysfunction and resultant immunosuppression.

The infection process takes three forms:
▶ immunodeficiency (opportunistic infections and unusual cancers)
▶ autoimmunity (lymphoid interstitial pneumonitis, arthritis, hypergammaglobulinemia, and production of autoimmune antibodies)
▶ neurologic dysfunction (AIDS dementia complex, HIV encephalopathy, and peripheral neuropathies).

HIV is transmitted by direct inoculation during intimate sexual contact — especially in receptive rectal intercourse; transfusion of contaminated blood or blood products (a risk that's been diminished by routine testing of all blood products); sharing of contaminated needles; or transplacental or postpartum transmission from infected mother to fetus (by cervical or blood contact at delivery and in breast milk).

Accumulating evidence suggests that HIV isn't transmitted by casual household or social contact.

Signs and symptoms

HIV infection manifests itself in many ways. After a high-risk exposure and inoculation, the infected person usually experiences a mononucleosis-like syndrome, which may be attributed to a flu or other virus and then may remain asymptomatic for years. In this latent stage, the only sign of HIV infection is laboratory evidence of seroconversion.

When symptoms appear, they may take many forms:
▶ persistent generalized adenopathy
▶ nonspecific symptoms (weight loss, fatigue, night sweats, fevers)
▶ neurologic symptoms resulting from HIV encephalopathy
▶ opportunistic infection or cancer.

In children with AIDS, the clinical course varies slightly. Apparently their incubation time is shorter, with a mean of

17 months. Signs and symptoms resemble those in adults, except for findings related to STDs. Children show virtually all of the opportunistic infections observed in adults, with a higher incidence of bacterial infections: otitis media, sepsis, chronic salivary gland enlargement, lymphoid interstitial pneumonia, *Mycobacterium avium* complex function, and pneumonias, including *Pneumocystis carinii.*

Diagnosis

The CDC defines AIDS as an illness characterized by one or more "indicator" diseases coexisting with laboratory evidence of HIV infection and other possible causes of immunosuppression. The CDC's current AIDS surveillance case definition requires laboratory confirmation of HIV infection in people who have a CD4+ T-cell count of 200 cells/l or who have an associated clinical condition or disease. HIV infection should be considered when there is a prolonged illness without ready explanation.

Antibody tests

The most commonly performed tests, antibody tests, indicate HIV infection indirectly, by revealing HIV antibodies. The recommended protocol requires initial screening of individuals and blood products with an enzyme-linked immunosorbent assay (ELISA) test. A positive ELISA test should be repeated and then confirmed by an alternate method, usually the Western blot or an immunofluorescence assay. However, antibody testing isn't always reliable. Because the body takes a variable amount of time to produce a detectable level of antibodies, a "window" varying from a few weeks to as long as 35 months (in one documented case) allows an HIV-infected person to test negative for HIV antibodies.

Antibody tests are also unreliable in neonates because transferred maternal antibodies persist for 6 to 10 months. To overcome these problems, direct testing is performed to detect HIV. Direct tests

A PROMISING H.I.V. VACCINE

The development of an effective HIV vaccine is a public health priority throughout the world. Currently the AIDSVAX Phase III clinical trial is being conducted among uninfected drug users in Thailand. Phase I and II trials have already demonstrated that the vaccine is safe for use and is capable of inducing antibodies against HIV infection. A similar trial is also being conducted in the United States with a version of the vaccine designed to protect against the HIV strains common in North America.

AIDSVAX uses a genetically engineered protein (gp120) from the surface of the human immunodeficiency virus. When injected into the body, it stimulates production of antibodies to attack any future invading HIV. Researchers hope the antibodies will prevent the virus from binding to, and infecting, healthy T-cells.

include antigen tests (p24 antigen), HIV cultures, nucleic acid probes of peripheral blood lymphocytes with determination of HIV-1 RNA levels, and the polymerase chain reaction.

Other tests

Additional tests to support the diagnosis and help evaluate the severity of immunosuppression include CD4+ and CD8+ T-lymphocyte subset counts, erythrocyte sedimentation rate (ESR), complete blood cell count, serum beta$_2$-microglobulin, p24 antigen, neopterin levels, and anergy testing. Because many opportunistic infections in AIDS patients are reactivations of previous infections, patients are also test-

ed for syphilis, hepatitis B, tuberculosis, toxoplasmosis and, in some areas, histoplasmosis.

Treatment

No cure has yet been found for AIDS; however, primary therapy for HIV infection includes three different types of antiretroviral agents:

▶ protease inhibitors (PIs), such as amprenavir, ritonavir, indinavir, nelfinavir, and saquinavir
▶ nucleoside reverse transcriptase inhibitors (NRTIs), such as zidovudine, didanosine, zalcitabine, lamivudine, abacavir, or stavudine
▶ nonnucleoside reverse transcriptase inhibitors (NNRTIs), such as efavirenz, nevirapine or delavirdine.

These agents, used in various combinations, are designed to inhibit HIV viral replication. Other potential therapies include immunomodulatory agents designed to boost the weakened immune system, and anti-infective and antineoplastic agents to combat opportunistic infections and associated cancers; some are used prophylactically to help patients resist opportunistic infections. A vaccine to prevent AIDS is currently under investigation. (See *A promising HIV vaccine.*)

Current treatment protocols combine two or more agents in an effort to gain the maximum benefit with the fewest adverse reactions. Such regimens often include one PI plus two NRTIs, one NNRTI plus two NRTIs, or three NRTIs. Many variations and drug interactions are under study. Combination therapy helps inhibit the production of resistant, mutant strains. Zidovudine, an NRTI, has been used as a single agent for pregnant HIV-positive women. Supportive treatments help maintain nutritional status and relieve pain and other distressing physical and psychological symptoms.

Many pathogens in AIDS respond to anti-infective drugs but tend to recur after treatment ends. For this reason, most patients need continuous anti-infective treatment, presumably for life or until the drug is no longer tolerated or effective.

Special considerations

▶ Be sure to use precautions in all situations that risk exposure to blood, body fluids, and secretions. Diligently practicing universal precautions can prevent the inadvertent transmission of AIDS, hepatitis B, and other infectious diseases transmitted by similar routes.

▶ Combination antiretroviral therapy aims to maximally suppress HIV replication, thereby improving survival. However, poor drug compliance may lead to resistance and treatment failure. Stress to patients that medication regimens must be followed closely and may be required for many years, if not throughout life.

▶ The immunosuppression caused by HIV disease makes patients vulnerable to additional infections and complications. All patients should undergo periodic screening tests for complications. (See *Suggested screening tests for infection.*)

▶ Recognize that a diagnosis of AIDS is profoundly distressing because of the disease's social impact and the discouraging prognosis. The patient may lose his job and financial security as well as the support of family and friends. Coping with an altered body image, the emotional burden of serious illness, and the threat of death may overwhelm the patient.

 PREVENTION TIP Prevention for HIV infection should include risk reduction counseling, particularly information on safe sex.

ACTINOMYCOSIS

Actinomycosis is a rare, slowly progressive bacterial infection primarily caused by the gram-positive anaerobic bacillus *Actinomyces israelii,* which produces granulomatous, suppurative lesions with abscesses. Common infection sites are the head, neck, thorax, and abdomen, but it

> ## SUGGESTED SCREENING TESTS FOR INFECTION
>
> In addition to standard health screening, the following tests are recommended:
> ▶ Cytomegalovirus antibody test
> ▶ Hepatitis B and C serologies
> ▶ Papanicolaou smear in women (1 to 2 times a year)
> ▶ Purified protein derivative test for TB (annually)
> ▶ *Toxoplasma gondii* serology
> ▶ Venereal Disease Research Laboratory flocculation test (VDRL) test for syphilis (annually in sexually active patients).

can spread to contiguous tissues, causing multiple draining sinuses.

Actinomycosis affects three times as many males as females, with peak incidence in middle decades. People with dental disease or human immunodeficiency virus infection are at increased risk.

Diffuse involvement of the maxillofacial subcutaneous tissue and sinuses is the typical complication of actinomycosis. Abscesses and fistulae may involve the brain or be aspirated and cause pneumonia and empyema.

Causes

A. israelii occurs as part of the normal flora of the mouth, lower gastrointestinal tract, and female genitourinary tract; infection results from traumatic introduction into body tissues.

Signs and symptoms

Symptoms appear from days to months after injury and may vary, depending on the site of infection.

In *cervicofacial actinomycosis* (lumpy jaw), painful, indurated swellings appear in the mouth or neck up to several weeks after dental extraction or trauma. They gradually enlarge and form fistulas that open onto the skin. Sulfur granules (yellowish gray masses that are actually colonies of *A. israelii*) appear in the exudate.

In *pulmonary actinomycosis,* aspiration of bacteria from the mouth into areas of the lungs already anaerobic from infection or atelectasis produces a fever and a cough that becomes productive and occasionally causes hemoptysis. Eventually, empyema follows, a sinus forms through the chest wall, and septicemia may occur.

In *GI actinomycosis,* ileocecal lesions are caused by swallowed bacteria, which produce abdominal discomfort, fever, sometimes a palpable mass, and an external sinus. This follows intestinal mucosa disruption, usually by surgery or an inflammatory bowel condition such as appendicitis.

Rare sites of actinomycotic infection are the bones, brain, liver, kidneys, and female reproductive organs. Symptoms reflect the organ involved.

Diagnosis

Isolation of *A. israelii in* exudate or tissue confirms actinomycosis.

Other tests that help identify this condition are:
▶ microscopic examination of sulfur granules
▶ immunofluorescence tests through the Centers for Disease Control and Prevention, a diagnostic alternative
▶ chest X-ray to show lesions in unusual locations, such as the shaft of a rib.

Treatment

Drug treatment of actinomycosis involves high-dose I.V. penicillin or tetracycline therapy for 2 to 6 weeks followed by oral therapy for 6 to 12 months. Surgical excision and drainage of abscesses may be performed, but medical therapy alone is sufficient if the patient isn't critically ill.

Special considerations

▶ Dispose of all dressings in a sealed plastic bag.
▶ After surgery, provide proper aseptic wound management.

▶ Administer antibiotics, as ordered. Before giving the first dose, obtain an accurate patient history of allergies. Watch for hypersensitivity reactions, such as rash, fever, itching, and signs of anaphylaxis. If the patient has a history of any allergies, keep epinephrine 1:1,000 and resuscitative equipment available.

 PREVENTION TIP Stress the importance of good oral hygiene and proper dental care. Stress the importance of continuing antibiotic therapy for the extended time to minimize relapse of the disease.

ADENOVIRUS INFECTION

Adenoviruses cause acute, self-limiting febrile infections, with inflammation of the respiratory or the ocular mucous membranes, or both.

Adenovirus has at least 47 known serotypes. Types 1, 2, 3, and 5 are seen most frequently in children, with 4 and 7 (also 3, 14, and 21) associated with outbreaks in military camps. Infections occur throughout the year but are most common from fall to spring. Nearly 100 % of adults have serum antibody to several serotypes.

Acute conjunctivitis, sinusitis, pharyngitis, and pneumonia are potential complications of adenoviral infections.

Causes

Adenovirus can be transmitted by direct inoculation into the eye, by the oral-fecal route (adenovirus may persist in the GI tract for years after infection), or by inhalation of an infected droplet.

Signs and symptoms

The incubation period—usually lasting less than 1 week—is followed by acute illness lasting less than 5 days. Clinical features vary, depending on the type of infection. Prolonged asymptomatic reinfection may occur. (See *Major adenovirus infections.*)

MAJOR ADENOVIRUS INFECTIONS

DISEASE	AGE GROUP	CLINICAL FEATURES
Acute febrile respiratory illness	Children	Nonspecific coldlike symptoms, similar to other viral respiratory illnesses: fever, pharyngitis, tracheitis, bronchitis, pneumonitis
Acute respiratory disease	Adults (usually military recruits)	Malaise, fever, chills, headache, pharyngitis, hoarseness, and dry cough
Viral pneumonia	Children and adults	Sudden onset of high fever, rapid infection of upper and lower respiratory tracts, rash, diarrhea, intestinal intussusception
Acute pharyngoconjunctival fever	Children (particularly after swimming in pools or lakes)	Spiking fever lasting several days, headache, pharyngitis, conjunctivitis, rhinitis, cervical adenitis
Acute follicular conjunctivitis	Adults	Unilateral tearing and mucoid discharge; later, milder symptoms in other eye
Epidemic keratoconjunctivitis	Adults	Unilateral or bilateral ocular redness and edema, preorbital swelling, local discomfort, superficial opacity of the cornea without ulceration
Hemorrhagic cystitis	Children	Adenovirus in urine, hematuria, dysuria, urinary frequency

Diagnosis

For definitive diagnosis, the virus must be isolated from respiratory or ocular secretions or fecal smears; during epidemics, however, typical symptoms alone can confirm the diagnosis. Other conditions to consider include infections caused by other respiratory agents and *Mycoplasma pneumoniae.*

Because adenoviral illnesses resolve rapidly, serum antibody titers aren't useful for diagnosis. Adenoviral diseases cause lymphocytosis in children. When they cause respiratory disease, chest X-ray may show pneumonitis.

Adenovirus types 40 and 41 (associated with diarrheal disease) require special tissue-culture cells for isolation and are most commonly detected by direct ELISA of stool.

Treatment

Supportive treatment includes bed rest, antipyretics, and analgesics. Ocular infections may require corticosteroids and direct supervision by an ophthalmologist. Hospitalization is required in cases of pneumonia (in infants) to prevent death and in epidemic keratoconjunctivitis (EKC) to prevent blindness.

Special considerations

▶ During the acute illness, monitor respiratory status, and intake and output. Give analgesics and antipyretics, as needed. Stress the need for bed rest.

 PREVENTION TIP To help minimize the incidence of adenoviral disease, instruct all patients in proper hand washing to reduce fecal-oral transmission. EKC can be prevented by sterilizing ophthalmic instruments, adequate chlorination in swimming pools, and avoiding swimming pools during EKC epidemics.

▶ Live vaccines have been developed against adenovirus types 4 and 7 and can prevent adenoviral infection. These vaccines are recommended for high-risk groups such as military recruits.

AMEBIASIS

Amebiasis, also known as amebic dysentery, is an acute or chronic protozoal infection caused by *Entamoeba histolytica*. This infection produces varying degrees of illness, from no symptoms at all or mild diarrhea to fulminant dysentery. Extraintestinal amebiasis can induce hepatic abscess and infections of the lungs, pleural cavity, pericardium, peritoneum and, rarely, the brain.

Amebiasis occurs worldwide but is most common in the tropics, subtropics, and other areas with poor sanitation and health practices. Incidence in the United States averages between 1% and 3% but may be higher among gay men and lesbians, and institutionalized people, in whom fecal-oral contamination is more common.

The prognosis is generally good, although complications — such as ameboma, intestinal stricture, hemorrhage or perforation, intussusception, or abscess — increase mortality. Brain abscess, a rare complication, is usually fatal.

Causes

E. histolytica exists in two forms: a cyst (which can survive outside the body) and a trophozoite (which can't survive outside the body). Transmission occurs through ingesting feces-contaminated food or water. The ingested cysts pass through the intestine, where digestive secretions break down the cysts and liberate the motile trophozoites within. The trophozoites multiply, and either invade and ulcerate the mucosa of the large intestine or simply feed on intestinal bacteria. As the trophozoites are carried slowly toward the rectum, they are encysted and then excreted in feces. Humans are the principal reservoir of infection.

Signs and symptoms

The clinical effects of amebiasis vary with the severity of the infestation. *Acute amebic dysentery* causes a sudden high temperature of 104° to 105° F (40° to 40.6° C) accompanied by chills and abdominal cramping; profuse, bloody, mucoid diarrhea with tenesmus; and diffuse abdominal tenderness due to extensive rectosigmoid ulcers.

Chronic amebic dysentery produces intermittent diarrhea that lasts for 1 to 4 weeks, and recurs several times a year. Such diarrhea produces 4 to 8 (or, in severe diarrhea, up to 18) foul-smelling mucus- and blood-tinged stools daily in a patient with a mild fever, vague abdominal cramps, possible weight loss, tenderness over the cecum and ascending colon and, occasionally, hepatomegaly. Amebic granuloma (ameboma), commonly mistaken for cancer, can be a complication of the chronic infection. Amebic granuloma produces blood and mucus in the stool and, when granulomatous tissue covers the entire circumference of the bowel, causes partial or complete obstruction.

Parasitic and bacterial invasion of the appendix may produce typical signs of subacute appendicitis (abdominal pain and tenderness). Occasionally, *E. histolytica* perforates the intestinal wall and spreads to the liver. When it perforates the liver and diaphragm, it spreads to the lungs, pleural cavity, peritoneum and, rarely, the brain.

Diagnosis

Isolating *E. histolytica* (cysts and trophozoites) in fresh feces or aspirates from abscesses, ulcers, or tissue confirms acute amebic dysentery.

Diagnosis must distinguish between cancer and ameboma with X-rays, sigmoidoscopy, stool examination for amebae, and cecum palpation. In those with amebiasis, exploratory surgery is hazardous; it can lead to peritonitis, perforation, and pericecal abscess.

Other laboratory tests that support the diagnosis of amebiasis include:
▶ indirect hemagglutination test — positive with current or previous infection
▶ complement fixation — usually positive only during active disease
▶ barium studies — rule out nonamebic causes of diarrhea, such as polyps and cancer
▶ sigmoidoscopy — detects rectosigmoid ulceration; a biopsy may be helpful.

Patients with amebiasis shouldn't have preparatory enemas because these may remove exudates and destroy the trophozoites, thus interfering with test results.

Other conditions to consider include:
▶ Infectious causes of colitis including shigellosis, *Campylobacter* infection, pseudomembranous colitis, salmonellosis, or *Yersinia* infection
▶ Noninfectious causes of colitis including ulcerative colitis, Crohn's disease, and ischemic colitis
▶ Hepatic amebiasis should be distinguished from pyrogenic liver abscess.

Treatment

Drugs used to treat mild to severe amebic dysentery include metronidazole at intestinal and extraintestinal sites and for amebic hepatic abscess, followed by iodoquinol, diloxanide, or paromomycin, effective amebicides also used for asymptomatic carriers.

Special considerations

 PREVENTION TIP Tell patients with amebiasis to avoid drinking alcohol when taking metronidazole. The combination may cause nausea, vomiting, and headache.

ASCARIASIS

Also known as roundworm infection, ascariasis is caused by the parasitic worm *Ascaris lumbricoides*. It occurs worldwide but is most common in tropical areas with poor sanitation and in areas where farmers use human stool as fertilizer. In the United States, it's more prevalent in the South, particularly among 4- to 12-year-olds. Ascariasis may lead to biliary or intestinal obstruction and pulmonary disease.

Causes

A. lumbricoides is a large roundworm resembling an earthworm. It's transmitted to humans by ingestion of soil contaminated with human stool that harbors the eggs of *A. lumbricoides*. Such ingestion may occur directly (by eating contaminated soil) or indirectly (by eating poorly washed raw vegetables grown in contaminated soil).

Ascariasis never passes directly from person to person. After ingestion, *A. lumbricoides* eggs hatch and release larvae, which penetrate the intestinal wall and reach the lungs through the bloodstream. After about 10 days in pulmonary capillaries and alveoli, the larvae migrate to the bronchioles, bronchi, trachea, and epiglottis. There they are swallowed and return to the intestine to mature into worms.

Signs and symptoms

Mild intestinal ascariasis may cause only vague stomach discomfort. The first clue may be vomiting a worm or passing a worm in the stool. Severe disease, however, causes stomach pain, vomiting, restlessness, disturbed sleep, and, in extreme cases, intestinal obstruction. Larvae migrating by the lymphatic and the circulatory systems cause symptoms that vary; for instance, when they invade the lungs, pneumonitis may result.

Diagnosis

Microscopic identification of eggs in the stool or observation of adult worms, which may be passed rectally or by mouth, confirms the diagnosis. When migrating larvae invade the alveoli, other conclusive tests include X-rays that show characteristic bronchovascular markings: infiltrates, patchy areas of pneumonitis, and widening of hilar shadows. In a patient with ascariasis, these findings usually accompany a complete blood count that shows eosinophilia.

Treatment

Drug therapy with mebendazole or albendazole is the primary treatment. The anthelmintic action inhibits uptake of glucose and other low-molecular-weight nutrients in susceptible helminths, depleting the glycogen stores they need for survival and reproduction. These drugs are contraindicated in pregnancy and in heavy infections, in which they may provoke ectopic migration. Pyrantel or piperazine, which temporarily paralyze the worms permitting peristalsis to expel them, are safe in pregnancy. These drugs are up to 95% effective, even after a single dose. In multiple helminth infection, one of these drugs must be the first treatment; using some other anthelmintic first may stimulate *A. lumbricoides* perforation into other organs. No specific treatment exists for migratory infection because anthelmintics affect only mature worms.

In intestinal obstruction, nasogastric (NG) suctioning controls vomiting. When suctioning can be discontinued, instill piperazine and clamp the tube. If vomiting doesn't occur, give a second dose of piperazine orally 24 hours later. If this is ineffective, treatment probably requires surgery.

Special considerations

▶ Isolation is unnecessary; proper disposal of stool and soiled linen, using standard precautions, should be adequate.

▶ If the patient is receiving NG suctioning, be sure to provide good mouth care.

 PREVENTION TIP Teach the patient to prevent reinfection by washing hands thoroughly, especially before eating and after defecation, and by bathing and changing his underwear and bed linens daily.

▶ Inform the patient of possible drug adverse reactions. Tell him that piperazine may cause stomach upset, dizziness, and urticaria.

▶ Be aware that piperazine is contraindicated in seizure disorders. Pyrantel produces red stool and vomit and may cause stomach upset, headache, dizziness, and skin rash; and mebendazole may cause abdominal pain and diarrhea.

ASPERGILLOSIS

Aspergillosis is an opportunistic, sometimes life-threatening infection caused by fungi of the genus *Aspergillus*, usually *A. fumigatus, A. flavus,* or *A. niger.* It occurs in four major forms:

▶ *aspergilloma,* which produces a fungus ball in the lungs (called a mycetoma)

▶ *allergic aspergillosis,* a hypersensitive asthmatic reaction to *Aspergillus* antigens

▶ *aspergillosis endophthalmitis,* an infection of the anterior and posterior chambers of the eye that can lead to blindness

▶ *disseminated aspergillosis,* an acute infection that produces septicemia, thrombosis, and infarction of virtually any organ, but especially the heart, lungs, brain, and kidneys.

Aspergillus may cause infection of the ear (otomycosis), cornea (mycotic keratitis), and prosthetic heart valves (endocarditis); pneumonia (especially in persons receiving immunosuppressive drugs, such as antineoplastic agents or high-dose steroids); sinusitis; and brain abscesses.

The prognosis varies with each form. Occasionally, aspergilloma causes fatal hemoptysis.

Causes

Aspergillus is found worldwide, often in fermenting compost piles and damp hay. It's transmitted by inhalation of fungal spores or, in aspergillosis endophthalmitis, by the invasion of spores through a wound or other tissue injury. It's a common laboratory contaminant.

Aspergillus produces clinical infection only in persons who become especially vulnerable to it. Such vulnerability can result from excessive or prolonged use of antibiotics, glucocorticoids, or other immunosuppressive agents; from radiation; from such conditions as acquired immunodeficiency syndrome, Hodgkin's disease, leukemia, azotemia, alcoholism, sarcoidosis, bronchitis, or bronchiectasis; from organ transplants; and, in aspergilloma, from tuberculosis or another cavitary lung disease.

Signs and symptoms

The incubation period in aspergillosis ranges from a few days to weeks. In aspergilloma, colonization of the bronchial tree with *Aspergillus* produces plugs and atelectasis and forms a tangled ball of hyphae (fungal filaments), fibrin, and exudate in a cavity left by a previous illness such as tuberculosis. Characteristically, aspergilloma either produces no symptoms or mimics tuberculosis, causing a productive cough and purulent or blood-tinged sputum, dyspnea, empyema, and lung abscesses.

Allergic aspergillosis causes wheezing, dyspnea, cough with some sputum production, pleural pain, and fever.

Aspergillosis endophthalmitis usually appears 2 to 3 weeks after an eye injury or surgery, and accounts for half of all cases of endophthalmitis. It causes clouded vision, eye pain, and reddened conjunctivae. Eventually, *Aspergillus* infects the anterior and posterior chambers, where it produces purulent exudate.

In disseminated aspergillosis, *Aspergillus* invades blood vessels, and causes thrombosis, infarctions, and the typical signs of septicemia (chills, fever, hypotension, delirium), with azotemia, hematuria, urinary tract obstruction, headaches, seizures, bone pain and tenderness, and soft-tissue swelling. This form of the disorder is rapidly fatal.

Diagnosis

In patients with aspergilloma, a chest X-ray reveals a crescent-shaped radiolucency surrounding a circular mass, but this isn't definitive for aspergillosis. In aspergillosis endophthalmitis, a history of ocular trauma or surgery and a culture or exudate showing *Aspergillus* is diagnostic. In allergic aspergillosis, sputum examination shows eosinophils. Culture of mouth scrapings or sputum showing *Aspergillus* is inconclusive because even healthy persons harbor this fungus. In disseminated aspergillosis, culture and microscopic examination of affected tissue can confirm the diagnosis, but this form is usually diagnosed at autopsy.

Treatment

Treatment of aspergilloma necessitates local excision of the lesion and supportive therapy, such as chest physiotherapy and coughing, to improve pulmonary function.

Allergic aspergillosis requires desensitization and, possibly, steroids.

Disseminated aspergillosis and aspergillosis endophthalmitis require a 2- to 3-week course of I.V. amphotericin B (as well as prompt cessation of immunosuppressive therapy). However, the disseminated form of aspergillosis often resists amphotericin B therapy and rapidly progresses to death.

Itraconazole may be useful in slowly progressing immunocompetent cases.

Special considerations

▶ Aspergillosis doesn't require isolation.

B

BLASTOMYCOSIS

Also called *Gilchrist's disease,* blastomycosis is caused by the yeastlike fungus
Blastomyces dermatitidis, which usually
infects the lungs and produces bronchopneumonia. Less frequently, this fungus
may spread through the blood and cause
osteomyelitis and central nervous system
(CNS), skin, and genital disorders.

Blastomycosis is generally found in
North America (where *B. dermatitidis* normally inhabits the soil) and is endemic to
the southeastern United States. Sporadic
cases have also been reported in Africa.
Blastomycosis usually infects men ages
30 to 50, but no occupational link has been
found.

Untreated blastomycosis is slowly progressive and usually fatal; however, spontaneous remissions occasionally occur.
With antifungal drug therapy and supportive treatment, the prognosis for patients with blastomycosis is good.

Blastomycosis can cause abscesses or
fistulas, meningitis, cerebral abscesses,
Addison's disease, pericarditis, and arthritis.

Causes
Blastomycosis is caused by the yeastlike
fungus *B. dermatitidis,* which is probably
inhaled by people who are in close contact with the soil. The incubation period
may range from weeks to months.

Signs and symptoms
Initial clinical indicators of pulmonary
blastomycosis mimic those of a viral upper respiratory infection. These findings

typically include a dry, hacking, or productive cough (occasionally hemoptysis),
pleuritic chest pain, fever, shaking, chills,
night sweats, malaise, anorexia, and weight
loss.

▶ Cutaneous blastomycosis causes small,
painless, nonpruritic, and nondistinctive
macules or papules on exposed body parts.
These lesions become raised and reddened,
and occasionally progress to draining skin
abscesses or fistulas.

▶ Skeletal involvement causes soft tissue
swelling, tenderness, and warmth over
bony lesions, which generally occur in the
thoracic, lumbar, and sacral regions; long
bones of the legs; and, in children, the
skull.

▶ Genital involvement produces painful
swelling of the testes, the epididymis, or
the prostate; deep perineal pain; pyuria;
and hematuria.

▶ CNS involvement causes meningitis or
cerebral abscesses, resulting in a decreased
level of consciousness (LOC), lethargy,
and change in mood or affect.

Other forms of dissemination may result in Addison's disease (adrenal insufficiency), pericarditis, and arthritis.

Diagnosis
Various tests may be ordered to diagnose
blastomycosis, including:

▶ culture of *B. dermatitidis* from skin lesions, pus, sputum, or pulmonary secretions

▶ biopsy of tissue from the skin or lungs,
or of bronchial washings, sputum, or pus,
as the doctor finds appropriate

▶ complement fixation testing. Although
such testing isn't conclusive, a high titer

in extrapulmonary disease is a poor prognostic sign.

▶ immunodiffusion testing. This specific study detects antibodies for the A and B antigen of blastomycosis.

Additionally, suspected pulmonary blastomycosis requires a chest X-ray, which may show pulmonary infiltrates. Other abnormal laboratory findings include an increased white blood cell count and erythrocyte sedimentation rate, slightly increased serum globulin levels, mild normochromic anemia and, with bone lesions, an increased alkaline phosphatase level.

Treatment
All forms of blastomycosis respond to amphotericin B. Ketoconazole or fluconazole may be used as alternatives. Patient care is mainly supportive.

Special considerations
▶ In severe pulmonary blastomycosis, check for hemoptysis. If the patient has a fever, provide a cool room and give tepid sponge baths.

▶ If blastomycosis causes joint pain or swelling, elevate the joint and apply heat.

▶ In CNS infection, watch the patient carefully for decreasing LOC and unequal pupillary response.

▶ In men with disseminated disease, watch for hematuria.

 ALERT Infuse I.V. amphotericin B slowly (a too-rapid infusion may cause circulatory collapse). During the infusion, monitor vital signs. (Temperature may rise but should subside within 1 to 2 hours.) Watch for decreased urine output and monitor laboratory results for increased blood urea nitrogen and serum creatinine levels and hypokalemia, which may indicate renal toxicity. Report any hearing loss, tinnitus, or dizziness immediately.

▶ To relieve adverse effects of amphotericin B, give antiemetics and antipyretics as needed.

BLEPHARITIS

A common inflammation, blepharitis produces a red-rimmed appearance on the margins of the eyelids. It is frequently chronic and bilateral and can affect both upper and lower lids. Seborrheic blepharitis is characterized by waxy scales and symptoms of burning and foreign body sensation. It is common in older adults and in persons with red hair. Staphylococcal (ulcerative) blepharitis is characterized by dry scales along the inflamed lid margins, which also have ulcerated areas. It's more common in females and may be associated with keratoconjunctivitis sicca (KCS), a dry eye syndrome. Both types may coexist. Blepharitis tends to recur and become chronic.

Causes
Seborrheic blepharitis may be seen in conjunction with seborrhea of the scalp, eyebrows, and ears; ulcerative blepharitis, from *Staphylococcus aureus* infection. (People with this infection may also tend to develop chalazions and styes.)

Signs and symptoms
Clinical features of blepharitis include itching, burning, foreign-body sensation, and sticky, crusted eyelids on waking. This constant irritation results in unconscious rubbing of the eyes (causing reddened rims) or continual blinking. Other signs include waxy scales in seborrheic blepharitis; flaky scales on lashes, loss of lashes, and ulcerated areas on lid margins in ulcerative blepharitis. In association with KCS, dry eyes may also be a problem.

Diagnosis
In blepharitis, diagnosis depends on the patient history and characteristic symptoms. In ulcerative blepharitis, a culture of the ulcerated lid margin shows *S. aureus.* Persistent inflammation and thickening of the eyelid margin may indicate squamous cell, basal cell, or sebaceous

cell carcinoma masquerading as blepharitis.

Treatment
The goals of therapy are to control the disease, maintain vision, and avoid secondary complications. In addition to warm compresses, treatment depends on the type of blepharitis:

❱ *seborrheic blepharitis:* daily lid hygiene (using a mild shampoo on a damp applicator stick or a washcloth) to remove scales from the lid margins; also, frequent shampooing of the scalp and eyebrows

❱ *ulcerative blepharitis:* warm compresses may be applied and an appropriate antibiotic eye ointment, such as erythromycin or tetracycline, may be used at bedtime. Additionally a combination antibiotic/steroid, such as prednisolone (Vasocidin or Blephamide, sulfa and steroid), may be used.

❱ *blepharitis resulting from pediculosis:* removal of nits (with forceps) or application of ophthalmic physostigmine or other ointment as an insecticide. (This may cause pupil constriction and possibly headache, conjunctival irritation, and blurred vision from the film of ointment on the cornea.)

Special considerations
❱ Instruct the patient to gently remove scales from the lid margins daily with an applicator stick or a clean washcloth.

❱ Teach the patient the following method for applying warm compresses: First, run warm water into a clean bowl. Then immerse a clean cloth in the water and wring it out. Place the warm cloth against the closed eyelid. (Be careful not to burn the skin.) Hold the compress in place until it cools. Continue this procedure for 15 minutes.

❱ Antibiotic ophthalmic ointment should be applied after a 15-minute application of warm compresses.

❱ Treatment of seborrheic blepharitis also requires attention to the face and scalp.

 PREVENTION TIP Teach your patients that frequent hand washing and general good hygiene can help prevent some cases of blepharitis. A hypoallergenic formula of eye makeup may help prevent blepharitis.

BOTULISM

A life-threatening paralytic illness, botulism results from an exotoxin produced by the gram-positive, anaerobic bacillus *Clostridium botulinum.* It occurs as botulism food poisoning, wound botulism, and infant botulism. Mortality from botulism is about 25%, with death most often caused by respiratory failure during the first week of illness.

Causes
Botulism is usually the result of ingesting inadequately cooked contaminated foods, especially those with low acid content, such as home-canned fruits and vegetables, sausages, and smoked or preserved fish or meat. Honey and corn syrup may contain *C. botulinum* spores and should not be fed to infants. Rarely, botulism results from wound infection with *C. botulinum.*

Botulism occurs worldwide and affects adults more often than children. Recently, studies have shown that an infant's GI tract can become colonized with *C. botulinum* from some unknown source, and then the exotoxin is produced within the infant's intestine. Incidence had been declining, but the current trend toward home canning has resulted in an upswing (approximately 250 cases per year in the United States) in recent years.

Signs and symptoms
The disease usually presents within 12 to 36 hours (range is 6 hours to 8 days) after the ingestion of contaminated food. The severity varies with the amount of toxin ingested and the patient's degree of immunocompetence. Generally, early on-

set (within 24 hours) signals critical and potentially fatal illness. Initial symptoms include dry mouth, sore throat, weakness, vomiting, and diarrhea.

The cardinal sign of botulism, though, is acute symmetrical cranial nerve impairment (ptosis, diplopia, dysarthria), followed by descending weakness or paralysis of muscles in the extremities or trunk, and dyspnea from respiratory muscle paralysis. Such impairment doesn't affect mental or sensory processes and is not associated with fever.

Infant botulism
Usually afflicting infants ages 3 to 20 weeks, infant botulism can produce hypotonic (floppy) infant syndrome. Symptoms are constipation, feeble cry, depressed gag reflex, and inability to suck. Cranial nerve deficits also occur in infants and are manifested by a flaccid facial expression, ptosis, and ophthalmoplegia. Infants also develop generalized muscle weakness, hypotonia, and areflexia. Loss of head control may be striking. Respiratory arrest is likely.

Diagnosis
Identification of the offending toxin in the patient's serum, stool, gastric content, or the suspected food confirms the diagnosis. An electromyogram showing diminished muscle action potential after a single supramaximal nerve stimulus is also diagnostic.

Diagnosis also must rule out other diseases often confused with botulism, such as Guillain-Barré syndrome, myasthenia gravis, cerebrovascular accident, staphylococcal food poisoning, tick paralysis, chemical intoxications, carbon monoxide poisoning, fish poisoning, trichinosis, and diphtheria.

Treatment
I.V. or I.M. administration of botulinum antitoxin (available through the Centers for Disease Control and Prevention) is the treatment of choice.

 ALERT Antibiotics and aminoglycosides should be avoided because of the risk of neuromuscular blockade. They should be used only to treat secondary infections.

Special considerations
If you suspect ingestion of contaminated food:
▶ Obtain a careful history of the patient's food intake for the past several days. Check to see if other family members exhibit similar symptoms and share a common food history.
▶ Observe carefully for abnormal neurologic signs. If the patient returns home, tell his family to watch for signs of weakness, blurred vision, and slurred speech, and to return the patient to the facility immediately if such signs appear.
▶ If ingestion has occurred within several hours, induce vomiting, begin gastric lavage, and give a high enema to purge any unabsorbed toxin from the bowel.
If clinical signs of botulism appear:
▶ Bring the patient to the intensive care unit, and monitor cardiac and respiratory function carefully.
▶ Administer botulinum antitoxin, as required, to neutralize any circulating toxin. Before giving antitoxin, obtain an accurate patient history of allergies, especially to horses, and perform a skin test.
▶ Serum samples should be collected to identify the toxin before antitoxin is administered.

 ALERT After administration of antitoxin, watch for anaphylaxis or other hypersensitivity, and serum sickness. Keep epinephrine 1:1,000 (for subcutaneous administration) and emergency airway equipment available.
▶ Closely observe and accurately record neurologic function, including bilateral motor status (reflexes, ability to move arms and legs).
▶ Give I.V. fluids as needed. Turn the patient often, and encourage deep-breathing exercises. Assisted respiration may be required. Isolation isn't required.

▶ Because botulism is sometimes fatal, keep the patient and his family informed about the course of the disease.

▶ Immediately notify local public health authorities of all cases of botulism.

 PREVENTION TIP To help prevent botulism, encourage patients to observe proper techniques in processing, preserving, and storing foods. Warn them to avoid even tasting food from a bulging can or one with a peculiar odor, and to sterilize by boiling any utensil that comes in contact with suspect food. Ingestion of even a small amount of food contaminated with botulism toxin can prove fatal.

BRAIN ABSCESS

Brain abscess is a free or encapsulated collection of pus that usually occurs in the temporal lobe, cerebellum, or frontal lobes. It can vary in size and may present singly or multilocularly. Brain abscess has a relatively low occurrence. Although it can occur at any age, it's most common in people ages 10 to 35 and is rare in older adults.

An untreated brain abscess is usually fatal; with treatment, the prognosis is only fair. About 30% of patients develop focal seizures. Multiple metastatic abscesses secondary to systemic or other infections have the poorest prognosis.

Causes

A brain abscess usually occurs secondary to some other infection, especially otitis media, sinusitis, dental abscess, and mastoiditis. Other causes include subdural empyema; bacterial endocarditis; human immunodeficiency virus infection; bacteremia; pulmonary or pleural infection; pelvic, abdominal, and skin infections; and cranial trauma, such as a penetrating head wound or compound skull fracture.

This condition also occurs in about 2% of children with congenital heart disease, possibly because the hypoxic brain is a good culture medium for bacteria. Common infecting organisms are pyogenic bacteria, such as *Staphylococcus aureus* and *Streptococcus viridans*. Penetrating head trauma or bacteremia usually leads to staphylococcal infection; pulmonary disease, to streptococcal infection.

Signs and symptoms

Onset varies with cause and location. Early symptoms are characteristic of a bacterial infection and include headache, chills, fever, malaise, confusion and drowsiness. The white blood cell count will be elevated with a differential indicating infection. As the lesion enlarges, it produces clinical effects similar to those of a brain tumor. At this time symptoms correlate with a disturbance of function in the invaded lobe.

Other features differ with the site of the abscess:

▶ *temporal lobe abscess:* auditory-receptive dysphasia, central facial weakness, hemiparesis

▶ *cerebellar abscess:* dizziness, coarse nystagmus, gaze weakness on lesion side, tremor, ataxia

▶ *frontal lobe abscess:* expressive dysphasia, hemiparesis with unilateral motor seizure, drowsiness, inattention, mental function impairment, seizures.

Diagnosis

A history of infection — especially of the middle ear, mastoid, nasal sinuses, heart, or lungs — or a history of congenital heart disease, along with a physical examination showing such characteristic clinical features as increased intracranial pressure (ICP), point to a brain abscess. An enhanced computed tomography (CT) scan and, occasionally, arteriography (which highlights the abscess by a halo) help locate the site.

Examination of cerebrospinal fluid can help confirm infection, but lumbar puncture is too risky because it can release the increased ICP and provoke cerebral herniation. A CT-guided stereotactic biopsy may be performed to drain and culture the abscess. Other tests include culture and sensitivity of drainage to identify the causative organism, skull X-rays, and a radioisotope scan.

Other conditions to be considered include brain tumors, stroke, resolving intracranial hemorrhage, subdural empyema, extradural abscess or encephalitis.

Treatment

Therapy consists of antibiotics to combat the underlying infection and surgical aspiration or drainage of the abscess. However, surgery is delayed until the abscess becomes encapsulated (a CT scan helps determine this) and is contraindicated in patients with congenital heart disease or another debilitating cardiac condition. Administration of a penicillinase-resistant antibiotic, such as nafcillin or methicillin, for at least 2 weeks before surgery can reduce the risk of spreading infection.

Other treatments during the acute phase are palliative and supportive; they include mechanical ventilation and administration of I.V. fluids with diuretics (urea, mannitol) and glucocorticoids (dexamethasone) to combat increased ICP and cerebral edema. Anticonvulsants, such as phenytoin and phenobarbital, help prevent seizures.

Special considerations

▶ The patient with an acute brain abscess requires intensive care monitoring.

 ALERT Frequently assess neurologic status, especially cognition and mentation, speech, and sensorimotor and cranial nerve function. Early increases in ICP can be detected by using such diagnostic tools as the mini-mental status exam, Glasgow Coma Scale, and National Institutes of Health (NIH) Stroke Scale. These highly sensitive tools facilitate recognition of early neurologic changes and may assist in retarding the increase of ICP. Once increased ICP results in abnormal pupils, depressed respirations, widened pulse pressure, and tachycardia or bradycardia, the cycle of increased ICP may not be reversible.

▶ Assess and record vital signs at least every hour.

▶ Monitor fluid intake and output carefully because fluid overload could contribute to cerebral edema.

▶ If surgery is necessary, explain the procedure to the patient and answer his questions.

▶ After surgery, continue frequent neurologic assessment. Monitor vital signs and intake and output.

▶ Watch for signs of meningitis (nuchal rigidity, headaches, chills, sweats), an ever-present threat.

▶ Change a damp dressing often. Never allow bandages to remain damp. Reinforce the dressing or change it as ordered. To promote drainage and prevent reaccumulation of the abscess, position the patient on the operative side. Measure drainage from Jackson-Pratt or other types of drains as instructed by the surgeon.

▶ If the patient remains stuporous or comatose for an extended period, give meticulous skin care to prevent pressure ulcers, and position him to preserve function and prevent contractures.

▶ If the patient requires isolation because of postoperative drainage, make sure he and his family understand why.

▶ Ambulate the patient as soon as possible to prevent immobility and encourage independence.

▶ Give prophylactic antibiotics as needed after a compound skull fracture or penetrating head wound.

 PREVENTION TIP To prevent brain abscess, stress the need for treatment of otitis media, mastoiditis, dental abscess, and other infections.

BRONCHIECTASIS

A condition marked by chronic abnormal dilation of bronchi and destruction of bronchial walls, bronchiectasis can occur throughout the tracheobronchial tree or can be confined to one segment or lobe. However, it is usually bilateral and in-

FORMS OF BRONCHIAL DILATATION

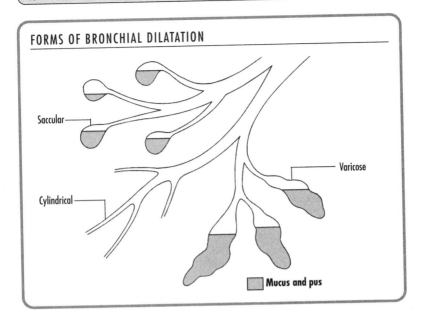

Saccular

Cylindrical

Varicose

■ Mucus and pus

volves the basilar segments of the lower lobes. This disease has three forms: cylindrical (fusiform), varicose, and saccular (cystic). It affects people of both sexes and all ages.

Because of the availability of antibiotics to treat acute respiratory tract infections, the incidence of bronchiectasis has dramatically decreased in the past 20 years. Incidence is highest among Eskimos and the Maoris of New Zealand. Bronchiectasis is irreversible once established.

Causes

The different forms of bronchiectasis may occur separately or simultaneously. In *cylindrical bronchiectasis,* the bronchi expand unevenly, with little change in diameter, and end suddenly in a squared-off fashion. In *varicose bronchiectasis,* abnormal, irregular dilation and narrowing of the bronchi give the appearance of varicose veins. In *saccular bronchiectasis,* many large dilations end in sacs. These sacs balloon into pus-filled cavities as they approach the periphery and are called saccules. (See *Forms of bronchial dilatation.*)

This disease results from conditions associated with repeated damage to bronchial walls and abnormal mucociliary clearance, which cause a breakdown of supporting tissue adjacent to airways. Such conditions include:
▶ cystic fibrosis
▶ immunologic disorders (agammaglobulinemia, for example)
▶ recurrent, inadequately treated bacterial respiratory tract infections, such as tuberculosis, and complications of measles, pneumonia, pertussis, or influenza
▶ obstruction (by a foreign body, tumor, or stenosis) in association with recurrent infection. (Foreign bodies are most common in children.)
▶ inhalation of corrosive gas or repeated aspiration of gastric juices into the lungs
▶ congenital anomalies (uncommon), such as bronchomalacia, congenital bronchiectasis, immotile-cilia syndrome, and Kartagener's syndrome (a variant of immotile-cilia syndrome characterized by situs inversus, bronchiectasis, and either nasal polyps or sinusitis).

In bronchiectasis, hyperplastic squamous epithelium denuded of cilia replaces ulcerated columnar epithelium. Abscess formation involving all layers of the bronchial wall produces inflammatory cells and fibrous tissue, resulting in both dilation and narrowing of the airways. Mucous plugs or fibrous tissue obliterates smaller bronchioles, while peribronchial lymphoid tissue becomes hyperplastic. Extensive vascular proliferation of bronchial circulation occurs and produces frequent hemoptysis.

Signs and symptoms

Initially, bronchiectasis may be asymptomatic. When symptoms do arise, they're often attributed to other illnesses. The patient usually complains of frequent bouts of pneumonia or hemoptysis. The classic symptom, however, is a chronic cough that produces foul-smelling, mucopurulent secretions in amounts ranging from less than 10 ml/day to more than 150 ml/day. This finding is observed in more than 90% of bronchiectasis patients. Characteristic findings include coarse crackles during inspiration over involved lobes or segments, occasional wheezing, dyspnea, sinusitis, weight loss, anemia, malaise, clubbing, recurrent fever, chills, and other signs of infection.

Advanced bronchiectasis may produce chronic malnutrition as well as right-sided heart failure and cor pulmonale due to hypoxic pulmonary vasoconstriction.

Diagnosis

A history of recurrent bronchial infections, pneumonia, and hemoptysis in a patient whose chest X-rays show peribronchial thickening, areas of atelectasis, and scattered cystic changes suggests bronchiectasis.

In recent years, computed tomography scanning has supplanted bronchography as the most useful diagnostic test for bronchiectasis. It is sometimes used with high-resolution techniques to better determine anatomic changes. Bronchoscopy does not establish the diagnosis of bron-

chiectasis, but it does help to identify the source of secretions. Bronchoscopy can also be instrumental in pinpointing the site of bleeding in hemoptysis.

Other helpful laboratory tests include:
▶ sputum culture and Gram stain to identify predominant organisms
▶ complete blood count to detect anemia and leukocytosis
▶ pulmonary function studies to detect decreased vital capacity, expiratory flow rate, and hypoxemia; these tests also help determine the physiologic severity of the disease and the effects of therapy, and help evaluate patients for surgery.

Evaluation may also include urinalysis and ECG. (The latter is normal unless cor pulmonale develops.) When cystic fibrosis is suspected as the underlying cause of bronchiectasis, a sweat electrolyte test is useful.

Other conditions to consider include chronic bronchitis, chronic obstructive pulmonary disease, cystic fibrosis, pulmonary tuberculosis, or allergic bronchopulmonary aspergillosis.

Treatment

Treatment includes antibiotics, given orally or I.V., for 7 to 10 days or until sputum production decreases. Long term antibiotic therapy is not appropriate because it may predispose the patient to serious Gram-negative infections. Bronchodilators, combined with postural drainage and chest percussion, help remove secretions if the patient has bronchospasm and thick, tenacious sputum. Bronchoscopy may be used to help mobilize secretions. Hypoxia requires oxygen therapy; severe hemoptysis commonly requires lobectomy, segmental resection, or bronchial artery embolization if pulmonary function is poor.

Special considerations

Provide supportive care and help the patient adjust to the permanent changes in lifestyle that irreversible lung damage necessitates. Thorough teaching is vital.

▶ Administer antibiotics, as ordered, and explain all diagnostic tests. Perform chest physiotherapy, including postural drainage and chest percussion designed for involved lobes, several times a day. The best times to do this are early morning and just before bedtime. Instruct the patient to maintain each position for 10 minutes; then perform percussion and tell him to cough. Show family members how to perform postural drainage and percussion. Also teach the patient coughing and deep-breathing techniques to promote good ventilation and the removal of secretions.

▶ Advise the patient to stop smoking, if appropriate, to avoid stimulating secretions and irritating the airways. Refer him to a local self-help group.

▶ Provide a warm, quiet, comfortable environment, and urge the patient to rest as much as possible. Encourage balanced, high-protein meals to promote good health and tissue healing, and plenty of fluids (2 to 3 qt [2 to 3 L]) per day to hydrate and thin bronchial secretions). Give frequent mouth care to remove foul-smelling sputum. Teach the patient to dispose of all secretions properly. Instruct the patient to seek prompt attention for respiratory infections.

▶ Tell the patient to avoid air pollutants and people with upper respiratory tract infections, and to take medications (especially antibiotics) exactly as prescribed.

 PREVENTION TIP To help prevent this disease, treat bacterial pneumonia vigorously and stress the need for immunization to prevent childhood diseases.

BRONCHIOLITIS OBLITERANS WITH ORGANIZING PNEUMONIA, IDIOPATHIC

Idiopathic bronchiolitis obliterans with organizing pneumonia (BOOP), also known as cryptogenic organizing pneumonia, is one of several types of bronchiolitis obliterans. "Bronchiolitis obliterans" is a generic term used to describe an inflammatory disease of the small airways. "Organizing pneumonia" refers to unresolved pneumonia, in which inflammatory alveolar exudate persists and eventually undergoes fibrosis.

Although BOOP was first described in 1901, confusing terminology and pathology that overlapped other diseases of the small airways kept it from being sufficiently recognized until the mid-1980s, when it was classified as a distinct clinical entity. Since that time, BOOP has been diagnosed with increasing frequency, although much debate still exists about the various pathologies and classifications of bronchiolitis obliterans.

Most patients with BOOP are between ages 50 and 60. Incidence is equally divided between men and women. A smoking history doesn't seem to increase the risk of developing BOOP.

Causes

BOOP has no known cause. However, other forms of bronchiolitis obliterans and organizing pneumonia may be associated with specific diseases or situations, such as bone marrow, heart, or heart-lung transplantation; collagen vascular diseases, such as rheumatoid arthritis and systemic lupus erythematosus; inflammatory diseases, such as Crohn's disease, ulcerative colitis, and polyarteritis nodosa; bacterial, viral, or mycoplasmal respiratory infections; inhalation of toxic gases; and drug therapy with amiodarone, bleomycin, penicillamine, or lomustine.

Signs and symptoms

The presenting symptoms of BOOP are usually subacute, with a flulike syndrome of fever, persistent and nonproductive cough, dyspnea (especially on exertion), malaise, anorexia, and weight loss lasting from several weeks to several months. Physical assessment findings may reveal dry crackles as the only abnormality. Less common symptoms include a productive cough, hemoptysis, chest pain, generalized aching, and night sweats.

Diagnosis

Diagnosis begins with a thorough patient history meant to exclude any known cause of bronchiolitis obliterans or diseases with a pathology that includes an organizing pneumonia pattern.

▶ Chest X-ray usually shows patchy, diffuse airspace opacities with a ground-glass appearance that may migrate from one location to another. High-resolution computed tomography scans show areas of consolidation. Except for the migrating opacities, these findings are nonspecific and present in many other respiratory disorders.

▶ Pulmonary function tests may be normal or show reduced capacities. The diffusing capacity for carbon monoxide (DLCO) is generally low.

▶ Arterial blood gas analysis usually shows mild to moderate hypoxemia at rest, which worsens with exercise.

▶ Blood tests reveal an increased erythrocyte sedimentation rate, increased C-reactive protein level, increased white blood cell count with a somewhat increased proportion of neutrophils, and a minor rise in eosinophils. Immunoglobulin (Ig)G and IgM levels are normal or slightly increased, and the IgE level is normal.

▶ Bronchoscopy reveals normal or slightly inflamed airways. Bronchoalveolar lavage fluid obtained during bronchoscopy shows a moderate elevation in lymphocytes and, sometimes, elevated neutrophil and eosinophil levels. Foamy-looking alveolar macrophages may also be found.

Lung biopsy, thoracoscopy, or bronchoscopy is required to confirm the diagnosis of BOOP. Pathologic changes in lung tissue include plugs of connective tissue in the lumen of the bronchioles, alveolar ducts, and alveolar spaces.

These changes may occur in other types of bronchiolitis and in other diseases that cause organizing pneumonia. They also differentiate BOOP from constrictive bronchiolitis, characterized by inflammation and fibrosis that surround and may narrow or completely obliterate the bronchiolar airways. Although the pathologic findings in proliferative and constrictive bronchiolitis are different, the causes and presentations may overlap. Any known cause of bronchiolitis obliterans or organizing pneumonia must be ruled out before the diagnosis of BOOP is made. Other conditions to consider include interstitial pneumonitis, tuberculosis, sarcoidosis, histoplasmosis, berylliosis, Goodpasture's syndrome, neoplasm, systemic lupus erythematosus, chronic eosinophilic pneumonia, or cryptogenic bronchiolitis.

Treatment

Corticosteroids are the current treatment for BOOP, although the ideal dosage and duration of treatment remain topics of discussion. In most cases, treatment begins with 1 mg/kg/day of prednisone for at least several days to several weeks; the dosage is then gradually reduced over several months to a year, depending on the patient's response. Relapse is common when steroids are tapered off or stopped but usually can be reversed when steroids are increased or resumed. Occasionally, a patient may need to continue corticosteroids indefinitely.

Immunosuppressive-cytotoxic drugs such as cyclophosphamide have been used in the few cases in which the patient could not tolerate or was unresponsive to corticosteroids.

Oxygen is used to correct hypoxemia. The patient may need either no oxygen or a small amount of oxygen at rest and a greater amount during exercise.

Other treatments vary, depending on the patient's symptoms, and may include inhaled bronchodilators, cough suppressants, and bronchial hygiene therapies.

BOOP is very responsive to treatment and usually can be completely reversed with corticosteroid therapy. However, a few deaths have been reported, particularly in patients who had more widespread pathologic changes in the lung or patients who developed opportunistic infections or other complications related to steroid therapy.

Special considerations

▶ Explain all diagnostic tests. The patient may experience anxiety and frustration because of the length of time and number of tests needed to establish the diagnosis.

▶ Explain the diagnosis to the patient and his family. This uncommon diagnosis may cause confusion and anxiety.

▶ Monitor the patient for adverse effects of corticosteroid therapy: weight gain, moon face, glucose intolerance, fluid and electrolyte imbalance, mood swings, cataracts, peptic ulcer disease, opportunistic infections, and osteoporosis leading to bone fractures. These effects may leave many patients unable to tolerate the treatment. Teach the patient and family about these adverse effects, emphasizing which reactions they should report to the doctor.

▶ Monitor oxygenation, both at rest and with exertion. The doctor will probably prescribe an oxygen flow rate for use when the patient is at rest and a higher one for exertion. Teach the patient how to increase the oxygen flow rate to the appropriate level for exercise.

 PREVENTION TIP Teach measures that may help prevent complications related to treatment, such as infection control and improved nutrition. Also teach breathing, relaxation, and energy conservation techniques to help the patient manage symptoms.

BRUCELLOSIS

Brucellosis (also known as undulant fever, Malta fever, or Bang's disease) is an acute febrile illness transmitted to humans from animals.

Brucellosis occurs throughout the world; however, such measures as pasteurization of dairy products and immunization of cattle have reduced the incidence of brucellosis in the U.S. population.

Sources of infection occur through travel abroad, consuming imported cheese, and occupation-related exposure. It's most common among farmers, stock handlers, butchers, and veterinarians.

The incubation period usually lasts from 5 to 35 days, but in some cases it can last for months. The prognosis is good. With treatment, brucellosis is seldom fatal, although complications can cause permanent disability.

Brucellosis can result in endocarditis, orchitis, persistent hepatosplenomegaly, and osteoarticular problems, such as arthritis and osteomyelitis. Skin manifestations, such as eczematous rashes, petechiae, and purpura, are possible, as is pulmonary involvement, including pleural effusions and pneumothorax.

Brucellosis can cause abscesses in the testes, ovaries, kidneys, spleen, liver, bone, and brain (meningitis and encephalitis). About 15% of patients with such brain abscesses develop hearing and visual disorders, hemiplegia, and ataxia.

Causes

Brucellosis is caused by the nonmotile, nonspore-forming, Gram-negative coccobacilli of the genus *Brucella*, notably *B. suis* (found in swine), *B. melitensis* (in goats), *B. abortus* (in cattle), and *B. canis* (in dogs).

The disease is transmitted through the consumption of unpasteurized dairy products, or uncooked or undercooked contaminated meat, and through contact with infected animals or their secretions or excretions.

Signs and symptoms

Onset of brucellosis is usually insidious, but the disease course falls into two distinct phases. Characteristically, the acute phase causes fever, chills, profuse sweating, fatigue, headache, backache, enlarged lymph nodes, hepatosplenomegaly, weight loss, and abscess and granuloma formulation in subcutaneous tissues, lymph nodes, liver, and spleen. Despite this disease's common name — undulant fever — few patients have a truly intermittent (undulant) fever; in fact, fever is commonly insignificant.

The chronic phase produces recurrent depression, sleep disturbances, fatigue, headache, sweating, and sexual impotence; hepatosplenomegaly and enlarged lymph nodes persist. Additionally, abscesses may form in the testes, ovaries, kidneys, and brain (meningitis and encephalitis). About 10% to 15% of patients with such brain abscesses develop hearing and visual disorders, hemiplegia, and ataxia. Other complications include osteomyelitis, orchitis and, rarely, subacute bacterial endocarditis, which is difficult to treat.

Diagnosis

In patients with characteristic clinical features, a history of exposure to animals suggests brucellosis. Multiple agglutination tests help to confirm the diagnosis. Approximately 90% of patients with brucellosis have agglutinin titers of 1:160 or more within 3 weeks of developing this disease. However, elevated agglutinin titers also follow vaccination against tularemia, *Yersinia* infection, or cholera; skin tests; or relapse. Agglutinin titers testing can also monitor effectiveness of treatment.

Multiple (three to six) cultures of blood and bone marrow and biopsies of infected tissue (for example, the spleen) provide a definite diagnosis. Culturing is best done during the acute phase.

Blood studies indicate increased erythrocyte sedimentation rate and normal or reduced white blood cell count. Diagnosis must rule out infectious diseases that produce similar symptoms, such as typhoid and malaria.

Treatment

Treatment consists of bed rest during the febrile phase. Antibiotic therapy includes a combination of doxycycline and an aminoglycoside such as streptomycin, gentamicin, or netilmicin for 4 weeks followed by the combination of doxycycline and rifampin for 4 weeks. In pregnancy, trimethoprim-sulfamethoxazole can be given along with rifampin. Heart surgery may be necessary in cases of *Brucella* endocarditis and aortic root abscess.

Special considerations

In suspected cases of brucellosis, take a full history. Ask the patient about his occupation and if he has recently traveled or eaten unprocessed food such as goat's milk.

❯ During the acute phase, monitor and record the patient's temperature every 4 hours. Be sure to use the same route (oral or rectal) every time. Provide between-meal milkshakes and other supplemental foods to counter weight loss. Watch for heart murmurs, muscle weakness, vision loss, and joint inflammation — which may signal complications.

❯ During the chronic phase, watch for depression and disturbed sleep patterns. Administer sedatives as ordered, and plan your care to allow adequate rest.

❯ Keep suppurative granulomas and abscesses dry. Double-bag and properly dispose of all secretions and soiled dressings. Reassure the patient that this infection is curable.

❯ Before discharge, stress the importance of continuing medication for the prescribed duration.

 PREVENTION TIP To prevent recurrence, advise the patient to cook meat thoroughly and avoid using unpasteurized milk. Warn meat packers and other people at risk of occupational exposure to wear rubber gloves and goggles.

C

CAMPYLOBACTERIOSIS

Campylobacteriosis is caused by bacteria of the genus *Campylobacter*. *C. jejuni is* the most common bacterial cause of diarrhea in the United States. Most cases occur as isolated, sporadic events; however, large outbreaks can occur. Over 10,000 cases are reported to the Centers for Disease Control and Prevention (CDC) each year, or about six cases per 100,000 persons. Because surveillance is limited, however, many more cases go undiagnosed or unreported, and campylobacteriosis is estimated to affect over 2 million persons each year— one percent of the population.

Campylobacteriosis occurs much more frequently in the summer than in the winter. *Campylobacter* is isolated predominantly from infants and young adults and from males more often than females. Although campylobacteriosis is rarely fatal, perhaps 500 persons with *Campylobacter* infections may die each year.

Causes

Campylobacteriosis is most often associated with handling raw poultry or eating raw or undercooked poultry meat. A single drop of water from raw chicken — or fewer than 500 *Campylobacter* microbes — can cause illness in humans. The microbes from raw meat can then spread to other foods. *Campylobacter* is not usually spread from person to person, but this can happen if the infected person is a small child or is producing a large volume of diarrhea. Larger outbreaks due to *Campylobacter* are not usually associated with raw poultry but are usually related to drinking unpasteurized milk or contaminated water. Animals can also be infected, and some people have acquired their infection from contact with the infected stool of an ill dog or cat.

Signs and symptoms

Although the infection may not produce symptoms, most people experience diarrhea, cramping, abdominal pain, and fever 2 to 5 days after exposure to the microbes. Diarrhea may be bloody and may be accompanied by nausea and vomiting. The illness typically lasts 1 week. In immunocompromised persons, *Campylobacter* may spread to the bloodstream and cause life-threatening sepsis. Others (about 1:1,000 cases) may develop arthritis or Guillain-Barré syndrome following campylobacteriosis.

Diagnosis

Microscopic examination of the stool may reveal many segmented neutrophils and, frequently, red blood cells. Visualization of *Campylobacter* in stool with Gram staining or phase-contrast or dark-field microscopy to identify the microbe's characteristic "darting" motility confirms the diagnosis.

Other conditions to consider include viral gastroenteritis, pseudomembranous colitis, other bacterial infections, and inflammatory or granulomatous bowel disease.

Treatment

Usually all persons infected with *Campylobacter* recover without specific treatment. Patients should drink plenty of fluids as long as the diarrhea lasts. In severe cases, antibiotics such as erythromycin or a fluoroquinolone should be given; these can shorten the duration of symptoms if given early in the illness.

Special considerations

▶ Help the patient maintain adequate hydration. Remember that dehydration occurs rapidly in elderly patients.

▶ Measure intake and output (including stools) carefully. Cleanse the perineum thoroughly to prevent skin breakdown.

▶ If possible, stool specimens should be chilled (not frozen) and sent to the laboratory within 24 hours of collection. Storing specimens in deep, airtight containers minimizes exposure to oxygen and desiccation. If a specimen cannot be processed within 24 hours or is likely to contain small numbers of organisms, a rectal swab placed in a specimen transport medium should be used.

▶ Follow standard precautions. Always wash your hands thoroughly before and after any contact with the patient, and advise others to do the same.

 PREVENTION TIP Teach the patient to use proper hand-washing technique, especially after defecating and before eating or handling food. Stress proper food handling techniques, especially the thorough cooking of all poultry and other meats, and instruct in common sense kitchen hygiene practices such as washing hands with soap before and after handling raw meat. Use separate cutting boards for foods of animal origin and other foods and carefully clean all cutting boards, countertops and utensils with soap and hot water after preparing raw food of animal origin. Tell patients to avoid drinking unpasteurized milk and untreated surface water.

CANDIDIASIS

Also called candidosis and moniliasis, candidiasis is usually a mild, superficial fungal infection caused by the genus *Candi-*

da. Most often, it infects the nails (onychomycosis), skin (diaper rash), or mucous membranes, especially the oropharynx (thrush), vagina (moniliasis), esophagus, and GI tract.

Rarely, these fungi enter the bloodstream and invade the kidneys, lungs, endocardium, brain, or other structures, causing serious infections. Such systemic infection is most prevalent among drug abusers and patients already hospitalized, particularly diabetics and immunosuppressed patients. The prognosis varies, depending on the patient's resistance.

Causes

Most cases of *Candida* infection result from *C. albicans.* Other infective strains include *C. parapsilosis, C. tropicalis,* and *C. krusei.* These fungi are part of the normal flora of the GI tract, mouth, vagina, and skin. They cause infection when some change in the body permits their sudden proliferation—rising glucose levels from diabetes mellitus; lowered resistance from a disease (such as cancer), an immunosuppressive drug, radiation, aging, or human immunodeficiency virus (HIV) infection; elevated estrogen levels during pregnancy; or when they're introduced systemically by I.V. or urinary catheters, drug abuse, hyperalimentation, or surgery.

However, the most common predisposing factor remains the use of broad-spectrum antibiotics, which depress normal flora and allow *Candida* microbes to proliferate. The infant of a mother with vaginal moniliasis can contract oral thrush while passing through the birth canal, although this is uncommon.

The incidence of candidiasis is rising because of wider use of I.V. therapy and a greater number of immunocompromised patients, especially those with HIV infection.

Signs and symptoms

Superficial candidiasis produces symptoms that correspond to the following sites of infection:

RECOGNIZING THRUSH

Candidiasis of the oropharyngeal mucosa (thrush) causes cream-colored or bluish white pseudomembranous patches on the tongue, mouth, or pharynx. Fungal invasion may extend to circumoral tissues.

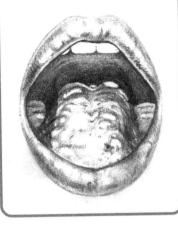

▶ *skin:* scaly, erythematous, papular rash, sometimes covered with exudate, appearing below the breast, between the fingers, and at the axillae, groin, and umbilicus; in diaper rash, papules appear at the edges of the rash.

▶ *nails:* red, swollen, darkened nailbed; occasionally, purulent discharge and the separation of a pruritic nail from the nailbed

▶ *oropharyngeal mucosa (thrush):* cream-colored or bluish-white patches of exudate on the tongue, mouth, or pharynx that reveal bloody engorgement when scraped. They may swell, causing respiratory distress in infants. They're only occasionally painful but cause a burning sensation in the throats and mouths of adults. (See *Recognizing thrush.*)

▶ *esophageal mucosa:* dysphagia, retrosternal pain, regurgitation and, occasionally, scales in the mouth and throat

▶ *vaginal mucosa:* white or yellow discharge, with pruritus and local excoriation; white or gray raised patches on vaginal walls, with local inflammation; dyspareunia

Systemic infection produces chills; high, spiking fever; hypotension; prostration; and occasional rash. Specific symptoms depend on the site of infection:

▶ *pulmonary system:* hemoptysis, fever, cough

▶ *renal system:* fever, flank pain, dysuria, hematuria, pyuria

▶ *brain:* headache, nuchal rigidity, seizures, focal neurologic deficits

▶ *endocardium:* systolic or diastolic murmur, fever, chest pain, embolic phenomena

▶ *eye:* endophthalmitis, blurred vision, orbital or periorbital pain, scotoma, exudate.

Diagnosis

Identification of superficial candidiasis depends on evidence of *Candida* on a Gram stain of skin, vaginal scrapings, or discharge, pus, or sputum or on skin scrapings prepared in potassium hydroxide solution. Systemic infections require obtaining a sample for blood or tissue culture.

Treatment

The first aim of treatment is to improve the underlying condition that predisposes the patient to candidiasis, such as controlling diabetes or discontinuing antibiotic therapy and catheterization, if possible.

Nystatin is an effective antifungal for superficial candidiasis. Clotrimazole, fluconazole, ketoconazole, and miconazole are effective in mucous-membrane and vaginal *Candida* infections. Ketoconazole or fluconazole is the treatment of choice for chronic candidiasis of the mucous membranes. Treatment for systemic infection may consist of I.V. fluconazole or I.V. amphotericin B with or without 5-fluorocytosine.

Special considerations

▶ Swab nystatin on the oral mucosa of an infant with thrush.

▶ Instruct a patient using nystatin solution to swish it around in his mouth for several minutes before he swallows the solution.

▶ Provide the patient with a nonirritating mouthwash to loosen tenacious secretions and a soft toothbrush to avoid irritation.

▶ Relieve the patient's mouth discomfort with a topical anesthetic, such as lidocaine, at least 1 hour before meals. (It may suppress the gag reflex and cause aspiration.)

▶ Provide a soft diet for the patient with severe dysphagia. Tell the patient with mild dysphagia to chew food thoroughly, and make sure he doesn't choke.

▶ Use cornstarch or dry padding in intertriginous areas of obese patients to prevent irritation.

▶ Note dates of insertion of I.V. catheters, and replace them according to your facility's policy to prevent phlebitis.

▶ Assess the patient with candidiasis for underlying causes such as diabetes mellitus. If the patient is receiving amphotericin B for systemic candidiasis, he may have severe chills, fever, anorexia, nausea, and vomiting. Premedicate with acetaminophen, antihistamines, or antiemetics to help reduce adverse reactions.

▶ Frequently check vital signs of patients with systemic infections. Provide appropriate supportive care.

▶ In patients with renal involvement, carefully monitor intake and output and urine blood and protein levels.

 PREVENTION TIP Check high-risk patients daily, especially those receiving antibiotics, for patchy areas, irritation, sore throat, bleeding of mouth or gums, or other signs of superinfection. Check for vaginal discharge; record the color and amount.

CELLULITIS

Cellulitis is an acute inflammatory process involving skin and subcutaneous tissues. It can occur on any part of the body and is common in the lower extremities, abdomen, and face. Bacteria enter the skin's protective outer layer, usually at a site of injury (surgery, trauma, ulceration, burn, and bite) or at the site of a surgical wound or I.V. catheter. For patients with peripheral vascular disease or diabetes, even minor injuries to the lower extremities can precipitate cellulitis. Cellulitis occurs in both sexes equally across all age groups.

Causes

Cellulitis can be caused by different bacteria depending on the circumstances surrounding the infection. The most common agents are *Streptococcus pyogenes* and *Staphylococcus aureus*. Other types of skin injuries may involve more unusual bacteria, such as *Pasteurella multocida* for cat and dog bites, *Aeromonas hydrophila* for fresh water injuries, *Pseudomonas aeruginosa* for deep puncture wounds through wet footwear, *Erysipelothrix rhusiopathiae* for injuries sustained while cleaning meat or fish, and *Mycobacterium marinum* for injuries exposed to aquarium or pool water. *Haemophilus influenzae* type B in non-immunized children causes periorbital cellulitis. *Streptococcus pneumoniae* is the most likely agent in *H. influenzae* type B immunized children. Many different species of bacteria can cause hospital-acquired cellulitis and may be especially difficult to treat. These bacteria have become increasingly antibiotic-resistant.

Signs and symptoms

The classic sign of cellulitis is sudden tenderness, edema, and erythema of the affected area. The skin may feel warm to the touch. Fever, chills, and general malaise may accompany skin findings, along with enlarged lymph nodes near the site of infection. Serious but rare complications include severe necrotizing subcutaneous infection and sepsis. Without treatment, some cases of superficial cellulitis spontaneously resolve. However, recurrences are common and can lead to serious damage to the lymph nodes. With antibiotics, such complications are uncommon.

Diagnosis

Diagnosis can be made based on the patient's history and clinical findings. The responsible microbe is difficult to identify unless there is drainage to culture. Blood tests such as titers of anti-DNAase B confirm streptococci, but are usually unnecessary. CBC, sedimentation rate, and blood cultures may be helpful.

Other conditions to consider include acute gout, fasciitis or myositis, thrombophlebitis, osteomyelitis, ruptured Baker's cyst, herpetic whitlow, cutaneous diphtheria, and pseudogout.

Treatment

Penicillin is the drug of choice for streptococcal cellulitis. In penicillin-allergic patients, erythromycin is effective for mild infections, and parenteral clindamycin for severe infections. Some doctors prefer using antibiotics that are also effective against *S. aureus:* dicloxacillin for mild infections, or oxacillin or nafcillin for severe infections. Vancomycin is indicated for those patients with suspected methicillin-resistant *S. aureus* infection.

Use warm, moist heat to relieve local tenderness. Elevate and immobilize the affected area to help reduce edema.

Special considerations

▶ Remind the patient to take the full course of antibiotics even if symptoms abate.
▶ Encourage the patient to rest and elevate the affected area.
▶ Be aware of allergies to antibiotics.
▶ Teach the patient skin hygiene and avoidance of skin trauma. Encourage the patient to report early skin changes to the doctor.

CHANCROID

Chancroid (also known as soft chancre) is a sexually transmitted disease (STD) characterized by painful genital ulcers and inguinal adenitis. This infection occurs worldwide but is particularly common in tropical countries; it affects more males than females. Chancroidal lesions may heal spontaneously and usually respond well to treatment in the absence of secondary infections. A high rate of human immunodeficiency virus (HIV) infection has been reported among patients with chancroid.

Causes

Chancroid results from *Haemophilus ducreyi,* a gram-negative streptobacillus, and is transmitted through sexual contact. Poor hygiene may predispose males (especially those who are uncircumcised) to this disease.

Signs and symptoms

After a 3- to 5-day incubation period, a small papule appears at the site of entry, usually the groin or inner thigh; in the male, it may appear on the penis; in the female, on the vulva, vagina, or cervix. Occasionally, this papule may erupt on the tongue, lip, breast, or navel. The papule rapidly ulcerates, becoming painful, soft, and malodorous; it bleeds easily and produces pus. It is gray and shallow, with irregular edges, and measures up to 1″ (2.5 cm) in diameter. Within 2 to 3 weeks, inguinal adenitis develops, creating suppurated, inflamed nodes that may rupture into large ulcers or buboes. Headache and malaise occur in 50% of patients. During the healing stage, phimosis may develop.

Diagnosis

Gram stain smears of ulcer exudate or bubo aspirate are 50% reliable; blood agar cultures are 75% reliable. Biopsy confirms the diagnosis but is reserved for resistant cases or cases in which cancer is suspected. Dark-field examination and serologic testing rule out other STDs that cause similar ulcers. Testing for HIV infection should be done at the time of diagnosis.

Treatment

The treatment of choice is azithromycin, orally in a single dose; erythromycin, for 7 days; or ceftriaxone, 250 mg I.M. in a single dose. Although ciprofloxacin may be prescribed, it should not be used by pregnant or lactating women or people ages 18 and younger. The safety of azithromycin for pregnant or lactating women has not been established. Aspiration of fluid-filled nodes helps prevent spreading the infection.

Special considerations

▶ Practice standard precautions.

▶ Make sure the patient is not allergic to any drug before giving the first dose.

▶ Instruct the patient not to apply lotions, creams, or oils on or near the genitalia or on other lesion sites.

▶ Tell the patient to abstain from sexual contact until healing is complete (usually about 2 weeks after treatment begins) and to wash the genitalia daily with soap and water. Instruct uncircumcised males to retract the foreskin for thorough cleaning.

 PREVENTION TIP To prevent chancroid, advise patients to avoid sexual contact with infected people, to use condoms during sexual activity, and to wash the genitalia with soap and water after sexual activity.

CHLAMYDIAL INFECTIONS

Urethritis in men and urethritis and cervicitis in women compose a group of infections that are linked to one organism: *Chlamydia trachomatis.* Chlamydial infections are the most common sexually transmitted diseases in the United States, affecting an estimated 4 million Americans each year.

Trachoma inclusion conjunctivitis, a chlamydial infection that occurs rarely in the United States, is a leading cause of blindness in Third World countries. Lymphogranuloma venereum, a rare disease in the United States, is also caused by *C. trachomatis.*

Untreated, chlamydial infections can lead to such complications as acute epididymitis, salpingitis, pelvic inflammatory disease and, eventually, sterility. Some studies show that chlamydial infections in pregnant women are associated with spontaneous abortion and premature delivery. Other studies haven't confirmed these findings.

Causes

Transmission of *C. trachomatis* primarily follows vaginal or rectal intercourse or oral-genital contact with an infected person. Because signs and symptoms of chlamydial infections commonly appear late in the course of the disease, sexual transmission of the organism typically occurs unknowingly.

Children born of mothers who have chlamydial infections may contract associated conjunctivitis, otitis media, and pneumonia during passage through the birth canal.

Signs and symptoms

Both men and women with chlamydial infections may be asymptomatic or may show signs of infection on physical examination. Individual signs and symptoms vary with the specific type of chlamydial infection and are determined by the organism's route of transmission to susceptible tissue. (See *Lymphogranuloma venereum,* page 58.)

Women who have cervicitis may develop cervical erosion, mucopurulent discharge, pelvic pain, and dyspareunia.

Women who have endometritis or salpingitis may experience signs of pelvic inflammatory disease, such as pain and tenderness of the abdomen, cervix, uterus, and lymph nodes; chills; fever; break-

LYMPHOGRANULOMA VENEREUM

A rare disease in the United States, lymphogranuloma vene-reum (LGV) is caused by serovars L_1, L_2, or L_3 of *Chlamydia trachomatis*. The most common clinical manifestations of LGV among heterosexuals, especially male patients, is enlarged inguinal lymph nodes (usually unilateral). These nodes may become fluctuant, tender masses. Regional nodes draining the initial lesion may enlarge and appear as a series of bilateral buboes. Untreated buboes may rupture and form sinus tracts that discharge a thick, yellow, granular secretion.

Women and homosexually active men may have proctocolitis or inflammatory involvement of perirectal or perianal lymphatic tissue, resulting in fistulas and strictures.

By the time patients seek treatment, the self-limited genital ulcer that sometimes occurs at the site of inoculation is no longer present. The diagnosis usually is made serologically and by excluding other causes of inguinal lymphadenopathy or genital ulcers.

The treatment of choice is doxycycline. Treatment cures infection and prevents ongoing tissue damage, although the patient may develop a scar or an indurated inguinal mass. Buboes may require aspiration or incision and drainage through intact skin.

Men who have urethritis may experience dysuria, erythema, tenderness of the urethral meatus, urinary frequency, pruritus, and urethral discharge. In urethritis, such discharge may be copious and purulent or scant and clear or mucoid.

Men with epididymitis may experience painful scrotal swelling and urethral discharge.

Men who have prostatitis may have lower back pain, urinary frequency, dysuria, nocturia, and painful ejaculation.

In proctitis, patients may have diarrhea, tenesmus, pruritus, bloody or mucopurulent discharge, and diffuse or discrete ulceration in the rectosigmoid colon.

Diagnosis

A swab from the site of infection (urethra, cervix, or rectum) establishes a diagnosis of urethritis, cervicitis, salpingitis, endometritis, or proctitis. A culture of aspirated material establishes a diagnosis of epididymitis.

Nucleic acid probes using polymerase chain reactions are the diagnostic method of choice. Antigen detection methods, including the enzyme-linked immunosorbent assay and the direct fluorescent antibody test, are older diagnostic tests for identifying chlamydial infection. Tissue cell cultures may also be used and are more sensitive and specific.

Treatment

The recommended first-line treatment for adults and adolescents who have chlamydial infections is drug therapy with oral doxycycline for 7 days or oral azithromycin in a single dose.

For pregnant women with chlamydial infections, azithromycin (Zithromax), in a single dose for both the male and female partners, is the treatment of choice.

Special considerations

▶ Practice universal precautions when caring for a patient with a chlamydial infection.

through bleeding; bleeding after intercourse; and vaginal discharge. They may also have dysuria.

Women with urethral syndrome may experience dysuria, pyuria, and urinary frequency.

▶ Make sure that the patient fully understands the dosage requirements of any prescribed medications for this infection.

▶ If required in your state, report all cases of chlamydial infection to the appropriate local public health authorities who will then conduct follow-up notification of the patient's sexual contacts.

▶ Suggest that the patient and his sexual partners receive testing for human immunodeficiency virus (HIV).

▶ Check newborns of infected mothers for signs of chlamydial infection. Obtain appropriate specimens for diagnostic testing.

CHOLERA

Cholera (also known as Asiatic cholera or epidemic cholera) is an acute enterotoxin-in-mediated GI infection caused by the gram-negative bacillus *Vibrio cholerae*. It produces profuse diarrhea, vomiting, massive fluid and electrolyte loss and, possibly, hypovolemic shock, metabolic acidosis, and death. A similar bacterium, *Vibrio parahaemolyticus,* causes food poisoning.

Even with prompt diagnosis and treatment, cholera is fatal in up to 2% of children; in adults, it is fatal in fewer than 1%. However, untreated cholera may be fatal in as many as 50% of patients. Cholera infection confers only transient immunity.

Cholera is most common in Africa, southern and Southeast Asia, and the Middle East, although outbreaks have occurred in Japan, Australia, and Europe.

Cholera occurs during the warmer months and is most prevalent among lower socioeconomic groups. In India, it's common among children ages 1 to 5, but in other endemic areas, it's equally distributed among all age groups. Susceptibility to cholera may be increased by a deficiency or an absence of hydrochloric acid.

In the United States, cholera has been virtually eliminated by modern sewage and water treatment systems. However, as a result of improved transportation, more persons from the United States travel to parts of Latin America, Africa, or Asia where epidemic cholera is occurring. U.S. travelers to areas with epidemic cholera may be exposed to the cholera bacterium. In addition, travelers may bring contaminated seafood back to the United States.

Causes

Humans are the only hosts and victims of *V. cholerae,* a motile, aerobic microbe. It's transmitted through food and water contaminated with fecal material from carriers or people with active infections.

Signs and symptoms

After an incubation period ranging from several hours to 5 days, cholera produces acute, painless, profuse, watery diarrhea and effortless vomiting (without preceding nausea). As diarrhea worsens, the stools contain white flecks of mucus (rice-water stools). Because of massive fluid and electrolyte losses from diarrhea and vomiting (fluid loss in adults may reach 1 L/hour), cholera causes intense thirst, weakness, loss of skin turgor, wrinkled skin, sunken eyes, pinched facial expression, muscle cramps (especially in the extremities), cyanosis, oliguria, tachycardia, tachypnea, thready or absent peripheral pulses, falling blood pressure, fever, and inaudible, hypoactive bowel sounds.

Patients usually remain oriented but apathetic, although small children may become stuporous or develop seizures. If complications don't occur, the symptoms subside and the patient recovers within a week. But if treatment is delayed or inadequate, cholera may lead to metabolic acidosis, uremia and, possibly, coma and death. About 3% of patients who recover continue to carry *V. cholerae* in the gallbladder; however, most patients are free from the infection after about 2 weeks.

Diagnosis

In endemic areas or during epidemics, typical clinical features strongly suggest cholera.

A culture of *V. cholerae* from feces or vomitus indicates cholera; however, definitive diagnosis requires agglutination and other clear reactions to group- and type-specific antisera.

A dark-field microscopic examination of fresh feces showing rapidly moving bacilli (like shooting stars) allows for a quick, tentative diagnosis. Immunofluorescence also allows rapid diagnosis. Diagnosis must rule out *Escherichia coli* infection, salmonellosis, and shigellosis.

Treatment

Improved sanitation and the administration of cholera vaccine to travelers in endemic areas can control this disease. Unfortunately, the vaccine now available confers only 60% to 80% immunity and is effective for only 3 to 6 months. Consequently, vaccination is impractical for residents of endemic areas.

Treatment requires rapid I.V. infusion of large amounts (50 to 100 ml/minute) of isotonic saline solution, alternating with isotonic sodium bicarbonate or sodium lactate. Potassium replacement may be added to the I.V. solution. Antibiotic therapy has not proved successful in shortening the course of infection, but in severe cases doxycycline has been prescribed.

When I.V. infusions have corrected hypovolemia, fluid infusion decreases to quantities sufficient to maintain normal pulse and skin turgor or to replace fluid loss through diarrhea. An oral glucose-electrolyte solution can substitute for I.V. infusions. In mild cholera, oral fluid replacement is adequate. If symptoms persist despite fluid and electrolyte replacement, treatment includes tetracycline.

Special considerations

A cholera patient requires enteric precautions, supportive care, and close observation during the acute phase.

▶ Wear a gown and gloves when handling feces-contaminated articles or when a danger of contaminating clothing exists, and wash your hands after leaving the patient's room.

▶ Monitor output (including stool volume) and I.V. infusion accurately. To detect overhydration, carefully observe neck veins, take serial patient weights, and auscultate the lungs. (Fluid loss in cholera is massive, and improper replacement may cause potentially fatal renal insufficiency.)

▶ Protect the patient's family by administering oral tetracycline, if ordered.

 PREVENTION TIP Advise anyone traveling to an endemic area to boil all drinking water and avoid eating uncooked vegetables and unpeeled fruits. If the doctor orders a cholera vaccine, tell the patient that he'll need a booster 3 to 6 months later for continuing protection.

CHRONIC FATIGUE SYNDROME

Persons with chronic fatigue syndrome (CFS) must often function at a greatly reduced level of activity than they were capable of before the onset of illness. In CFS, debilitating fatigue typically is not relieved by bedrest, and the fatigue may be aggravated by physical or mental activity. In addition to these key defining characteristics, nonspecific symptoms include weakness, muscle pain, impaired memory or mental concentration or both, insomnia, and post-exertional fatigue lasting more than 24 hours. In some patients, CFS can persist for years. It commonly occurs in adults under age 45, primarily in women.

Causes

Chronic fatigue syndrome has no known single cause. Conditions thought to trigger the development of CFS include viral infection or other transient traumatic conditions, stress, and toxins.

Signs and symptoms

The characteristic symptom of CFS is prolonged, often overwhelming fatigue that's commonly associated with a varying complex of other symptoms. To aid identification of the disease, the Centers for Disease Control and Prevention (CDC) uses a "working case definition" to group symptoms and severity. (See *CDC criteria for diagnosing CFS.*)

Diagnosis

No single test unequivocally confirms CFS. Therefore, the diagnosis is based on the patient's history and the CDC criteria. Because these criteria are admittedly a working concept that may not include all forms of CFS and are based on symptoms that can result from other diseases, a diagnosis is difficult and uncertain. Considerable overlap exists between CFS and fibromyalgia syndrome, myalgic encephalomyelitis, neurasthenia, multiple chemical sensitivities, and chronic mononucleosis.

The following serologic tests are typically performed to exclude other causes of fatiguing illness: alanine aminotransferase (ALT), albumin, alkaline phosphatase (ALP), blood urea nitrogen (BUN), calcium, complete blood count, creatinine, electrolytes, erythrocyte sedimentation rate (ESR), globulin, glucose, phosphorus, thyroid stimulating hormone (TSH), total protein, transferrin saturation, and urinalysis.

Further testing may be required to confirm a diagnosis for illness other than CFS. For example, kidney disease would be suspected if a patient has low serum albumin levels together with above-normal BUN levels. If autoimmune disease is suspected on the basis of initial testing and physical examination, the doctor may request additional tests such as for antinuclear antibodies.

Treatment

No therapy is known to cure CFS. Treatment of symptoms may include tricyclic antidepressants (doxepin), histamine$_2$-blocking agents (cimetidine), nonsteroidal anti-inflammatory agents (naproxen, ibuprofen, or piroxicam) and antianxiety agents (alprazolam). In some patients, avoidance of environmental irritants and certain foods may help to relieve symptoms. (See *Investigational treatments for CFS,* page 62.)

C.D.C. CRITERIA FOR DIAGNOSING C.F.S.

To meet the case definition established by the Centers for Disease Control and Prevention (CDC) for chronic fatigue syndrome (CFS), a patient must be clinically evaluated and found to meet both of the following criteria:

▶ Clinically evaluated, unexplained persistent or relapsing chronic fatigue that is of new or definite onset (not lifelong), is not the result of ongoing exertion, is not substantially alleviated by rest, and results in substantial reduction in previous levels of occupational, educational, social, or personal activities.

▶ The concurrent occurrence of four or more of the following symptoms:
– substantial impairment in short-term memory or concentration
– sore throat
– tender lymph nodes
– muscle pain
– multi-joint pain without swelling or redness
– headaches of a new type, pattern, or severity
– unrefreshing sleep
– post-exertional malaise lasting more than 24 hours.

These symptoms must have persisted or recurred during 6 or more consecutive months of illness and must not have predated the fatigue.

INVESTIGATIONAL TREATMENTS FOR C.F.S.

Ampligen is a synthetic nucleic acid product that stimulates the production of interferons, a family of immune response modifiers that are also known to have anti-viral activity. One report of a double-blinded, placebo-controlled study of CFS patients documented modest improvements in cognition and performance among Ampligen recipients compared with the placebo group.

Dehydroepiandrosterone (DHEA) was reported in preliminary studies to improve symptoms in some patients; however, this finding has not been confirmed and the use of DHEA in patients should be regarded as experimental.

Gamma globulin (Gammar) is pooled human immune globulin. Its use with CFS patients is experimental and based on the unsubstantiated hypothesis that CFS is related to an underlying immune disorder.

Special considerations

▶ Refer the patient to the CFS Association for information as well as to local support groups; supportive contact with others who share this disease may benefit the patient.
▶ If appropriate, suggest psychological counseling.

CHRONIC MUCOCUTANEOUS CANDIDIASIS

Chronic mucocutaneous candidiasis is a form of candidiasis (moniliasis) that usually develops during the first year of life but occasionally occurs as late as the 20s.

Affecting males and females, it's characterized by repeated infection with *Candida albicans* that may result from an inherited defect in cell-mediated (T-cell) immunity. (Humoral [B-cell] immunity remains intact and provides a normal antibody response to *C. albicans*.) In some patients, an autoimmune response affecting the endocrine system may induce various endocrinopathies.

Despite chronic candidiasis, these patients seldom die of systemic infection. Instead, they usually die of hepatic or endocrine failure. The prognosis for chronic mucocutaneous candidiasis depends on the severity of the associated endocrinopathy. Patients with associated endocrinopathy seldom live beyond their 30s.

Causes

No characteristic immunologic defects have been identified in this infection, but many patients have a diminished response to various antigens or to *Candida* alone. In some patients, anergy may result from deficient migration inhibition factor, a mediator normally produced by lymphocytes.

Signs and symptoms

Chronic candidal infections can affect the skin, mucous membranes, nails, and vagina, usually causing large, circular lesions. These infections seldom produce systemic symptoms, but in late stages may be associated with recurrent respiratory tract infections. Other associated conditions include severe viral infections that may precede the onset of endocrinopathy and, sometimes, hepatitis. Involvement of the mouth, nose, and palate may cause speech and eating difficulties.

Symptoms of endocrinopathy are peculiar to the organ involved. Tetany and hypocalcemia are most common and are associated with hypoparathyroidism. Addison's disease, hypothyroidism, diabetes, and pernicious anemia are also connected with chronic mucocutaneous candidiasis. Psychiatric disorders are likely because of disfigurement and multiple endocrine aberrations.

Diagnosis

Laboratory findings usually show a normal circulating T-cell count, although it may be decreased. Skin tests don't usually show delayed hypersensitivity to *Candida,* even during the infectious stage. Migration inhibiting factor that indicates the presence of activated T cells may not respond to *Candida.*

Nonimmunologic abnormalities resulting from endocrinopathy may include hypocalcemia, abnormal hepatic function studies, hyperglycemia, iron deficiency, and abnormal vitamin B_{12} absorption (pernicious anemia). Diagnosis must rule out other immunodeficiency disorders associated with chronic *Candida* infection, especially DiGeorge syndrome, ataxia-telangiectasia, and severe combined immunodeficiency disease, all of which produce severe immunologic defects. After diagnosis, the patient needs evaluation of adrenal, pituitary, thyroid, gonadal, pancreatic, and parathyroid function as well as careful follow-up. The disease is progressive, and most patients eventually develop endocrinopathy.

Treatment

Treatment aims to control infection but is not always successful. Topical antifungal agents are often ineffective against chronic mucocutaneous candidiasis. Miconazole and nystatin are sometimes useful but ultimately fail to control this infection.

Systemic infections may not be fatal, but they're serious enough to warrant vigorous treatment. Oral ketoconazole and injected thymosin and levamisole have had some positive effect. Oral or I.M. iron replacement may also be necessary. Treatment may also include plastic surgery, when possible, and counseling to help patients cope with their disfigurement.

 PREVENTION TIP Teach the patient about the progressive manifestations of the disease, and emphasize the importance of seeing an endocrinologist for regular checkups.

CLONORCHIASIS

Clonorchiasis is an infection of the biliary system caused by a worm, *Clonorchis sinensis,* or the Oriental liver fluke. Infection follows the consumption of raw, dried, salted or pickled fish from areas where the worm breeds. It is endemic in the Far East, especially Korea, Japan, Taiwan, and southern China. In some areas, most of the population is infected but asymptomatic. Up to 26% of immigrants from China to the United States have been found to be infected with *C. sinensis.* The rate of infection is not related to gender or years since immigration. Prognosis is good with treatment.

Causes

Humans become infected after ingesting metacercariae in poorly cooked fish. The metacercariae exist in the small intestine and migrate through the ampulla of Vater into the biliary ducts, where they mature in 3 to 4 weeks and subsequently release eggs. Adult flukes can survive for 20 to 25 years.

Signs and symptoms

Light infections are usually asymptomatic. More heavily infected persons report vague complaints such as fever, chills, anorexia, diarrhea, and epigastric pain, which begin 10 to 26 days after eating inadequately cooked infected fish. Symptoms generally last 2 to 4 weeks. In chronic infections, chronic cholangitis may progress to portal fibrosis and may be associated with portal hypertension, cirrhosis, and atrophy of liver parenchyma. Jaundice is usually caused by biliary obstruction due to a mass of flukes or to formation of stones.

Other complications include cholangio-carcinoma, suppurative cholangitis, and chronic pancreatitis.

Diagnosis

The diagnosis is established when *Clonorchis* eggs are found in feces; therefore, three samples of stool for ova and parasites should be obtained. Adult flukes may be found in the gallbladder or bile ducts during exploratory surgery for biliary tract disease. Endoscopic retrograde cholangiopancreatography may reveal stones, dilated ducts, or both. Alkaline phosphatase and bilirubin levels may be elevated. Complete blood count may reveal eosinophilia and leukocytosis.

The differential diagnosis of the acute phase of *C. sinensis* infection includes acute schistosomiasis.

Treatment

The treatment of choice is oral praziquantel taken after each meal in one day. Albendazole can also be used, but a 7-day treatment course is required.

Special considerations

▶ There should be a high index of suspicion when diagnosing Asian immigrants and those who prepare fish imported from endemic areas.

▶ Help the patient maintain adequate nutrition and hydration through the acute phase of the infection.

▶ Explain procedures and support the patient and family through possible diagnostic tests such as ultrasound, endoscopic retrograde cholangiopancreatography, and percutaneous transhepatic cholangiography.

 PREVENTION TIP Encourage careful preparation and cooking of freshwater fish, crustaceans, and vegetables. Also advise patients to avoid eating raw, pickled, or smoked freshwater fish from endemic areas.

CLOSTRIDIUM DIFFICILE INFECTION

Clostridium difficile is a gram-positive anaerobic bacterium most often associated with antibiotic-associated colitis and diarrhea. Symptoms ranging from asymptomatic carrier states to severe pseudomembranous colitis are caused by exotoxins produced by the microbe: toxin A (an enterotoxin) and toxin B (a cytotoxin). Complications include electrolyte abnormalities, hypovolemic shock, anasarca (caused by hypoalbuminemia), sepsis, and hemorrhage. Rarely, death may result.

Causes

Although *C. difficile* colitis can be caused by almost any antibiotic that disrupts the intestinal flora, it's classically associated with clindamycin use. Additional factors that alter normal intestinal flora include enemas and intestinal stimulants. Patients at high risk for this disorder include those taking many kinds of antibiotics or antineoplastic agents that have antibiotic activity; candidates for abdominal surgery; immunocompromised individuals; pediatric patients (infections are common in day-care centers); and nursing-home patients.

C. difficile may be transmitted directly from patient to patient via contaminated hands of personnel (most common), or indirectly through contaminated equipment such as bedpans, urinals, call bells, rectal thermometers, and NG tubes, and surfaces of bed rails, floors, and toilet seats.

Signs and symptoms

Risk of *C. difficile* infection begins 1 to 2 days after antibiotic therapy is started and persists for as long as 2 to 3 months after the last dose. The patient may be asymptomatic, or may present any of the following symptoms: soft, unformed stool or watery diarrhea (more than 3 evacuations in 24 hours) that may be foul-smelling or grossly bloody; abdominal pain, cramping, or tenderness; and fever. The white blood cell count may be elevated to 20,000/L. In severe cases, toxic megacolon, colonic perforation, and peritonitis may develop.

Diagnosis

C. difficile infection is confirmed by identification of the exotoxins, using one of the following methods:

◗ *cell cytotoxin test:* highly sensitive and specific for toxins A and B of *C. difficile;* results available in 2 days.

◗ *enzyme immunoassays:* slightly less sensitive than the cell cytotoxin test, but results are obtained in a few hours; specificity is excellent.

◗ *stool culture:* most sensitive, with 2-day turnaround. Nontoxin-producing strains of *C. difficile* can be easily identified using 3 separate stool samples to test for the presence of the toxin.

◗ *endoscopy (flexible sigmoidoscopy):* may be used in patients who present with an acute abdomen but no diarrhea, making it difficult to obtain a stool specimen. If pseudomembranes are seen, treatment for *C. difficile* is usually initiated.

Treatment

Withdrawing the causative antibiotic (if possible) resolves symptoms in patients who are mildly symptomatic. This is usually the only treatment required.

For more severe cases, metronidazole 250 mg by mouth (P.O.) four times daily or 500 mg P.O. three times daily, or vancomycin 125 mg P.O. four times daily for 10 days are effective therapies, with metronidazole being the preferred treatment. Retesting for *C. difficile* is unnecessary if symptoms resolve.

In 10% to 20% of patients, *C. difficile* may recur within 14 to 30 days of treatment. Beyond 30 days, it's questionable whether the recurrence is a relapse or reinfection with *C. difficile.* If metronidazole was the initial treatment, low-dose vancomycin, given 125 mg P.O. four times daily for 21 days, may be effective. Alternatively, give vancomycin (125 mg P.O. four times daily) in combination with rifampin (600 mg P.O. twice daily) for 10 days.

Special considerations

◗ Patients with known or suspect *C. difficile* diarrhea who are unable to practice good hygiene should be placed in a single room or with other patients with the same infection and no other infections.

◗ Follow standard precautions and contact precautions for contact with blood and body fluids for all direct patient contact and contact with the patient's immediate environment. Use good hand-washing technique with antiseptic soap.

◗ Reusable equipment must be disinfected before use on another patient.

◗ Patients who are asymptomatic, without diarrhea or fecal incontinence for 72 hours, and who are able to practice good hygiene may be transferred out of single rooms.

◗ Preventive strategies include careful selection of antibiotic therapy, use of single antibiotics when possible, avoiding antibiotics when they're not absolutely necessary, and limiting the duration of the antibiotic treatment regimen.

◗ Because spores of *C. difficile* are resistant to most commonly used stool disinfectants, the patient's room may be contaminated even after the patient is discharged. The immediate environment must be thoroughly cleaned and disinfected with 0.5% sodium hypochlorite.

COCCIDIOIDOMYCOSIS

Also known as valley fever and San Joaquin Valley fever, coccidioidomycosis is caused by the fungus *Coccidioides immitis.* It is primarily a respiratory infection, although generalized dissemination may occur.

The primary pulmonary form is usually self-limiting and rarely fatal. The rare secondary (progressive, disseminated) form produces abscesses throughout the body and carries a mortality of up to 60%, even with treatment. Such dissemination is more common in dark-skinned men, pregnant women, and patients who are receiving immunosuppressants.

Coccidioidomycosis is endemic to the southwestern United States, especially between the San Joaquin Valley in California and southwestern Texas. It's also found in Mexico, Guatemala, Honduras, Venezuela, Colombia, Argentina, and Paraguay. Because of population distribution and an occupational link (it's common in migrant farm laborers), coccidioidomycosis generally strikes Filipino Americans, Mexican Americans, Native Americans, and blacks. In primary infection, the incubation period is from 1 to 4 weeks.

Causes

Coccidioidomycosis may result from inhalation of *C. immitis* spores found in the soil in endemic areas or from inhalation of spores from dressings or plaster casts of infected persons. It's most prevalent during warm, dry months.

Signs and symptoms

Chronic pulmonary cavitation can occur in both the primary and the disseminated forms of coccidioidomycosis, causing hemoptysis with or without chest pain. Other signs and symptoms vary with the form of the disease.

Primary coccidioidomycosis

Acute or subacute respiratory symptoms (dry cough, pleuritic chest pain, pleural effusion), fever, sore throat, chills, malaise, headache, and an itchy macular rash usually accompany the primary form of the disease. Occasionally, the sole symptom is a fever that persists for weeks. From 3 days to several weeks after onset, some patients, particularly white women, may develop tender red nodules (erythema nodosum) on their legs, especially the shins, with joint pain in the knees and ankles. Generally, the primary form heals spontaneously within a few weeks.

Disseminated coccidioidomycosis

In rare cases, coccidioidomycosis spreads to other organs several weeks or months after the primary infection. Disseminated coccidioidomycosis causes fever and abscesses throughout the body, especially in skeletal, central nervous system (CNS), splenic, hepatic, renal, and subcutaneous tissues. Depending on the location of these abscesses, disseminated coccidioidomycosis may cause bone pain and meningitis.

Diagnosis

Typical clinical features and skin and serologic studies confirm the diagnosis. The primary form — and sometimes the disseminated form — produces a positive coccidioidin skin test. In the first week of illness, complement fixation for immunoglobulin G antibodies or, in the first month, positive serum precipitins (immunoglobulins) also establish this diagnosis.

Examination or immunodiffusion testing of sputum, pus from lesions, and a tissue biopsy may show *C. immitis* spores. The presence of antibodies in pleural and joint fluid, and a rising serum or body fluid antibody titer indicate dissemination.

Other abnormal laboratory results include an increased white blood cell (WBC) count, eosinophilia, increased erythrocyte sedimentation rate, and a chest X-ray showing bilateral diffuse infiltrates.

In coccidioidal meningitis, examination of cerebrospinal fluid shows the WBC count increased to more than $500/mm^3$ (primarily because of mononuclear leukocytes) and increased protein and decreased glucose levels. Ventricular fluid obtained from the brain may contain complement fixation antibodies.

After the diagnosis has been reached, the results of serial skin tests, blood cultures, and serologic testing may document the effectiveness of therapy.

Treatment

Usually, mild primary coccidioidomycosis requires only bed rest and relief of symptoms. Severe primary disease and dissemination, however, also require long-term I.V. infusion or, in CNS dissemination, intrathecal administration of amphotericin B and, possibly, excision or drainage of lesions. Severe pulmonary lesions may require lobectomy. Miconazole and ketoconazole suppress *C. immitis* but don't eradicate it.

Special considerations

▶ Don't wash off the circle marked on the skin for serial skin tests; this aids in reading test results.

▶ In mild primary disease, encourage bed rest and adequate fluid intake. Record the amount and color of sputum. Watch for shortness of breath that may point to pleural effusion. In patients with arthralgia, provide analgesics.

▶ Coccidioidomycosis requires strict secretion precautions if the patient has draining lesions. A no-touch dressing technique and careful hand washing are essential. No specific isolation precautions are required.

▶ In CNS dissemination, monitor the patient carefully for a decreased level of consciousness or a change in mood or affect.

▶ Before intrathecal administration of amphotericin B, explain the procedure to the patient, and reassure him that he'll receive analgesics before a lumbar puncture.

▶ In patients receiving amphotericin B, watch for decreased urinary output, and monitor laboratory results for elevated blood urea nitrogen and creatinine levels and hypokalemia. Tell patients to immediately report hearing loss, tinnitus, dizziness, and all signs of toxicity. To ease adverse reactions, give antiemetics and antipyretics.

COLORADO TICK FEVER

Colorado tick fever is a benign infection that results from the Colorado tick fever arbovirus and is transmitted to humans by a tick. Colorado tick fever occurs in the Rocky Mountain region of the United States, mostly in April and May at lower altitudes and in June and July at higher altitudes. Because of occupational or recreational exposure, it's more common in men than in women. Colorado tick fever apparently confers long-lasting immunity against reinfection.

Causes

Colorado tick fever is transmitted to humans by a hard-shelled wood tick, *Dermacentor andersoni*. The adult tick acquires the virus when it bites infected rodents and remains permanently infective.

Signs and symptoms

After a 3- to 6-day incubation period, Colorado tick fever begins abruptly with chills; temperature of 104° F (40° C); severe aching of back, arms, and legs; lethargy; and headache with eye movement. Photophobia, abdominal pain, nausea, and vomiting may occur. Rare effects include petechial or maculopapular rashes and CNS involvement. Symptoms subside after several days but return within 2 to 3 days and continue for 3 more days before slowly disappearing. Complete recovery usually follows.

Diagnosis

A history of recent exposure to ticks along with moderate to severe leukopenia, complement fixation tests, or virus isolation confirm the diagnosis.

Treatment

After correct removal of the tick, supportive treatment focuses on relieving symptoms, combating secondary infection, and maintaining fluid balance.

Special considerations

▶ Carefully remove the tick by grasping it with forceps or gloved fingers and pulling gently. Be careful not to crush the tick's body. Keep it for identification. Thoroughly wash the wound with soap and water. If the tick's head remains embedded, surgical removal is necessary. Give a tetanus-diphtheria booster, as ordered.

▶ Be alert for secondary infection.

▶ Monitor fluid and electrolyte balance, and provide replacement accordingly.

▶ Reduce fever with antipyretics and tepid sponge baths.

 PREVENTION TIP To prevent tick-borne infection, tell the patient to avoid tick bites by wearing protective clothing (long pants tucked into boots) and carefully checking his body and scalp for ticks several times a day whenever in infested areas.

COMMON COLD

The common cold — an acute, usually afebrile viral infection — causes inflammation of the upper respiratory tract. It accounts for more time lost from school or work than any other cause and is the most common infectious disease. Although it's benign and self-limiting, it can lead to secondary bacterial infections.

The common cold is more prevalent in children than in adults; in adolescent boys than in girls; and in women than in men. In temperate zones, it occurs more often in the colder months; in the tropics, during the rainy season.

Causes

About 90% of colds stem from a viral infection of the upper respiratory passages and consequent mucous membrane inflammation; occasionally, colds result from a mycoplasmal infection.

Over a hundred viruses can cause the common cold. Major offenders include rhinoviruses, coronaviruses, myxoviruses, adenoviruses, coxsackieviruses, and echoviruses.

Transmission occurs through airborne respiratory droplets, contact with contaminated objects, and hand-to-hand transmission. Children acquire new strains from their schoolmates and pass them on to family members. Fatigue or drafts don't increase susceptibility. (See *What happens in the common cold.*)

Signs and symptoms

After a 1- to 4-day incubation period, the common cold produces pharyngitis, nasal congestion, rhinitis, headache, and burning, watery eyes; there may be fever (in children), chills, myalgia, arthralgia, malaise, lethargy, and a hacking, nonproductive, or nocturnal cough.

As the cold progresses, clinical features develop more fully. After a day, symptoms include a feeling of fullness with a copious nasal discharge that often irritates the nose, adding to discomfort. About 3 days after onset, major signs diminish, but the "stuffed-up" feeling often persists for a week.

Reinfection (with productive cough) is common, but complications (sinusitis, otitis media, pharyngitis, lower respiratory tract infection) are rare. A cold is communicable for 2 to 3 days after the onset of symptoms.

Diagnosis

No explicit diagnostic test exists to isolate the specific organisms responsible for the common cold. Consequently, the diagnosis rests on a cold's typically mild, localized, and afebrile upper respiratory symptoms. Despite infection, white blood cell count and differential are within normal limits.

A diagnosis must rule out allergic rhinitis, measles, rubella, and other disorders that produce similar early symptoms. A fever higher than 100.4° F (38° C), severe malaise, anorexia, tachycardia, exudate on the tonsils or throat, petechiae, and tender lymph glands may point to more serious disorders and require additional diagnostic tests.

Treatment

The primary treatment — aspirin or acetaminophen, fluids, and rest — is purely symptomatic, as the common cold has no known cure. Aspirin eases myalgia and headache; fluids help loosen accumulat-

WHAT HAPPENS IN THE COMMON COLD

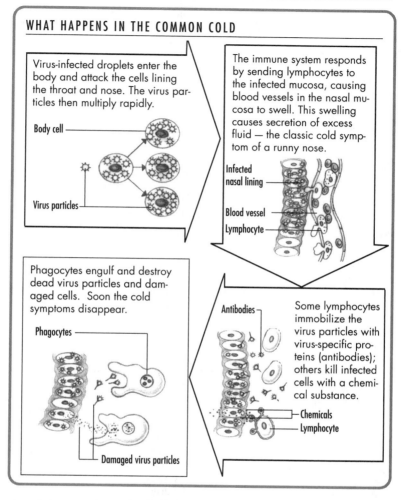

Virus-infected droplets enter the body and attack the cells lining the throat and nose. The virus particles then multiply rapidly.

Body cell

Virus particles

The immune system responds by sending lymphocytes to the infected mucosa, causing blood vessels in the nasal mucosa to swell. This swelling causes secretion of excess fluid — the classic cold symptom of a runny nose.

Infected nasal lining

Blood vessel

Lymphocyte

Phagocytes engulf and destroy dead virus particles and damaged cells. Soon the cold symptoms disappear.

Phagocytes

Damaged virus particles

Some lymphocytes immobilize the virus particles with virus-specific proteins (antibodies); others kill infected cells with a chemical substance.

Antibodies

Chemicals

Lymphocyte

ed respiratory secretions and maintain hydration; and rest combats fatigue and weakness. In a child with a fever, acetaminophen is the drug of choice, as aspirin has been associated with the onset of Reyes' syndrome.

Decongestants can relieve congestion. Throat lozenges relieve soreness. Steam encourages expectoration. In infants, saline nose drops and mucus aspiration with a bulb syringe may be beneficial.

Nasal douching, sinus drainage, and antibiotics aren't necessary except in complications or chronic illness. Pure anti-

tussives relieve severe coughs but are contraindicated with productive coughs, when cough suppression is harmful. The role of vitamin C and zinc remain controversial.

Currently, no known measure can prevent the common cold. (See *Experimental treatment for the common cold,* page 70.)

Special considerations

▶ Emphasize that antibiotics don't cure the common cold and generally are not indicated unless signs and symptoms of bacterial infection are present.

EXPERIMENTAL TREATMENT FOR THE COMMON COLD

A new drug, Pleconaril, is now in Phase III clinical trials as a treatment for the common cold. The drug inhibits capsid function in picornaviruses. The capsid is essential for the virus to infect healthy cells. In Phase II trials, patients receiving Pleconaril experienced a statistically significant reduction of their disease.

▶ Tell the patient to maintain bed rest if feasible during the first few days, to use a lubricant on his nostrils to decrease irritation, to relieve throat irritation with hard candy or cough drops, to increase his fluid intake, and have him eat light meals.
▶ Inform the patient that warm baths or heating pads can reduce aches and pains but won't hasten a cure. Suggest hot or cold steam vaporizers. Commercial expectorants are available, but their effectiveness is unproven.
▶ Advise the patient against overuse of nose drops or sprays; these may cause rebound congestion.

 PREVENTION TIP To help prevent colds, warn the patient to minimize contact with people who have colds. To avoid spreading colds, teach the patient to wash his hands often, to cover coughs and sneezes, and to avoid sharing towels and drinking glasses.

CONJUNCTIVITIS

Hyperemia of the conjunctiva from infection, allergy, or chemical reactions characterizes conjunctivitis. Bacterial and viral conjunctivitis are highly contagious, but are also self-limiting after a couple of weeks' duration. Chronic conjunctivitis may result in degenerative changes to the eyelids. In the Western hemisphere, conjunctivitis is probably the most common eye disorder.

Causes

The most common causative organisms are the following:
▶ *bacterial: Staphylococcus aureus, Streptococcus pneumoniae, Neisseria gonorrhoeae, Neisseria meningitidis*
▶ *chlamydial: Chlamydia trachomatis* (inclusion conjunctivitis)
▶ *viral:* adenovirus types 3, 7, and 8; herpes simplex virus, type 1.

Other causes include allergic reactions to pollen, grass, topical medications, air pollutants, and smoke; occupational irritants (acids and alkalies); rickettsial diseases (Rocky Mountain spotted fever); parasitic diseases caused by *Phthirus pubis, Schistosoma haematobium;* and, rarely, fungal infections.

Vernal conjunctivitis is a severe IgE-mediated mast cell hypersensitivity reaction. This form of conjunctivitis is bilateral; onset is between 3 to 5 years of age and persists for about 10 years. It's sometimes associated with other signs and symptoms of allergy commonly related to pollens, asthma, and allergic rhinitis.

Epidemic keratoconjunctivitis (EKC) is an acute, highly contagious, viral conjunctivitis. Health care professionals must be careful to use gloves, wash their hands, and disinfect instruments to prevent the spread of this disease.

Signs and symptoms

Conjunctivitis commonly produces hyperemia of the conjunctiva, sometimes accompanied by discharge and tearing. It generally doesn't affect vision unless there's corneal involvement, which also causes pain and photophobia. Conjunctivitis usually begins in one eye and rapidly spreads to the other by contamination of towels, washcloths, or the patient's own hand.

In acute bacterial conjunctivitis (pink-eye), the infection usually lasts only 2 weeks. The patient typically complains of burning and the sensation of a foreign body in his eye. The eyelids show a crust of sticky, mucopurulent discharge. If the disorder stems from *N. gonorrhoeae,* however, the patient exhibits a profuse, purulent discharge.

Viral conjunctivitis produces copious tearing with minimal exudate, and enlargement of the preauricular lymph node. Some viruses follow a chronic course and produce severe disabling disease; others last 2 to 3 weeks.

Diagnosis

Physical examination reveals peripheral injection of the bulbar conjunctival vessels. In children, possible systemic symptoms include sore throat or fever if the conjunctivitis is suspected of being from an adenoviral origin.

Lymphocytes are predominant in stained smears of conjunctival scrapings if conjunctivitis is caused by a virus. Polymorphonuclear cells (neutrophils) predominate if conjunctivitis stems from bacteria; eosinophils, if it's allergy-related. Culture and sensitivity tests identify the causative bacterial organism and indicate appropriate antibiotic therapy.

Treatment

The cause of conjunctivitis dictates the treatment. Bacterial conjunctivitis requires topical application of the appropriate broad-spectrum antibiotic.

Although viral conjunctivitis resists treatment, broad-spectrum antibiotic eyedrops may prevent secondary infection.

Herpes simplex infection generally responds to treatment with trifluridine drops, vidarabine ointment, or oral acyclovir, but the infection may persist for 2 to 3 weeks. Treatment of vernal conjunctivitis includes administration of corticosteroid drops followed by cromolyn sulfate and cold compresses to relieve itching and, occasionally, oral antihistamines.

Instillation of a one-time dose of erythromycin into the eyes of newborns prevents gonococcal and chlamydial conjunctivitis.

Special considerations

▶ Apply warm compresses and therapeutic ointment or drops. Don't irrigate the eye; this will only spread infection. Have the patient wash his hands before he uses the medication, and use clean washcloths or towels frequently so he doesn't infect his other eye.

▶ Notify public health authorities if cultures show *N. gonorrhoeae.*

▶ If ointments are prescribed, remind the patient that ointment blurs vision.

 PREVENTION TIP Teach proper handwashing technique because bacterial and viral forms of conjunctivitis are highly contagious. Stress the risk of spreading infection to family members by sharing washcloths, towels, and pillows. Warn against rubbing the infected eye, which can spread the infection to the other eye and to other persons.

▶ Teach the patient to instill eyedrops and ointments correctly — without touching the bottle tip to his eye or lashes. Stress the importance of safety glasses for the patient who works near chemical irritants.

CONJUNCTIVITIS, INCLUSION

Inclusion conjunctivitis is an acute ocular inflammation resulting from infection by the bacterium *Chlamydia trachomatis.* Although inclusion conjunctivitis occasionally becomes chronic, the prognosis is generally good with treatment. If untreated, the disease may run a course of 3 to 9 months.

Causes

C. trachomatis is a bacterium of the lymphogranuloma venereum serotype D to K that is sexually transmitted. Secondary eye involvement in adults occurs in 1 out of 300 genital cases.

Because contaminated cervical secretions infect the eyes of the neonate during birth, inclusion conjunctivitis is an important cause of ophthalmia neonatorum.

Signs and symptoms
Inclusion conjunctivitis develops 5 to 12 days after contamination. (It takes longer to develop than gonococcal ophthalmia.) In a neonate, the eyelids redden and tearing with moderate mucoid discharge is a presenting symptom. Also, in neonates, pseudomembranes may form, which can lead to conjunctival scarring. In adults, follicles appear inside the lower eyelids; such follicles don't form in infants because the lymphoid tissue isn't yet well developed. Children and adults also develop preauricular lymphadenopathy and, as complications, otitis media and occasionally interstitial pneumonia. Inclusion conjunctivitis may persist for weeks or months, possibly with superficial corneal involvement

Diagnosis
Clinical features and a history of sexual contact with an infected person suggest inclusion conjunctivitis. Examination of Giemsa-stained conjunctival scraping showing cytoplasmic inclusion bodies in conjunctival epithelial cells is effective in detecting neonatal and infant chlamydial infections. The direct fluorescent monoclonal antibody (DFA) test and enzyme-linked immunosorbent assay (ELISA) test are more effective in adults.

Treatment
Because treatment is not limited to the eye in either neonates, infant, or adults, systemic antimicrobial treatment is necessary. Administration of erythromycin base for neonates and infants is fairly effective — 80% for the first course of treatment. Sometimes a second course of erythromycin is needed.

Tetracycline may be given to adults and children over age 8. Erythromycin base is used in the treatment of younger children and pregnant women. The patient's sexual partner should also be examined.

Special considerations
▶ Keep the patient's eyes as clean as possible, using aseptic technique. Clean the eyes from the inner to the outer canthus. Record the amount and color of drainage. Apply warm soaks as needed.
▶ Remind the patient not to rub his eyes, which can irritate them and possible spread the infection.
▶ If the patient's eyes are sensitive to light, keep the room dark or suggest that he wear dark glasses.
▶ To prevent further spread of inclusion conjunctivitis, wash your hands thoroughly before and after administering eye medications.
▶ Suggest a pelvic examination for the mother of an infected neonate or for any woman who has inclusion conjunctivitis.
▶ Obtain a history of recent sexual contacts so they can be examined and, if necessary, treated for chlamydial infection.

CREUTZFELDT-JAKOB DISEASE

Creutzfeldt-Jakob disease (CJD) is a rapidly progressive viral disease that attacks the central nervous system, causing dementia accompanied by neurologic symptoms such as myoclonic jerking, ataxia, aphasia, visual disturbances, and paralysis. It generally affects adults aged 40 to 65 and is found in over 50 countries, affecting males and females equally. Higher incidences of CJD have been found among Libyan Jewish immigrants to Israel, residents of Czechoslovakia, and North African immigrants to France. The annual incidence is 1 case per 1 million. Most die of pneumonia within 3 to 12 months of onset of symptoms; 5 to 10 per-

SYMPTOMS OF C.J.D.

The symptoms of Creutzfeldt-Jakob disease (CJD) vary with the stage of the disease. The chart below identifies common symptoms for each stage.

STAGE 1	STAGE 2	STAGE 3
▶ Impaired judgment ▶ Forgetfulness ▶ Lassitude ▶ Cognitive difficulties ▶ Personality and behavior changes ▶ Mood swings ▶ Sleep disturbances ▶ Difficulty with calculation ▶ Gait disorders ▶ Dementia ▶ Heightened startle reaction ▶ Loss of short-term memory ▶ Agitation ▶ Paranoid ideation ▶ Impaired balance	▶ Spasticity ▶ Clonus ▶ Rigidity ▶ Tremors ▶ Asymmetrical, myoclonic jerks ▶ Ataxia ▶ Dysarthria ▶ Agnosia ▶ Sleep disturbances ▶ Incoordination ▶ Further mental status changes	▶ Epileptic seizures ▶ Decorticate posturing ▶ Complete mental and physical dysfunction

Adapted with permission from *Journal of Gerontological Nursing,* 19(11):20, October 1999.

cent survive for 2 years or more. A new variant of CJD emerged in Europe in 1996.

Causes

The causative organism is difficult to identify because no foreign RNA or DNA has been linked to the disease. CJD is believed to be caused by a specific protein called a prion, which lacks nucleic acids, resists proteolytic digestion, and spontaneously aggregates in the brain. Prions are also associated with several other degenerative brain diseases, notably Alzheimer's disease and Kuru. Most cases are sporadic; 5% to 15% are familial with an autosomal dominant pattern of inheritance. Although CJD is not transmitted by normal casual contact, human-to-human transmission has occurred inadvertently as a result of certain medical procedures, such as corneal and cadaveric dura mater grafts.

Isolated cases have been attributed to treatment during childhood with growth hormone prepared from cadaveric human pituitary glands, and to improperly decontaminated neurosurgical instruments and brain electrodes.

Signs and symptoms

The disease is divided in three stages. The progression from stage 1 to stage 2 may only be several weeks. Usually the progression from stage 2 to stage 3 is from 6 to 18 months. Sometimes symptoms from all stages occur simultaneously. (See *Symptoms of CJD.*) Early signs of mental impairment may be manifested as slowness in thinking, difficulty concentrating, impaired judgment, and memory loss. Muscle twitching occurs within 6 months after symptoms begin, along with trembling, clumsiness, peculiar body movements, and visual disturbances. Specific clinical manifestations have been described depending on the predominant involvement of certain regions of the brain (occipital, thalamic, and cerebellar types.)

Diagnosis

CJD must be considered for anyone presenting with signs of progressive dementia. Neurological examination remains the most effective tool in diagnosing CJD. Difficulty with rapid alternating movements and point to point examinations are often evident early in the disease. Other findings may include difficulty in tandem, heel-to-toe, and normal walking; Romberg's sign; altered muscle tonicity; loss of sensation; exaggerated deep tendon reflexes of the arms and legs; nonelicitable ankle reflexes; negative abdominal reflexes; and a positive Babinski's sign.

An EEG may also be performed to assess typical changes in brain wave activity. Initially, the EEG is normal but eventually develops a characteristic pattern of slow wave activity and rhythmic, periodic bursts of high voltage, diphasic, or triphasic sharp wave complexes intervening with periods of electrical silence.

Other causes of dementia, such as tumors, must be ruled out using CT scans or MRI of the brain. Lumbar puncture should be done to rule out bacterial infection of the brain and central nervous system. Definitive diagnosis is usually not obtained until an autopsy is done and brain tissue is examined. Care must be taken by the pathologist and anyone else in potential contact with the cadaveric materials due to the risk of infection.

Alzheimer's disease, Gerstmann-Sträussler-Scheinker disease, fatal familial insomnia, and Kuru are other conditions to consider.

Treatment

There is no cure for CJD and its progress cannot be slowed. Palliative care is given to make the patient comfortable and to treat the symptoms.

Special considerations

▶ Direct the patient and family to CJD support groups and encourage participation.
▶ Allow for and assist the patient and family through the grieving process.

 PREVENTION TIP To prevent disease transmission, use caution when handling fluids and other materials from patients suspected of having CJD.

CROUP

This severe inflammation and obstruction of the upper airway can occur as acute laryngotracheobronchitis (most common), laryngitis, and acute spasmodic laryngitis; it must always be distinguished from epiglottitis.

Croup is a childhood disease affecting boys more often than girls (typically between ages 3 months and 3 years) that usually occurs during the winter. Up to 15% of patients have a strong family history of croup. Recovery is usually complete.

Causes

Croup usually results from a viral infection. Parainfluenza viruses cause two-thirds of such infections; adenoviruses, respiratory syncytial virus (RSV), influenza and measles viruses, and bacteria (pertussis, diphtheria, and mycoplasma) account for the rest.

Signs and symptoms

The onset of croup usually follows an upper respiratory tract infection. Clinical features include inspiratory stridor, hoarse or muffled vocal sounds, varying degrees of laryngeal obstruction and respiratory distress, and a characteristic sharp, barking, seal-like cough. These symptoms may last only a few hours or persist for a day or two.

As croup progresses, it causes inflammatory edema and, possibly, spasm, which can obstruct the upper airway and severely

HOW CROUP AFFECTS THE UPPER AIRWAY

In croup, inflammatory swelling and spasms constrict the larynx, thereby reducing airflow. This cross-sectional drawing (from chin to chest) shows the upper airway changes caused by croup. Inflammatory changes almost completely obstruct the larynx (which includes the epiglottis) and significantly narrow the trachea.

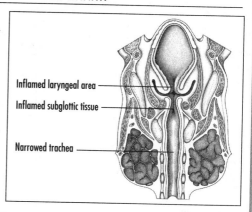

Inflamed laryngeal area

Inflamed subglottic tissue

Narrowed trachea

compromise ventilation. (See *How croup affects the upper airway*.)

Each form of croup has additional characteristics:

In *laryngotracheobronchitis*, the symptoms seem to worsen at night. Inflammation causes edema of the bronchi and bronchioles, and increasingly difficult expiration, which frightens the child. Other characteristic features include fever, diffusely decreased breath sounds, expiratory rhonchi, and scattered crackles.

Laryngitis, which results from vocal cord edema, is usually mild and produces no respiratory distress except in infants. Early indications include a sore throat and cough that, rarely, may progress to marked hoarseness, suprasternal and intercostal retractions, inspiratory stridor, dyspnea, diminished breath sounds, and restlessness. In later stages, severe dyspnea and exhaustion may result.

Acute spasmodic laryngitis affects children between ages 1 and 3, particularly those with allergies and a family history of croup. It typically begins with mild to moderate hoarseness and nasal discharge, followed by the characteristic cough and noisy inspiration (which often awakens the child at night), labored breathing with retractions, rapid pulse, and clammy skin. The child understandably becomes anxious, which may lead to increasing dyspnea and transient cyanosis. These severe symptoms diminish after several hours but reappear in a milder form on the next one or two nights.

Diagnosis

The clinical features are very characteristic so that the diagnosis should be suspected immediately. When bacterial infection is the cause, throat cultures may identify organisms and their sensitivity to antibiotics as well as rule out diphtheria. A posterior-anterior X-ray of the chest may reveal narrowing at the upper airway (steeple sign). Laryngoscopy may reveal inflammation and obstruction in epiglottal and laryngeal areas.

In evaluating the patient, consider foreign body obstruction (a common cause of croupy cough in young children) as well as masses and cysts.

Treatment

For most children with croup, home care with rest, cool humidification during sleep, and antipyretics such as acetaminophen relieve symptoms. However, respiratory distress that interferes with oral hydration requires hospitalization and parenteral fluid replacement to prevent dehydration.

If bacterial infection is the cause, antibiotic therapy is necessary. Oxygen therapy may also be required.

Special considerations

▶ Monitor and support respiration, and control fever. Because croup is so frightening to the child and his family, also provide support and reassurance.

▶ Carefully monitor cough and breath sounds, hoarseness, severity of retractions, inspiratory stridor, cyanosis, respiratory rate and character (especially prolonged and labored respirations), restlessness, fever, and cardiac rate.

▶ Keep the child as quiet as possible, but avoid sedation, which can depress respiration.

▶ If the patient is an infant, position him in an infant seat or prop him up with a pillow.

▶ Place an older child in Fowler's position. If an older child requires a cool mist tent to help him breathe, explain why it's needed.

▶ Isolate patients suspected of having RSV and parainfluenza infections, if possible. Wash your hands carefully before leaving the room to avoid transmission to other children, particularly infants. Instruct parents and others involved in the care of these children to take similar precautions.

▶ Control fever with sponge baths and antipyretics. Keep a hypothermia blanket on hand for temperatures above 102° F (38.9° C). Watch for seizures in infants and young children with high fevers. Give I.V. antibiotics as necessary.

▶ Relieve sore throat with soothing, water-based ices, such as fruit sherbet and ice pops. Avoid thicker, milk-based fluids if the child is producing heavy mucus or has great difficulty in swallowing.

▶ Apply petroleum jelly or another ointment around the nose and lips to soothe irritation from nasal discharge and mouth breathing.

▶ Maintain a calm, quiet environment and offer reassurance. Explain all procedures and answer any questions.

 ALERT To relieve croupy spells, tell parents to carry the child into the bathroom, shut the door, and turn on the hot water. Breathing in warm, moist air quickly eases an acute spell of croup. Suggest the use of a cool mist humidifier (vaporizer). Warn parents that ear infections and pneumonia are complications of croup, which may appear about 5 days after recovery. Stress the importance of reporting earache, productive cough, high fever, or increased shortness of breath immediately.

CRYPTOCOCCOSIS

The fungus *Cryptococcus neoformans* causes this disease, also called torulosis and European blastomycosis. Cryptococcosis usually begins as an asymptomatic pulmonary infection but disseminates to extrapulmonary sites, usually to the central nervous system (CNS), but also to the skin, bones, prostate gland, liver, or kidneys.

Cryptococcosis is most prevalent in men, usually those between ages 30 and 60, and is rare in children. It's especially likely to develop in immunocompromised patients, such as those with Hodgkin's disease, sarcoidosis, leukemia, or lymphoma and those who are receiving immunosuppressive agents. Currently, patients with acquired immunodeficiency syndrome (AIDS) are by far the most commonly affected group.

With appropriate treatment, the prognosis in pulmonary cryptococcosis is good. CNS infection, however, can be fatal, but treatment dramatically reduces mortality.

Causes

Transmission is through inhalation of *C. neoformans* in particles of dust contaminated by pigeon stool that harbors this microbe. Therefore, cryptococcosis is primarily an urban infection.

Signs and symptoms

Typically, pulmonary cryptococcosis is asymptomatic. Onset of CNS involvement is gradual (cryptococcal meningitis), and causes progressively severe frontal and temporal headache, diplopia, blurred vision, dizziness, ataxia, aphasia, vomiting, tinnitus, memory changes, inappropriate behavior, irritability, psychotic symptoms, convulsions, and fever.

If untreated, symptoms progress to coma and death, usually as a result of cerebral edema or hydrocephalus. Complications include optic atrophy, ataxia, hydrocephalus, deafness, paralysis, chronic brain syndrome, and personality changes.

Skin involvement produces red facial papules and other skin abscesses, with or without ulcerations; bone involvement produces painful osseous lesions of the long bones, skull, spine, and joints.

Diagnosis

A routine chest X-ray showing a pulmonary lesion may point to pulmonary cryptococcosis. However, this infection usually escapes diagnosis until it disseminates.

A firm diagnosis requires identification of *C. neoformans* by culture of sputum, urine, prostatic secretions, bone marrow aspirate or biopsy, or pleural biopsy; and, in CNS infection, by an India ink preparation of cerebrospinal fluid (CSF) and culture. Blood cultures are positive only in severe infection. Biopsy of skin lesions may also be diagnostic.

Supportive values include an increased antigen titer in serum and CSF in disseminated infection; increased CSF pressure, protein, and white blood cell count in CNS infection; and moderately decreased CSF glucose in about half of these patients. The diagnosis must rule out cancer and tuberculosis.

Treatment

The patient with pulmonary cryptococcosis will require close medical observation for a year after diagnosis. Treatment is unnecessary unless extrapulmonary lesions develop or pulmonary lesions progress.

Treatment of disseminated infection calls for I.V. amphotericin B or fluconazole. Patients with AIDS will also need long-term therapy, usually with oral fluconazole.

Special considerations

▶ Cryptococcosis doesn't require isolation.
▶ Check the patient's vital functions, and note any changes in mental status, orientation, pupillary response, and motor function.
▶ Watch for headache, vomiting, and nuchal rigidity.
▶ Before giving I.V. amphotericin B, check for phlebitis. Infuse slowly and dilute — rapid infusion may cause circulatory collapse.
▶ Before beginning therapy, draw blood for a serum electrolyte analysis to determine baseline renal status.
▶ During drug therapy, watch for decreased urine output, elevated blood urea nitrogen and creatinine levels, and hypokalemia.
▶ Monitor results of complete blood count, urinalysis, magnesium and potassium levels, and hepatic function tests. Ask the patient to report hearing loss, tinnitus, or dizziness.
▶ Give analgesics, antihistamines, and antiemetics for fever, chills, nausea, and vomiting.
▶ Provide psychological support to help the patient cope with long-term hospitalization.

CRYPTOSPORIDIOSIS

Caused by the protozoan *Cryptosporidium parvum*, cryptosporidiosis is a highly infectious enteric microbe that causes an acute, self-limiting diarrheal illness. It is identified in up to 5% of all cases of gastroenteritis in both industrialized and developing countries. At high risk for developing this disease are children — particularly those who are not toilet trained; child care workers; travelers to foreign countries; immunocompromised patients; medical personnel caring for patients with cryptosporidiosis; dairy farmers; persons exposed to human feces via sexual contact; and those who come into contact with any water source contaminated by *Cryptosporidium*.

In daycare settings, outbreaks of cryptosporidiosis are most common during the late summer and early fall. Cryptosporidiosis has been increasingly recognized as a cause of life-threatening, intractable diarrhea in HIV-infected patients; the annual rate of crytosporidial infection among patients with AIDS may approach 5% to 10%.

Causes

Transmission of cryptosporidia oocytes occurs primarily via the oral-fecal route, including hand contact with the stool of infected humans or animals or with objects contaminated with stool. Ingestion of food or water contaminated with stool, including water in recreational water parks and swimming pools, is also a common mode of transmission. Once ingested, the protozoa replicate intracellularly in the brush border of the small intestine. Infective oocysts are then shed and passed in the feces. The number of oocysts needed to cause infection is very low, perhaps as few as 2 to 10. Stools may contain active oocysts for up to 2 months after symptoms resolve.

Signs and symptoms

Clinical illness occurs in over 80% of infected people. Most patients experience acute onset of watery diarrhea, stomach cramps and, less often, upset stomach and fever. Some infected persons may be asymptomatic. Occasionally, infected persons can have severe diarrhea and weight loss. Symptoms appear 2 to 10 days after infection and persist for 1 to 2 weeks. The symptoms can be more severe in immunocompromised patients and the infection cannot be cleared unless the underlying immune defect is corrected; intractable diarrhea may continue for life.

Diagnosis

Fecal examination is performed to identify oocysts. Acid-fast or immunofluorescence staining usually confirms identification of oocysts. Intestinal biopsy can also be done.

Other conditions to be considered are amebiasis, giardiasis, and viral gastroenteritis.

Treatment

No drug has been found to cure cryptosporidiosis. Paromomycin may reduce symptoms and is used in immunocompromised individuals. Treatment includes supportive care with replacement of fluids and electrolytes and administration of antidiarrheal agents.

Special considerations

▶ Help patient maintain adequate hydration. Parenteral rehydration and hyperalimentation may be required in immunocompromised persons.

▶ Cleanse the perineum thoroughly to prevent skin breakdown.

 PREVENTION TIP Follow standard precautions. Stools of patients with cryptosporidiosis are highly infectious. Always wash your hands thoroughly before and after any contact with the patient, and advise others to do the same.

▶ Cryptosporidiosis is not bloodborne.

▶ Be aware that chlorine does not kill cryptosporidia. A 3% solution of hydrogen peroxide is an effective disinfectant.

▶ Cases of cryptosporidiosis in children who attend daycare should be reported to the local health department; evidence of negative stool cultures may be required prior to their readmission to daycare.

▶ A CD4 cell count of less than 200 signals the likelihood of a severe, long-lasting, and possibly deadly bout of cryptosporidiosis for HIV-infected individuals.

 PREVENTION TIP To prevent or reduce the risk of infection, instruct patients about proper hand washing, especially after defecating and before eating or handling food. Also, stress the importance of washing hands after touching anything that might have had contact with even the smallest amounts of human or animal stool, even if gloves were worn. Because of the waterborne transmission, special attention should be directed toward drinking safe water. Boiling water is the most reliable decontamination method and only filters with absolute pore sizes of 1 micron, that say "reverse osmosis" or that indicate tested and certified by NSF – an independent testing group. Standard 53 for cyst removal or cyst reduction on the label, should be used. Warn those who swim or use hot tubs to avoid swallowing water. Advise parents of children who are not toilet trained to change diapers away from pool areas: the child's genitals should be thoroughly cleansed with soap and water before re-entering the pool. If appropriate, advise patients to avoid any sexual practices that involve contact with the rectal area. Instruct patients to avoid touching the stool of any animal. Since cryptosporidiosis is common in puppies and kittens less than 6 months old, they should be tested by a veterinarian. Advise travelers to developing countries to avoid foods and drinks such as raw fruits and vegetables, tap water, unpasteurized milk or dairy products, and items purchased from street vendors.

CUTANEOUS LARVA MIGRANS

Cutaneous larva migrans, also known as creeping eruption, is a skin reaction to infestation by nematodes (hookworms or roundworms) that usually infect dogs and cats. This parasitic infection usually affects people who come in contact with infected soil or sand, such as children and farmers. Eruptions associated with cutaneous larva migrans clear completely with treatment.

Causes

Under favorable conditions — warmth, moisture, sandy soil — hookworm or roundworm ova present in feces of affected animals (such as dogs and cats) hatch into larvae, which can then burrow into human skin on contact. The larva becomes trapped under the skin, unable to reach the intestines to complete its normal life cycle. The parasite then begins to move, producing the peculiar, tunnel-like lesions that delineate the nematode's persistent and unsuccessful attempts to escape the body.

Signs and symptoms

A transient rash or, possibly, a small vesicle appears at the point of penetration, usually on an exposed area that has come in contact with the ground, such as the feet, legs, or buttocks. The incubation period may be weeks or months, or the parasite may be active almost as soon as it enters the skin.

As the parasite migrates, it etches a noticeable thin, raised, red line on the skin, which may become vesicular and encrusted. Pruritus quickly develops, often with crusting and secondary infection following excoriation. Onset is usually characterized by slight itching that develops into intermittent stinging pain as the thin, red lines develop. The larva's apparently random path can cover from 1 mm to 1 cm a day. Penetration by more than one larva may involve a much larger area of the skin, marking it with many tracks.

Diagnosis
Characteristic migratory lesions strongly suggest cutaneous larva migrans. A thorough patient history usually reveals contact with warm, moist soil within the past several months.

Treatment
Cutaneous larva migrans infections may require administration of thiabendazole orally for 2 to 3 days. Tell the patient that adverse effects of systemic thiabendazole include nausea, vomiting, abdominal pain, and dizziness. Topical thiabendazole may also be effective.

Special considerations
▶ Reassure the patient that larva migrans lesions usually clear 1 to 2 weeks after treatment, especially if he is sensitive about his appearance. Stress the importance of adhering to the treatment regimen exactly as ordered.

▶ Have the patient's nails cut short to prevent skin breaks and secondary bacterial infection from scratching. Apply cool, moist compresses to alleviate itching.

▶ Be alert for possible adverse reactions associated with systemic thiabendazole treatment, including nausea, vomiting, abdominal pain, and dizziness.

▶ Encourage the patient to verbalize feelings about the infestation, including embarrassment, fear of rejection by others, and body image disturbance.

 PREVENTION TIP Prevention requires patient teaching about the existence of these parasites, sanitation of beaches and sandboxes, and proper pet care. Instruct the patient and his family in good hand-washing technique, and stress the importance of preventing the spread of the infection among family members.

CYTOMEGALOVIRUS INFECTION

Also called generalized salivary gland disease and cytomegalic inclusion disease, cytomegalovirus (CMV) infection is caused by the cytomegalovirus, a deoxyribonucleic acid, ether-sensitive virus belonging to the herpes family. The disease occurs worldwide and is transmitted by human contact.

About four out of five people over age 35 have been infected with CMV, usually during childhood or early adulthood. In most of these people, the disease is so mild that it's overlooked. CMV infection during pregnancy can be hazardous to the fetus, possibly leading to stillbirth, brain damage, and other birth defects or to severe neonatal illness.

Causes
CMV has been found in the saliva, urine, semen, breast milk, stool, blood, and vaginal and cervical secretions of infected persons. The virus is usually transmitted by contact with these infected secretions, which harbor the virus for months or even years.

The virus may be transmitted by sexual contact and can travel across the placenta, causing a congenital infection. Immunosuppressed patients, especially those who have received transplanted organs, run a 90% chance of contracting CMV infection. Recipients of blood transfusions from donors with positive CMV antibodies are at some risk.

Signs and symptoms
CMV probably spreads through the body in lymphocytes or mononuclear cells to the lungs, liver, GI tract, eyes, and central nervous system, where it often produces inflammatory reactions.

Most patients with CMV infection have mild, nonspecific complaints, or none at all, even though antibody titers indicate infection. In these patients, the disease usually runs a self-limiting course.

Immunodeficient patients, such as those with acquired immunodeficiency syndrome (AIDS), and those receiving immunosuppressants may develop pneumonia or other secondary infections. AIDS patients may also develop disseminated CMV infection, which may cause chorioretinitis (resulting in blindness), colitis, or encephalitis.

Infected infants ages 3 to 6 months usually appear asymptomatic but may develop hepatic dysfunction, hepatosplenomegaly, spider angiomas, pneumonitis, and lymphadenopathy.

Congenital CMV infection is seldom apparent at birth, although the infant's urine contains CMV. About 1% of all newborns have CMV.

The virus can cause brain damage that may not show up for months after birth. Occasionally, it produces a rapidly fatal neonatal illness characterized by jaundice, petechial rash, hepatosplenomegaly, thrombocytopenia, hemolytic anemia, microcephaly, psychomotor retardation, mental deficiency, and hearing loss.

In some adults, CMV may cause cytomegalovirus mononucleosis, with 3 weeks or more of irregular, high fever.

Other findings may include a normal or elevated white blood cell (WBC) count, lymphocytosis, and increased atypical lymphocytes.

Diagnosis
Although virus isolation in urine is the most sensitive laboratory method, a diagnosis can also rest on virus isolation from saliva, throat, cervix, WBC, and biopsy specimens.

Other laboratory tests support the diagnosis, including complement fixation studies, hemagglutination inhibition antibody tests and, for congenital infections, indirect immunofluorescent tests for CMV immunoglobulin M antibody.

Treatment
Because CMV infection is usually self-limiting, treatment aims to relieve symptoms and prevent complications. In the immunosuppressed patient, however, CMV is treated with ganciclovir and foscarnet, combined with anti-CMV immune globulin for pneumonitis and possible GI disease. A new oral agent, famciclovir, has a limited role.

Special considerations
▶ Provide parents of children with severe congenital CMV infection with counseling to help them cope with the possibility of brain damage or death.
▶ Observe standard precautions when handling body secretions.

 PREVENTION TIP To help prevent CMV infection, warn immunosuppressed patients and pregnant women to avoid exposure to confirmed or suspected CMV infection. Tell pregnant patients that maternal CMV infection can cause serious fetal abnormalities. Urge patients with CMV infection — especially young children — to wash their hands thoroughly to prevent spreading it.

D

DACRYOCYSTITIS

Dacryocystitis is an infection of the lacrimal sac. In infants, it results from congenital atresia of the nasolacrimal duct. In adults, it results from an obstruction (dacryostenosis) of the nasolacrimal duct (most often in women over age 40). Dacryocystitis can be acute or chronic.

Causes

Dacryocystitis in infants occurs as a result of atresia of the nasolacrimal ducts due to failure of canalization or, in the first few months of life, from blockage when the membrane that separates the lower part of the nasolacrimal duct and the inferior nasal meatus fails to open spontaneously before tear secretion. Bony obstruction of the duct may also occur.

In adults, dacryocystitis can be caused by microbes infecting the lacrimal sac. In acute dacryocystitis, *Staphylococcus aureus* and, occasionally, beta-hemolytic streptococci are the cause. In chronic dacryocystitis, *Streptococcus pneumoniae* or, sometimes, a fungus — such as *Actinomyces* or *Candida albicans* — is the causative organism. Primary and secondary tumors of the sinus, nose, and orbits also may cause dacryocystitis.

Signs and symptoms

The hallmark of both the acute and chronic forms of dacryocystitis is constant tearing. Other symptoms of dacryocystitis include inflammation and tenderness over the nasolacrimal sac; pressure over this area may fail to produce purulent discharge from the punctum. Acute dacryocystitis is extremely painful.

Diagnosis

Clinical features and a physical examination suggest dacryocystitis. Culture of the discharged material demonstrates *S. aureus* and, occasionally, beta-hemolytic streptococci in acute dacryocystitis, and *S. pneumoniae* or *C. albicans* in the chronic form. The white blood cell count may be elevated in the acute form; in the chronic form, it's generally normal. An X-ray after injection of a radiopaque medium (dacryocystography) locates the atresia in infants.

Treatment

Treatment of acute dacryocystitis consists of warm compresses, topical and systemic antibiotic therapy and, occasionally, incision and drainage. Chronic dacryocystitis may eventually require dacryocystorhinostomy.

Therapy for nasolacrimal duct obstruction in an infant consists of careful massage of the area over the lacrimal sac four times a day for 6 to 9 months. If this fails to open the duct, dilation of the punctum and probing of the duct are necessary.

Special considerations

▶ Check the patient history for possible allergy to antibiotics before administration. Emphasize the importance of precise compliance with the prescribed antibiotic regimen.
▶ Tell the adult patient what to expect after surgery: He'll have ice compresses over

the surgical site and will have bruising and swelling.

▶ Monitor blood loss by counting dressings used to collect the blood.

▶ Apply ice compresses postoperatively. A small adhesive bandage may be placed over the suture line to protect it from damage.

DERMATOPHYTOSIS

Also called tinea or ringworm, dermatophytosis is a disease that can affect the scalp (tinea capitis), body (tinea corporis), nails (tinea unguium), feet (tinea pedis), groin (tinea cruris), and bearded skin (tinea barbae).

Tinea infections are quite prevalent in the United States and are usually more common in males than in females. With effective treatment, the cure rate is very high, although about 20% of persons with infected feet or nails develop chronic conditions.

Causes

Tinea infections (except for tinea versicolor) result from dermatophytes (fungi) of the genera *Trichophyton, Microsporum,* and *Epidermophyton.*

Transmission can occur directly (through contact with infected lesions) or indirectly (through contact with contaminated articles, such as shoes, towels, or shower stalls). Some cases come from contact with animals or soil.

Signs and symptoms

Lesions vary in appearance and duration with the type of infection.

Tinea capitis, which mainly affects children, is characterized by round erythematous patches on the scalp, causing hair loss with scaling. In some children, a hypersensitivity reaction develops, leading to boggy, inflamed, often pus-filled lesions (kerions).

Tinea corporis produces flat lesions on the skin at any site except the scalp, bearded skin, groin, palms, or soles. These lesions may be dry and scaly or moist and crusty; as they enlarge, their centers heal, causing the classic ring-shaped appearance.

Tinea unguium (onychomycosis) infection typically starts at the tip of one or more toenails (fingernail infection is less common) and produces gradual thickening, discoloration, and crumbling of the nail, with accumulation of subungual debris. Eventually, the nail may be destroyed completely.

Tinea pedis causes scaling and blisters between the toes. Severe infection may result in inflammation, with severe itching and pain on walking. A dry, squamous inflammation may affect the entire sole.

Tinea cruris (jock itch) produces red, raised, sharply defined, itchy lesions in the groin that may extend to the buttocks, inner thighs, and the external genitalia. Warm weather and tight clothing encourage fungus growth.

Tinea barbae is an uncommon infection that affects the bearded facial area of men.

Diagnosis

Microscopic examination of lesion scrapings prepared in potassium hydroxide solution usually confirms tinea infection. Other diagnostic procedures include Wood's light examination (which is useful in only about 5% of cases of tinea capitis) and culture of the infecting organism.

Treatment

Tinea infections usually respond to topical agents such as imidazole cream or to oral griseofulvin, which is especially effective in tinea infections of the skin and hair. Oral terbinafine or itraconazole is helpful in nail infections. However, topical therapy is ineffective for tinea capitis; oral griseofulvin for 1 to 3 months is the treatment of choice. Griseofulvin is contraindicated in the patient with porphyria, and it may necessitate an increase in dosage during anticoagulant (warfarin) therapy.

In addition to imidazole, other antifungals include naftifine, ciclopirox, terbinafine, haloprogin, and tolnaftate. Topical treatments should continue for 2 weeks after lesions resolve.

Supportive measures include open wet dressings, removal of scabs and scales, and application of keratolytics such as salicylic acid to soften and remove hyperkeratotic lesions of the heels or soles.

Special considerations

▶ For all tinea infections except those of the hair and nails, apply topical agents, watch for sensitivity reactions and secondary bacterial infections, and provide patient teaching.

▶ Monitor liver function of patients on long-term griseofulvin therapy.

▶ For *tinea capitis,* use good hand-washing technique, and teach the patient to do the same. To prevent spreading infection to others, advise washing towels, bedclothes, and combs frequently in hot water and to avoid sharing them. Suggest that family members be checked for tinea capitis.

▶ For *tinea corporis,* use abdominal pads between skin folds for the patient with excessive abdominal girth; change pads frequently. Check the patient daily for excoriated, newly denuded areas of skin. If the involved area is moist, apply open wet dressings two or three times daily to decrease inflammation and help remove scales.

▶ For *tinea unguium,* keep the patient's nails short and straight. Gently remove debris under the nails with an emery board.

▶ For *tinea pedis,* encourage the patient to expose feet to air whenever possible and to wear sandals or leather shoes and clean cotton socks. Instruct the patient to wash the feet twice daily and, after drying them thoroughly, to apply the antifungal cream followed by antifungal powder to absorb perspiration and prevent excoriation.

▶ For *tinea cruris,* instruct the patient to dry the affected area thoroughly after bathing and to evenly apply antifungal powder after applying the topical antifungal agent. Advise wearing loose-fitting clothing, which should be changed frequently and washed in hot water.

▶ For *tinea barbae,* suggest that the patient let his beard grow. (Whiskers should be trimmed with scissors, not a razor.) If the patient insists that he must shave, advise him to use an electric razor instead of a blade.

DIENTAMOEBA FRAGILIS INFECTION

Dientamoeba fragilis is an intestinal flagellate that lives in the large intestine. Infection occurs worldwide and is common in the United States. Those at greatest risk are people who live in poor sanitary conditions or travelers visiting developing countries. Prognosis is good for complete resolution of infection with treatment.

Causes

The infection is caused by the parasite *D. fragilis* and is thought to be transmitted through the oral-fecal route. The life cycle of this parasite hasn't been determined.

Signs and symptoms

Many people with this infection are asymptomatic. The most common symptoms are loose stools, intermittent diarrhea, and abdominal cramping. Anorexia, fatigue, weight loss, and abdominal tenderness may also occur.

Diagnosis

The diagnosis is made by detection of trophozoites of *D. fragilis* in permanently stained fecal smears. Several samples obtained on alternate days are helpful in increasing the rate of detection. Fecal samples should be preserved immediately after collection.

Other infections to consider are cyclosporiasis, microsporidiosis, balantidiasis, amebiasis, and giardiasis.

Treatment
Antimicrobial agents such as iodoquinol, paromomycin, or tetracycline are appropriate for treatment.

Special considerations
▶ Follow standard precautions. Thorough hand washing before and after any contact with the patient is a must. Advise others such as family members to do the same. Teach the patient to use proper hand-washing technique, especially after defecating and before eating or handling food.
▶ Store stool specimens in airtight containers to minimize exposure to oxygen and desiccation. Specimens should be submitted to a laboratory within 24 hours of collection.

 PREVENTION TIP To prevent acquiring or spreading *D. fragilis,* stress the importance of washing hands with soap and warm water for 20 seconds, especially after using the toilet, changing baby diapers, and before preparing foods.

DIPHTHERIA

Diphtheria is an acute, highly contagious toxin-mediated infection caused by *Corynebacterium diphtheriae,* a gram-positive rod that usually infects the respiratory tract, primarily the tonsils, nasopharynx, and larynx, usually producing a membranous pharyngitis. GI and urinary tracts, conjunctivae, and ears are rarely involved.

Thanks to effective immunization, diphtheria is rare in many parts of the world, including the United States. Since 1972, the incidence of cutaneous diphtheria has been increasing, especially in the Pacific Northwest and the Southwest, in areas where crowding and poor hygienic conditions prevail. Most victims are children under age 15; about 10% of patients die. Recent outbreaks have occurred in the newly independent states adjacent to the former Soviet Union.

Causes
Transmission usually occurs through intimate contact or by airborne respiratory droplets from asymptomatic carriers or convalescing patients; many more people carry this disease than contract active infection. Diphtheria is more prevalent during the colder months because of closer person-to-person contact indoors. But it may be contracted at any time during the year. Humans are the only known reservoir for this bacteria.

Signs and symptoms
Most infections go unrecognized, especially in partially immunized individuals. After incubation of less than 1 week, clinical cases of diphtheria characteristically show a thick, patchy, grayish-green membrane over the mucous membranes of the pharynx, larynx, tonsils, soft palate, and nose; fever; sore throat; a rasping cough, hoarseness, and other symptoms similar to croup. Attempts to remove the membrane usually cause bleeding, which is highly characteristic of diphtheria. If this membrane causes airway obstruction (especially likely in laryngeal diphtheria), signs include tachypnea, stridor, possibly cyanosis, suprasternal retractions, and suffocation, if untreated. In cutaneous diphtheria, skin lesions resemble impetigo.

Complications include thrombocytopenia, myocarditis, neurologic involvement (primarily affecting motor fibers but possibly also sensory neurons), renal involvement, and pulmonary involvement (bronchopneumonia) due to *C. diphtheriae* or other superinfecting microbes.

Diagnosis
Examination showing the characteristic membrane and a throat culture, or culture

of other suspect lesions growing *C. diphtheriae,* confirm this diagnosis.

Treatment

Treatment must not wait for confirmation by culture. Standard treatment includes diphtheria antitoxin administered I.M. or I.V.; antibiotics, such as penicillin or erythromycin, to eliminate the microbes from the upper respiratory tract and other sites, to terminate the carrier state; measures to prevent complications; and possible tracheotomy if airway obstruction occurs.

Diphtheria infection doesn't confer immunity, therefore diphtheria immunization should be given during convalescence.

Special considerations

▶ Serial ECGs should be performed twice weekly for 4 to 6 weeks to watch for myocarditis.

 PREVENTION TIP To prevent spread of this disease, stress the need for strict isolation. Teach proper disposal of nasopharyngeal secretions. Maintain infection precautions until after three consecutive negative cultures at least 24 hours apart, with the first culture being at least 24 hours after the completion of antimicrobial therapy. Treatment of exposed individuals with antitoxin remains controversial. Suggest that family members later receive diphtheria toxoid if they haven't been immunized.

▶ Give drugs as ordered. Although time-consuming and risky, desensitization should be attempted if tests are positive because diphtheria antitoxin is the only specific treatment available. Because mortality increases directly with delay in antitoxin administration, the antitoxin is given before laboratory confirmation of diagnosis if sensitivity tests are negative. Before giving diphtheria antitoxin, which is made from horse serum, obtain eye and skin tests to determine sensitivity. After giving antitoxin or penicillin, be alert for anaphylaxis; keep epinephrine 1:1,000 and

resuscitation equipment handy. In patients who receive erythromycin, watch for thrombophlebitis.

▶ Monitor respirations carefully, especially in laryngeal diphtheria (usually, such patients are in a high-humidity or croup tent). Watch for signs of airway obstruction, and be ready to give immediate life support, including intubation and tracheotomy.

▶ Watch for signs of shock, which can develop suddenly.

▶ Obtain cultures as ordered.

▶ If neuritis develops, tell the patient it's usually transient. Be aware that peripheral neuritis may not develop until 2 to 3 months after onset of illness.

▶ Assign a primary nurse to increase the effectiveness of isolation. Give reassurance that isolation is temporary.

▶ Stress the need for childhood immunizations to all parents. Report all cases of diphtheria to local public health authorities.

 ALERT Be alert for signs of myocarditis, such as development of heart murmurs or ECG changes. Ventricular fibrillation is a common cause of sudden death in diphtheria patients.

EBOLA VIRUS INFECTION

One of the most frightening viruses to come out of the African subcontinent, the Ebola virus first appeared in 1976. More than 400 persons in Zaire (now known as Democratic Republic of Congo) and the neighboring Sudan died due to the hemorrhagic fever that the virus causes. Ebola virus has been responsible for several outbreaks since then, including another in Zaire in the summer of 1995.

An unclassified ribonucleic acid (RNA) virus, Ebola virus is morphologically similar to the Marburg virus. Both viruses cause headache, malaise, myalgia, and high fever, progressing to severe diarrhea, vomiting, and internal and external hemorrhage.

Four strains of the Ebola virus are known to exist: Ebola Zaire, Ebola Sudan, Ebola Tai, and Ebola Reston. All four types are structurally similar but have different antigenic properties. One type, Ebola Reston, affects only monkeys; the other three types affect humans.

The prognosis for Ebola virus disease is extremely poor, with a mortality rate as high as 90%. The incubation period ranges from 2 to 21 days.

Causes

Ebola virus disease is caused by an unclassified RNA virus that is transmitted by direct contact with infected blood, body secretions, or organs. Nosocomial and community-acquired transmission can occur. Transmission through semen may occur up to 7 weeks after clinical recovery.

The virus remains contagious even after the patient has died.

Signs and symptoms

The patient's health history usually reveals contact with an infected person. However, no clear line of infection may be apparent at the beginning of an Ebola virus outbreak. The patient usually complains of flulike signs and symptoms (such as headache, malaise, myalgia, fever, cough, and sore throat), that first appear within 3 days of infection.

As the virus spreads through the body, inspection reveals bruising as capillaries rupture and dead blood cells infiltrate the skin. A maculopapular eruption appears after the 5th day of infection. The patient may also display melena, hematemesis, epistaxis, and bleeding gums. As the infection progresses, severe complications, including liver and kidney dysfunction, dehydration, and hemorrhage, may develop. In pregnant women, Ebola virus disease leads to abortion and massive hemorrhage.

In the final stages of the disease, the skin blisters and sloughs off, blood seeps from all body orifices, and the patient begins vomiting his liquefied internal organs. Death usually results during the 2nd week of illness from organ failure or hemorrhage.

Diagnosis

Specialized laboratory tests reveal specific antigens or antibodies and may show the isolated virus. As with other types of hemorrhagic fever, tests also demonstrate neutrophil leukocytosis, hypofibrinogenemia, thrombocytopenia, and microangiopathic hemolytic anemia.

Treatment

No cure exists for Ebola virus disease; treatment consists mainly of intensive supportive care. The administration of I.V. fluids helps offset the effects of severe dehydration. The patient may receive replacement of plasma heparin before the onset of clinical shock.

Experimental treatments include administration of plasma that contains Ebola virus-specific antibodies. Although this treatment has reduced levels of Ebola virus in the body, further evaluation is needed.

Throughout treatment, the patient should remain in isolation. If diagnostic tests indicate that the patient is free from the virus, which typically occurs 21 days after onset in those few who survive, the patient can be released.

Special considerations

▶ Follow the guidelines for strict isolation precautions formulated by the Centers for Disease Control and Prevention (CDC) when assessing a patient who may have Ebola virus disease. Any patient confirmed to have Ebola virus disease should be reported to the CDC.
▶ Check the results of complete blood count and coagulation studies for signs of blood loss and coagulopathy.
▶ Assess the patient daily for petechiae, ecchymoses, and oozing blood. Note and document the size of ecchymoses at least every 24 hours.
▶ Protect all areas of petechiae and ecchymoses from further injury.
▶ Test stools, urine, and vomitus for occult blood.
▶ Watch for frank bleeding, including GI bleeding and, in women, menorrhagia. Note and document the amount of bleeding every 24 hours or more often.
▶ Monitor the patient's family and other close contacts for fever and other signs of infection.

▶ Provide emotional support for the patient and family during the course of this devastating disease. Encourage them to ask questions and discuss any concerns they have about the disease and its treatment.

The CDC recommends the following guidelines to help prevent the spread of this deadly disease:
▶ Keep the patient in isolation throughout the course of the disease.
▶ If possible, place the patient in a negative pressure room at the beginning of hospitalization to avoid the need for transfer as the disease progresses.
▶ Restrict nonessential staff members from entering the patient's room.
▶ Make sure that anyone who enters the patient's room wears gloves and a gown to prevent contact with any surface in the room that may have been soiled.
▶ Use barrier precautions to prevent skin and mucous membrane exposure to blood or other body fluids, secretions, or excretions when caring for the patient.
▶ If you must come within 3' (1 m) of the patient, also wear a face shield or a surgical mask and goggles or eyeglasses with side shields.
▶ Don't reuse gloves or gowns unless they have been completely disinfected.
▶ Make sure any patient who dies of the disease is promptly buried or cremated. Precautions to avoid contact with the patient's body fluids and secretions should continue even after the patient's death.

EHRLICHIOSIS

The human ehrlichioses are considered emerging zoonotic diseases (diseases that can be passed from animals to man). There are two distinct forms of illness: human monocytic ehrlichiosis (HME) and human granulocytic ehrlichiosis (HGE). Since these diseases are newly recognized and there is no national surveillance program yet, national incidence rates are not available. However, hundreds of cases have been reported in 30 states, predominantly in the south-central, southeastern and mid-Atlantic regions. One-third of persons who seroconvert actually become ill. A majority of documented cases require hospitalization and a small percentage die.

Causes

Human monocytic ehrlichiosis is caused by *Ehrlichia chaffeensis* and an agent similar to the veterinary microbe *E. equi*, while *E. phagocytophilia* causes human granulocytic ehrlichiosis. The bacteria are transmitted to humans through tick bites. The lone star tick carries *E. chaffeensis* and is common in the southeastern United States. The black-legged tick transmits *E. phagocytophilia* in the northeastern United States and the western black-legged tick in the western coastal United States.

Signs and symptoms

The most common symptoms of both HME and HGE are nonspecific and include fever, headache, myalgia, thrombocytopenia, leukopenia, and elevated liver enzyme levels. A rash develops in approximately one-third of patients with HME but is rare in patients with HGE. Complications such as adult respiratory distress syndrome, renal failure, neurologic disorders, and disseminated intravascular coagulation can occur.

Diagnosis

To diagnose ehrlichiosis, the doctor must have a high index of suspicion when presented with the above symptoms and a history of recent exposure to ticks in an endemic area during the previous 3 weeks. Laboratory results showing leukopenia and thrombocytopenia are used to support clinical findings. Indirect immunofluorescence assay and polymerase chain reaction are used to confirm the diagnosis.

Differential diagnoses include rickettsial diseases such as Rocky Mountain spotted fever, eastern tick-borne rickettsioses, rick-

ettsialpox, and Q fever. Other infectious diseases to consider are meningococcemia and rubeola. Until a rash appears, it may be difficult to differentiate; however, treatment of suspected ehrlichiosis should not be delayed.

Treatment

Tetracycline or doxycycline can be given orally or I.V. Chloramphenicol can also be used but may not be as effective.

Special considerations

▶ Stress the importance of completing the full course of antibiotic therapy even if symptoms resolve.
▶ Provide appropriate comfort measures.
▶ Observe for signs and symptoms of any developing complications and respond appropriately.

 PREVENTION TIP Advise patients that the best way to prevent Ehrlichiosis is to avoid being bitten by ticks. Instruct patients on proper precautions in endemic areas, such as wearing protective clothing, using tick repellent, and careful, prompt removal of ticks found on the body.

EMPYEMA

Empyema is the accumulation of pus and necrotic tissue in the pleural space. Normally, this space contains a small amount of extracellular fluid that lubricates the pleural surfaces. Empyema typically is a complication of pneumonia but may result from penetrating chest trauma, esophageal rupture, or inoculation of the pleural cavity after thoracentesis or chest tube placement. The prognosis for empyema with treatment is generally good.

Causes

Empyema is usually associated with infection in the pleural space, which may be idiopathic or related to pneumonitis,

EMPYEMA FLUID CHARACTERISTICS

Empyema is indicated by the following fluid analysis:
▶ pH less than 7
▶ Glucose less than 40 mg/dl
▶ LDH greater than 1000 IU/dl
▶ Positive Gram stain
▶ Positive culture (50%)
▶ Specific gravity greater than 1.018
▶ WBC greater than 500 cells/mm^3
▶ Protein greater than 2.5 g/dl

carcinoma, perforation, or esophageal rupture.

Signs and symptoms
Most patients experience fever, malaise, shortness of breath, night sweats, anorexia, and pleuritic chest pain. Physical findings include tachypnea, and decreased breath sounds; percussion over the effused area, detects dullness, which doesn't change with breathing.

Diagnosis
Chest X-ray is done to differentiate between pneumonia, pulmonary abscess, and empyema. A computed tomography scan or ultrasound of the chest may be needed to help localize the fluid collection. The most useful test is thoracentesis and aspiration of pus for analysis. (See *Empyema fluid characteristics.*)

Treatment
Treatment of empyema requires insertion of one or more chest tubes after thoracentesis to allow drainage of purulent material, and possibly decortication (surgical removal of the thick coating over the lung) or rib resection to allow open drainage and lung expansion. Empyema also requires parenteral antibiotics. Asso-

ciated hypoxia requires oxygen administration.

Special considerations
▶ Explain thoracentesis to the patient. Before the procedure, tell the patient to expect a stinging sensation from the local anesthetic and a feeling of pressure when the needle is inserted. Instruct him to tell you immediately if he feels uncomfortable or has trouble breathing during the procedure.
▶ Reassure the patient during thoracentesis. Remind him to breathe normally and avoid sudden movements, such as coughing or sighing.

 ALERT Monitor vital signs, and watch for syncope. If fluid is removed too quickly, the patient may suffer bradycardia, hypotension, pain, pulmonary edema, or even cardiac arrest. Watch for respiratory distress or pneumothorax (sudden onset of dyspnea, and cyanosis) after thoracentesis.
▶ Administer oxygen and antibiotics, as ordered.
▶ Encourage the patient to do deep-breathing exercises to promote lung expansion. Use an incentive spirometer to promote deep breathing.
▶ Provide meticulous chest tube care, and use aseptic technique for changing dressings around the tube insertion site in empyema. Ensure tube patency by watching for fluctuations of fluid in the underwater seal chamber. Watch for bubbling in the water-seal chamber, indicating the presence of air in the pleural spaces. Record the amount, color, and consistency of any tube drainage.
▶ If the patient has open drainage through a rib resection or intercostal tube, use hand and dressing precautions.
▶ Because weeks of such drainage are usually necessary to obliterate the space, make visiting nurse referrals for patients who will be discharged with the tube in place.

ENCEPHALITIS

A severe inflammation of the brain, encephalitis is usually caused by a mosquito-borne or (in some areas) a tick-borne virus. The virus may also be transmitted through ingestion of infected goat's milk and accidental injection or inhalation of the virus. In encephalitis, intense lymphocytic infiltration of brain tissues and the leptomeninges causes cerebral edema, degeneration of the brain's ganglion cells, and diffuse nerve cell destruction. Eastern equine encephalitis may produce permanent neurologic damage and is often fatal. (See also "West Nile encephalitis.")

Causes

Encephalitis generally results from infection with arboviruses specific to rural areas. In urban areas, it's most frequently caused by enteroviruses (coxsackievirus, poliovirus, and echovirus).

Other causes include herpesvirus, mumps virus, human immunodeficiency virus, adenoviruses, and demyelinating diseases following measles, varicella, rubella, or vaccination.

Between World War I and the Depression, a type of encephalitis known as lethargic encephalitis, von Economo's disease, or sleeping sickness occurred with some regularity. The causative virus was never clearly identified, and the disease is rare today. Even so, the term sleeping sickness persists and is often mistakenly used to describe other types of encephalitis as well.

The prognosis depends on factors such as immune status, pre-existing neurologic conditions, and extremes of age (very young or elderly) as well as the virulence of the virus.

Signs and symptoms

All viral forms of encephalitis have similar clinical features, although certain differences do occur.

Usually, the acute illness begins with sudden onset of fever, headache, and vomiting and progresses to include signs and symptoms of meningeal irritation (stiff neck and back) and neuronal damage (drowsiness, coma, paralysis, seizures, ataxia, and organic psychoses). After the acute phase of the illness, coma may persist for days or weeks.

The severity of arbovirus encephalitis may range from subclinical to rapidly fatal necrotizing disease. Herpes encephalitis also produces signs and symptoms that vary from subclinical to acute and often fatal fulminating disease. Associated effects include disturbances of taste or smell.

Diagnosis

During an encephalitis epidemic, diagnosis is easily based on clinical findings and patient history. Sporadic cases are difficult to distinguish from other febrile illnesses, such as gastroenteritis and meningitis. When possible, identification of the virus in cerebrospinal fluid (CSF) or blood confirms the diagnosis.

The common viruses that also cause herpes, measles, and mumps are easier to identify than arboviruses. Arboviruses and herpesviruses can be isolated by inoculating young mice with specimens taken from patients. In herpes encephalitis, serologic studies may show rising titers of complement-fixing antibodies.

In all forms of encephalitis, CSF pressure is elevated, and despite inflammation, the fluid is often clear. White blood cell and protein levels in CSF are slightly elevated, but the glucose level remains normal. An EEG reveals abnormalities. Occasionally, a computed tomographic scan may be ordered to rule out cerebral hematoma.

Treatment

The antiviral agents acyclovir and foscarnet are effective only against herpes encephalitis. Treatment of all other forms of encephalitis is entirely supportive.

PERFORMING A RAPID NEUROLOGIC EXAMINATION

To assess neurologic function in the patient with encephalitis, include the following:

▶ *Orientation:* patient's knowledge of where he is, the year, season, date, day, and month

▶ *Registration and recall:* patient's ability to recall three objects that you name

▶ *Attention and calculation:* patient's ability to focus on what you're saying

▶ *Language:* patient's ability to name objects, repeat word clearly, read, follow a written command

▶ *Focus on recall of recent events:* patient's ability to recall your name, what he had for breakfast, who came to visit.

As you elicit answers, be particularly concerned about the restless patient and the patient who requires more stimulation to provide the same responses to the points listed above than required at previous checks.

Drug therapy includes phenytoin or another anticonvulsant, usually given I.V.; glucocorticoids to reduce cerebral inflammation and edema; furosemide or mannitol to reduce cerebral swelling; sedatives for restlessness; and aspirin or acetaminophen to relieve headache and reduce fever.

Other supportive measures include adequate fluid and electrolyte intake to prevent dehydration and antibiotics for an associated infection such as pneumonia. Isolation is unnecessary.

Special considerations

During the acute phase of the illness:

▶ Assess neurologic function often. Observe the patient's mental status and cognitive abilities by performing a rapid neurologic examination. (See *Performing a rapid neurologic examination.*) If the tissue within the brain becomes edematous, changes will occur in the patient's mental status and cognitive abilities.

▶ Assessment should focus on early changes in intracranial dynamics. Continued swelling may result in cranial nerve compression, causing changes in pupillary reaction to light, ptosis, eyelid droop, and an eye rotating outward.

▶ Monitor for signs of progression of a herniation pattern (abnormal posturing movements, such as decerebration, decortication, and flaccidity, to noxious stimuli).

▶ Watch for cranial nerve involvement (ptosis, strabismus, diplopia), abnormal sleep patterns, and behavioral changes.

▶ Maintain adequate fluid intake to prevent dehydration, but avoid fluid overload, which may increase cerebral edema. Measure and record intake and output accurately.

▶ Give acyclovir by slow I.V. infusion only. The patient must be well hydrated and the infusion given over 1 hour to avoid kidney damage. Watch for adverse effects, such as nausea, diarrhea, pruritus, and rash, and adverse effects of other drugs. Check the infusion site often to avoid infiltration and phlebitis.

▶ Carefully position the patient to prevent joint stiffness and neck pain, and turn him often. Assist with range-of-motion exercises.

▶ Maintain adequate nutrition. It may be necessary to give the patient small, frequent meals or to supplement meals with nasogastric tube or parenteral feedings.

▶ To prevent constipation and minimize the risk of increased intracranial pressure from straining during defecation, give a mild laxative or stool softener.

▶ Provide good mouth care.

▶ Maintain a quiet environment. Darkening the room may decrease photophobia and headache. If the patient naps during the day and is restless at night, plan daytime activities to minimize napping and promote sleep at night.

▶ Provide emotional support and reassurance because the patient is apt to be frightened by the illness and frequent diagnostic tests.

▶ If the patient is delirious or confused, attempt to reorient him often. Providing a calendar or a clock in the patient's room may be helpful.

▶ Reassure the patient and his family that behavioral changes caused by encephalitis usually disappear. If a neurologic deficit is severe and appears permanent, refer the patient to a rehabilitation program as soon as the acute phase has passed.

ENDOCARDITIS

Also called infective endocarditis and bacterial endocarditis, endocarditis is an infection of the endocardium, heart valves, or a cardiac prosthesis, resulting from bacterial or fungal invasion. This invasion produces vegetative growths on the heart valves, the endocardial lining of a heart chamber, or the endothelium of a blood vessel that may embolize to the spleen, kidneys, central nervous system, and lungs.

In endocarditis, fibrin and platelets aggregate on the valve tissue and engulf circulating bacteria or fungi that flourish and produce friable verrucous vegetations. Such vegetations may cover the valve surfaces, causing ulceration and necrosis; they may also extend to the chordae tendineae, leading to their rupture and subsequent valvular insufficiency. (See *Degenerative changes in endocarditis*.)

Untreated endocarditis is usually fatal, but with proper treatment, about 70% of patients recover. The prognosis is worst when endocarditis causes severe valvular damage, leading to insufficiency and heart failure, or when it involves a prosthetic valve.

DEGENERATIVE CHANGES IN ENDOCARDITIS

This illustration shows typical vegetation on the endocardium produced by fibrin and platelet deposits on infection sites.

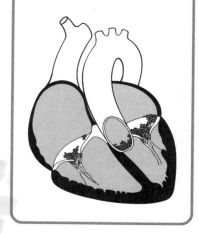

Causes

Most commonly, endocarditis occurs in I.V. drug abusers, patients with prosthetic heart valves, and those with mitral valve prolapse (especially males with a systolic murmur). These conditions have surpassed rheumatic heart disease as the leading risk factor.

Other predisposing conditions include coarctation of the aorta; tetralogy of Fallot; subaortic and valvular aortic stenosis; ventricular septal defects; pulmonary stenosis; Marfan's syndrome; degenerative heart disease, especially calcific aortic stenosis; and, rarely, syphilitic aortic valve. Some patients with endocarditis have no underlying heart disease.

Microbes that cause infection differ among patient groups. In patients with native valve endocarditis who aren't I.V. drug abusers, causative organisms usually include, in order of frequency, streptococci (especially *Streptococcus viridans*), staphylococci, and enterococci. Although many other bacteria occasionally cause the disorder, fungal causes are rare in this group. The mitral valve is involved most commonly, followed by the aortic valve.

In patients who are I.V. drug abusers, *Staphylococcus aureus* is the most common infecting organism. Less frequently, streptococci, enterococci, gram-negative bacilli, or fungi cause the disorder. Most often the tricuspid valve is involved, followed by the aortic valve and then the mitral valve.

In patients with prosthetic valve endocarditis, early cases (those that develop within 60 days of valve insertion) are usually due to staphylococcal infection. Gram-negative aerobic organisms, fungi, streptococci, enterococci, or diphtheroids may also cause the disorder. The course of the infection is often fulminating and associated with a high mortality rate. Late cases (those that develop after 60 days) present similarly to native valve endocarditis.

Signs and symptoms

Early clinical features of endocarditis are usually nonspecific and include malaise, weakness, fatigue, weight loss, anorexia, arthralgia, night sweats, chills, valvular insufficiency and, in 90% of patients, an intermittent fever that may recur for weeks. A more acute onset is associated with highly pathogenic organisms such as *S. aureus*.

Endocarditis often causes a loud, regurgitant murmur that is typical of the underlying heart lesion. A suddenly changing murmur or the discovery of a new murmur in the presence of fever is a classic physical sign of endocarditis.

In about 30% of patients, embolization from vegetating lesions or diseased valvular tissue may produce the following features of splenic, renal, cerebral, or pulmonary infarction or peripheral vascular occlusion:

▶ *splenic infarction:* pain in the left upper quadrant, radiating to the left shoulder; abdominal rigidity

▶ *renal infarction:* hematuria, pyuria, flank pain, decreased urine output

▶ *cerebral infarction:* hemiparesis, aphasia, or other neurologic deficits

▶ *pulmonary infarction* (most common in right-sided endocarditis, which usually occurs in I.V. drug abusers and after cardiac surgery): cough, pleuritic pain, pleural friction rub, dyspnea, hemoptysis

▶ *peripheral vascular occlusion:* numbness and tingling in an arm or a leg, finger, or toe or signs of impending peripheral gangrene.

Other signs include splenomegaly; petechiae of the skin (especially common on the upper anterior trunk) and the buccal, pharyngeal, or conjunctival mucosa; and splinter hemorrhages under the nails. Rarely, endocarditis produces Osler's nodes (tender, raised subcutaneous lesions on the fingers or toes), Roth's spots (hemorrhagic areas with white centers on the retina), and Janeway lesions (purplish macules on the palms or soles).

Diagnosis

Three or more blood cultures in a 24- to 48-hour period (each from a separate site) identify the causative microbe in up to 90% of patients. The remaining 10% may have negative blood cultures, possibly suggesting fungal infection or infections that are difficult to diagnose, such as *Haemophilus parainfluenzae*. Research has supported the use of guidelines commonly referred to as the Duke criteria. The Duke approach distinguishes between major and minor criteria. (See *Duke criteria for diagnosing infective endocarditis.*)

Other abnormal but nonspecific laboratory test results include:
▶ normal or elevated white blood cell count
▶ abnormal histiocytes (macrophages)
▶ elevated erythrocyte sedimentation rate
▶ normocytic, normochromic anemia (in 70% to 90% of endocarditis cases)
▶ positive serum rheumatoid factor (in about one-half of all patients with endocarditis after the disease is present for 3 to 6 weeks).

DUKE CRITERIA FOR DIAGNOSING INFECTIVE ENDOCARDITIS

A patient who has 2 major criteria, 1 major and 3 minor, or 5 minor criteria has a definite case of infective endocarditis (IE). Patients whose criteria don't add up to a definite diagnosis, but don't exclude it, has a possible case of IE. A diagnosis of IE is ruled out in a patient whose manifestations of IE resolve in 4 or fewer days of antibiotic therapy.

MAJOR CRITERIA:

▶ Isolation of an infective organism in a patient with persistent bacteremia in 2 blood cultures separated by 12 or more hours, or
▶ Isolation of an infective organism in a patient with persistent bacteremia in 3 to 4 blood cultures with the passage of at least 1 hour between the first and last culture.
▶ Evidence of myocardial involvement as demonstrated by an echocardiogram with any of the following positive findings for IE:
– oscillating vegetation
– intracardiac abscess
– prosthetic valve instability

MINOR CRITERIA:

▶ Predisposition: Predisposing heart condition or intravenous drug abuse
▶ Fever: fever greater than or equal to 100.4° F (38° C)
▶ Vascular phenomena: major arterial emboli, septic pulmonary infarcts, mycotic aneurysm, intracranial hemorrhage, conjunctival hemorrhages, Janeway lesions
▶ Immunologic phenomena: Glomerulonephritis, Osler's nodes, Roth's spots, rheumatoid factor
▶ Microbiologic evidence: Positive blood culture but not meeting major criteria or serologic evidence of active infection with organism consistent with IE
▶ Echocardiogram: Consistent with IE but not meeting major criteria.

Adapted from Durack, D.T.; Lukes, A.S.; Bright, D.K.; and The Duke Endocarditis Service, "New criteria for diagnosis of infective endocarditis: Utilization of specific endocardiographic findings," *American Journal of Medicine* 96:200-209, 1994, with permission from Excerpta Medica, Inc.

Echocardiography may identify valvular damage; electrocardiography may show atrial fibrillation and other arrhythmias that accompany valvular disease.

Transesophageal echocardiography (TEE) is extremely sensitive and specific for detecting perivalvular extensions of infection.

Treatment

The goal of treatment is to eradicate the infecting organism. Antimicrobial therapy should start promptly and continue over 4 to 6 weeks. Selection of an antibiotic is based on identification of the infecting microbe and on sensitivity studies. While awaiting test results or if blood cultures are negative, empiric antimicrobial therapy is based on the likely infecting microbe.

Supportive treatment includes bed rest, aspirin for fever and aches, and sufficient fluid intake. Severe valvular damage, especially aortic or mitral insufficiency, may necessitate corrective surgery if refractory heart failure develops or in cases in which an infected prosthetic valve must be replaced.

Special considerations

▶ Watch for signs of embolization (hematuria, pleuritic chest pain, left upper quad-

ment. Tell the patient to watch for and report these signs, which may indicate impending peripheral vascular occlusion or splenic, renal, cerebral, or pulmonary infarction.

❚ Monitor the patient's renal status (blood urea nitrogen levels, creatinine clearance, and urine output) to check for signs of renal emboli or evidence of drug toxicity.

❚ Observe for signs of heart failure, such as dyspnea, tachycardia, crackles, neck vein distention, edema, and weight gain.

❚ Provide reassurance by teaching the patient and his family about this disease and the need for prolonged treatment. Suggest quiet diversionary activities to prevent excessive physical exertion.

 PREVENTION TIP Tell the patient and his family to watch closely for fever, anorexia, and other signs of relapse about 2 weeks after treatment stops. Make sure a susceptible patient understands the need for prophylactic antibiotics before, during, and after dental work, childbirth, and genitourinary, GI, or gynecologic procedures. Teach the patient how to recognize symptoms of endocarditis, and tell him to notify the doctor immediately if they occur.

ENTEROBIASIS

Enterobiasis (also called pinworm, seatworm, or threadworm infection, or oxyuriasis) is a benign intestinal disease caused by the nematode *Enterobius vermicularis*. Found worldwide, even in temperate regions with good sanitation, it's the most prevalent helminthic infection in the United States.

Enterobiasis infection and reinfection occur most often in children between ages 5 and 14 and in certain institutionalized groups because of poor hygiene and frequent hand-to-mouth activity. Crowded living conditions increase the likelihood of its spreading to family members.

Causes

Adult pinworms live in the intestine; female worms migrate to the perianal region to deposit their ova. *Direct transmission* occurs when the patient's hands transfer infective eggs from the anus to the mouth. *Indirect transmission* occurs when the patient comes in contact with contaminated articles, such as linens and clothing.

Signs and symptoms

Asymptomatic enterobiasis is commonly overlooked. However, intense perianal pruritus may occur, especially at night, when the female worm leaves the anus to deposit ova. Pruritus causes irritability, scratching, skin irritation and, sometimes, vaginitis. Enuresis and insomnia may also result because of the night activity. Rarely, complications include appendicitis, salpingitis, and pelvic granuloma.

Diagnosis

A history of anal pruritus suggests enterobiasis; identification of *Enterobius* ova recovered from the perianal area with a cellophane tape swab confirms it.

This test must be repeated three times and is done before the patient bathes and defecates in the morning. A stool sample is usually ova- and worm-free because the worms deposit ova outside the intestine and die after return to the anus.

Treatment

Drug therapy with pyrantel, piperazine, or mebendazole destroys the causative parasites. Effective eradication requires simultaneous treatment of family members and, in institutions, other patients.

Special considerations

❚ If the patient receives pyrantel, tell him and his family that this drug colors the stool bright red and may cause vomiting (vomitus will also be red). The tablet form of this drug is coated with aspirin and shouldn't be given to aspirin-sensitive patients.

▶ Before giving piperazine, obtain a history of seizure disorders; this drug is contraindicated in patients with such a history.

 PREVENTION TIP To help prevent this disease, tell parents to bathe children daily (showers are preferable to tub baths) and to change underwear and bed linens daily. Educate children in proper personal hygiene, and stress the need for hand washing after defecation and before handling food. Discourage nail biting. If the child can't stop, suggest that he wear gloves until the infection clears.

▶ Report all outbreaks of enterobiasis to school authorities.

▶ Tell parents to strictly adhere to the prescribed drug dosage as directed by a doctor.

ENTEROVIRAL DISEASES (NONPOLIO)

Enteroviral diseases are a group of syndromes caused by enteroviruses. Sixty-three nonpolio enteroviruses such as coxsackieviruses are very common and cause an estimated 30 million or more infections a year in the United States. Infants, children, and adolescents are most susceptible to infection and illness from these viruses. Long-term complications are rare and symptoms usually resolve spontaneously.

Causes

Numerous serotypes of coxsackie A and coxsackie B, echoviruses, and four other enteroviruses cause a variety of diseases such as herpangina, hand-foot-and-mouth disease, epidemic pleurodynia, aseptic meningitis, paralysis, myocarditis, pericarditis, respiratory disease, diarrhea, and conjunctivitis.

Signs and symptoms

Symptoms of nonpolio enteroviral syndromes are usually non-specific, and commonly include fever, flu-like illness, rash, and mild upper respiratory symptoms are common. Less often, specific viruses cause aseptic meningitis. Rarely the heart and brain are affected, as in myocarditis, pericarditis, and encephalitis.

Diagnosis

Isolation of the causative microbe in cell culture is the most common procedure for diagnosing the infection. Throat and nasopharyngeal secretions, stool, cerebrospinal fluid, and serum are most often cultured depending on the presenting symptoms. Cultures are more likely to be positive earlier than later in the course of infection.

Several other conditions associated with the particular system affected need to be considered such as: herpetic stomatitis, recurrent aphthae and Bednar's aphthae; poliomyelitis, myocardial infarction, spontaneous pneumothorax, acute appendicitis, pancreatitis, costochondritis, perforated viscus, or an influenza-like respiratory infection.

Treatment

For most presenting illnesses, treatment is symptomatic. The infections are usually mild and resolve spontaneously. Cardiac, hepatic, or CNS disease may need intensive supportive care. Immunoglobulin has been used with some success in treatment of certain enterovirus infections, especially in neonates.

Special considerations

▶ Use good hand-washing technique to prevent disease transmission.

▶ Use gown and gloves in the clinical setting to prevent nosocomial spread of enteroviruses during epidemics.

▶ Use enteric precautions for 7 days after the onset of enterovirus infections.

 PREVENTION TIP Teach proper hand-washing technique to patients and family members and stress the importance of washing hands after any contact with secretions from an infected person, contaminated surfaces, or changing diapers. Also encourage the patient and family to maintain a clean environment.

EPIDIDYMITIS

This infection of the epididymis, the testicle's cordlike excretory duct, is one of the most common infections of the male reproductive tract. It usually affects adults and is rare before puberty. Epididymitis may spread to the testicle itself, causing orchitis; bilateral epididymitis may cause sterility.

Causes

Epididymitis usually results from pyogenic organisms, such as Enterobacteriaceae and *Pseudomonas*. Epididymitis can result from an existing urinary tract infection or prostatitis and reach the epididymis through the lumen of the vas deferens.

Rarely, epididymitis is secondary to a distant infection, such as pharyngitis or tuberculosis, that spreads through the lymphatics or, less commonly, the bloodstream.

Other causes include trauma, gonorrhea, syphilis, and a chlamydial infection. Trauma may reactivate a dormant infection or initiate a new one. Epididymitis is a complication of prostatectomy and may also result from chemical irritation by extravasation of urine through the vas deferens.

Signs and symptoms

The key symptoms are pain, extreme tenderness, and swelling in the groin and scrotum. Other clinical effects include high fever, malaise, and a characteristic waddle — an attempt to protect the groin and scrotum during walking. Symptoms of a urinary tract infection may also be present. An acute hydrocele may also occur as a reaction to the inflammatory process.

Diagnosis

Clinical features suggest epididymitis, but the actual diagnosis is made with the aid of the following laboratory tests:
▶ Urinalysis shows an increased white blood cell (WBC) count, indicating infection.
▶ Urine culture and sensitivity tests may identify the causative microbe.
▶ Serum WBC count of more than 10,000/μl indicates infection.
▶ Scrotal ultrasonography may help differentiate acute epididymitis from other conditions such as testicular torsion, a surgical emergency.

Treatment

The goal of treatment is to reduce pain and swelling and combat infection. Therapy must begin immediately, particularly in the patient with bilateral epididymitis, because sterility is always a threat.

During the acute phase, treatment consists of bed rest, scrotal elevation with towel rolls or adhesive strapping, broad-spectrum antibiotics, and analgesics.

An ice bag applied to the area may reduce swelling and relieve pain. (Heat is contraindicated because it may damage germinal cells, which are viable only at or below normal body temperature.) When pain and swelling subside and allow walking, an athletic supporter may prevent pain.

Occasionally, corticosteroids may be prescribed to help counteract inflammation, but their use is controversial.

Special considerations

▶ Watch closely for abscess formation (a localized hot, red, tender area) and extension of the infection into the testes. Closely monitor temperature, and ensure adequate fluid intake.
▶ Because the patient is usually uncomfortable, administer analgesics as necessary. During bed rest, check often for proper scrotum elevation.
▶ Before discharge, emphasize the importance of completing the prescribed an-

tibiotic therapy, even after symptoms subside.

▶ If the patient faces the possibility of sterility, suggest supportive counseling, as necessary.

EPIGLOTTITIS

Acute epiglottitis is an inflammation of the epiglottis that tends to cause airway obstruction. It typically strikes children ages 2 to 8. A critical emergency, epiglottitis can prove fatal in 8% to 12% of victims unless it's recognized and treated promptly.

Causes
Epiglottitis usually results from infection with the bacterium *Haemophilus influenzae* type B, and, occasionally, pneumococci and group A streptococci.

Signs and symptoms
Sometimes preceded by an upper respiratory tract infection, epiglottitis may progress to complete upper airway obstruction within 2 to 5 hours. Laryngeal obstruction results from inflammation and edema of the epiglottis. Accompanying symptoms include high fever, stridor, sore throat, dysphagia, irritability, restlessness, and drooling.

To relieve severe respiratory distress, the child with epiglottitis may hyperextend his neck, sit up, and lean forward with his mouth open, tongue protruding, and nostrils flaring as he tries to breathe. He may develop inspiratory retractions and rhonchi.

Diagnosis
In acute epiglottitis, throat examination reveals a large, edematous, bright red epiglottis. Such examination should follow lateral neck X-rays and, generally, should not be performed if the suspected obstruction is large.

When examining the patient, have special equipment (a laryngoscope and endotracheal [ET] tubes) available because a tongue depressor can cause sudden, complete airway obstruction. Trained personnel (such as an anesthesiologist) should be on hand during throat examination to secure an emergency airway.

Treatment
 ALERT A child with acute epiglottitis and airway obstruction requires emergency hospitalization; he may need emergency endotracheal intubation or a tracheotomy and should be monitored in an intensive care unit.

Respiratory distress that interferes with swallowing necessitates parenteral fluid administration to prevent dehydration.

A patient with acute epiglottitis should always receive a 10-day course of parenteral antibiotics — usually a second- or third-generation cephalosporin. (If the child is allergic to penicillin, a quinolone or sulfa drug may be substituted.) Oxygen therapy and arterial blood gas monitoring may be desirable.

Special considerations
▶ Keep the following equipment available in case of sudden, complete airway obstruction: a tracheotomy tray, ET tubes, a handheld resuscitation bag, oxygen equipment, and a laryngoscope with blades of various sizes. Monitor arterial blood gas levels for hypoxia and hypercapnia.

▶ Watch for increasing restlessness, rising heart rate, fever, dyspnea, and retractions, which may indicate the need for an emergency tracheotomy.

▶ After tracheotomy, anticipate the patient's needs because he won't be able to cry or call out, and provide emotional support. Reassure the patient and his family that the tracheotomy is a short-term intervention (usually from 4 to 7 days).

▶ Monitor the patient for rising temperature and pulse rate and for hypotension — signs of secondary infection.

ERYSIPELAS

Erysipelas is a skin infection, caused by Group A streptococci, involving the dermis and lymphatics. It's a more superficial subcutaneous infection of the skin than cellulitis. The affected area is well demarcated, erythematous, edematous, indurated, and warm. Often very painful, erysipelas commonly occurs on the face, lower extremities, and in areas of pre-existing edema. Without prompt treatment erysipelas can be life-threatening due to the spread of the infection; treatment usually controls the disease within 1 week.

Causes

Group A beta-hemolytic streptococci are the most common cause of erysipelas. It may also be caused by group B, C, and G streptococci and, rarely, staphylococci. The microbes enter the skin through a wound such as abrasions, trauma, insect bites, and skin ulcers.

Signs and symptoms

This disease is marked by abrupt onset of fever, chills, and bright red skin rash with sharp, distinct borders, usually appearing on the face, arms or legs. The affected area may feel warm or hot to the touch. The rash may spread or enlarge noticeably and blisters may develop. The patient may also complain of joint stiffness, muscle aches, headache, nausea, vomiting and loss of appetite, and malaise.

Diagnosis

Diagnosis is based on clinical findings. The causative microbe is difficult to culture from the rash but may be cultured from blood in 5% of cases. The white blood cell count is increased with a leftward shift and erythrocyte sedimentation rate may be elevated. The diagnosis should rule out early stages of contact dermatitis, giant urticaria, and prevesicular herpes zoster.

Treatment

Depending on the severity, treatment involves either oral or I.V. antibiotics — usually penicillin or erythromycin. Analgesics and antipyretics are given for pain and fever. Nondrug treatments include rest and immobilization and elevation of the affected area. Warm, moist compresses increase circulation in the area and promote healing.

Special considerations

❱ Remind the patient to finish the full course of antibiotics even if symptoms abate.

❱ Encourage the patient to rest and elevate the affected area.

❱ Be aware of allergies to antibiotics.

 PREVENTION TIP Instruct the patient about good skin hygiene and avoidance of skin traumas. Encourage the patient to report any skin changes to the doctor.

ERYTHEMA INFECTIOSUM (FIFTH DISEASE)

Erythema infectiosum, commonly known as fifth disease, is an acute parvovirus infection that occurs mostly in children but can affect adults as well. Infection is most likely at 4 to 12 years of age , but nearly 60% of the population is seropositive by adulthood. During outbreaks in schools, 10% to 60% of students may be infected. Fifth disease occurs most often during late winter or early spring. It is known worldwide. Although highly contagious, fifth disease resolves spontaneously in 7 to 10 days without serious complications in healthy individuals. It can, however, cause serious illness in persons with sickle cell disease or similar forms of chronic anemia; once the infection is controlled, the anemia resolves. It can also cause serious illness in those with leukemia or cancer, in those who have received an organ transplant, and in those with human immunodeficiency virus (HIV). Fifth disease causes the majority of episodes of transient aplastic crisis (TAC) in persons with chronic hemolytic anemia. Occasionally, serious complications may develop from parvovirus B19 infection during pregnancy.

Causes

The disease is caused by human parvovirus B19 and is transmitted via respiratory secretions. The incubation period is usually 4 to 10 days.

Signs and symptoms

The classic sign of fifth disease is erythema over the cheeks (slapped-cheek appearance) and a lacy red rash on the trunk and limbs. Low-grade fever, malaise, or upper respiratory symptoms develop a few days before the rash appears. In adults, mild joint pain and swelling occurs (usually in the hands, wrists, and knees) and can last or recur for weeks to months.

Diagnosis

Diagnosis is usually made from the typical appearance and pattern of spread of the rash. Light and electron microscopy are also helpful in detecting B19 infections. The IgM-antibody assay test detects antibodies to parvovirus and can be performed when it is important to confirm the diagnosis.

Other conditions to consider are rubella, enteroviral disease, systemic lupus erythematosus, drug reaction, Lyme disease, and rheumatoid arthritis. Parvovirus B19 infection should be included in the differential diagnosis of chronic anemia in immunodeficient patients.

Treatment

Symptomatic treatment of fever, pain, or itching is all that is required. Adults with joint involvement should rest, restrict activities, and take anti-inflammatory medications (aspirin or ibuprofen.) Those with severe anemia may require blood transfusions and those with immune deficien-

cies may be treated with immune globulin.

Special considerations

▶ Follow standard precautions. Always wash your hands thoroughly before and after any contact with patients.

▶ Patients with TAC or chronic B19 infection should be considered infectious and placed on isolation precautions in private rooms for the duration of their illness or until the infection has cleared. B19-infected patients may share a room if there are no other contraindications. Persons in close contact with these individuals should wear masks, gowns if soiling is likely, and gloves.

▶ To avoid the risk of fetal loss and other complications of parvovirus infection, pregnant health care workers should consult their health care professional if there is an outbreak in the workplace.

▶ Because persons with fifth disease were already contagious before their rash appeared, it is not necessary to exclude them from work, school, or child care centers.

▶ Instruct patients with chronic hemolytic diseases to be aware of the risk of aplastic crisis if exposed to erythema infectiosum.

 PREVENTION TIP Teach patients that frequent and proper hand washing helps reduce the risk of becoming infected with fifth disease.

ESCHERICHIA COLI AND OTHER ENTEROBACTERIACEAE INFECTIONS

Enterobacteriaceae—a group of mostly aerobic gram-negative bacilli—cause local and systemic infections, including an invasive diarrhea that resembles *Shigella* and, more often, a noninvasive toxin-mediated diarrhea that resembles cholera. (See *Enterobacterial infections,* page 102.)

ENTEROBACTERIAL INFECTIONS

The Enterobacteriacae include *Escherichia, Arizona, Citrobacter, Enterobacter, Erwinia, Hafnia, Klebsiella, Morganella, Proteus, Providencia, Salmonella, Serratia, Shigella,* and *Yersinia.*

Enterobacterial infections are exogenous (from other people or the environment), endogenous (from one part of the body to another), or a combination of both. Enterobacteriaceae infections may cause any of a long list of bacterial diseases: bacterial (gram-negative) pneumonia, empyema, endocarditis, osteomyelitis, septic arthritis, urethritis, cystitis, bacterial prostatitis, urinary tract infection, pyelonephritis, perinephric abscess, abdominal abscesses, cellulitis, skin ulcers, appendicitis, gastroenterocolitis, diverticulitis, eyelid and periorbital cellulitis, corneal conjunctivitis, meningitis, bacteremia, and intracranial abscesses.

Appropriate antibiotic therapy depends on the results of culture and sensitivity tests. Generally, the aminoglycosides, cephalosporins, and penicillins — such as ampicillin, mezlocillin, and piperacillin — are most effective.

Escherichia coli and other Enterobacteriaceae cause most nosocomial infections. Noninvasive, enterotoxin-producing *E. coli* infections may be a major cause of diarrheal illness in children in the United States.

The prognosis in mild to moderate infection is good. Severe infection requires immediate fluid and electrolyte replacement to avoid fatal dehydration — especially among children, whose mortality may be quite high.

Causes

Although some strains of *E. coli* exist as part of the normal GI flora, infection usually results from certain non-native strains. For example:

Noninvasive diarrhea results from two toxins produced by strains called enterotoxic or enteropathogenic *E. coli.* These toxins interact with intestinal juices and promote excessive loss of chloride and water.

In the invasive form, *E. coli* directly invades the intestinal mucosa without producing enterotoxins, thereby causing local irritation, inflammation, and diarrhea. Normal strains can cause infection in immunocompromised patients.

Transmission can occur directly from an infected person or indirectly by ingestion of contaminated food or water or contact with contaminated utensils. Incubation takes 12 to 72 hours.

The incidence of *E. coli* infection is highest among travelers returning from other countries, particularly Mexico, Southeast Asia, and South America. *E. coli* infection also induces other diseases, especially in people whose resistance is low. Another strain, *E. coli 0157:H7,* has been reported. It's associated with undercooked hamburger.

Signs and symptoms

Effects of noninvasive diarrhea depend on the causative toxin but may include the abrupt onset of watery diarrhea with cramping abdominal pain and, in severe illness, acidosis. Invasive infection produces chills, abdominal cramps, and diarrheal stools that contain blood and pus.

Infantile diarrhea from an *E. coli* infection is usually noninvasive; it begins with loose, watery stools that change from yellow to green and contain little mucus or blood. Vomiting, listlessness, irritability, and anorexia often precede diarrhea.

This condition can progress to fever, severe dehydration, acidosis, and shock. Bloody diarrhea may occur from an *E. coli 0157:H7* infection.

Diagnosis

Because certain strains of *E. coli* normally reside in the GI tract, culturing is of little value; a working diagnosis depends on clinical observation alone.

A firm diagnosis requires sophisticated identification procedures, such as bioassays, that are expensive, time-consuming and, consequently, not widely available. The diagnosis must rule out salmonellosis and shigellosis, other common infections that produce similar signs and symptoms.

Treatment

Effective treatment consists of isolation, correction of fluid and electrolyte imbalance and, in an infant, I.V. antibiotics based on the microbe's drug sensitivity. For cramping and diarrhea, bismuth subsalicylate may be given.

Special considerations

▶ Keep accurate intake and output records. Measure stool volume and note the presence of blood and pus. Replace fluids and electrolytes as needed, monitoring for decreased serum sodium and chloride levels and signs of gram-negative shock. Watch for signs of dehydration, such as poor skin turgor and dry mouth.

▶ For infants, provide isolation, give nothing by mouth, administer antibiotics, and maintain body warmth.

To prevent the spread of this infection:

▶ Screen all hospital personnel and visitors for diarrhea, and prevent them from making direct patient contact during epidemics.

▶ Report cases to the local public health authorities.

▶ Use proper hand-washing technique. Teach personnel, patients, and their families to do the same.

▶ Use standard precautions: private room, gown and gloves while handling feces, and hand washing before entering and after leaving the patient's room.

▶ To prevent the accumulation of these water-loving microbes, discard suction bottles, irrigating fluid, and open bottles of saline solution every 24 hours. Be sure to change I.V. tubing according to facility policy, and empty the ventilator water reservoirs before refilling them with sterile water. Remember to use suction catheters only once.

 PREVENTION TIP Advise travelers to foreign countries to avoid unbottled water and uncooked vegetables.

F

FOLLICULITIS, FURUNCLES, AND CARBUNCULOSIS

A bacterial infection of the hair follicle, folliculitis causes the formation of a pustule. The infection can be superficial (follicular impetigo or Bockhart's impetigo) or deep (sycosis barbae).

Furuncles, commonly known as boils, are another form of deep folliculitis. Carbuncles are a group of interconnected furuncles. The prognosis depends on the severity of the infection and the patient's physical condition and ability to resist infection. (See *Forms of bacterial skin infection.*)

Causes

The most common cause of folliculitis, furuncles, or carbuncles is coagulase-positive *Staphylococcus aureus.* Predisposing factors include an infected wound, poor hygiene, debilitation, diabetes, alcoholism, occlusive cosmetics, tight clothes, friction, chafing, incorrect shaving technique, exposure to chemicals, treatment of skin lesions with tar or with occlusive therapy, and immunosuppressive therapy.

Signs and symptoms

Folliculitis, furuncles, and carbuncles have different signs and symptoms. *Folliculitis* pustules usually appear on the scalp, arms, and legs in children and on the trunk, buttocks, bearded face and legs in adults. *Furuncles* are hard, painful nodules that commonly develop on the neck, face, axillae, and buttocks. For several days, these nodules enlarge and then rupture, discharging pus and necrotic material. After the nodules rupture, pain subsides, but erythema and edema may persist for days or weeks. *Carbuncles* are extremely painful, deep abscesses that drain through multiple openings onto the skin surface, usually around several hair follicles. Fever and malaise may accompany these lesions, which are now rather rare.

Diagnosis

The obvious skin lesion confirms folliculitis, furuncles, or carbuncles. Wound culture usually shows *S. aureus.* In carbuncles, patient history reveals preexistent furuncles. A complete blood count may show an elevated white blood cell count (leukocytosis).

The differential diagnosis for folliculitis includes pustular miliaria, varicella, and eczema with folliculitis. The differential diagnosis for furuncles includes necrotic herpes simplex and hidradenitis suppurativa.

Treatment

Folliculitis is treated by cleaning the infected area thoroughly with antibacterial soap and water; applying warm, wet compresses to promote vasodilation and drainage from the lesions; applying topical antibiotics, such as mupirocin ointment or clindamycin or erythromycin solution; and, in extensive infection, administering systemic antibiotics (a cephalosporin or dicloxacillin).

Furuncles may require incision and drainage of ripe lesions after application of warm, wet compresses and systemic antibiotics after drainage.

FORMS OF BACTERIAL SKIN INFECTION

The degree of hair follicle involvement in bacterial skin infection ranges from superficial erythema and pustule of a single follicle to deep abscesses (carbuncles) involving several follicles.

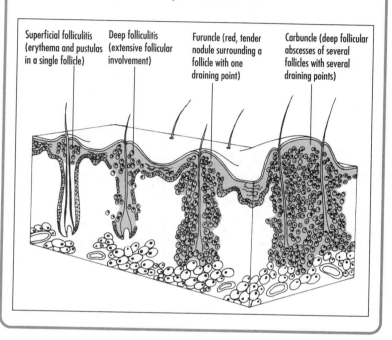

Superficial folliculitis (erythema and pustulas in a single follicle)

Deep folliculitis (extensive follicular involvement)

Furuncle (red, tender nodule surrounding a follicle with one draining point)

Carbuncle (deep follicular abscesses of several follicles with several draining points)

Carbuncles require systemic antibiotic therapy as well as incision and drainage.

Special considerations

Care for folliculitis, furuncles, and carbuncles is basically supportive and emphasizes teaching the patient scrupulous personal and family hygiene measures. Taking the necessary precautions to prevent spreading infection is also an important part of care.

PREVENTION TIP Caution the patient never to squeeze a boil because this may cause it to rupture into the surrounding area. To avoid spreading bacteria to family members, urge the patient not to share towels or washcloths. Tell him that these items should be washed in hot water before being reused. The patient should change clothes and bedsheets daily, and they also should be washed in hot water. Encourage the patient to change dressings frequently and to discard them promptly in paper bags. Advise the patient with recurrent furuncles to have a physical examination because an underlying disease, such as diabetes, may be present. Instruct men to use disposable razors to help decrease the spread of infection.

G

GAS GANGRENE

Local infection with the anaerobic, spore-forming, gram-positive rod *Clostridium perfringens* (or another clostridial species) causes gas gangrene. It occurs in devitalized tissues and results from compromised arterial circulation after trauma or surgery.

This rare infection carries a high mortality unless therapy begins immediately. With prompt treatment, 80% of patients with gas gangrene of the extremities survive; the prognosis is poorer for gas gangrene in other sites, such as the abdominal wall and the bowel. The incubation period is usually 1 to 4 days but can vary from 3 hours to 6 weeks or longer.

Causes

C. perfringens is a normal inhabitant of the GI and female genital tracts; it's also prevalent in soil. The microbe is typically transmitted during trauma or surgery. Because *C. perfringens* is anaerobic, gas gangrene occurs most often in deep wounds, especially those in which tissue necrosis further reduces oxygen supply.

When *C. perfringens* invades soft tissues, it produces thrombosis of regional blood vessels, tissue necrosis, and localized edema. Such necrosis releases both carbon dioxide and hydrogen subcutaneously, producing interstitial gas bubbles. Gas gangrene occurs most commonly in the extremities and in abdominal wounds and less frequently in the uterus. (See *Growth cycle of* Clostridium perfringens.)

Signs and symptoms

True gas gangrene produces myositis and another form of this disease, involving only soft tissue, called anaerobic cellulitis. Most signs of infection develop within 72 hours of trauma or surgery. The hallmark of gas gangrene is crepitation, a result of carbon dioxide and hydrogen accumulation as a metabolic byproduct in necrotic tissues.

Other typical indications are severe localized pain, swelling, and discoloration (often dusky brown or red), with formation of bullae and necrosis within 36 hours from the onset of symptoms. Soon the skin over the wound may rupture, revealing dark red or black necrotic muscle, a foul-smelling watery or frothy discharge, intravascular hemolysis, thrombosed blood vessels, and evidence of infection spread.

In addition to these local symptoms, gas gangrene produces early signs of toxemia and hypovolemia (tachycardia, tachypnea, and hypotension) and a moderate fever that usually doesn't exceed 101° F (38.3° C). Although pale, prostrate, and motionless, most patients remain alert and oriented and are extremely apprehensive.

Usually death occurs suddenly, often during surgery for removal of necrotic tissue. Less often, death is preceded by delirium and coma, sometimes accompanied by vomiting, profuse diarrhea, and circulatory collapse.

Diagnosis

A history of recent surgery or a deep puncture wound and the rapid onset of pain and crepitation around the wound suggest gas gangrene. It's confirmed by anaerobic cultures of wound drainage showing *C. perfringens;* a Gram stain of wound drainage showing large, gram-positive, rod-shaped bacteria; X-rays showing gas in tissues; and blood studies showing leukocytosis and, later, hemolysis.

The diagnosis must rule out synergistic gangrene and necrotizing fasciitis; unlike gas gangrene, both of these disorders anesthetize the skin around the wound.

Treatment

Effective treatment includes careful observation for signs of myositis and cellulitis, immediate treatment if these signs appear, and immediate wide surgical excision of all affected tissues and necrotic muscle in myositis. Delayed or inadequate surgical excision is a fatal mistake.

Treatment also includes I.V. administration of high-dose penicillin, adequate debridement, and hyperbaric oxygenation. If a hyperbaric chamber is available, the patient is placed in the chamber for 1 to 3 hours every 6 to 8 hours and exposed to pressures designed to increase oxygen tension and prevent multiplication of the anaerobic microbes. Surgery may be done within the hyperbaric chamber if the chamber is large enough.

Special considerations

Before diagnosis:
▶ Look for signs of ischemia: cool skin; pallor or cyanosis; sudden, severe pain; sudden edema; and loss of pulses in the involved limb.

After diagnosis:
▶ Throughout this illness, provide adequate fluid replacement and assess pulmonary and cardiac functions often. Maintain airway and ventilation.
▶ To prevent skin breakdown and further infection, give good skin care. After surgery, provide meticulous wound care.
▶ Before administering penicillin, obtain a patient history of allergies; afterward, watch closely for signs of hypersensitivity.

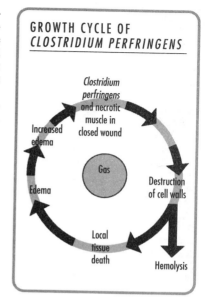

GROWTH CYCLE OF *CLOSTRIDIUM PERFRINGENS*

Clostridium perfringens and necrotic muscle in closed wound

Increased edema

Edema

Local tissue death

Gas

Destruction of cell walls

Hemolysis

▶ Provide psychological support. This is critical because these patients can remain alert until death, knowing that death is imminent and unavoidable.
▶ Deodorize the room to control foul odor from the wound. Prepare the patient emotionally for a large wound after surgical excision, and refer him for physical rehabilitation as necessary.
▶ Institute wound precautions. Dispose of drainage material properly (double-bag dressings in plastic bags for incineration), and wear sterile gloves when changing dressings. No special cleaning measures are required after the patient is discharged.
▶ Take measures to prevent gas gangrene. Routinely take precautions to render all wound sites unsuitable for growth of microbes by attempting to keep granulation tissue viable; adequate debridement is imperative to reduce anaerobic growth conditions.
▶ Be alert for devitalized tissues.
▶ Position the patient to facilitate drainage, and eliminate all dead spaces in closed wounds.

GASTROENTERITIS

Also called intestinal flu, traveler's diarrhea, viral enteritis, and food poisoning, gastroenteritis is a self-limiting disorder characterized by diarrhea, nausea, vomiting, and abdominal cramping. It occurs in all age-groups and is a major cause of morbidity and mortality in developing countries.

In the United States, gastroenteritis ranks second to the common cold as a cause of lost work time and fifth as the cause of death among young children. It also can be life-threatening in elderly and debilitated people.

Causes

Gastroenteritis has many possible causes, including the following:

▶ bacteria (responsible for acute food poisoning): *Staphylococcus aureus, Salmonella, Shigella, Clostridium botulinum, Escherichia coli, Clostridium perfringens*
▶ amoebae: especially *Entamoeba histolytica*
▶ parasites: *Ascaris, Enterobius, Trichinella spiralis*
▶ viruses (may be responsible for traveler's diarrhea): adenovirus, echovirus, or coxsackievirus
▶ ingestion of toxins: plants or toadstools (mushrooms)
▶ drug reactions: antibiotics
▶ enzyme deficiencies
▶ food allergens.

The bowel reacts to any of these enterotoxins with hypermotility, producing severe diarrhea and secondary depletion of intracellular fluid.

Signs and symptoms

Clinical manifestations vary, depending on the pathogen and the level of GI tract involved. Gastroenteritis in adults is usually a self-limiting, nonfatal disease that produces diarrhea, abdominal discomfort (ranging from cramping to pain), nausea,

and vomiting. Other possible symptoms include fever, malaise, and borborygmi.

In children and elderly and debilitated people, gastroenteritis produces the same symptoms, but the inability of these patients to tolerate electrolyte and fluid losses leads to a higher mortality.

Diagnosis

Patient history can aid diagnosis of gastroenteritis. A stool culture as well as stool examination for ova and parasites should be obtained. Blood cultures are indicated in febrile patients.

Treatment

Usually supportive, treatment consists of nutritional support and increased fluid intake. An episode of acute gastroenteritis is self-limiting. When an episode is severe and produces symptoms for more than 3 or 4 days and the patient is a young child or an elderly or debilitated person, hospitalization may be necessary. Treatment may include fluid and electrolyte replacement, antibiotic therapy, and antiemetics.

Special considerations

▶ Administer medications; correlate dosages, routes, and times appropriately with the patient's meals and activities; for example, give antiemetics 30 to 60 minutes before meals.
▶ If the patient is unable to tolerate food, replace lost fluids and electrolytes with clear liquids and sports-type drinks. Vary the diet to make it more enjoyable, and allow some choice of foods. Instruct the patient to avoid milk and milk products, which may exacerbate the condition.
▶ Record intake and output carefully. Watch for signs of dehydration, such as dry skin and mucous membranes, fever, and sunken eyes.
▶ Wash your hands thoroughly after giving care to avoid spreading infection.

▶ Instruct the patient to take warm sitz baths three times a day to relieve anal irritation.

▶ If food poisoning is probable, contact public health authorities to interview patients and food handlers, and take samples of the suspected contaminated food.

 PREVENTION TIP Teach good hygiene to prevent recurrence. Instruct patients to thoroughly cook foods, especially meat, poultry, eggs, and shellfish; to refrigerate perishable foods, such as milk, mayonnaise, potato salad, and cream-filled pastry; and to always wash their hands with warm water and soap before handling food, especially after using the bathroom. Additionally, teach patients to clean utensils thoroughly, to avoid drinking water or eating raw fruit or vegetables when visiting a foreign country, and to eliminate flies and roaches in the home.

GENITAL HERPES

Genital herpes is an acute inflammatory disease of the genitalia. The prognosis varies, depending on the patient's age, the strength of his immune defenses, and the infection site. Primary genital herpes usually is self-limiting but may cause painful local or systemic disease. In newborns and immunocompromised patients, such as those with acquired immunodeficiency syndrome, genital herpes is commonly severe, resulting in complications and a high mortality.

Causes

Genital herpes usually is caused by infection with herpes simplex virus Type 2, but some studies report increasing incidence of infection with herpes simplex virus Type 1. This disease typically is transmitted through sexual intercourse, orogenital sexual activity, kissing, and hand-to-body contact. Pregnant women may transmit the infection to newborns during vaginal delivery if they have an active infection and are shedding virus. Such transmitted infection may be localized (for instance, in the eyes) or disseminated and may be associated with central nervous system involvement. (See *Understanding the genital herpes cycle,* page 110.)

Signs and symptoms

After a 3- to 7-day incubation period, fluid-filled vesicles appear, usually on the cervix (the primary infection site) and possibly on the labia, perianal skin, vulva, or vagina of the female and on the glans penis, foreskin, or penile shaft of the male. Extragenital lesions may appear on the mouth or anus. In both males and females, the vesicles, usually painless at first, will rupture and develop into extensive, shallow, painful ulcers, with redness, marked edema, tender inguinal lymph nodes, and the characteristic yellow, oozing centers.

Other features of initial mucocutaneous infection include fever, malaise, dysuria and, in females, leukorrhea. Rare complications (generally from extragenital lesions) include herpetic keratitis, which may lead to blindness, and potentially fatal herpetic encephalitis.

Diagnosis

Diagnosis is based on the physical examination and patient history. Helpful (but nondiagnostic) measures include laboratory data showing increased antibody titers, smears of genital lesions showing atypical cells, and cytologic preparations (Tzanck test) that reveal giant cells. Diagnosis can be confirmed by demonstration of the herpes simplex virus in vesicular fluid, using tissue culture techniques, or by antigen tests that identify specific antigens.

Treatment

Acyclovir has proved to be an effective treatment for genital herpes. I.V. administration may be required for patients who are hospitalized with severe genital her-

UNDERSTANDING THE GENITAL HERPES CYCLE

After a patient is infected with genital herpes, a latency period follows. The virus takes up permanent residence in the nerve cells surrounding the lesions, and intermittent viral shedding may take place.

Repeated outbreaks may develop at any time, again followed by a latent stage during which the lesions heal completely. Outbreaks may recur as often as three to eight times yearly.

Although the cycle continues indefinitely, some people remain symptom-free for years.

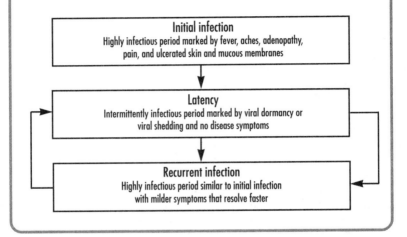

Initial infection
Highly infectious period marked by fever, aches, adenopathy, pain, and ulcerated skin and mucous membranes

Latency
Intermittently infectious period marked by viral dormancy or viral shedding and no disease symptoms

Recurrent infection
Highly infectious period similar to initial infection with milder symptoms that resolve faster

pes or for those who are immunocompromised and have a potentially life-threatening herpes infection. Oral acyclovir may be prescribed for patients with first-time infections or recurrent outbreaks; newer agents include famcyclovir and valacyclovir. Daily prophylaxis with acyclovir reduces the frequency of recurrences by at least 50%, but this is only appropriate for patients with frequent outbreaks, and it may not decrease transmission rates of the disease.

Special considerations
▶ Practice standard precautions.
▶ Encourage the patient to get adequate rest and nutrition and to keep the lesions dry.

▶ Advise the patient to avoid sexual intercourse during the active stage of this disease (while lesions are present) and to use condoms during all sexual exposures. Urge him to have his sexual partners seek medical examination.
▶ Advise the female patient to have a Papanicolaou test as recommended by her gynecologist.
▶ Explain to the pregnant patient with an active herpes infection about the risk to her newborn from vaginal delivery. Advise her that a cesarean delivery may help reduce the risk of passing the infection to her infant.
▶ Refer patients to the Herpes Resource Center, which has local chapters nationwide.

GENITAL WARTS

Also called venereal warts and condylomata acuminata, genital warts consist of papillomas with fibrous tissue overgrowth from the dermis and thickened epithelial coverings. They are uncommon before puberty and after menopause. Certain types of human papillomavirus (HPV) infections have been strongly associated with genital dysplasia and, over a period of years, cervical neoplasia (depending on the viral strain).

Causes

Infection with one of the more than 60 known strains of HPV causes genital warts. Transmission occurs through sexual contact. The warts grow rapidly in the presence of heavy perspiration, poor hygiene, and pregnancy and often accompany other genital infections.

Signs and symptoms

After a 1- to 6-month incubation period (usually 2 months), genital warts develop on moist surfaces: in men, on the subpreputial sac, within the urethral meatus and, less commonly, on the penile shaft; in women, on the vulva and on vaginal and cervical walls.

Genital warts can develop years after the first contact. In both sexes, papillomas spread to the perineum and the perianal area. These painless warts start as tiny red or pink swellings that grow (sometimes to 4" [10 cm]) and become pedunculated. Typically, multiple swellings give them a cauliflower-like appearance. If infected, the warts become malodorous. Most patients report no symptoms; a few complain of itching or pain.

Diagnosis

Dark-field examination of scrapings from wart cells reveals marked vascularization of epidermal cells, which helps to differentiate genital warts from condylomata lata, which are associated with second-stage syphilis. Histologic examinations of biopsies of warts are done for classification and to assess cancer risk. Applying 5% acetic acid (white vinegar) to the warts turns them white. In general, warts are easily diagnosed on visual inspection, with biopsy indicated only when neoplasia is strongly suspected.

The differential diagnoses include syphilis and vulvar/vaginal cancer (for example, verrucous carcinoma).

Treatment

Treatment is, for the most part, for cosmetic reasons and should be guided by patient preference. Topical drug therapy, such as trichloroacetic acid 85%, is applied weekly to external areas, or podophyllum resin may be applied topically to the wart, also weekly. (Podophyllum is contraindicated in pregnancy.) Warts that are larger than 1" (2.5 cm) are generally removed by carbon dioxide laser treatment, cryosurgery, or electrocautery. Treatment aims to remove exophytic warts and to ameliorate signs and symptoms. No therapy has proved effective in eradicating HPV. Relapse is common. Other treatments include interferon (intralesional), Podofilox (patient-applied), Imiquimod (patient-applied), and combined laser and interferon therapy.

Special considerations

▶ Use standard precautions.
▶ Recommend that the patient abstain from sexual intercourse or use a condom until healing is complete.
▶ Encourage the patient's sexual partners to be examined for HPV, human immunodeficiency virus, and other sexually transmitted diseases.
▶ Encourage female patients to get annual Papanicolaou tests, and recommend that men be examined by a urologist because cancer of the penis can develop.
▶ Recommend the use of condoms.

GENITOURINARY INFECTIONS, NONSPECIFIC

Nonspecific genitourinary infections, including nongonococcal urethritis (NGU) in males and mild vaginitis and cervicitis in females, are a group of infections with similar manifestations that are not linked to a single organism. These sexually transmitted infections have become more prevalent since the mid-1960s. They are more widespread than gonorrhea and may be the most common sexually transmitted diseases in the United States. The prognosis is good if sexual partners are treated simultaneously.

Causes

Nonspecific genitourinary infections are spread primarily through sexual intercourse. In males, NGU commonly results from infection with *Chlamydia trachomatis* or *Ureaplasma urealyticum*. Less frequently, infection may be related to preexisting strictures, neoplasms, or chemical or traumatic inflammation. Some cases remain unexplained.

Although less is known about nonspecific genitourinary infections in females, chlamydial organisms may also cause these infections. A thin vaginal epithelium may predispose prepubertal and postmenopausal females to nonspecific vaginitis.

Signs and symptoms

Nongonococcal urethritis occurs 1 week to 1 month after coitus, with scant or moderate mucopurulent urethral discharge, variable dysuria, and occasional hematuria. If untreated, NGU may lead to acute epididymitis. Subclinical urethritis may be found on physical examination, especially if the sex partner has a positive diagnosis.

Females with nonspecific genitourinary infections may experience persistent vaginal discharge, acute or recurrent cystitis for which no underlying cause can be found, or cervicitis with inflammatory erosion.

Both males and females with nonspecific genitourinary infections may be asymptomatic but show signs of urethral, vaginal, or cervical infection on physical examination.

Diagnosis

In males, microscopic examination of smears of prostatic or urethral secretions shows excess polymorphonuclear leukocytes but few, if any, specific microbes.

In females, cervical or urethral smears also reveal excess leukocytes and no specific microbes. "Clue cells" (normal epithelial cells covered with bacteria that appear stippled) are diagnostic.

Differential diagnoses include gonorrhea and urinary tract infection.

Treatment

Therapy for both sexes consists of a single 1-g oral dose of azithromycin (Zithromax) or doxycycline 100 mg orally twice a day for 7 days. If the infection recurs or persists, metronidazole 2 g orally as a single dose with erythromycin for 7 days is recommended. For females, treatment may also include application of a sulfa vaginal cream.

Special considerations

▶ Tell female patients to clean the pubic area before applying vaginal medication and to avoid using tampons during treatment.
▶ Make sure the patient clearly understands and strictly follows the dosage schedule for all prescribed medications.

GIARDIASIS

Also known as *Giardia* enteritis and lambliasis, giardiasis is an infection of the small bowel caused by the symmetrical flagellate protozoan *Giardia lamblia*. Giardiasis occurs worldwide but is most common in developing countries and other areas where sanitation and hygiene are poor. In the United States, giardiasis is most common in travelers who have recently returned from endemic areas and in campers who drink unpurified water from contaminated streams. Probably because of frequent hand-to-mouth activity, children are more likely to become infected with *G. lamblia* than adults. Hypogammaglobulinemia may also predispose people to this disorder.

Causes

G. lamblia has two stages: the cystic stage and the trophozoite stage. Ingestion of *G. lamblia* cysts in fecally contaminated water or the fecal-oral transfer of cysts by an infected person results in giardiasis.

When cysts enter the small bowel, they become trophozoites and attach themselves with their sucking disks to the bowel's epithelial surface. Then the trophozoites encyst again, travel down the colon, and are excreted. Unformed stool that passes quickly through the intestine may contain trophozoites as well as cysts.

Signs and symptoms

A mild infection may not produce intestinal symptoms. In untreated giardiasis, symptoms wax and wane; with treatment, recovery is complete. Attachment of *G. lamblia* to the intestinal lumen causes superficial mucosal invasion as well as destruction, inflammation, and irritation. All these destructive effects decrease food transit time through the small intestine and result in malabsorption. Such malabsorption results in chronic GI complaints — such as abdominal cramps — and pale, loose, greasy, malodorous, frequent stools (from 2 to 10 daily) with concurrent nausea. Stools may contain mucus but not pus or blood. Chronic giardiasis may produce fatigue and weight loss in addition to these typical signs and symptoms.

Diagnosis

Suspect giardiasis when travelers to endemic areas or campers who may have drunk unpurified water develop symptoms.

Actual diagnosis requires laboratory examination of a fresh stool specimen for cysts or examination of duodenal aspirate for trophozoites. An antibody test of the stool for giardiasis is also very effective in diagnosis. A barium X-ray of the small bowel may show mucosal edema and barium segmentation. Diagnosis must also rule out other causes of diarrhea and malabsorption.

Treatment

Giardiasis responds readily to a 10-day course of metronidazole or a 7-day course of quinacrine and oral furazolidone. Severe diarrhea may require parenteral fluid replacement to prevent dehydration if oral fluid intake is inadequate.

Special considerations

▶ If hospitalization is required, apply standard precautions. The patient requires a private room if he's a child or an incontinent adult.

▶ When caring for such a patient, pay strict attention to hand washing, particularly after handling stool. Quickly dispose of fecal material. (Normal sewage systems can adequately remove and process infected stool.)

▶ Report epidemic situations to the public health authorities.

▶ Teach patients about possible drug reactions and about how to avoid spreading or contracting giardiasis.

▶ Warn against drinking alcoholic beverages, which may provoke a disulfiram-like reaction in the patient receiving metronidazole.

▶ If the patient is a woman, ask if she's pregnant because metronidazole is contraindicated during pregnancy.

▶ Giardiasis does not confer immunity, so reinfections may occur.

 PREVENTION TIP Warn travelers to endemic areas not to drink water or eat uncooked or unpeeled fruits or vegetables, which may have been rinsed in contaminated water. Advise campers to purify all stream water before drinking it.

GINGIVITIS IN WOMEN

Women encounter changes in their gums at different periods of their life. The table below describes these changes:

PUBERTY

Increased levels of sex hormones cause increased blood circulation to the gums. The gums may become swollen, red, and tender.

MENSTRUATION

Menstruation gingivitis results in gingival bleeding, redness, and swelling, with sores sometimes appearing on the inside of the cheek. Symptoms normally occur right before the onset of a woman's period and disappear once her period has begun.

PREGNANCY

Pregnancy gingivitis appears at the beginning of the second or third month of pregnancy, gradually becoming more severe through the eighth month. Studies have shown a possible link between periodontal disease and pre-term, low-birth-weight babies.

Women who use oral contraceptives may be more susceptible to gingivitis.

MENOPAUSE AND POSTMENOPAUSE

Dry mouth, pain, and burning sensations in the gum tissue and altered taste (especially salty, peppery or sour) occur at this time. Because bone loss is associated with periodontal disease and osteoporosis, hormone replacement therapy may help to relieve these symptoms.

GINGIVITIS

Gingivitis is an infectious disease of the gums which, if left untreated, can progress to periodontal disease. In a recent National Institutes of Health survey, 47% of men and 37% of women aged 18-64 exhibited some symptoms of gingivitis. Although 70% of adult tooth loss is due to chronic, progressive gingivitis, the prognosis is generally favorable with appropriate treatment.

Causes

Bacterial plaque — a sticky, colorless film that constantly forms on teeth — is the primary cause of gum disease. If plaque isn't removed each day by brushing and flossing the teeth, it hardens into a rough, porous substance called calculus or tartar. Toxins produced and released by the bacteria in the plaque irritate the gums. These toxins cause the breakdown of the fibers that hold the gums tightly to the teeth, thereby creating pockets which subsequently become filled with more bacteria. As the bacterial pockets deepen, the bone holding the teeth in place is destroyed. Secondary contributing factors include malocclusion, food impaction, faulty dental restorations, xerostomia, uncontrolled diabetes, immunosuppression, and tobacco use.

Signs and symptoms

Gums become swollen, red, tender and bleed during flossing or brushing. There is a mouth odor along with a change of normal gum contours. Calculus is seen on tooth surfaces. Some people may experience pain with chewing and teeth may be sensitive. Pus may be present around the teeth and gums. A change in the fit of partial dentures or a change in the way teeth fit together when biting are also indicators of gingivitis. In severe cases, teeth may be loose or absent.

Diagnosis

A dental professional diagnoses gingivitis through observation of signs and symptoms. Gingivitis of diabetes mellitus, gingivitis of pregnancy, desquamative gingivitis, gingivitis in leukemia, phenytoin gingivitis, pericoronitis, and human immunodeficiency virus (HIV) are other conditions to consider.

Treatment

Daily brushing and flossing and routine cleaning by a dentist or hygienist at regular intervals controls simple gingivitis. Causative factors should be corrected. Severe infections may require antibiotics, commonly penicillin. If left untreated, simple gingivitis may progress to periodontitis, necrotizing ulcerative gingivitis or glossitis (inflammation of the tongue.)

Special considerations

▶ Be aware that gingivitis may be an early sign of a systemic disorder, such as primary herpes simplex, hypovitaminosis, diabetes mellitus or debilitating disease.

 PREVENTION TIP Good oral hygiene with daily brushing and flossing and cleaning by a dentist or hygienist every 6 months or sooner is essential in preventing gingivitis. Encourage nutritionally balanced meals and avoidance of smoking and chewing tobacco. Advise women about their special oral health needs. (See *Gingivitis in women.*)

GLOMERULONEPHRITIS, ACUTE POSTSTREPTOCOCCAL

Acute poststreptococcal glomerulonephritis (APSGN), also called acute glomerulonephritis and acute nephrotic syndrome, is a relatively common bilateral inflammation of the glomeruli. It follows a streptococcal infection of the respiratory tract or, less often, a skin infection, such as impetigo.

APSGN is most common in boys ages 6 to 10 but can occur at any age. Up to 95% of children and up to 70% of adults with APSGN recover fully; the remainder

of patients may progress to chronic renal failure within months.

Causes

APSGN results from the entrapment and collection of antigen-antibody complexes (produced as an immunologic mechanism in response to streptococci) in the glomerular capillary membranes, inducing inflammatory damage and impeding glomerular function. Sometimes the immune complement further damages the glomerular membrane. The damaged and inflamed glomerulus loses the ability to be selectively permeable and allows red blood cells (RBCs) and proteins to filter through as the glomerular filtration rate (GFR) falls. Uremic poisoning may result.

Signs and symptoms

APSGN begins within 1 to 3 weeks after untreated pharyngitis. Symptoms are mild to moderate edema, oliguria (400 ml/24 hours), proteinuria, azotemia, hematuria, and fatigue. Mild to severe hypertension may result from either sodium or water retention (due to decreased GFR) and inappropriate renin release. Heart failure from hypervolemia leads to pulmonary edema.

Diagnosis

A detailed patient history, assessment of clinical symptoms, and laboratory tests are needed to diagnose this disease. The following tests support the diagnosis:
▶ Urinalysis typically reveals proteinuria and hematuria. RBCs, white blood cells, and mixed cell casts are common findings in urinary sediment.
▶ Blood tests show elevated serum creatinine levels, low creatinine clearance, and impaired glomerular filtration.
▶ Elevated antistreptolysin-O titers (in 80% of patients), elevated streptozyme and anti-DNAse B titers, and low serum complement levels verify recent streptococcal infection.

▶ Throat culture may also show group A beta-hemolytic streptococci.

▶ Renal ultrasonography may show a normal or slightly enlarged kidney.

▶ Renal biopsy may confirm the diagnosis in a patient with APSGN or may be used to assess renal tissue status.

Other conditions to consider include membranoproliferative glomerulonephritis, other postinfective glomerulonephritis, systemic lupus erythematosus, IgA nephropathy, anaphylactoid purpura, and rapidly progressive glomerulonephritis.

Treatment

The goals of treatment are relief of symptoms and prevention of complications. Vigorous supportive care includes bed rest, fluid and dietary sodium restrictions, and correction of electrolyte imbalances (possibly with dialysis, although this is seldom necessary).

Therapy may include diuretics, such as metolazone and furosemide, to reduce extracellular fluid overload and an antihypertensive such as hydralazine. The use of antibiotics to prevent secondary infection or transmission to others is controversial.

Special considerations

▶ APSGN usually resolves within 2 weeks, so patient care is primarily supportive.

▶ Check vital signs and electrolyte values. Monitor intake and output and daily weight. Assess renal function daily through serum creatinine and blood urea nitrogen levels and urine creatinine clearance. Watch for signs of acute renal failure (oliguria, azotemia, and acidosis).

▶ Consult the dietitian to provide a diet high in calories and low in protein, sodium, potassium, and fluids.

▶ Protect the debilitated patient against secondary infection by providing good nutrition, using good hygienic technique, and preventing contact with infected people.

▶ Bed rest is necessary during the acute phase. Encourage the patient to gradually resume normal activities as symptoms subside.

▶ Provide emotional support for the patient and family. If the patient is on dialysis, explain the procedure fully.

▶ Advise the patient with a history of chronic upper respiratory tract infections to immediately report signs of infection (fever, sore throat).

▶ Tell the patient that follow-up examinations are necessary to detect chronic renal failure. Stress the need for regular blood pressure, urinary protein, and renal function assessments during the convalescent months to detect recurrence. After APSGN, gross hematuria may recur during nonspecific viral infections; abnormal urinary findings may persist for years (microhematuria, especially after strenuous exercise).

▶ Encourage pregnant women with a history of APSGN to have frequent medical evaluations because pregnancy further stresses the kidneys and increases the risk of chronic renal failure.

GONORRHEA

A common sexually transmitted disease, gonorrhea is an infection of the genitourinary tract (especially the urethra and cervix) and, occasionally, the rectum, pharynx, and eyes. Untreated gonorrhea can spread through the blood to the joints, tendons, meninges, and endocardium; in females, it can also lead to chronic pelvic inflammatory disease (PID) and sterility. After adequate treatment, the prognosis in both males and females is excellent, although reinfection is common. Gonorrhea is especially prevalent among young people and in people with multiple sexual partners, particularly those between ages 19 and 25.

Causes

Transmission of *Neisseria gonorrhoeae,* the microbe that causes gonorrhea, almost exclusively follows sexual contact with an infected person. Children born of infected mothers can contract gonococcal ophthalmia neonatorum during passage

WHAT HAPPENS IN GONORRHEA

After exposure to *Neisseria gonorrhoeae,* the epithelial cells at the infection site become infected; then the disease begins to spread locally. The disease pattern depends on the individual infected and the site of infection.

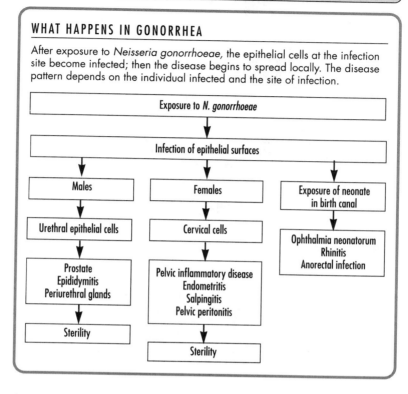

through the birth canal. Children and adults with gonorrhea can contract gonococcal conjunctivitis by touching their eyes with contaminated hands. (See *What happens in gonorrhea.*)

Signs and symptoms

Although many infected males are asymptomatic, after a 3- to 6-day incubation period, some develop symptoms of urethritis, including dysuria and purulent urethral discharge, with redness and swelling at the site of infection. Most infected females remain asymptomatic but may develop inflammation and a greenish yellow discharge from the cervix — the most common gonorrheal symptoms in females.

Other clinical features vary according to the site involved:

◗ *urethra:* dysuria, urinary frequency and incontinence, purulent discharge, itching, red and edematous meatus

◗ *vulva:* occasional itching, burning, and pain due to exudate from an adjacent infected area. Vulval symptoms are more severe before puberty and after menopause.

◗ *vagina* (most common site in children over age 1): engorgement, redness, swelling, and profuse purulent discharge

◗ *pelvis:* severe pelvic and lower abdominal pain, muscle rigidity, tenderness, and abdominal distention. As the infection spreads, nausea, vomiting, fever, and tachycardia may develop in patients with salpingitis or PID.

◗ *liver:* right upper quadrant pain in patients with perihepatitis.

Other possible symptoms include pharyngitis, tonsillitis, rectal burning and itching, and bloody mucopurulent discharge.

Gonococcal septicemia is more common in females than in males. Its characteristic signs include tender papillary skin lesions on the hands and feet; these lesions may be pustular, hemorrhagic, or necrotic. It may also produce migratory polyarthralgia and polyarthritis and tenosynovitis of the wrists, fingers, knees, and ankles. Untreated septic arthritis leads to progressive joint destruction.

Signs of *gonococcal ophthalmia neonatorum* include lid edema, bilateral conjunctival infection, and abundant purulent discharge 2 to 3 days after birth. Adult conjunctivitis, most common in men, causes unilateral conjunctival redness and swelling. Untreated gonococcal conjunctivitis can progress to corneal ulceration and blindness.

Diagnosis

A culture from the site of infection (urethra, cervix, rectum, or pharynx), grown on a Thayer-Martin or Transgrow medium, usually establishes the diagnosis by isolating *N. gonorrhoeae.* DNA probe analysis (which can also detect *Chlamydia*) has become the diagnostic method of choice. A Gram stain showing gram-negative diplococci supports the diagnosis and may be sufficient to confirm gonorrhea in males.

Confirmation of gonococcal arthritis requires identification of gram-negative diplococci on smears made from joint fluid and skin lesions. Complement fixation and immunofluorescent assays of serum reveal antibody titers four times the normal rate. Culture of conjunctival scrapings confirms gonococcal conjunctivitis.

Treatment

For adults and adolescents, the recommended treatment for uncomplicated gonorrhea caused by susceptible non-penicillinase-producing *N. gonorrhoeae* is a single 125-mg dose of ceftriaxone I.M. or a single oral dose of cefixime 400 mg P.O. Ciprofloxacin 500 mg P.O., or ofloxacin 400 mg P.O. are also recommended by the Centers for Disease Control and Prevention (CDC) for single dose oral therapy for gonorrhea. For presumptive treatment of concurrent *Chlamydia trachomatis* infection, the treatment is 100 mg of doxycycline P.O. twice daily for 7 days or azithromycin (Zithromax) 1 g P.O. in a single dose.

A single dose of ceftriaxone and erythromycin for 7 days is recommended for pregnant patients and those allergic to penicillin.

The recommended initial regimen for disseminated gonococcal infection in adults and adolescents is 1 g of ceftriaxone I.M. or I.V. every 24 hours or, for patients allergic to beta-lactam antibiotics, 2 g of spectinomycin I.M. every 12 hours.

All regimens should be continued for 24 to 48 hours after improvement begins; then therapy may be switched to one of the following regimens to complete 1 full week of antimicrobial therapy: 400 mg of cefixime P.O. twice daily or 500 mg of ciprofloxacin P.O. twice daily. Ciprofloxacin is contraindicated in children, adolescents, and pregnant or lactating women. Gonorrhea may also be treated with a single 1-g dose of azithromycin (Zithromax), per CDC guidelines.

Treatment of gonococcal conjunctivitis requires a single 1-g dose of ceftriaxone I.M. and lavage of the infected eye once with normal saline solution.

Routine instillation of 1% silver nitrate drops, or erythromycin ointment, or tetracycline ointment into neonates' eyes has greatly reduced the incidence of gonococcal ophthalmia neonatorum.

Special considerations

▸ Before treatment, establish whether the patient has any drug sensitivities, and watch closely for adverse effects during therapy.
▸ Warn the patient that until cultures prove negative, he's still infectious and can transmit gonococcal infection.
▸ Practice standard precautions.
▸ In the patient with gonococcal arthritis, apply moist heat to ease pain in affected joints.

▶ Urge the patient to inform sexual contacts of his infection so that they can seek treatment, even if cultures are negative. Advise them to avoid sexual intercourse until treatment is complete.

▶ Report all cases of gonorrhea to local public health authorities for follow-up on sexual contacts. Examine and test all people exposed to gonorrhea as well as newborn infants of infected mothers.

▶ Report all cases of gonorrhea in children to child abuse authorities.

▶ Routinely instill two drops of 1% silver nitrate, or erythromycin ointment, or tetracycline ointment in the eyes of all neonates immediately after birth. Check newborn infants of infected mothers for signs of infection. Take specimens for culture from the infant's eyes, pharynx, and rectum.

 PREVENTION TIP To prevent gonorrhea, tell patients to avoid anyone even *suspected* of being infected, to use condoms during intercourse, to wash their genitalia with soap and water before and after intercourse, and to avoid sharing washcloths or douche equipment.

GRANULOMA INGUINALE

Granuloma inguinale (also known as Donovanosis, lupoid ulceration granuloma of the pudenda, granuloma contagiosa and granuloma venereum) is a chronic, sexually transmitted disease caused by the bacterium *Calymmatobacterium granulomatis*. It is rarely seen in the United States, where fewer than 100 cases are diagnosed each year; however, it is endemic to tropical and subtropical areas of the world such as Southeast India, Guyana, and New Guinea. Granuloma inguinale affects men more often than women (2.5 to 1). It is primarily found among black and homosexual men; heterosexual partners of the infected rarely contract the bacterium. Peak incidence occurs between the ages of 20 and 45.

Causes

Infection occurs from ingestion of contaminated food or water and inoculation through skin abrasions or mucous membranes. Person-to-person transmission occurs through anal intercourse. Granuloma inguinale is mildly to moderately contagious, and is most often transmitted in its early stages before symptoms are noticed.

Signs and symptoms

Granuloma inguinale is characterized by painless, irregularly-shaped, beefy-red open sores on a cobblestone base. Initially, the lesions begin as indurated papules which slowly ulcerate. The lesions, which appear anywhere from one week to 3 months after infection, occur primarily on the skin and mucous membranes of the genital area, although self-infection to other body parts is possible. Subcutaneous granulomas in the inguinal areas may also develop, but the lymph nodes are not usually affected. Left untreated, the lesions enlarge, causing mutilation and destruction of the genitals. Disseminated infection may result in death secondary to complications such as heart failure, pneumonia or hemorrhage.

Diagnosis

The diagnosis of granuloma inguinale is made through visual observation of the lesions, sexual history, and microscopic examination of cells obtained from the borders of the sores. The presence of enlarged mononuclear cells with intracytoplasmic vacuoles containing Donovan bodies (Gram-negative rods which exhibit bipolar staining, giving a safety pin-like appearance) confirms the diagnosis. No serologic tests are currently available. Punch biopsy may be necessary.

In its earliest stages, granuloma inguinale must be distinguished from other sexually transmitted diseases such as chancroid and syphilis. Extensive lesions should be differentiated from advanced genital cancers, lymphogranuloma venereum, and anogenital amebiasis.

Treatment

Treatment of granuloma inguinale consists of a 2- to 3-week course of antibiotic therapy with tetracycline, doxycycline, minocycline, erythromycin, sulfamethoxazole or ciprofloxin. Lesions remain infectious as long as bacteria are present. Response to treatment occurs in as little as one week; complete healing of the sores may take as long as 5 weeks. If treated early, no tissue destruction or scarring should result.

Special considerations

▶ Monitor lesions for signs and symptoms of secondary bacterial infection.

▶ Be aware that the lesions bleed easily if traumatized. Gloves should be worn before any contact with lesions, followed by good hand washing.

▶ Genital scarring, depigmentation, and edema may occur even with successful treatment.

▶ Annual follow-up visits are advised because the disease can reappear after an apparently successful cure. Additionally, scars left by the lesions are considered to be precancerous and warrant regular observation.

▶ Advise patients with granuloma inguinale to abstain from sexual activity for at least one week after initiation of antibiotic treatment, preferably until the infection is cured.

▶ All sexual contacts of the infected patient should be notified so that they may obtain appropriate medical care.

▶ Patients should be made aware that past infection with this disorder does not confer immunity.

GUILLAIN-BARRÉ SYNDROME

Also known as infectious polyneuritis, Landry-Guillain-Barré syndrome, and acute idiopathic polyneuritis, Guillain-Barré syndrome is an acute, rapidly progressive, and potentially fatal form of polyneuritis that causes muscle weakness and mild distal sensory loss. This syndrome can occur at any age but is most common between ages 30 and 50; it affects both sexes equally. Recovery is spontaneous and complete in about 95% of patients, although mild motor or reflex deficits in the feet and legs may persist. The prognosis is best when symptoms clear between 15 and 20 days after onset.

Causes

The precise cause of Guillain-Barré syndrome is unknown, but it may be a cell-mediated immune response with an attack on peripheral nerves in response to a virus. The major pathologic effect is segmental demyelination of the peripheral nerves. Because this syndrome causes inflammation and degenerative changes in both the posterior (sensory) and the anterior (motor) nerve roots, signs of sensory and motor losses occur simultaneously.

About 50% of patients with Guillain-Barré syndrome have a recent history of minor febrile illness, usually an upper respiratory tract infection or, less often, gastroenteritis. When infection precedes the onset of Guillain-Barré syndrome, signs of infection subside before neurologic features appear. Other possible precipitating factors include surgery, rabies or swine influenza vaccination, viral illness, Hodgkin's disease, or some other malignant disease, and systemic lupus erythematosus.

Signs and symptoms

Muscle weakness, the major neurologic sign, usually appears in the legs first (ascending type) and then extends to the arms and facial nerves within 24 to 72 hours. Sometimes muscle weakness develops in the arms first (descending type) or in the arms and legs simultaneously. In milder forms of the disease, muscle weakness may affect only the cranial nerves or not occur.

Paresthesia, another common neurologic sign, sometimes precedes muscle weakness but vanishes quickly. Some patients with the disorder never develop this symptom.

Other clinical features include facial diplegia (possibly with ophthalmoplegia [ocular paralysis]), dysphagia or dysarthria and, less often, weakness of the muscles supplied by cranial nerve XI (spinal accessory nerve). Muscle weakness develops so quickly that muscle atrophy doesn't occur, but hypotonia and areflexia do. Stiffness and pain in the form of a severe charley horse often occur.

The clinical course of Guillain-Barré syndrome is divided into three phases:

▶ The *initial phase* begins when the first definitive symptom develops; it ends 1 to 3 weeks later, when no further deterioration is noted.

▶ The *plateau phase* lasts several days to 2 weeks.

▶ The *recovery phase* is believed to coincide with remyelination and axonal process regrowth. This phase extends over 4 to 6 months; patients with severe disease may take up to 2 years to recover, and recovery may not be complete.

Significant complications of Guillain-Barré syndrome include mechanical ventilatory failure, aspiration pneumonia, sepsis, joint contractures, and deep vein thrombosis. Unexplained autonomic nervous system involvement may cause sinus tachycardia or bradycardia, hypertension, orthostatic hypotension, and loss of bladder and bowel sphincter control.

Diagnosis

A history of preceding febrile illness (usually a respiratory tract infection) and typical clinical features suggest Guillain-Barré syndrome. Several days after onset of signs and symptoms, the cerebrospinal fluid (CSF) protein level begins to rise, peaking in 4 to 6 weeks, probably as a result of widespread inflammatory disease of the nerve roots. The CSF white blood cell count remains normal, but in severe disease, CSF pressure may rise above normal.

Probably because of predisposing infection, the complete blood count shows leukocytosis with the presence of immature forms early in the illness, but blood study results soon return to normal. Electromyography may show repeated firing of the same motor unit, instead of widespread sectional stimulation. Nerve conduction velocities are slowed soon after paralysis develops. The diagnosis must rule out similar diseases such as acute poliomyelitis.

Treatment

Primarily supportive, treatment consists of endotracheal intubation or tracheotomy if the patient has difficulty clearing secretions.

A trial dose of prednisone may be given if the course of the disease is relentlessly progressive. If prednisone produces no noticeable improvement after 7 days, the drug is discontinued. Plasmapheresis is useful during the initial phase but offers no benefit if begun 2 weeks after onset.

Special considerations

▶ Watch for ascending sensory loss, which precedes motor loss. Also, monitor vital signs and level of consciousness.

▶ Assess and treat respiratory dysfunction. If respiratory muscles are weak, take serial vital capacity recordings. Use a respirometer with a mouthpiece or a face mask for bedside testing.

▶ Obtain arterial blood gas measurements. Because neuromuscular disease results in primary hypoventilation with hypoxemia and hypercapnia, watch for a partial pressure of arterial oxygen (PaO_2) below 70 mm Hg, which signals respiratory failure. Be alert for signs of a rising partial pressure of carbon dioxide (confusion, tachypnea).

▶ Auscultate for breath sounds, turn and reposition the patient regularly, and encourage coughing and deep breathing.

▶ Begin respiratory support at the first sign of dyspnea (in adults, a vital capacity of less than 800 ml; in children, less than 12 ml/kg of body weight) or a decreasing PaO_2.

▶ If respiratory failure becomes imminent, establish an emergency airway with an endotracheal tube.

▶ Give meticulous skin care to prevent skin breakdown and contractures.

▶ Establish a strict turning schedule; inspect the skin (especially the sacrum, heels, and ankles) for breakdown, and reposition the patient every 2 hours.

▶ After each position change, stimulate circulation by carefully massaging pressure points. Also, use foam, gel, or alternating-pressure pads at points of contact.

▶ Perform passive range-of-motion exercises within the patient's pain limits, perhaps using a Hubbard tank. Remember that the proximal muscle groups of the thighs, shoulders, and trunk will be the most tender and cause the most pain on passive movement and turning.

▶ When the patient's condition stabilizes, change to gentle stretching and active assistance exercises.

▶ Assess the patient for signs of dysphagia: coughing, choking, "wet"-sounding voice, increased presence of rhonchi after feeding, drooling, delayed swallowing, regurgitation of food, and weakness in cranial nerves V, VII, IX, X, XI, or XII.

▶ Take measures to minimize aspiration: elevate the head of the bed, position the patient upright and leaning forward when eating, feed semisolid food, and check the mouth for food pockets.

▶ Encourage the patient to eat slowly and remain upright for 15 to 20 minutes after eating.

▶ A speech pathologist and modified video fluoroscopy can assist in identifying the best feeding strategies.

▶ If aspiration cannot be minimized by diet and position modification, nasogastric feeding is recommended.

▶ As the patient regains strength and can tolerate a vertical position, be alert for orthostatic hypotension. Monitor blood pressure and pulse rate during tilting periods, and if necessary, apply toe-to-groin elastic bandages or an abdominal binder to prevent orthostatic hypotension.

▶ Inspect the patient's legs regularly for signs of thrombophlebitis (localized pain, tenderness, erythema, edema, positive Homans' sign), a common complication of Guillain-Barré syndrome.

▶ To prevent thrombophlebitis, apply antiembolism stockings and give prophylactic anticoagulants, as needed.

▶ If the patient has facial paralysis, give eye and mouth care every 4 hours.

▶ Protect the corneas with isotonic eyedrops and conical eye shields.

▶ Encourage adequate fluid intake (2,000 ml/day), unless contraindicated.

▶ Watch for urine retention. Measure and record intake and output every 8 hours, and offer the bedpan every 3 to 4 hours.

▶ If urine retention develops, begin intermittent catheterization, as needed. Because the abdominal muscles are weak, the patient may need manual pressure on the bladder (Credé's method) before he can urinate.

▶ To prevent and relieve constipation, offer prune juice and a high-bulk diet. If necessary, give daily or alternate-day suppositories (glycerin or bisacodyl) or Fleet enemas.

▶ Before discharge, prepare a home care plan. Teach the patient how to transfer from bed to wheelchair and from wheelchair to toilet or tub and how to walk short distances with a walker or cane.

▶ Teach the family how to help the patient eat, compensating for facial weakness, and how to help him avoid skin breakdown. Stress the need for a regular bowel and bladder routine.

▶ Refer the patient for physical therapy, occupational therapy, and speech therapy, as needed.

HAEMOPHILUS INFLUENZAE INFECTION

A small, gram-negative, pleomorphic aerobic bacillus, *Haemophilus influenzae* causes diseases in many organ systems but most frequently attacks the respiratory system. In exudates, this organism predominantly resembles a coccobacillus.

H. influenzae is a common cause of epiglottitis, laryngotracheobronchitis, pneumonia, bronchiolitis, otitis media, and meningitis. Less often, it causes bacterial endocarditis, conjunctivitis, facial cellulitis, septic arthritis, and osteomyelitis.

H. influenzae pneumonia is an increasingly common nosocomial infection. It infects about one-half of all children before age 1 and virtually all children by age 3, although a new vaccine given at ages 2, 4, and 6 months has reduced this number.

Signs and symptoms

H. influenzae provokes a characteristic tissue response — acute suppurative inflammation. When *H. influenzae* infects the larynx, trachea, and bronchial tree, it leads to mucosal edema and thick exudate; when it invades the lungs, it leads to bronchopneumonia. In the pharynx, *H. influenzae* usually produces no remarkable changes, except when it causes epiglottitis, which generally affects both the laryngeal and the pharyngeal surfaces. The pharyngeal mucosa may be reddened, rarely with soft yellow exudate. More commonly, it appears normal or shows only slight diffuse redness, even while severe pain makes swallowing difficult or impossible. These infections typically cause high fever and generalized malaise.

Diagnosis

Isolation of the organism, usually with a blood culture, confirms *H. influenzae* infection. Other laboratory findings include:
▶ polymorphonuclear leukocytosis (15,000 to 30,000/μl)
▶ leukopenia (2,000 to 3,000/μl) in young children with severe infection
▶ *H. influenzae* bacteremia, found frequently in patients with meningitis.

Treatment

H. influenzae infections usually respond to a 2-week course of ampicillin, but 30% of strains are resistant. Ceftriaxone, cefotaxime, or chloramphenicol is used concurrently until sensitivities are identified. Rifampin should be given before discharge to assure treatment success.

Special considerations

▶ Maintain adequate respiratory function through proper positioning, humidification for children, and suctioning, as needed.
▶ Monitor the rate and type of respirations.
▶ Watch for signs of cyanosis and dyspnea, which necessitate intubation or a tracheotomy.
▶ For home treatment, suggest that the patient use a room humidifier or breathe moist air from a shower or bath, as necessary.
▶ Check the patient's history for drug allergies before giving antibiotics.

▶ Monitor the complete blood count for signs of bone marrow depression when therapy includes chloramphenicol.

▶ Monitor intake (including I.V. infusions) and output. Watch for signs of dehydration, such as decreased skin turgor, parched lips, concentrated urine, decreased urine output, and increased pulse rate.

▶ Take preventive measures, such as giving the *H. influenzae* vaccine to children ages 2 (or younger) to 6, maintaining respiratory isolation, using proper hand-washing technique, properly disposing of respiratory secretions, placing soiled tissues in a plastic bag, and decontaminating all equipment.

HANTAVIRUS PULMONARY SYNDROME

Mainly occurring in the southwestern United States, hantavirus pulmonary syndrome was first reported in May 1993. The syndrome, which rapidly progresses from flu-like symptoms to respiratory failure and, possibly, death, is known for its high mortality.

Causes

A member of the Bunyaviridae family, the genus *Hantavirus* is responsible for hantavirus pulmonary syndrome. However, the hantavirus strain that causes disease in Asia and Europe — mainly hemorrhagic fever and kidney disease — is distinctly different from the one described in North America. In the United States, most disease is caused by the strain called *sin nombre* virus.

The disease is transmitted by infected rodents, the primary reservoir for this virus. Data suggest that the deer mouse is the main source, but piñon mice, brush mice, and western chipmunks in proximity to humans in rural areas are also sources. Infected rodents are asymptomatic but shed the virus in feces, urine, and saliva.

Human infection may occur from inhalation, ingestion of contaminated food or water, contact with rodent excrement, or rodent bites. Transmission from person to person or by mosquitos, fleas, or other arthropod vectors has not been reported.

Hantavirus infections have been documented in people whose activities are associated with rodent contact, such as farming, hiking, or camping in rodent-infested areas, and occupying rodent-infested dwellings.

Signs and symptoms

Noncardiogenic pulmonary edema distinguishes the syndrome. Common chief complaints include myalgia, fever, headache, nausea, vomiting, and cough. Respiratory distress typically follows the onset of a cough. Fever, hypoxia and, in some patients, serious hypotension typify the hospital course.

Other signs and symptoms include a rising respiratory rate (28 breaths per minute) and an increased heart rate (120 beats per minute).

Diagnosis

Despite efforts to identify clinical and laboratory features that distinguish hantavirus pulmonary syndrome from other infections with similar features, diagnosis is based on clinical suspicion along with a process of elimination developed by the Centers for Disease Control and Prevention (CDC) with the Council of State and Territorial Epidemiologists. (See *Screening for hantavirus pulmonary syndrome.*)

Note: The CDC and state health departments can perform definitive testing for hantavirus exposure and antibody formation.

Laboratory tests usually reveal an elevated white blood cell count with a predominance of neutrophils, myeloid precursors, and atypical lymphocytes; elevated hematocrit; decreased platelet count; prolonged partial thromboplastin time; and a normal fibrinogen level. Usually, laboratory findings demonstrate only minimal abnormalities in renal function, with serum creatinine levels no higher than

SCREENING FOR HANTAVIRUS PULMONARY SYNDROME

The Centers for Disease Control and Prevention (CDC) has developed a screening procedure to track cases of hantavirus pulmonary syndrome. The screening criteria identify potential and actual cases.

POTENTIAL CASES

For a diagnosis of possible hantavirus pulmonary syndrome, a patient must have one of the following:

▶ a febrile illness (temperature equal to or above 101° F [38.3° C]) occurring in a previously healthy person and characterized by unexplained adult respiratory distress syndrome

▶ bilateral interstitial pulmonary infiltrates that develop within 1 week of hospitalization with respiratory compromise that requires supplemental oxygen

▶ an unexplained respiratory illness resulting in death and autopsy findings demonstrating noncardiogenic pulmonary edema without an identifiable specific cause of death.

EXCLUSIONS

Of the patients who meet the criteria for having potential hantavirus pulmonary syndrome, the CDC excludes those who have any of the following:

▶ a predisposing underlying medical condition (for example, severe underlying pulmonary disease, solid tumors or hematologic cancers, congenital or acquired immunodeficiency disorders, or medical conditions or treatments — such as rheumatoid arthritis or organ transplantation — requiring immunosuppressive drug therapy (for example, steroids or cytotoxic chemotherapy)

▶ an acute illness that provides a likely explanation for the respiratory illness (for example, a recent major trauma, burn, or surgery; recent seizures or history of aspiration; bacterial sepsis; another respiratory disorder such as respiratory syncytial virus in young children; influenza, or *Legionella* pneumonia).

CONFIRMED CASES

Cases of confirmed hantavirus pulmonary syndrome must include the following:

▶ at least one serum or tissue specimen available for laboratory testing for evidence of hantavirus infection

▶ in a patient with a compatible clinical illness, serologic evidence (presence of hantavirus-specific immunoglobulin G), polymerase chain reaction for hantavirus ribonucleic acid, or positive immunohistochemistry for hantavirus antigen.

2.5 mg/dl. Chest X-rays eventually show bilateral diffuse infiltrates in almost all patients (findings consistent with adult respiratory distress syndrome).

Treatment

Primarily supportive, treatment consists of maintaining adequate oxygenation, monitoring vital signs, and intervening to stabilize the patient's heart rate and blood pressure.

Drug therapy includes administering vasopressors, such as dopamine or epinephrine, for hypotension. Fluid volume replacement may also be ordered (with precautions not to overhydrate the patient). Intravenous ribavirin early in the illness has shown benefit.

Special considerations

▶ Assess the patient's respiratory status and arterial blood gas values often.

▶ Monitor the patient's serum electrolyte levels, and correct imbalances as appropriate.

▶ Maintain a patent airway by suctioning. Ensure adequate humidification, and check ventilator settings frequently.

❥ In patients with hypoxemia, assess neurologic status frequently along with heart rate and blood pressure.

❥ Administer drug therapy, and monitor the patient's response.

❥ Provide I.V. fluid therapy based on the results of hemodynamic monitoring.

❥ Provide emotional support for the patient and his family.

❥ Report cases of hantavirus pulmonary syndrome to the state health department.

 PREVENTION TIP Provide prevention guidelines. Until more is known about hantavirus pulmonary syndrome, preventive measures focus on rodent control.

HELICOBACTER PYLORI INFECTION

Manifesting as either an acute or chronic illness, *Helicobacter pylori* is an infectious disease responsible for more than 90% of duodenal ulcers and 80% of gastric ulcers. It is also responsible for atrophic gastritis and infected persons have a 2- to 6-fold increase in their risk of developing gastric cancer and mucosal-associated-lymphoid-type (MALT) lymphoma. *H. pylori* is probably the most chronic infection in human beings; approximately two-thirds of the world's population is infected with the bacterium. In the United States, it is estimated that 10% of Americans suffer from peptic ulcer disease (PUD). *H. pylori* is most prevalent among older adults, African Americans, Hispanics, and lower socioeconomic groups. Incidence occurs earlier and at increased rates in developing countries; however, prevalence of infection is probably decreasing in developed countries.

Causes

H. pylori is a gram-negative, spiral microaerophilic bacterium that occurs in the gastric mucus layer or the epithelial lining of the stomach. Transmission is be-lieved to be via an oral-oral or fecal-oral route, but the exact source remains unknown. Humans are the only known reservoirs; however, infected water sources may also be implicated. Iatrogenic infection via contaminated endoscopes has also been documented.

Signs and symptoms

Although *H. pylori* infections are widespread, not all infected persons become symptomatic. Acute infection is characterized by gnawing or burning epigastric pains, which typically occur when the stomach is empty, between meals, and in the early morning hours. The pain, which may persist for minutes to hours, is often partially relieved by eating or taking antacids and H_2 blockers. Other symptoms may include nausea, vomiting, loss of appetite, and bleeding — which can manifest as hematemesis, hematochezia or melena. Severe or prolonged bleeding can cause anemia, fatigue, and weakness and hypotension. Comorbid conditions such as cardiopulmonary disease may be exacerbated by significant blood loss. Chronic infection may result in the finding of gastric carcinoma or MALT lymphoma.

Diagnosis

H. pylori can be diagnosed through serologic tests that measure *H. pylori* antibodies in the blood. The ^{13}C-urea breath test, involving the drinking of a special carbon-labeled urea formula and subsequent measuring of expired CO_2 levels, is also available. Upper endoscopy is the diagnostic test of choice; histological identification of the bacterium via tissue biopsy remains the gold standard. The biopsy urease test, based on the bacterium's ability to produce urease, may also be undertaken and provides for rapid identification at the time of biopsy. The ^{13}C-urea breath test is more reliable than serology for the detection of active *H. pylori* infection in children. Below 10 years of age, serology is insufficiently sensitive for clinical purposes, whereas the ^{13}C-urea breath test remains a reliable test.

Differential diagnoses to consider include: functional gastrointestinal disorder, viral gastroenteritis, pancreatic disease, and gastric cancer.

Treatment

Anyone with active PUD, a documented history of PUD, early gastric cancer or MALT lymphoma should be tested for *H. pylori* infection and treated if found to be infected. *H. pylori* can be effectively eradicated with antibiotics. Currently, there are five Food and Drug Administration (FDA) approved treatment regimens consisting of 1 to 2 weeks of one or more antibiotics such as tetracycline, metronidazole or clarithromycin, plus either ranitidine bismuth citrate, bismuth subsalicylate, or a proton pump inhibitor. (See *FDA-approved treatment options for* Helicobacter pylori.) Treatment regimes for children have not yet been formalized. Eradication rates range from 70% to 90%, depending upon the regimen used, antibiotic resistance patterns, and patient compliance.

Conditions resulting from substantial bleeding, such as hypotension, anemia, and cardiopulmonary complications should also be treated accordingly. Retesting after treatment may also be prudent in cases of complicated PUD.

Special considerations

▶ Monitor for signs and symptoms of bleeding, such as hypotension, tachycardia, dyspnea, fecal occult blood, occult blood in vomitus, and decreased hemoglobin values.
▶ Be aware that tarry black stools may result from bismuth and iron preparations and do not indicate gastric bleeding.
▶ Active gastric bleeding may require insertion of a nasogastric tube; the patient may be unable to take oral nutrition during the acute episode.
▶ Discontinue nonsteroidal anti-inflammatory drugs.

FDA-APPROVED TREATMENT OPTIONS FOR *HELICOBACTER PYLORI*

Currently, five *H. pylori* treatment regimens (listed below) are approved by the Food and Drug Administration; however, several other combinations have been used successfully.
▶ Omeprazole 40 mg q.d. + clarithromycin 500 mg t.i.d. x 2 weeks, then omeprazole 20 mg q.d. x 2 weeks
   OR
▶ Ranitidine bismuth citrate (RBC) 400 mg b.i.d. + clarithromycin 500 mg t.i.d. x 2 weeks then RBC 400 mg b.i.d. x 2 weeks
   OR
▶ Bismuth subsalicylate (Pepto Bismol) 525 mg q.i.d. + metronidazole 250 mg q.i.d. + tetracycline 500 mg q.i.d.* x 2 weeks + H$_2$ receptor antagonist therapy as directed x 4 weeks
   OR
▶ Lansoprazole 30 mg b.i.d. + amoxicillin 1 g b.i.d. + clarithromycin 500 mg b.i.d. x 14 days
   OR
▶ Lansoprazole 30 mg t.i.d. + amoxicillin 1 g t.i.d. x 14 days**

* Although not FDA approved, amoxicillin has been substituted for tetracycline for patients in whom tetracycline is not recommended.
**This dual therapy regimen has restrictive labeling. It is indicated for patients who are either allergic or intolerant to clarithromycin or for infections with known or suspected resistance to clarithromycin.

▶ Utilize appropriate personal protective gear when performing patient care activities that may result in soiling with bodily discharges, such as blood, feces, or vomitus.

▶ Advise patients that past infection with *H. pylori* does not confer immunity.

 PREVENTION TIP Since the mode of transmission of *H. pylori* is unknown, stress the importance of thorough hand washing after using the toilet and before eating.

HENDRA VIRUS

Hendra virus, formerly called equine morbillivirus, is named after the Australian suburb in which the first known outbreak occurred in 1994. It is a newly recognized genus within the Paramyxovirus family that includes the measles, human parainfluenza, rinderpest, canine distemper, and respiratory syncytial viruses. The enveloped, negative-stranded RNA Hendra virus is a hyperacute respiratory disease which remains isolated and rare, with only three human and 14 equine deaths confirmed in Australia. All three of the human subjects had had direct physical contact with the infected horses. Although the virus is not considered to be highly contagious, it is lethal.

Causes

Hendra virus is not host-specific, meaning it can infect more than one species of animal. Current research indicates that four species of Australian fruit bats carry antibodies to Hendra virus and act as the natural host. The mode of transmission between bats and horses is unclear, but researchers believe infected bat urine, aborted fetuses, or reproductive fluids may be involved. Scientists have demonstrated that horses can be infected by eating material contaminated with the virus. Studies have not found evidence of infection between humans and fruit bats. Horse-to-human transmission is believed to occur via close contact with the body fluids of infected animals, suggesting that rigorous stable hygiene and personal protective clothing for horse handlers could help prevent or contain future outbreaks. There is no evidence of viral transmission to humans through the breath of horses, which may account for its limited incidence. Human-to-human transmission has not been reported.

Signs and symptoms

In humans and horses, signs and symptoms of Hendra virus include respiratory distress, high fever, and blood-tinged, foamy oral and nasal secretions signifying pulmonary edema. Additionally, encephalitis can occur in humans as long as a year after initial infection. Signs and symptoms of encephalitis include nuchal rigidity, high fever, headache, photophobia, confusion, drowsiness, irritability, loss of consciousness, seizures, and muscle weakness.

Diagnosis

Several recently developed diagnostic tests include an enzyme-linked immunosorbent assay Hendra IgM test, an immunoperoxidase test for use on formalin-fixed tissue, virus isolation, and virus neutralization tests to detect antibodies. In cases of encephalitis, a lumbar puncture is indicated.

Other conditions to consider include influenza, pneumonia, *Legionella*, respiratory syncytial virus, pulmonary edema, Hantavirus, encephalitis, rabies, Dengue fever, and Nipah virus.

Because the virus is thus far confined to Australia, the suspicion of Hendra virus should be limited to those patients who have traveled to Australia within the past year, had close contact with horses while there, and who exhibit severe influenza-like symptoms, pulmonary edema, pneumonia or encephalitis.

Treatment

There are no known medical treatments for Hendra virus at this time. Due to its lethal nature and the lack of experience with the virus, supportive measures may offer only a minimal chance of survival.

Special considerations

▶ Be prepared to provide emotional support to the patient and family members during this usually fatal illness.

▶ Because little is known of the disease, isolation precautions are advisable. Wear gloves for any contact with body fluids. Wash hands before and after all patient contact.

▶ Be on the alert for new information regarding Hendra virus or emerging treatment modalities. The Centers for Disease Control and Prevention (CDC) is a reliable source for up-to-date information.

HEPATITIS, NONVIRAL

Classified as toxic or drug-induced (idiosyncratic) hepatitis, nonviral hepatitis is an inflammation of the liver. Most patients recover from this illness, although a few develop fulminating hepatitis or cirrhosis.

Causes

Nonviral hepatitis results from various causes:

▶ *Alcohol overuse:* may lead to inflammation of the liver; continued alcohol intake can have severe effects, such as cirrhosis and liver failure.

▶ *Direct hepatotoxicity:* hepatocellular damage and necrosis, usually caused by toxins. It is dose-dependent and primarily caused by acetaminophen overdose.

▶ *Idiosyncratic hepatotoxicity:* typically follows a sensitization period of several weeks; caused by hypersensitivity to medications (for example, isoniazid, methyldopa, mercaptopurine, lovastatin, pravastatin, dipyridamole, and halothane)

▶ *Cholestatic reactions:* lack of bile excretion; possibly direct hepatotoxicity from oral contraceptives or anabolic steroids; hypersensitivity to phenothiazine derivatives such as chlorpromazine, antibiotics, thyroid medications, antidiabetic drugs; and cytotoxic drugs

▶ *Metabolic and autoimmune disorders:* acute exacerbations of subclinical liver disease, such as autoimmune hepatitis and Wilson's disease

▶ *Infectious agents:* systemic viruses, such as cytomegalovirus, mononucleosis or Epstein-Barr virus, measles virus, varicella zoster, adenovirus, herpes simplex virus, coxsackievirus, and human immunodeficiency virus; spirochetes such as those that cause syphilis and leptospirosis.

Signs and symptoms

Clinical features of toxic and drug-induced hepatitis vary with the severity of liver damage and the causative agent. In most patients, symptoms resemble those of viral hepatitis: anorexia, nausea, vomiting, jaundice, dark urine, hepatomegaly, possibly abdominal pain (with acute onset and massive necrosis), clay-colored stools, and, in the cholestatic form of hepatitis, pruritus.

Carbon tetrachloride poisoning also produces headache, dizziness, drowsiness, and vasomotor collapse; halothane-related hepatitis produces fever, moderate leukocytosis, and eosinophilia; chlorpromazine produces a rash, abrupt fever, arthralgias, lymphadenopathy, and epigastric or right-upper-quadrant pain.

Diagnosis

Diagnostic findings include elevations in serum aspartate aminotransferase, alanine aminotransferase, total and direct bilirubin (with cholestasis), and alkaline phosphatase levels; elevated white blood cell (WBC) count; and elevated eosinophil count (possible in the drug-induced type). A liver biopsy may help identify the underlying pathology, especially infiltration with WBCs and eosinophils. Liver function tests have limited value in distinguishing between nonviral and viral hepatitis.

Treatment

Effective treatment must remove the causative agent by lavage, catharsis, or hyperventilation, depending on the route of exposure. Acetylcysteine may serve as an antidote for toxic hepatitis caused by acetaminophen poisoning but doesn't prevent drug-induced hepatitis caused by other substances.

Corticosteroids may be prescribed for patients with drug-induced hepatitis.

 PREVENTION TIP To prevent nonviral hepatitis, teach the patient the proper use of drugs and the proper handling of cleaning agents and solvents.

HEPATITIS, VIRAL

A fairly common systemic disease, viral hepatitis is marked by hepatocellular destruction, necrosis, and autolysis, leading to anorexia, jaundice, and hepatomegaly. In most patients, hepatic cells eventually regenerate with little or no residual damage. Old age and serious underlying disorders make complications more likely. The prognosis is poor if edema and endstage liver disease develop.

There are five types of hepatitis:

▶ *Type A (infectious or short-incubation hepatitis)* is rising among homosexuals and in people with immunosuppression related to human immunodeficiency virus (HIV) infection. It's usually self-limiting and without a chronic form. About 40% of cases in the United States result from hepatitis A virus.

▶ *Type B (serum or long-incubation hepatitis)* also is increasing among HIV-positive individuals. Hepatitis B is now considered a sexually transmitted disease because of its high incidence and rate of transmission by this route.

Routine screening of donor blood for the hepatitis B surface antigen (HBsAg)

has decreased the incidence of posttransfusion cases, but transmission by needles shared by drug abusers remains a major problem. Acute signs and symptoms usually begin insidiously and last for 1 to 4 weeks. Urticaria or arthralgia that is experienced before any signs of jaundice is highly suggestive of hepatitis B infection. A chronic, potentially infectious state develops in about 10% of infected adults and in 70% to 90% of infected infants. This chronic state is associated with progressive liver disease in some individuals. Fulminant hepatitis can ensue, and there is an increased risk of primary hepatocellular carcinoma.

▶ *Type C hepatitis* accounts for about 20% of all viral hepatitis cases and is primarily transmitted through blood and body fluids or obtained during tattooing.

▶ *Type D (delta hepatitis)* is responsible for about 50% of all cases of fulminant hepatitis, which has a high mortality. Developing in 1% of patients, fulminant hepatitis causes unremitting liver failure with encephalopathy. It progresses to coma and commonly leads to death within 2 weeks. In the United States, type D hepatitis is confined to people who are frequently exposed to blood and blood products, such as I.V. drug users and hemophiliacs. It is transmitted parenterally and, less commonly, sexually.

▶ *Type E* (formerly grouped with type C under the name non-A, non-B hepatitis) occurs primarily in people who have recently returned from an endemic area (such as India, Africa, Asia, or Central America). It's more common in young adults and more severe in pregnant women.

Causes

The five major forms of viral hepatitis result from infection with the causative viruses: A, B, C, D, or E.

Type A hepatitis

Highly contagious, hepatitis A is usually transmitted by the fecal-oral route. It may also be transmitted parenterally. Hepatitis A usually results from ingestion of contaminated food, milk, or water. Outbreaks of this type are often traced to ingestion of seafood from polluted water. I.V. drug abusers and recipients of multiple blood product transfusions are at increased risk for hepatitis A.

Type B hepatitis

Once thought to be transmitted only by the direct exchange of contaminated blood, hepatitis B is now also known to be transmitted by contact with human secretions and stool passed by health care workers, recipients of plasma-derived products, and hemodialysis patients. As a result, nurses, doctors, laboratory technicians, and dentists are frequently exposed to type B hepatitis, often as a result of wearing defective gloves. Transmission also occurs during intimate sexual contact and through perinatal transmission.

Type C hepatitis

Although hepatitis C viruses have been isolated, only a small percentage of patients have tested positive for them, perhaps reflecting the test's poor specificity. Usually, this type of hepatitis is transmitted through transfused blood from asymptomatic donors and from receiving tattoos. Most patients with hepatitis C are asymptomatic. The virus is associated with a high rate of chronic liver disease (chronic hepatitis, cirrhosis, and an increased risk of hepatocellular carcinoma), which develops in 50% to 80% of those infected. People with chronic hepatitis C are considered infectious.

Type D hepatitis

Hepatitis D is found only in patients with an acute or a chronic episode of hepatitis B and requires the presence of hepatitis B surface antigen (HBsAg). The type D virus depends on the double-shelled type B virus to replicate. For this reason, a type D infection can't outlast a type B infection.

Hepatitis D is rare in the United States, except in I.V. drug abusers.

Type E hepatitis

Hepatitis E is transmitted enterically (oralfecal and waterborne routes), much like type A. Because this virus is inconsistently shed in feces, detection is difficult.

Signs and symptoms

Assessment findings are similar for the different types of hepatitis. Typically, signs and symptoms progress in three stages: prodromal (preicteric), clinical (icteric), and recovery (posticteric).

Prodromal stage

In this stage, the patient typically complains of easy fatigue, anorexia (possibly with mild weight loss), generalized malaise, depression, headache, weakness, arthralgia, myalgia, photophobia, and nausea with vomiting. The patient also may describe changes in senses of taste and smell.

Assessment of vital signs may reveal a temperature of 100° to 102° F (37.8° to 38.9° C). As the prodromal stage draws to a close — usually 1 to 5 days before the onset of the clinical jaundice stage — inspection of urine and stool specimens may reveal dark-colored urine and clay-colored stools.

Clinical stage

If the patient has progressed to the clinical jaundice stage, he may report pruritus, abdominal pain or tenderness, and indigestion. Early in this stage, he may complain of anorexia; later, his appetite may return. Inspection of the sclerae, mucous membranes, and skin may reveal jaundice, which can last for 1 to 2 weeks. Jaundice indicates that the damaged liver is unable to remove bilirubin from the blood, but it doesn't indicate the severity of the disease. Occasionally, hepatitis occurs without jaundice.

During the clinical jaundice stage, inspection of the skin may detect rashes, erythematous patches, and urticaria, especially if the patient has hepatitis B or C. Palpation may disclose abdominal tenderness in the right upper quadrant, an enlarged and tender liver and, in some cases, splenomegaly and cervical adenopathy.

Recovery stage

During the recovery stage, most of the patient's symptoms decrease or subside. On palpation, a decrease in liver enlargement may be noted. The recovery phase commonly lasts from 2 to 12 weeks, although sometimes this phase lasts longer in patients with hepatitis B, C, or E.

Diagnosis

In suspected viral hepatitis, a hepatitis profile is routinely performed. This study identifies antibodies specific to the causative virus, establishing the type of hepatitis as follows:

▶ *Type A:* Detection of an antibody to hepatitis A confirms the diagnosis.

▶ *Type B:* The presence of HBsAg and hepatitis B antibodies confirms the diagnosis.

▶ *Type C:* The diagnosis depends on serologic testing for the specific antibody 1 or more months after the onset of acute hepatitis. Until then, the diagnosis is established primarily by obtaining negative test results for hepatitis A, B, and D.

▶ *Type D:* The detection of intrahepatic delta antigens or immunoglobulin M (IgM) antidelta antigens in acute disease (or IgM and IgG in chronic disease) establishes the diagnosis.

▶ *Type E:* Detection of hepatitis E antigens supports the diagnosis; the diagnosis may also be determined by ruling out hepatitis C.

Additional findings from liver function studies support the diagnosis:

▶ Serum aspartate aminotransferase and serum alanine aminotransferase levels are increased in the prodromal stage of acute viral hepatitis.

▶ Serum alkaline phosphatase levels are slightly increased.

▶ Serum bilirubin levels are elevated. Levels may continue to be high late in the disease, especially in severe cases.

▶ Prothrombin time (PT) is prolonged. (More than 3 seconds longer than normal indicates severe liver damage.)

▶ White blood cell counts commonly reveal transient neutropenia and lymphopenia followed by lymphocytosis.

▶ Liver biopsy is performed if chronic hepatitis is suspected. (It's performed for acute hepatitis only if the diagnosis is questionable.)

Treatment

No specific drug therapy has been developed for hepatitis, with the exception of hepatitis C, which has been treated somewhat successfully with interferon alfa-2B. Instead, the patient is advised to rest in the early stages of the illness and to combat anorexia by eating small, high-protein meals. The largest meal should be eaten in the morning because nausea tends to intensify as the day progresses. Protein intake should be reduced if signs of precoma — lethargy, confusion, and mental changes — develop.

In acute viral hepatitis, hospitalization usually is required only for patients with severe symptoms (severe nausea, vomiting, change in mental status, and PT greater than 3 seconds above normal) or complications. Parenteral nutrition may be required if the patient experiences persistent vomiting and is unable to maintain oral intake.

Antiemetics (diphenhydramine or prochlorperazine) may be given 30 minutes before meals to relieve nausea and prevent vomiting; phenothiazines have a cholestatic effect and should be avoided. For severe pruritus, the resin cholestyramine may be given.

Special considerations

▶ Enteric precautions are used when caring for patients with type A or E hepatitis. Practice standard precautions for all patients.

▶ Stress the importance of thorough hand washing.

▶ Inform visitors about isolation precautions.

▶ Provide rest periods throughout the day. Schedule treatments and tests so the patient can rest between bouts of activity.

▶ Because inactivity may make the patient anxious, include diversional activities as part of his care. Gradually add activities as the patient begins to recover.

▶ Encourage the patient to eat. Provide small, frequent meals. Minimize medications.

▶ Force fluids (at least 4,000 ml/day). Encourage the anorectic patient to drink fruit juices. Also offer chipped ice and effervescent soft drinks to maintain hydration without inducing vomiting.

▶ Administer supplemental vitamins and commercial feedings. If symptoms are severe and the patient can't tolerate oral intake, provide parenteral nutrition and hydration.

▶ Monitor the patient's weight daily, and record intake and output. Observe stools for color, consistency, and amount, and record the frequency of bowel movements.

▶ Watch for signs of fluid shift, such as weight gain and orthostasis.

▶ Watch for signs of hepatic coma, dehydration, pneumonia, vascular problems, and pressure ulcers.

▶ In fulminant hepatitis, maintain electrolyte balance and a patent airway, prevent infections, and control bleeding. Correct hypoglycemia and any other complications while awaiting liver regeneration and repair.

▶ Before the patient is discharged, discuss restrictions and how to prevent a recurrence of hepatitis. (See *Preventing a recurrence of hepatitis.*)

PREVENTING A RECURRENCE OF HEPATITIS

▶ Before discharge, emphasize the importance of having regular medical checkups for at least 1 year. The patient will have an increased risk of developing hepatocellular cancer.

▶ Warn the patient against using any alcohol or nonprescription drugs for 1 year.

▶ Teach the patient to recognize the signs of recurrence.

▶ Encourage appropriate vaccinations.

▶ Discuss the use of medications.

▶ Teach the patient how to protect himself against other viruses.

▶ Stress the need for personal safety.

HERPANGINA

Herpangina is an acute viral infection which typically produces vesicular lesions on the mucous membranes of the soft palate, tonsillar pillars, and throat. Herpangina usually affects children under age 10 (except newborns because of maternal antibodies), and generally subsides in 4 to 7 days. It's slightly more common in late summer and fall, and can be sporadic, endemic, or epidemic.

Causes

Herpangina is caused by group A coxsackieviruses (usually types 1 through 10, 16, and 23) and, less commonly, by group B coxsackieviruses and echoviruses. The main mode of transmission of herpangina is fecal-oral transfer.

Signs and symptoms

After a 2- to 9-day incubation period, herpangina begins abruptly with a sore throat, pain on swallowing, a temperature of 100°

to 104° F (37.8° to 40° C) that persists for 1 to 4 days and may cause seizures, headache, anorexia, vomiting, malaise, diarrhea, and pain in the stomach, back of the neck, legs, and arms. After this, up to 12 grayish white papulovesicles appear on the soft palate and, less commonly, on the tonsils, uvula, tongue, and larynx. These lesions grow from 1 to 2 mm in diameter to large, punched-out ulcers surrounded by small, inflamed margins.

Diagnosis
Characteristic oral lesions suggest this diagnosis; isolation of the virus from mouth washings or feces, and elevated specific antibody titer confirm it. Other routine test results are normal except for slight leukocytosis. Diagnosis requires distinguishing the mouth lesions in herpangina from those in streptococcal tonsillitis (no ulcers; lesions confined to tonsils).

Treatment
Treatment for herpangina is entirely symptomatic, emphasizing measures to reduce fever and prevent seizures and possible dehydration. Herpangina doesn't require isolation or hospitalization but does require careful hand washing and sanitary disposal of excretions.

Special considerations
▶ Teach parents to give adequate fluids, enforce bed rest, and administer tepid sponge baths and antipyretics.

HERPES SIMPLEX

A widespread, recurrent viral infection, herpes simplex affects the skin and mucous membranes and commonly produces cold sores and fever blisters. There are two strains of herpes simplex, Type 1 and Type 2. Herpes Type 1 typically affects the oral mucous membranes, while herpes Type 2 primarily affects the genital area.

Herpes is equally common in males and females. It occurs worldwide and is most prevalent among children in lower socioeconomic groups who live in crowded environments. Primary *Herpes virus hominis* (HVH) is the leading cause of gingivostomatitis in children ages 1 to 3. It causes the most common nonepidemic encephalitis and is the second most common viral infection in pregnant women. If viremia is present the virus can pass to the fetus transplacentally and, in early pregnancy, may cause spontaneous abortion or premature birth.

Causes
Herpes simplex infection is caused by HVH. Herpes Type 1 is transmitted by oral and respiratory secretions; herpes Type 2 is transmitted by sexual contact. Cross-infection may result from orogenital sex. Saliva, stool, urine, skin lesions, and purulent eye exudate are potential sources of infection.

Signs and symptoms
About 85% of all HVH infections are subclinical. The others produce localized lesions and systemic reactions. After the first infection, a patient is a carrier susceptible to recurrent infections, which may be provoked by fever, menses, stress, heat, and cold. In recurrent infections, the patient usually has no constitutional signs and symptoms.

In neonates, HVH symptoms usually appear 1 to 2 weeks after birth. They range from localized skin lesions to a disseminated infection of such organs as the liver, lungs, and brain. Common complications include seizures, mental retardation, blindness, chorioretinitis, deafness, microcephaly, diabetes insipidus, and spasticity. Neonates with disseminated disease have a high mortality rate. Primary infection in childhood may be generalized or localized.

Generalized infection
After an incubation period of from 2 to 12 days, onset of generalized infection begins with fever, pharyngitis, erythema, and

edema. After brief prodromal tingling and itching, typical primary lesions erupt as vesicles on an erythematous base, eventually rupturing and leaving a painful ulcer, followed by a yellowish crust. Healing begins 7 to 10 days after onset and is complete in 3 weeks.

Vesicles may form on any part of the oral mucosa, especially the tongue, gingiva, and cheeks. In generalized infection, vesicles occur with submaxillary lymphadenopathy, increased salivation, halitosis, anorexia, and a temperature as high as 105° F (40.6° C). Herpetic stomatitis may lead to severe dehydration in children.

A generalized infection usually runs its course in 4 to 10 days. In this form, virus reactivation causes cold sores — single or grouped vesicles in and around the mouth.

Localized infection

Genital herpes usually affects adolescents and young adults. Typically painful, the initial attack produces fluid-filled vesicles that ulcerate and heal in 1 to 3 weeks. Fever, regional lymphadenopathy, and dysuria may also occur.

HVH can also affect the eye. Usually, herpetic keratoconjunctivitis is unilateral and causes only local symptoms: conjunctivitis, regional adenopathy, blepharitis, and vesicles on the lid. Other ocular symptoms may be excessive lacrimation, edema, chemosis, photophobia, and purulent exudate.

Both types of HVH can cause acute sporadic encephalitis with an altered level of consciousness, personality changes, and seizures. Other effects include smell and taste hallucinations and neurologic abnormalities, such as aphasia.

Herpetic whitlow, an HVH finger infection, commonly affects health care workers. First the finger tingles and then it becomes red, swollen, and painful. Vesicles with a red halo erupt and may ulcerate or coalesce. Other effects may include satellite vesicles, fever, chills, malaise, and a red streak up the arm.

Diagnosis

Typical lesions may suggest HVH infection. Confirmation requires isolation of the virus from local lesions in specialized culture tubes. As the lesions are often pathognomonic and frequently painful, a biopsy is rarely necessary. A rise in antibodies and moderate leukocytosis may support the diagnosis, although such testing is not generally required for diagnosis.

Treatment

Symptomatic and supportive therapy is essential. Generalized primary infection usually requires an analgesic-antipyretic to reduce fever and relieve pain. Anesthetic mouthwashes such as viscous lidocaine may reduce the pain of gingivostomatitis, enabling the patient to eat and preventing dehydration. Topical lidocaine may relieve the pain of vulvovaginal herpes.

Refer patients with eye infections to an ophthalmologist. Topical corticosteroids are contraindicated in active infection, but idoxuridine, trifluridine, and vidarabine are appropriate.

Acyclovir and its variants may be useful for a primary herpetic outbreak by reducing viral shedding and decreasing the duration of the episode. It has not been shown to be beneficial for future outbreaks. For patients who suffer frequent outbreaks — generally defined as more than 6 episodes annually — chronic suppression with oral acyclovir may be indicated.

A 5% acyclovir ointment may bring relief to patients with genital herpes or to immunosuppressed patients with HVH skin infections. Intravenous acyclovir helps treat more severe infections, such as herpetic encephalitis.

Special considerations

▶ Abstain from direct patient care if you have herpetic whitlow.
▶ Patients with central nervous system infection alone need no isolation.

▶ Teach patients to use warm compresses or take sitz baths several times a day, to increase fluid intake, and to avoid unprotected intercourse during the active stage.

 PREVENTION TIP Instruct patients with herpetic whitlow not to share towels or utensils with uninfected people. Tell patients with cold sores not to kiss infants or people with eczema. Patients should not be made to feel guilty; herpes is a chronic but manageable disease in most instances.

HERPES ZOSTER

Also called shingles, herpes zoster is an acute unilateral and segmental inflammation of the dorsal root ganglia caused by infection with the herpesvirus varicella-zoster, which also causes chickenpox. Herpes zoster is found primarily in adults, especially those older than age 50. It seldom recurs. It produces localized vesicular skin lesions confined to a dermatome and severe neuralgic pain in peripheral areas innervated by the nerves arising in the inflamed root ganglia.

The prognosis is good unless the infection spreads to the brain. Eventually, most patients recover completely, except for possible scarring and, in corneal damage, visual impairment. Occasionally, neuralgia may persist for months or years.

Causes

Herpes zoster results from reactivation of varicella virus that has lain dormant in the cerebral ganglia (extramedullary ganglia of the cranial nerves) or the ganglia of posterior nerve roots since a previous episode of chickenpox. Exactly how or why this reactivation occurs isn't clear. Some believe that the virus multiplies as it is reactivated and that it is neutralized by antibodies remaining from the initial infection. But if effective antibodies aren't present, the virus continues to multiply in the ganglia, destroy the host neuron, and spread down the sensory nerves to the skin.

Signs and symptoms

Herpes zoster usually runs a typical course with classic signs and symptoms. Serious complications sometimes occur. Herpes zoster begins with fever and malaise. Within 2 to 4 days, severe deep pain, pruritus, and paresthesia or hyperesthesia develop, usually on the trunk and occasionally on the arms and legs in a dermatomal distribution. Pain may be continuous or intermittent and usually lasts from 1 to 4 weeks.

Up to 2 weeks after the first symptoms, small, red, nodular skin lesions erupt on the painful areas. These lesions commonly spread unilaterally around the thorax or vertically over the arms or legs. Sometimes nodules don't appear, but when they do, they quickly become vesicles filled with clear fluid or pus.

About 10 days after they appear, the vesicles dry and form scabs. (See *Skin lesions in herpes zoster.*) When they rupture, such lesions often become infected and, in severe cases, may lead to the enlargement of regional lymph nodes; they may even become gangrenous. Intense pain may occur before the rash appears and after the scabs form.

Occasionally, herpes zoster involves the cranial nerves, especially the trigeminal and geniculate ganglia or the oculomotor nerve. Geniculate zoster may cause vesicle formation in the external auditory canal, ipsilateral facial palsy, hearing loss, dizziness, and loss of taste. Trigeminal ganglion involvement causes eye pain and, possibly, corneal and scleral damage and impaired vision. Rarely, oculomotor involvement causes conjunctivitis, extraocular weakness, ptosis, and paralytic mydriasis.

In rare cases, herpes zoster leads to generalized central nervous system infection, muscle atrophy, motor paralysis (usually transient), acute transverse myelitis, and ascending myelitis. More often, generalized infection causes acute retention of urine and unilateral paralysis of the diaphragm. In postherpetic neuralgia, a complication most common in elderly patients, intractable neuralgic pain may persist for years. Scars may be permanent.

Diagnosis

A positive diagnosis of herpes zoster usually isn't possible until the characteristic skin lesions develop. Before then, the pain may mimic that of appendicitis, pleurisy, or other conditions. Diagnostic test results include the following:

▶ Examination of vesicular fluid and infected tissue shows eosinophilic intranuclear inclusions and varicella virus.

▶ Lumbar puncture shows increased cerebrospinal fluid pressure; examination of cerebrospinal fluid shows increased protein levels and, possibly, pleocytosis.

▶ Staining antibodies from vesicular fluid and identification under fluorescent light differentiate herpes zoster from localized herpes simplex.

Treatment

No specific treatment exists. The primary goal of supportive treatment is to relieve itching and neuralgic pain with calamine lotion or another antipruritic; aspirin, possibly with codeine or another analgesic; and, occasionally, collodion or tincture of benzoin applied to unbroken lesions. If bacteria have infected ruptured vesicles, treatment usually includes an appropriate systemic antibiotic. Trigeminal zoster with corneal involvement calls for instillation of idoxuridine ointment or another antiviral agent.

To help a patient cope with the intractable pain of postherpetic neuralgia, administer a systemic corticosteroid, such as cortisone or, possibly, corticotropin, to reduce inflammation, as well as tranquilizers, sedatives, or tricyclic antidepressants with phenothiazines.

Acyclovir seems to stop progression of the rash and prevent visceral complications. In immunocompromised patients — both children and adults — acyclovir therapy may be administered I.V. The drug

SKIN LESIONS IN HERPES ZOSTER

The characteristic skin lesions in herpes zoster are fluid-filled vesicles that dry and form scabs after about 10 days.

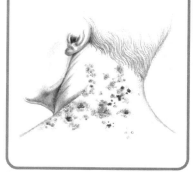

appears to prevent disseminated, life-threatening disease in some patients. Acyclovir and famciclovir shorten the duration of pain and symptoms in normal adults.

Special considerations

▶ Keep the patient comfortable, maintain meticulous hygiene, and prevent infection. During the acute phase, encourage him to get adequate rest and give supportive care to promote proper healing of lesions.

▶ Apply calamine lotion liberally to the lesions. If lesions are severe and widespread, apply a wet dressing.

▶ Instruct the patient to avoid scratching the lesions.

▶ If vesicles rupture, apply a cold compress.

▶ To decrease the pain of oral lesions, tell the patient to use a soft toothbrush, eat a soft diet, and use saline mouthwash.

▶ To minimize neuralgic pain, never withhold or delay administration of analgesics. Give them exactly on schedule because the pain of herpes zoster can be severe. In

postherpetic neuralgia, avoid narcotic analgesics because of the danger of addiction.
▶ Repeatedly reassure the patient that herpetic pain will eventually subside. Provide the patient with diversionary activity to take his mind off the pain and pruritus.

HISTOPLASMOSIS

Also called Ohio Valley disease, Central Mississippi Valley disease, Appalachian Mountain disease, and Darling's disease, histoplasmosis is a fungal infection caused by *Histoplasma capsulatum.* In the United States, it occurs in three forms: primary acute histoplasmosis, progressive disseminated histoplasmosis (acute disseminated or chronic disseminated disease), and chronic pulmonary (cavitary) histoplasmosis, which produces cavitations in the lung similar to those in pulmonary tuberculosis. A fourth form, African histoplasmosis, is caused by the fungus *Histoplasma capsulatum* var. *duboisii.*

Histoplasmosis occurs worldwide, especially in the temperate areas of Asia, Africa, Europe, and North and South America. In the United States, it is most prevalent in the central and eastern states, especially in the Mississippi and Ohio river valleys. Probably because of occupational exposure, histoplasmosis is more common in men. Fatal disseminated disease is more common in infants and elderly men.

The prognosis varies with each form. The primary acute disease is benign; the progressive disseminated disease is fatal in about 90% of patients; without proper chemotherapy, chronic pulmonary histoplasmosis is fatal in 50% of patients within 5 years.

Causes
H. capsulatum is found in the feces of birds and bats or in soil contaminated by their feces, such as that near roosts, chicken coops, barns, and caves and under bridges. Transmission is through inhala-tion of *H. capsulatum* or *H. duboisii* spores or through the invasion of spores after minor skin trauma. The incubation period is 5 to 18 days, although chronic pulmonary histoplasmosis may progress slowly for many years.

Signs and symptoms
Symptoms vary with each form of this disease:
▶ *Primary acute histoplasmosis* may be asymptomatic or cause symptoms of a mild respiratory illness similar to those that accompany a severe cold or influenza. Typical symptoms include fever, malaise, headache, myalgia, anorexia, cough, and chest pain.
▶ *Progressive disseminated histoplasmosis* causes hepatosplenomegaly, general lymphadenopathy, anorexia, weight loss, fever and, possibly, ulceration of the tongue, palate, epiglottis, and larynx with resulting pain, hoarseness, and dysphagia. It may also cause endocarditis, meningitis, pericarditis, and adrenal insufficiency.
▶ *Chronic pulmonary histoplasmosis* mimics pulmonary tuberculosis and causes a productive cough, dyspnea, and occasional hemoptysis. Eventually, it produces weight loss, extreme weakness, breathlessness, and cyanosis.
▶ *African histoplasmosis* produces lymphadenopathy, lesions of the skull and long bones, visceral involvement without pulmonary lesions, cutaneous nodules, papules, and ulcers.

Diagnosis
A history of exposure to contaminated soil in an endemic area, miliary calcification in the lungs or spleen, and a positive histoplasmin skin test indicate exposure to *H. capsulatum.* Rising complement fixation and agglutination titers (more than 1:32) strongly suggest the diagnosis. A urinary antigen test for histoplasmosis is now used for diagnosis.

The diagnosis of histoplasmosis requires morphologic examination of a tissue biopsy and culture of *H. capsulatum* from sputum in acute primary and chronic pulmonary histoplasmosis and from bone marrow, lymph nodes, blood, and infection sites in disseminated histoplasmosis. Cultures take several weeks to grow these organisms.

A faster diagnosis is possible with stained biopsies. Findings must rule out tuberculosis and other diseases that produce similar symptoms. The diagnosis of histoplasmosis caused by *H. duboisii* necessitates examination of a tissue biopsy and culture of the affected site.

Treatment

Histoplasmosis treatment consists of antifungal therapy, surgery, and supportive care. Antifungal therapy is most important. Except for asymptomatic primary acute histoplasmosis (which resolves spontaneously) and the African form, histoplasmosis requires high-dose or long-term (10-week) therapy with amphotericin B or fluconazole. For a patient who also has acquired immunodeficiency syndrome, lifelong therapy with fluconazole is indicated.

Supportive care usually includes oxygen for respiratory distress, glucocorticoids for adrenal insufficiency, and parenteral fluids for dysphagia due to oral or laryngeal ulcerations.

Histoplasmosis doesn't require the patient to be isolated.

Special considerations

▶ Administer medications, and teach patients about possible adverse effects. Because amphotericin B may cause chills, fever, nausea, and vomiting, give appropriate antipyretics and antiemetics.

▶ Patients with chronic pulmonary or disseminated histoplasmosis also need psychological support because of long-term hospitalization.

▶ As needed, refer the patient to a social worker or an occupational therapist. Help parents of children with this disease arrange for a visiting teacher.

 PREVENTION TIP To help prevent histoplasmosis, teach people in endemic areas to watch for early signs of this infection and to seek treatment promptly. Instruct people who risk occupational exposure to contaminated soil to wear face masks.

HOOKWORM DISEASE

Also known as uncinariasis, hookworm disease is an infection of the upper intestine caused by *Ancylostoma duodenale* (found in the eastern hemisphere) or *Necator americanus* (in the western hemisphere). Sandy soil, high humidity, a warm climate, and failure to wear shoes all favor its transmission.

In the United States, hookworm disease is most common in the southeast. Although this disease can cause cardiopulmonary complications, it's seldom fatal, except in debilitated people and infants under age 1.

Causes

Both forms of hookworm disease are transmitted to humans through direct skin penetration (usually in the foot) by hookworm larvae in soil contaminated with feces that contain hookworm ova. These ova develop into infectious larvae in 1 to 3 days.

Larvae travel through the lymphatics to the pulmonary capillaries, where they penetrate alveoli and move up the bronchial tree to the trachea and epiglottis. There they are swallowed and enter the GI tract. When they reach the small intestine, they mature, attach to the jejunal mucosa, and suck blood, oxygen, and glucose from the intestinal wall. These mature worms then deposit ova, which are excreted in stools, starting the cycle anew. Hookworm larvae mature in about 5 to 6 weeks.

Signs and symptoms

Most cases of hookworm disease produce few symptoms and may be overlooked until worms are passed in stools. The earliest signs and symptoms include irritation, pruritus, and edema at the site of entry, which are sometimes accompanied by secondary bacterial infection with pustule formation.

When the larvae reach the lungs, they may cause pneumonitis and hemorrhage with fever, sore throat, crackles, and cough. Finally, intestinal infection may cause fatigue, nausea, weight loss, dizziness, melena, and uncontrolled diarrhea.

In severe and chronic infection, anemia from blood loss may lead to cardiomegaly (a result of increased oxygen demands), heart failure, and generalized massive edema.

Diagnosis

Identification of hookworm ova in stools confirms the diagnosis. Anemia suggests severe chronic infection. In infected patients, blood studies show:
▶ hemoglobin level of 5 to 9 g/dl (in severe cases)
▶ leukocyte count as high as 47,000/μl
▶ eosinophil count of 500 to 700/μl.

Treatment

The usual treatment for hookworm infection includes administering an anthelmintic, such as mebendazole, albendazole, levamisole, or pyrantel, and providing an iron-rich diet or iron supplements to prevent or correct anemia. Stool examinations are repeated in 2 weeks. The patient may be retreated if indicated.

Special considerations

▶ Obtain a complete history, with special attention to travel or residency in endemic areas. Note the sequence and onset of symptoms. Interview the family and other close contacts to see if they too have any symptoms.
▶ Carefully assess the patient, noting signs of entry, lymphedema, and respiratory status.

If the patient has confirmed hookworm infestation:
▶ Segregate the incontinent patient.
▶ Wash your hands thoroughly after every patient contact.
▶ For severe anemia, administer oxygen at a low to moderate flow rate. Make sure the oxygen is humidified because the patient may already have upper airway irritation from the parasites.
▶ Encourage coughing and deep breathing to stimulate removal of blood or secretions from involved lung areas and to prevent secondary infection.
▶ Allow frequent rest periods because the patient may tire easily.
▶ If anemia causes immobility, reposition the patient often to prevent skin breakdown.
▶ Closely monitor intake and output. Note the quantity and frequency of diarrheal stools. Dispose of stools promptly, and wear gloves when doing so.
▶ To help assess nutritional status, weigh the patient daily.
▶ To combat malnutrition, emphasize the importance of good nutrition, with particular attention to foods high in iron and protein. If the patient receives iron supplements, explain that they will darken stools.
▶ Administer anthelmintics on an empty stomach but without a purgative.

 PREVENTION TIP To help prevent reinfection, educate the patient in proper hand-washing technique and sanitary disposal of feces. Tell him to wear shoes in endemic areas.

IJ

IMPETIGO

A contagious, superficial skin infection, impetigo (also known as impetigo contagiosa) occurs in nonbullous and bullous forms. This vesiculopustular eruptive disorder spreads most easily among infants, young children, and elderly people.

Predisposing factors such as poor hygiene, anemia, malnutrition, and a warm climate favor outbreaks of this infection, most of which occur during the late summer and early fall. Impetigo can complicate chickenpox, eczema, and other skin conditions marked by open lesions.

Causes

Coagulase-positive *Staphylococcus aureus* and, less commonly, group A beta-hemolytic streptococci usually produce nonbullous impetigo; *S. aureus* (especially of bacteriophage type 71) generally causes bullous impetigo.

Signs and symptoms

Common nonbullous impetigo typically begins with a small red macule that turns into a vesicle, becoming pustular with a honey-colored crust within hours. When the vesicle breaks, a thick yellow crust forms from the exudate. Autoinoculation may cause satellite lesions. Other features include pruritus, burning, and regional lymphadenopathy. In bullous impetigo, a thin-walled vesicle opens and a thin, clear crust forms on the subsequent eruption. It commonly appears on exposed areas.

A rare but serious complication of streptococcal impetigo is glomerulonephritis.

Diagnosis

Characteristic lesions suggest impetigo. (See *Recognizing impetigo,* page 142.) Microscopic visualization of the causative organism in a Gram stain of vesicle fluid usually confirms *S. aureus* infection and justifies antibiotic therapy. Culture and sensitivity testing of fluid or denuded skin may indicate the most appropriate antibiotic, but therapy shouldn't be delayed for laboratory results, which can take 3 days.

The differential diagnosis includes herpes simplex, infected eczema, varicella, and herpes zoster.

Treatment

Generally, treatment consists of systemic antibiotics (usually a pencillinase-resistant penicillin, cephalosporin, or erythromycin) for 10 days. A topical antibiotic such as mupirocin ointment may be used for minor infections.

Therapy also includes removal of the exudate by washing the lesions two or three times a day with soap and water or, for stubborn crusts, using warm soaks or compresses of normal saline or a diluted soap solution.

Special considerations

▶ Urge the patient not to scratch because this spreads impetigo. Advise parents to cut the child's fingernails.
▶ Give medications as necessary; remember to check for penicillin allergy. Stress the need to continue prescribed medications for 7 to 10 days, even after the lesions have healed.

RECOGNIZING IMPETIGO

In impetigo, when the vesicles break, crust forms from the exudate. This infection is especially contagious among young children.

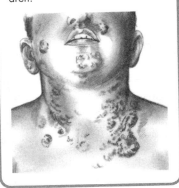

▶ Check family members for impetigo. If this infection is present in a schoolchild, notify the school.

 PREVENTION TIP Teach the patient or family how to care for the lesions. To prevent further spread of this highly contagious infection, encourage frequent bathing using a bactericidal soap. Tell the patient not to share towels, washcloths, or bed linens with family members. Emphasize the importance of following proper hand-washing technique.

INFLUENZA

Also called the grippe or the flu, influenza is an acute, highly contagious infection of the respiratory tract that results from three types of *Myxovirus influenzae*. It occurs sporadically or in epidemics (usually during the colder months). Epidemics tend to peak within 2 to 3 weeks after initial cases and subside within 1 month.

Although influenza affects all age-groups, its incidence is highest in school-children. Its severity is greatest in the very young, elderly people, and those with chronic diseases. In these groups, influenza may even lead to death. The catastrophic pandemic of 1918 was responsible for an estimated 20 million deaths. The most recent pandemics — in 1957, 1968, and 1977 — began in mainland China.

Causes

Transmission of influenza occurs through inhalation of a respiratory droplet from an infected person or by indirect contact, such as the use of a contaminated drinking glass. The influenza virus then invades the epithelium of the respiratory tract, causing inflammation and desquamation.

One of the remarkable features of the influenza virus is its capacity for antigenic variation. Such variation leads to infection by strains of the virus to which little or no immunologic resistance is present in the population at risk. Antigenic variation is characterized as *antigenic drift* (minor changes that occur yearly or every few years) and *antigenic shift* (major changes that lead to pandemics). Influenza viruses are classified into three groups:

▶ Type A, the most prevalent, strikes every year, with new serotypes causing epidemics every 3 years.

▶ Type B also strikes annually, but only causes epidemics every 4 to 6 years.

▶ Type C is endemic and causes only sporadic cases.

Signs and symptoms

After an incubation period of 24 to 48 hours, flu symptoms begin to appear: the sudden onset of chills, a temperature of 101° to 104° F (38.3° to 40° C), headache, malaise, myalgia (particularly in the back and limbs), a nonproductive cough and, occasionally, laryngitis, hoarseness, conjunctivitis, rhinitis, and rhinorrhea.

These symptoms usually subside in 3 to 5 days, but cough and weakness may persist. Fever is usually higher in children than in adults. Also, cervical adenopathy and croup are likely to be associated with influenza in children. In some patients (especially elderly ones), lack of energy and easy fatigability may persist for several weeks.

Fever that persists longer than 3 to 5 days signals the onset of complications. The most common complication is pneumonia, which can be primary influenza viral pneumonia or secondary to bacterial infection. Influenza may also cause myositis, exacerbation of chronic obstructive pulmonary disease, Reye's syndrome and, rarely, myocarditis, pericarditis, transverse myelitis, and encephalitis.

Diagnosis
At the beginning of an influenza epidemic, early cases are usually mistaken for other respiratory disorders. Because signs and symptoms are not pathognomonic, isolation of *M. influenzae* through the inoculation of chicken embryos (with nasal secretions from infected patients) is essential at the first sign of an epidemic. In addition, nose and throat cultures and increased serum antibody titers help confirm this diagnosis. After these measures confirm an influenza epidemic, diagnosis requires only observation of clinical signs and symptoms. Uncomplicated cases show a decreased white blood cell count with an increase in lymphocytes.

Treatment
Uncomplicated influenza is treated with bed rest, adequate fluid intake, aspirin or acetaminophen (in children) to relieve fever and muscle pain, and guaifenesin or another expectorant to relieve nonproductive coughing. Prophylactic antibiotics are not recommended because they have no effect on the influenza virus.

Amantadine, oseltamivir phosphate, and zanamivir (antiviral agents) have proved to be effective in reducing the duration of signs and symptoms in influenza A infection. In influenza complicated by pneumonia, supportive care (fluid and electrolyte supplements, oxygen, assisted ventilation) and treatment of bacterial superinfection with appropriate antibiotics are necessary. No specific therapy exists for cardiac, central nervous system, or other complications.

Special considerations
▶ Advise the patient to use mouthwashes and increase fluid intake. Warm baths or heating pads may relieve myalgia. Provide nonnarcotic analgesics and antipyretics as needed.

▶ Screen visitors to protect the patient from bacterial infection and the visitor from influenza. Use respiratory precautions.

▶ Teach the patient proper disposal of tissues and proper hand-washing technique to prevent the virus from spreading.

▶ Watch for signs and symptoms of developing pneumonia, such as crackles, another temperature rise, and coughing accompanied by purulent or bloody sputum. Assist the patient in a gradual return to normal activities.

 PREVENTION TIP Educate patients about influenza immunizations. For high-risk patients and health care personnel, suggest annual inoculations at the start of the flu season (late autumn). The vaccine administered is based on the previous year's virus and is usually about 75% effective. Remember that such vaccines are made from chicken embryos and must not be given to people who are hypersensitive to eggs, feathers, or chickens. All people receiving the vaccine should be made aware of possible adverse effects (discomfort at the vaccination site, fever, malaise and, rarely, Guillain-Barré syndrome). Although the vaccine has not been proven harmful to the fetus, it's not recommended for pregnant women during the first trimester. Children older than 8 months may safely receive the vaccine in reduced doses. For people who are hypersensitive to eggs, amantadine is an effective alternative to the vaccine.

KERATITIS

Keratitis, infection of the cornea, may occur as a result of bacterial, fungal or viral invasion. Infection of the cornea is a sight-threatening process.

Causes

The most common cause of keratitis is infection by herpes simplex virus, Type 1 (known as dendritic because of the characteristic branching lesion that occurs). Bacterial corneal ulcers frequently occur as a result of an infected corneal abrasion or contaminated contact lens. Fungal keratitis is more frequently encountered in tropical climates. Poor lid closure can result in exposure keratitis. Chemicals splashed in the eye can also produce keratitis.

Signs and symptoms

Usually unilateral, a patient presents with decreased vision, discomfort ranging from mild irritation to acute pain, tearing, and photophobia. When keratitis results from exposure, it usually affects the lower portion of the cornea. Visual acuity may be decreased if the lesion is central. On gross examination with a pen light, the corneal light reflex might be distorted.

Diagnosis

A slit-lamp examination confirms keratitis. Staining the eye with a sterile fluorescein strip enables the examiner to discern the extent and depth of the corneal lesion. Patient history may reveal a recent infection of cold sores, or eye irritation while wearing contact lenses.

Treatment

In acute keratitis due to herpes simplex virus (HSV), treatment consists of trifluridine eyedrops or vidarabine ointment. A broad-spectrum antibiotic may prevent secondary bacterial infection. HSV keratitis is treated in a doctor's office. Dendritic keratitis may become chronic, with recurrent episodes. Long-term topical therapy may be necessary. (Corticosteroid therapy is contraindicated in dendritic keratitis or any other viral or fungal disease of the cornea.)

Bacterial corneal ulcers require intense topical eye drop instillation every ½ hour for the first 48 hours with two broad-spectrum antibiotics. Treatment for fungal keratitis consists of natamycin. Bacterial and fungal corneal ulcers are treated in hospital.

Exposure keratitis is treated with application of ointment at night and frequent instillation of artificial tears during daytime. A plastic bubble shield may prevent tear evaporation. Vision may be restored by penetrating keratoplasty (corneal transplant) when blindness results from corneal scarring.

Special considerations

▶ Be aware that the patient with a red eye may have keratitis. Check for a history of contact lens wear, cold sores, or recent foreign body sensation. Refer patient for slit-lamp examination as soon as possible for treatment.
▶ Protect the exposed corneas of unconscious patients by cleaning the eyes daily, applying moisturizing ointment, or covering the eyes with an eye shield.

LABYRINTHITIS

An inflammation of the labyrinth of the inner ear, labyrinthitis frequently incapacitates the patient by producing severe vertigo that lasts for 3 to 5 days; symptoms gradually subside in 3 to 6 weeks. Associated symptoms include tinnitus and hearing loss. This disorder is rare, although viral labyrinthitis is often associated with upper respiratory tract infections.

Causes

Labyrinthitis is usually caused by viral infection. It may be a primary infection; the result of trauma; or a complication of influenza, otitis media, or meningitis. In chronic otitis media, cholesteatoma formation erodes the bone of the labyrinth, allowing bacteria to enter from the middle ear. Ototoxic drugs (particularly aminoglycosides) or toxic drug ingestion are other possible causes of labyrinthitis. (See *Otitis media: Genetic link?* page 146.)

Signs and symptoms

Because the inner ear controls both hearing and balance, this infection typically produces severe vertigo (with any movement of the head) and sensorineural hearing loss. Vertigo begins gradually but peaks within 48 hours, causing loss of balance and falling in the direction of the affected ear. Other associated signs and symptoms include spontaneous nystagmus, with jerking movements of the eyes toward the unaffected ear; nausea, vomiting, and giddiness; with cholesteatoma, signs of middle ear disease; and with severe bacterial infection, purulent drainage. To minimize symptoms such as giddiness and nystagmus, the patient may assume a characteristic posture — lying on the side of the unaffected ear and looking in the direction of the affected ear.

Diagnosis

A typical clinical picture and history of upper respiratory tract infection suggest labyrinthitis. Common diagnostic measures include culture and sensitivity testing to identify the infecting microbe if purulent drainage is present, and audiometric testing. When an infectious etiology can't be found, additional testing must be done to rule out a brain lesion or Ménière's disease. Differential diagnoses include benign positional vertigo, vestibular neuronitis, Ménière's disease, acoustic neuroma and other tumors of the cerebellopontine angle, and basilar insufficiency.

Treatment

Symptomatic treatment includes bed rest, with the head immobilized between pillows; oral meclizine to control vertigo; and massive doses of antibiotics to combat diffuse purulent labyrinthitis. Oral fluids can prevent dehydration from vomiting; for severe nausea and vomiting, I.V. fluids may be necessary. When conservative management fails, surgical excision of the cholesteatoma and drainage of the infected areas of the middle and inner ear may be done.

 PREVENTION TIP Inform patients that labyrinthitis can be prevented by early and vigorous treatment of

OTITIS MEDIA: GENETIC LINK?

A study involving 168 same-sex twins and 7 triplet sets, recruited within the first two months of life, revealed that prolonged and recurrent episodes of otitis media may be genetically based. Further study will need to identify which genes are specifically implicated; however, identification could lead to earlier intervention and decrease the incidence of other diseases related to otitis media, such as labyrinthitis.

predisposing conditions, such as otitis media and any local or systemic infection. In patients with chronic or recurrent vertigo, exercise is an important therapeutic modality, and should be encouraged once nausea and vomiting recedes. Exercise augments the central nervous system's ability to compensate for labyrinthine dysfunction.

Special considerations
▶ Keep the side rails up to prevent falls.
▶ If vomiting is severe, administer antiemetics. Record intake and output, and give I.V. fluids as necessary.
▶ Tell the patient that recovery may take as long as 6 weeks. During this time, the patient should limit activities that vertigo may make hazardous.
▶ If recovery doesn't occur within 4 to 6 weeks, a computed tomography scan should be performed to rule out an intracranial lesion.

LARYNGITIS

A common disorder, laryngitis is acute or chronic inflammation of the vocal cords and is characterized by hoarseness. Acute laryngitis may occur as an isolated infection or as part of a generalized bacterial or viral upper respiratory tract infection. Repeated attacks of acute laryngitis cause inflammatory changes associated with chronic laryngitis.

Causes
Acute laryngitis usually results from infection (primarily viral) or excessive use of the voice, an occupational hazard in certain vocations (teaching, public speaking, singing), and occasionally allergy (hay fever). It may also result from leisure-time activities (such as cheering at a sporting event), inhalation of smoke or fumes, or aspiration of caustic chemicals. It may also be associated with group A streptococcus and *Moraxella catarrhalis*. Causes of *chronic laryngitis* include chronic upper respiratory tract disorders (sinusitis, bronchitis, nasal polyps, allergy); mouth breathing; smoking; constant exposure to dust or other irritants; and alcohol abuse.

 ALERT Chronic laryngitis due to infection is rare and requires prompt evaluation to rule out possible cancer-related causes.

Reflux laryngitis is caused by regurgitation of gastric acid into the hypopharynx. Carcinoma of the larynx, tumor-associated damage to the recurrent laryngeal nerve, and other serious conditions may be responsible.

Tuberculosis may also cause a form of laryngitis, and may be mistaken for laryngeal cancer. In this case, fever and night sweats are possible symptoms, with chest radiography revealing apical thickening and fibrosis. Biopsy reveals granulomas with acid-fast bacilli. The diagnosis is confirmed by culture and sensitivity testing.

Fungal infections causing laryngitis include histoplasmosis, blastomycosis, and candidiasis in immunocompromised patients or in those with chronic mucocutaneous candidiasis.

Signs and symptoms

Acute laryngitis typically begins with hoarseness, ranging from mild to complete loss of voice. Associated clinical features include pain (especially when swallowing or speaking), dry cough, fever, laryngeal edema, and malaise. In chronic laryngitis, persistent hoarseness is usually the only symptom. In reflux laryngitis, hoarseness and dysphagia are present but heartburn is not.

Diagnosis

The initial work-up and evaluation of the patient with hoarseness is guided by the chronicity of the condition, so a comprehensive history is essential, as is examination of the larynx. Indirect laryngoscopy with a head light and a warmed laryngeal mirror provides the quickest and best view of the hypopharynx and larynx. This may be difficult for the primary care provider, so referral to otolaryngology may be necessary. Hoarseness lasting more than 3 weeks without a history of acute infection warrants referral and further evaluation.

Indirect laryngoscopy confirms the diagnosis by revealing red, inflamed and, occasionally, hemorrhagic vocal cords, with round, rather than sharp, edges and exudate. Bilateral swelling may be present. In severe cases, or if toxicity is a concern, a culture of the exudate is obtained.

Other pertinent physical examination includes the oropharynx, thyroid, and cervical lymph nodes. If there is an unexplained neck mass or suspicious lymph node, careful evaluation may include assessment of thyroid-stimulating hormone if hypothyroidism is suspected, and small-needle biopsy of any questionable mass.

The differential diagnosis of hoarseness should be evaluated in terms of acute and chronic etiologies. Acute hoarseness differential diagnoses include acute laryngitis, acute laryngeal edema, and acute epiglottitis. Chronic hoarseness may point to chronic laryngitis (such as vocal abuse, allergy), laryngeal carcinoma, lesions of the vocal cords, trauma to the vocal cords, systemic disease (such as hypothyroidism, rheumatoid arthritis, virilization), or psychogenic disorder.

Treatment

Primary treatment consists of resting the voice. When required to speak, the patient should use a moderate voice and not whisper. Hot tea with sugar and lemon may be helpful. For viral infection, symptomatic care includes analgesics and throat lozenges for pain relief. Humidity (such as a hot steam shower, or breathing through a hot, moist towel) may also be beneficial. Occasionally, a vasoconstricting spray and analgesics are used by professionals when use of their voice is absolutely necessary. Bacterial infection requires antibiotic therapy. Severe, acute laryngitis may necessitate hospitalization. When laryngeal edema results in airway obstruction, tracheotomy may be necessary. In chronic laryngitis, effective treatment must eliminate the underlying cause. In reflux laryngitis, postural and dietary changes along with antacids and H_2 antagonists combine for effective treatment.

Special considerations

▶ Explain to the patient why he shouldn't talk, and place a sign over the bed to remind others of this restriction. Provide a Magic Slate or a pad and pencil for communication. Mark the intercom panel so other facility personnel are aware that the patient can't answer.
▶ Minimize the need to talk by trying to anticipate the patient's needs.
▶ Urge him to complete the course of prescribed antibiotics.
▶ Obtain a detailed patient history to help determine the cause of chronic laryngitis. Encourage modification of predisposing habits.

 PREVENTION TIP Suggest that the patient maintain adequate humidification by using a vaporizer or humidifier during the winter and by avoiding air conditioning during the summer (because it dehumidifies). Suggest using medicated throat lozenges.

 PREVENTION TIP If pertinent, all patients with hoarseness who smoke or chew tobacco should be strongly encouraged to quit.

LASSA FEVER

Lassa fever is an epidemic hemorrhagic fever caused by the Lassa virus, an extremely virulent arenavirus. As many as 100 cases occur annually in western Africa; the disease is rare in the United States. This highly fatal disorder kills 10% to 50% of its victims, but those who survive its early stages usually recover and acquire immunity to secondary attacks.

Causes

A chronic infection in rodents, Lassa virus is transmitted to humans by contact with infected rodent urine, feces, and saliva. (This is why Lassa fever sometimes strikes laboratory workers.) Then the virus enters the bloodstream, lymph vessels, and respiratory and digestive tracts. After this, it multiplies in cells of the reticuloendothelial system. In the early stages of this illness, when the virus is in the throat, human transmission may occur through inhalation of infected droplets.

Signs and symptoms

After a 7- to 18-day incubation period, this disease produces a fever that persists for 2 to 3 weeks, exudative pharyngitis, oral ulcers, lymphadenopathy with swelling of the face and neck, purpura, conjunctivitis, and bradycardia. Severe infection may also cause hepatitis, myocarditis, pleural infection, encephalitis, and permanent unilateral or bilateral deafness. Virus multiplication in reticuloendothelial cells causes capillary lesions that lead to erythrocyte and platelet loss, mild to moderate thrombocytopenia (with a tendency to bleeding), and secondary bacterial infection. Capillary lesions also cause focal hemorrhage in the stomach, small intestine, kidneys, lungs, and brain and, possibly, hemorrhagic shock and peripheral vascular collapse.

 ALERT To prevent the spread of this contagious disease, carefully dispose of or disinfect all materials contaminated with the infected patient's urine, feces, respiratory secretions, or exudates.

Diagnosis

Isolation of the Lassa virus from throat washings, pleural fluid, or blood confirms the diagnosis. Recent travel to an endemic area and specific antibody titer support the diagnosis. Differential diagnoses include malaria, shigellosis, typhoid, leptospirosis, and rickettsial disease.

Treatment

Treatment of Lassa fever includes I.V. ribavirin, I.V. colloids for shock, analgesics for pain, and antipyretics for fever.

Special considerations

▶ Carefully monitor fluid and electrolyte status, vital signs, and intake and output.
▶ Watch for and immediately report signs of infection or shock.
▶ Strict isolation is necessary for at least 3 weeks, until the patient's throat washings and urine are free from the virus. Watch known contacts closely for at least 3 weeks for signs of the disease.
▶ Provide good mouth care. Remember to clean the patient's mouth with a soft-bristled toothbrush to avoid irritating his mouth ulcers. Ask your facility's dietary department to supply a soft, bland, non-irritating diet.
▶ Immediately report all cases of Lassa fever to the public health authorities in your area.

 ALERT Immediately contact the Viral Diseases Division of the Centers for Disease Control and Prevention in Atlanta to get specific guidelines for managing suspected or confirmed cases of Lassa fever.

LEGIONNAIRES' DISEASE

An acute bronchopneumonia, Legionnaires' disease is produced by a fastidious gram-negative bacillus. It derives its name and notoriety from the peculiar, highly publicized disease that struck 182 people (29 of whom died) at an American Legion convention in Philadelphia in July of 1976. This disease may occur epidemically or sporadically, usually in late summer or early fall. Its severity ranges from a mild illness, with or without pneumonitis, to multilobar pneumonia with a mortality rate as high as 15%. A milder, self-limiting form (Pontiac syndrome) subsides within a few days but leaves the patient fatigued for several weeks; this form mimics Legionnaires' disease but produces few or no respiratory symptoms, no pneumonia, and no fatalities.

Cause

The causative agent of Legionnaires' disease, *Legionella pneumophila,* is an aerobic, gram-negative bacillus that is probably transmitted by an airborne route. In past epidemics, it has spread through cooling towers or evaporation condensers in air conditioning systems. However, *Legionella* bacilli also flourish in soil and excavation sites. The disease does not spread from person to person. Legionnaires' disease occurs more often in men than in women and is most likely to affect:

▶ middle-aged to elderly people
▶ immunocompromised patients (particularly those receiving corticosteroids; for example, after a transplant), or those with lymphoma or other disorders associated with delayed hypersensitivity
▶ patients with a chronic underlying disease, such as diabetes, chronic renal failure, or chronic obstructive pulmonary disease
▶ alcoholics
▶ cigarette smokers (three to four times more likely to develop Legionnaires' disease than nonsmokers).

Signs and symptoms

The multisystem clinical features of Legionnaires' disease follow a predictable sequence, although onset of the disease may be gradual or sudden. After a 2- to 10-day incubation period, nonspecific, prodromal signs and symptoms appear, including diarrhea, anorexia, malaise, diffuse myalgias and generalized weakness, headache, recurrent chills, and an unremitting fever, which develops within 12 to 48 hours with a temperature that may reach 105° F (40.5° C). A cough then develops that initially is nonproductive but eventually may produce grayish, nonpurulent and, occasionally, blood-streaked sputum. Other characteristic features include nausea, vomiting, disorientation, mental sluggishness, confusion, mild temporary amnesia, pleuritic chest pain, tachypnea, dyspnea, fine crackles and, in 50% of patients, bradycardia. Patients who develop pneumonia may also experience hypoxia. Other complications include hypotension, delirium, heart failure, dysrhythmias, acute respiratory failure, renal failure, and shock (usually fatal).

Diagnosis

The patient history focuses on possible sources of infection and predisposing conditions. In addition, a chest X-ray shows patchy, localized infiltration, which progresses to multilobar consolidation (usually involving the lower lobes), pleural effusion and, in fulminant disease, opacification of the entire lung. Auscultation reveals fine crackles, progressing to coarse crackles as the disease advances.

Abnormal test findings include leukocytosis, an increased erythrocyte sedimentation rate, an increase in liver enzyme levels (alanine aminotransferase, aspartate aminotransferase, alkaline phosphatase), hyponatremia, decreased PaO_2 and, initially, decreased $PaCO_2$. Bronchial washings, blood, pleural fluid, and sputum tests rule out other infections.

Definitive tests include direct immunofluorescence of respiratory tract secretions and tissue, a culture of *L. pneumophila*, and indirect fluorescent antibody testing of serum comparing acute samples with convalescent samples drawn at least 3 weeks later. A urine specimen for *L. pneumophila* antigen may also be performed. A convalescent serum showing a fourfold or greater rise in antibody titer for *Legionella* confirms this diagnosis.

Differential diagnoses for Legionnaires' disease includes other atypical pneumonias caused by organisms such as *Chlamydia pneumoniae, C. psittaci, Mycoplasma pneumoniae,* and *Coxiella burnetti.*

Treatment

Antibiotic treatment begins as soon as Legionnaires' disease is suspected and diagnostic material is collected.

 ALERT Practitioners shouldn't wait for laboratory confirmation before beginning antibiotic therapy.

Erythromycin is the drug of choice, but if it's not effective alone, rifampin can be added to the regimen. If erythromycin is contraindicated, rifampin or rifampin with tetracycline may be used. Supportive therapy includes administration of antipyretics, fluid replacement, circulatory support with pressor drugs if necessary, and oxygen administration by mask, cannula, or mechanical ventilation.

Special considerations

▶ Closely monitor the patient's respiratory status. Evaluate chest wall expansion, depth and pattern of respirations, cough, and chest pain.

▶ Watch for restlessness, which may indicate that the patient is hypoxemic and requires suctioning, repositioning, or more aggressive oxygen therapy.

▶ Continually monitor the patient's vital signs, pulse oximetry or arterial blood gas values, level of consciousness, and dryness and color of the lips and mucous membranes. Watch for signs of shock (decreased blood pressure, thready pulse, diaphoresis, clammy skin).

▶ Keep the patient comfortable; avoid chills and exposure to drafts. Provide mouth care frequently. If necessary, apply soothing cream to the nostrils.

▶ Replace fluid and electrolytes as needed. The patient with renal failure may require dialysis.

▶ Provide mechanical ventilation and other respiratory therapy as needed. Teach the patient how to cough effectively, and encourage deep-breathing exercises. Stress the need to continue these measures until recovery is complete.

▶ Give antibiotics as necessary, and observe carefully for adverse effects.

LEISHMANIASIS

Prevalent on four continents, leishmaniasis refers to various clinical syndromes caused by a vector-borne protozoan and characterized by cutaneous lesions, weight loss, cough, fever, diarrhea, lethargy, and splenomegaly. It's endemic to subtropical countries, particularly those undergoing economic development and man-made environmental changes. Previously regarded as a rural disease, outbreaks of leishmaniasis have been reported in large cities and suburbs of Brazil due to favorable epidemiological conditions, malnutrition, poor sanitation, and population migration.

While leishmaniasis is associated with low mortality, it has a high morbidity rate. It is estimated that 350 million people are exposed to the disease and approximately 12 million are afflicted worldwide. The global annual incidence is estimated at 1.5 to 2 million new cases per year; however, it's now generally accepted that leishmaniasis is grossly underreported. It's considered to be an emerging disease in developed countries, where Leishmaniasis/human immunodeficiency virus (HIV) co-infection is becoming more prevalent due to the acquired immunodeficiency syndrome (AIDS) pandemic and expanded international travel.

Causes

Leishmania, responsible for human leishmaniasis, is a genus of protozoans that have a dimorphic life cycle. They occur in mononuclear phagocytes in the body's defense system and multiply intracellularly, resulting in lysis of host cells and infection of other phagocytes. *Leishmania* has also been located in macrophages throughout the reticuloendothelial system in cases of visceral leishmaniasis. Macrophages in skin lesions reveal *Leishmania* in cutaneous leishmaniasis.

Leishmaniasis is transmitted by small, biting sand flies, which are infected with *Leishmania* and inhabit moist soil, forests, caves, and rodent burrows. Although small rodents and mammals, dogs, foxes, chickens, horses, and humans serve as host reservoirs, the domestic dog is considered to be the principal reservoir. The protozoan is transmitted from one mammalian host to another by the bite of the sand fly, an avid feeder. It strikes humans primarily at night. Fast urbanization, invasion of primary forests, dramatic reductions in the vector's natural ecological space, drought, famine, poor sanitation, overcrowding, and the practice of harboring animal hosts, particularly dogs, close to human domiciles are among the main causes of exposure to and subsequent infection by the *Leishmania* vector.

Signs and symptoms

Leishmaniasis can be divided into four major clinical forms: cutaneous leishmaniasis (CL), mucocutaneous leishmaniasis (ML), diffuse cutaneous leishmaniasis (DCL), and visceral leishmaniasis (VL). Additionally, the first three forms are further classified as New World or Old World, depending on the clinical presentation, species of infective parasite, and geographic location.

Cutaneous leishmaniasis, the most common form of infection, manifests as single or multiple ulcerating papules which heal after a few weeks or months, leaving flat, atrophic scars. Regional lymphadenopathy usually accompanies the lesions; fever, malaise, anorexia, and weight loss may also occur. The incubation period for CL may range from two weeks to several months. Resistance to reinfection by the same species of protozoa often occurs.

Mucocutaneous leishmaniasis begins with simple cutaneous lesions which progress to form hideously disfiguring lesions of the nose, mouth or pharynx months or years after primary cutaneous infection. ML is responsible for soft tissue, cartilage, and bone destruction, which can lead to nasal obstruction, congestion, discharge, or epistaxis.

Diffuse cutaneous leishmaniasis, which closely resembles leprosy and is the most difficult to treat, is the anergic variant of CL. It is characterized by large numbers of parasites in multiple, ulcerating nodules found on the face and extremities. The syndrome may persist for more than 20 years, as the body fails to mount a cell-mediated immune response.

Left untreated, *visceral leishmaniasis* is the deadliest form of *Leishmania.* VL leishmaniasis symptoms include diarrhea, hepatosplenomegaly, lethargy, weight loss, cough, and fever. Some or all of these symptoms may be present, giving the disease a wide range of presentations. In general, symptoms manifest in three to eight months; however, incubation may occur in as little as ten days or extend as long as 34 months. Onset of symptoms may be sudden or gradual.

Diagnosis

Diagnosis of all forms of leishmaniasis is most accurately accomplished via staining and identification of the parasite from specimens obtained from skin punch biopsy or scrapings from the base of an ulcer, spleen and bone marrow aspirates, and lymph node biopsy. Specific antibodies may be detected via the indirect immunofluorescent test (IFAT), the enzyme-linked immunosorbent assay (ELISA), and

NEW TREATMENTS FOR LEISHMANIASIS

Investigational drugs for the treatment of cutaneous leishmaniasis include using interleukin-2 in combination with pentavalent antimony, and using cytokines, such as granulocyte macrophage colony-stimulating factor (GM-CSF) and interleukin-12, as vaccine adjuvants. Topical and intralesional treatments are also being studied.

the direct agglutination test (DAT). Occasionally, skin testing with leishmanial antigens may be employed. Polymerase chain reaction has proven to be highly sensitive and specific as well. Staining tissue with monoclonal antibodies is species-specific; however, it is available only in research laboratories.

The differential diagnoses to consider include: sporotrichosis, chromomycosis, lobomycosis, cutaneous tuberculosis, atypical mycobacterial infection, syphilis, yaws, leprosy, sarcoidosis, neoplasm, malaria, typhoid fever, typhus, acute Chagas' disease, acute schistosomiasis, miliary tuberculosis, amebic liver abscess, brucellosis, histoplasmosis, infectious mononucleosis, leukemia, lymphoma, agnogenic myeloid metaplasia, hepatosplenic schistomiasis, prolonged *Salmonella* bacteremia, and tropical splenomegaly from chronic malaria. Leishmaniasis can be safely excluded from those who are not international travelers or immigrants of endemic areas.

Treatment
Pentavalent antimonial compounds are the drugs of choice for treating visceral and cutaneous leishmaniasis. The drug must be obtained from the Drug Service of the Centers for Disease Control and Prevention (CDC). It is administered I.M. or I.V. over a 5- to 28-day period, depending on the type of leishmaniasis as well as the presence of drug-related signs of toxicity. Amphotericin B is employed in cases of resistant strains of VL. Pentamidine is considered a second-line agent, due to increasing resistance and prolonged course of therapy. (See *New treatments for leishmaniasis.*)

Special considerations
❱ Monitor skin lesions for signs and symptoms of bacterial infection.
❱ Utilize appropriate personal protective gear.
❱ Instruct patients to avoid touching skin lesions to avoid complications.
❱ Monitor for adverse effects of pentavalent antimonial agents, such as arthralgia, myalgia, nausea, vomiting, abdominal pain, headache, rash, pancreatitis, anemia, leukopenia, thrombocytopenia, and renal insufficiency.
❱ Monitor weekly transaminase, lipase, complete blood count (CBC), and creatinine levels. Transaminase levels greater than or equal to 4 to 5 times the upper limits of normal necessitate discontinuation of pentavalent antimonial therapy.
❱ Monitor weekly electrocardiograms for QT interval prolongation, T-wave inversions, or significant dysrhythmia with pentavalent antimonials.
❱ Observe for adverse effects of amphotericin therapy, which include nausea, vomiting, malaise, anemia, hypokalemia, hypomagnesemia, and nephrotoxicity. Be prepared to monitor frequent CBCs, potassium and magnesium levels, and blood urea nitrogen and creatinine levels.
❱ Monitor the patient for side effects of pentamidine therapy, which include hypoglycemia followed by diabetes, hypotension with too rapid infusion, nausea, vomiting, abdominal pain, and headache.
❱ Be prepared to provide emotional support for coinfected HIV/VL patients as their prognosis is poor.

PREVENTION TIP In the absence of prophylactic drug treatment for leishmaniasis, the best treatment is prevention. Instruct travelers to endemic areas to minimize sand fly exposure by avoiding outdoor activities when sand flies are most active (dusk to dawn); covering all exposed skin with netting; applying repellants such as DEET, lemon essential oils, or 2% neem oil to the skin and under the edges of clothing; and using permethrin-impregnated clothing.

LEPROSY

Leprosy, also known as Hansen's disease, is a chronic, systemic infection characterized by progressive cutaneous lesions. Leprosy occurs in three distinct forms:

▶ *Lepromatous leprosy,* the most serious type, causes damage to the upper respiratory tract, eyes, and testes as well as the nerves and skin.

▶ *Tuberculoid leprosy* affects peripheral nerves and sometimes the surrounding skin, especially on the face, arms, legs, and buttocks.

▶ *Borderline (dimorphous) leprosy* has characteristics of both lepromatous and tuberculoid leprosies. Skin lesions in this type of leprosy are diffuse and poorly defined.

Causes

Leprosy is caused by *Mycobacterium leprae,* an acid-fast bacillus that attacks cutaneous tissue and peripheral nerves, producing skin lesions, anesthesia, infection, and deformities. Contrary to popular belief, leprosy is not highly contagious but actually has a low rate of infectivity. Continuous, close contact is needed to transmit it. In fact, 9 out of 10 persons have a natural immunity to it. Susceptibility appears highest during childhood and seems to decrease with age. Presumably, transmission occurs through airborne respiratory droplets containing *M. leprae* or by inoculation through skin breaks (with a contaminated hypodermic or tattoo needle, for example). The incubation period is unusually long — 6 months to 8 years. Leprosy is most prevalent in the underdeveloped areas of Asia (especially India and China), Africa, South America, and the islands of the Caribbean and Pacific. About 11 million people worldwide suffer from this disease; approximately 4,000 are in the United States, mostly in California, Texas, Louisiana, Florida, New York, and Hawaii.

Signs and symptoms

M. leprae attacks the peripheral nervous system, especially the ulnar, radial, posterior-popliteal, anterior-tibial, and facial nerves. The central nervous system appears highly resistant. When the bacilli damage the skin's fine nerves, they cause anesthesia, anhidrosis, and dryness; if they attack a large nerve trunk, motor nerve damage, weakness, and pain occur, followed by peripheral anesthesia, muscle paralysis, or atrophy.

In later stages, clawhand, footdrop, and ocular complications — such as corneal insensitivity and ulceration, conjunctivitis, photophobia, and blindness — can occur. Injury, ulceration, infection, and disuse of deformed parts cause scarring and contracture. Neurologic complications occur in both lepromatous and tuberculoid leprosy but are less extensive and develop more slowly in the lepromatous form. Lepromatous leprosy can invade tissue in virtually every organ of the body, but the organs generally remain functional.

The lepromatous and tuberculoid forms affect the skin in markedly different ways. In lepromatous disease, early lesions are multiple, symmetrical, and erythematous, sometimes appearing as macules or papules with smooth surfaces. Later, they enlarge and form plaques or nodules called lepromas on the earlobes, nose, eyebrows, and forehead, giving the patient a characteristic leonine appearance. In advanced stages, *M. leprae* may infiltrate the entire skin surface. Lepromatous leprosy also causes loss of eyebrows, eyelashes, and sebaceous and sweat gland function; and, in advanced stages, conjunctival and scleral nodules. Upper respiratory lesions cause epistaxis, ulceration of the uvula and tonsils, septal perforation, and nasal collapse. Lepromatous leprosy can lead to hepatosplenomegaly and orchitis. Fingertips and toes deteriorate as bone resorption follows trauma and infection in these insensitive areas.

When tuberculoid leprosy affects the skin (sometimes its effect is strictly neural), it produces raised, large, erythematous plaques or macules with clearly defined borders. As they grow, they become rough, hairless, hypopigmented, and leave anesthetic scars.

In borderline leprosy, skin lesions are numerous, but smaller, less anesthetic, and less sharply defined than tuberculoid lesions. Untreated, borderline leprosy may deteriorate into lepromatous disease.

Occasionally, acute episodes intensify leprosy's slowly progressing course. Whether such exacerbations are part of the disease process or a reaction to therapy remains controversial. Erythema nodosum leprosum (ENL), seen in lepromatous leprosy, produces fever, malaise, lymphadenopathy, and painful red skin nodules, usually during antimicrobial treatment, although it may occur in untreated people. In Mexico and other Central American countries, some patients with lepromatous disease develop Lucio's phenomenon, which produces generalized punched-out ulcers that may extend into muscle and fascia. Leprosy may also lead to tuberculosis, malaria, secondary bacterial infection of skin ulcers, and amyloidosis.

Diagnosis

Early clinical indications of skin lesions and muscular and neurologic deficits are usually sufficiently diagnostic in patients from endemic areas. Biopsies of skin lesions are also diagnostic. Biopsies of peripheral nerves or smears of the skin or of ulcerated mucous membranes help confirm the diagnosis. Blood tests show increased erythrocyte sedimentation rate; decreased albumin, calcium, and cholesterol levels; and, possibly, anemia. Differential diagnoses include many skin and systemic diseases, such as lupus erythematosus, lupus vulgaris, sarcoidosis, yaws, and dermal leishmaniasis.

Treatment

Treatment consists of antimicrobial therapy using sulfones, primarily oral dapsone, which may cause hypersensitivity reactions.

 ALERT Hepatitis and exfoliative dermatitis, although uncommon, are especially dangerous reactions. If these reactions do occur, sulfone therapy should be stopped immediately.

Failure to respond to sulfones or the occurrence of respiratory involvement or other complications requires alternative therapy, such as rifampin in combination with clofazimine or ethionamide. Clawhand, wristdrop, or footdrop may require surgical correction.

When a patient's disease becomes inactive, as determined by the morphologic and bacterial index, treatment is discontinued according to the following schedule: tuberculoid, 3 years; borderline, depends on the severity of the disease but may be as long as 10 years; lepromatous, lifetime therapy.

Because ENL is commonly considered to be a sign that the patient is responding to treatment, antimicrobial therapy should be continued. Thalidomide and clofazimine have been used successfully to treat ENL at the National Hansen's Disease Center (NHDC); however, this treatment requires a signed consent form and strict adherence to established NHDC protocols. Corticosteroids may also be given as part of ENL therapy. With timely and correct treatment, leprosy has a good prognosis and is seldom fatal. Untreated, however, it can cause severe disability. The lepromatous type may lead to blindness and deformities.

Any patient suspected of having leprosy may be referred to the Gillis W. Long Hansen's Disease Center in Carville, Louisiana, or to a regional center. At this international research and educational center, patients undergo diagnostic studies and treatment and are educated about their disease. Patients are encouraged to return home as soon as their medical condition permits. The federal government pays the full cost of their medical and nursing care.

Special considerations

Patient care is supportive and consists of measures to control acute infection, prevent complications, speed rehabilitation and recovery, and provide psychological support.

▶ Give antipyretics, analgesics, and sedatives, as needed. Watch for and report ENL or Lucio's phenomenon.

▶ Use proper infection precautions when handling clothing or articles that have been in contact with open skin lesions.

▶ Patients with borderline or lepromatous leprosy may suffer associated eye complications, such as iridocyclitis and glaucoma. Decreased corneal sensation and lacrimation may also occur, requiring patients to use a tear substitute daily and protect their eyes to prevent corneal irritation and ulceration.

▶ Stress the importance of adequate nutrition and rest. Watch for fatigue, jaundice, and other signs of anemia and hepatitis.

▶ Tell the patient to be careful not to injure an anesthetized leg by putting too much weight on it. Advise testing bath water carefully to prevent scalding. To prevent ulcerations, suggest the use of sturdy footwear and soaking feet in warm water after any kind of exercise, even a short walk. Advise rubbing the feet with petroleum jelly, oil, or lanolin.

▶ For patients with deformities, an interdisciplinary rehabilitation program employing a physiotherapist and plastic surgeon may be necessary. Teach the patient and help him with prescribed therapies.

▶ Provide emotional support throughout treatment. Communicating accurate information about leprosy to the general public, and especially to health care professionals, is a function of primary importance for the entire staff at the NHDC.

 PREVENTION TIP Although leprosy isn't highly contagious, take precautions against the possible spread of infection. Tell patients to cover coughs or sneezes with a paper tissue and to dispose of it properly.

LEPTOSPIROSIS

First isolated in 1916 by a team of Japanese researchers, Leptospirosis is a group of bacterial diseases caused by antigenically distinct members of the bacteria *Leptospira interogans*. It is also known as Red Water Disease in cattle, and Weil's or Swineherd's disease in humans. It is primarily an animal pathogen, affecting both domestic and wild animals, and causes significant losses in the livestock industry. In humans, leptospirosis causes a flu-like illness ranging in severity from asymptomatic to fatal. Leptospirosis is the most widespread zoonotic disease in the world. In the United States, approximately 100 to 200 cases are identified annually; of these, 50% occur in Hawaii. The disease tends to occur most often in the summer and early autumn months. Those most likely to suffer infection include farmers, sewer workers, veterinarians, commercial fishery workers, dairy and pig farmers, military personnel, slaughterhouse workers, and meat inspectors. Campers and those who participate in outdoor sports, particularly if water is involved, are also at risk in contaminated areas.

Causes

Leptospire organisms tend to thrive in the kidneys and are released through urination, resulting in transmission of the microbes to humans and animals. Human exposure to leptospirosis occurs primarily through recreational swimming in urine-contaminated water and by occupational exposure to infected animal urine. The mucous membranes of the eye, nose, and mouth, as well as abraded skin, serve as portals of entry. Leptospires can survive several weeks outside the body in moist, alkaline soil and in stagnant or slow-moving, slightly alkaline water.

Signs and symptoms

The time between exposure and manifestation of clinical symptoms varies from two days to four weeks. Initial symptoms include abrupt onset of fever, headache, muscle aches, vomiting, conjunctivitis, and weakness. Diarrhea, abdominal pain, jaundice, and hemorrhagic rash may also be present. Symptoms typically last four to seven days, though some patients may be asymptomatic. The disease is often biphasic. If a second phase occurs it is more severe; kidney or liver failure, vasculitis, or meningitis complicates recovery. This phase, known as Weil's disease, accounts for approximately 10% of leptospirosis cases and can be fatal. Illness may last three or more weeks with treatment and several months without treatment.

Diagnosis

Diagnosis is based upon a combination of clinical signs and laboratory tests. Microscopically, leptospirosis is an aerobic, gram-negative spirochete tightly coiled around an axial filament. These motile spirochetes are often bent at one or both ends, producing a hook-like appearance. Examination of body fluids and tissues under dark-field microscopy, utilizing Warthin-Starry or Geimsa stains, will reveal the leptospire spirochete. Fluorescent antibody and microscopic and macroscopic agglutination tests are serologic methods of detection. Blood, cerebrospinal fluid, urine, or tissues can be successfully cultured during, or immediately after, the acute phase of the disease. Differential diagnoses include influenza, malaria, rickettsial disease, dengue, viral gastroenteritis, bacterial enteritis, or nephritis; aseptic, viral, or bacterial meningitis; and hepatitis. The variability of the signs and symptoms and the biphasic nature of the disease may complicate the differential diagnosis.

Treatment

Pharmacological treatment is accomplished with antibiotics such as doxycycline, penicillin, and streptomycin during the acute phase of the illness. For severe cases, I.V. penicillin is the recommended treatment. Fluid therapy to prevent dehydration and electrolyte imbalances may be required. In severe cases, dialysis and life-support measures may be instituted. Prophylactic therapy consists of doxycycline 200 mg once weekly, beginning one week prior to anticipated exposure.

Special considerations

▶ Although human-to-human transmission has not been documented, gloves should be worn when handling body fluids, particularly urine. Teach the patient to thoroughly wash hands after toileting.
▶ Intake and output should be accurately monitored and adequate hydration maintained.
▶ Monitor laboratory test results, such as blood urea nitrogen, creatinine, liver function tests, and bleeding times.
▶ Nationally, leptospirosis is not currently a reportable disease, although several states, including Hawaii, do require the reporting of suspected cases for surveillance purposes. Contact your state department of health for updates involving reportable diseases. An emerging trend is

the association of leptospirosis with flooding and urbanization.

▶ Recovery from leptospirosis confers immunity to that particular serovar; however, Leptospirosis serovars number 183.

▶ Patients who have been infected with leptospirosis should not donate blood for at least twelve months after recovery.

 PREVENTION TIP Advise persons at risk for occupational exposure to prevent infection by using waterproof aprons, gloves, and boots. Additionally, any breaks in the skin should be sealed with waterproof dressings; the dressing should be replaced after known or suspected contamination. Good personal hygiene, with particular attention to the faces of those with beards or mustaches, should be practiced. Advise those at risk for infection via recreational exposure to avoid swimming in stock ponds or slow-moving streams frequented by domestic or wild animals. Warn domestic pet owners to contain their pets away from pools, marshes, and streams. Advise them to consult their veterinarians regarding immunizing pets against leptospire infection in areas where the spirochete is present.

LISTERIOSIS

Listeriosis is an infection caused by the weakly hemolytic, gram-positive bacillus *Listeria monocytogenes*. It occurs most commonly in fetuses, in neonates (during the first 3 weeks of life), older patients, or immunosuppressed adults. The infected fetus is usually stillborn or is born prematurely, almost always with lethal listeriosis. This infection produces milder illness in pregnant women and varying degrees of illness in older and immunosuppressed patients; their prognoses depend on the severity of underlying illness.

Causes

The primary method of person-to-person transmission is neonatal infection in utero (through the placenta) or during passage through an infected birth canal. Other modes of transmission may include inhaling contaminated dust; drinking contaminated, unpasteurized milk; and coming in contact with infected animals, contaminated sewage or mud, or soil contaminated with feces containing *L. monocytogenes*.

 PREVENTION TIP Dietary recommendations for prevention of food-borne listeriosis include:

▶ Thoroughly cooking all raw food from animal sources

▶ Keeping uncooked meats separate from vegetables and from cooked, ready-to-eat foods

▶ Washing raw vegetables thoroughly

▶ Avoiding raw, unpasteurized milk

▶ Washing hands, cutting boards, and knives after handling uncooked foods.

Signs and symptoms

Contact with *L. monocytogenes* commonly causes a transient asymptomatic carrier state, though sometimes it produces bacteremia and a febrile, generalized illness. In pregnant women, especially during the third trimester, listeriosis causes a mild illness with malaise, chills, fever, and back pain. However, the fetus may suffer severe uterine infection, abortion, premature delivery, or stillbirth. Transplacental infection may also cause early neonatal death or granulomatosis infantiseptica, which produces organ abscesses in infants. Infection with *L. monocytogenes* commonly causes meningitis, resulting in tense fontanels, irritability, lethargy, seizures, and coma in neonates, and low-grade fever and personality changes in adults. Fulminant manifestations with coma are rare.

Diagnosis

L. monocytogenes is identified by its diagnostic tumbling motility on a wet mount of the culture. Other supportive diagnostic results include positive culture of blood, spinal fluid, drainage from cervical or vaginal lesions, or lochia from a mother with an infected infant, but isolation of the organism from these specimens is generally difficult. Listeriosis also causes monocytosis. Differential diagnoses include group B streptococcus infections, congenital syphilis, and toxoplasmosis.

Treatment

The treatment of choice is ampicillin or penicillin I.V. for 3 to 6 weeks, possibly with gentamicin to increase its effectiveness. Alternate treatments include erythromycin, chloramphenicol, tetracycline, or co-trimoxazole.

Ampicillin or penicillin G is best for treating meningitis due to *L. monocytogenes* because these antibiotics more easily cross the blood-brain barrier.

 ALERT Pregnant women require prompt, vigorous treatment to combat fetal infection.

Special considerations

▶ Deliver specimens to the laboratory promptly. Because few microbes may be present, take at least 10 ml of spinal fluid for culture.

▶ Use secretion precautions until a series of cultures are negative. Be especially careful when handling lochia from an infected mother and secretions from her infant's eyes, nose, mouth, and rectum, including meconium.

▶ Evaluate neurologic status at least every 2 hours. In an infant, check fontanels for bulging. Maintain adequate I.V. fluid intake; measure intake and output accurately.

▶ If the patient has central nervous system depression and becomes apneic, provide respiratory assistance, monitor respirations, and obtain frequent arterial blood gas measurements.

▶ Provide adequate nutrition by total parenteral nutrition, nasogastric tube feedings, or a soft diet, as ordered.

▶ Allow parents to see and, if possible, hold their infant in the intensive care unit. Be flexible about visiting privileges. Keep parents informed of the infant's status and prognosis at all times.

▶ Reassure parents of an infected newborn who may feel guilty about the infant's illness.

 PREVENTION TIP Educate pregnant women to avoid infective materials on farms where listeriosis is endemic among livestock.

LIVER ABSCESS

A liver abscess occurs when bacteria or protozoa destroy hepatic tissue, producing a cavity, which fills with infectious organisms, liquefied liver cells, and leukocytes. Necrotic tissue then walls off the cavity from the rest of the liver. Liver abscess occurs equally in men and women, usually in those over age 50. Death occurs in 15% of affected patients despite treatment.

Causes

Underlying causes of liver abscess include benign or malignant biliary obstruction along with cholangitis, extrahepatic abdominal sepsis, and trauma or surgery to the right upper quadrant. Liver abscesses also occur from intra-arterial chemoembolizations or cryosurgery in the liver, which causes necrosis of tumor cells and potential infection.

The method by which bacteria reach the liver reflects the underlying causes. Biliary tract disease is the most common cause of liver abscess. Liver abscess after intra-abdominal sepsis (such as with diverticulitis) is most likely to be caused by hematogenous spread through the portal bloodstream. Hematogenous spread by hepatic arterial flow may occur in infectious endocarditis.

Abscesses arising from hematogenous transmission are usually caused by a single pathogen; those arising from biliary obstruction are usually caused by a mixed flora. Patients with metastatic cancer to the liver, diabetes mellitus, and alcoholism are more likely to develop a liver abscess.

The organisms that predominate in liver abscess are gram-negative aerobic bacilli, enterococci, streptococci, and anaerobes. Amebic liver abscesses are caused by *E. histolytica.*

Signs and symptoms

The clinical manifestations of a liver abscess depend on the degree of involvement. Some patients are acutely ill; in others, the abscess is recognized only at autopsy, after death from another illness.

The onset of symptoms of a pyogenic abscess is usually sudden; in an amebic abscess, the onset is more insidious. Common signs include abdominal pain, weight loss, fever, chills, diaphoresis, nausea, vomiting, and anemia. Signs of right pleural effusion, such as dyspnea and pleural pain, develop if the abscess extends through the diaphragm. Liver damage may cause jaundice.

Diagnosis

Ultrasonography and computed tomography (CT) scan with contrast medium can accurately define intrahepatic lesions and allow assessment of intra-abdominal pathology. Percutaneous needle aspiration of the abscess can also be performed with diagnostic tests to identify the causative organism. Contrast-aided magnetic resonance imaging may become an accurate method for diagnosing hepatic abscesses.

Abnormal laboratory values include: elevated levels of serum aspartate aminotransferase, alanine aminotransferase, alkaline phosphatase, and bilirubin; an increased white blood cell count; and decreased serum albumin levels. In pyogenic abscess, a blood culture can identify the bacterial agent; in amebic abscess, a stool culture and serologic and hemagglutination tests can isolate *E. histolytica.*

Treatment

 ALERT Before the causative organism is identified, antibiotics should be started to treat aerobic gram-negative bacilli, streptococci, and anaerobic bacilli, including *Bacteroides* species.

Antibiotic therapy, along with drainage, is the preferred treatment for most hepatic abscesses. Percutaneous drainage, either with ultrasound or CT guidance, is usually sufficient to evacuate pus. Surgery may be performed to drain pus in unstable patients with continued sepsis (despite attempted nonsurgical treatment) and for patients with persistent fevers (lasting longer than 2 weeks) after percutaneous drainage and appropriate antibiotic therapy. A common combination is ampicillin, an aminoglycoside, and either metronidazole or clindamycin. Third-generation cephalosporins can be substituted for the aminoglycosides in patients at risk for renal toxicity. When the causative organisms are identified, the antibiotic regimen should be modified to match the patient's sensitivities. I.V. antibiotics should be administered for 14 days and then replaced with oral preparations to complete a 6-week course. Surgery is reserved for bowel perforation and rupture into the pericardium.

Special considerations

▶ Provide supportive care, monitor vital signs (especially temperature), and maintain fluid and nutritional intake.

▶ Administer anti-infectives and antibiotics as necessary, and watch for possible adverse effects. Stress the importance of compliance with therapy.

▶ Explain diagnostic and surgical procedures.

▶ Watch carefully for complications of abdominal surgery, such as hemorrhage or sepsis.

▶ Prepare the patient for I.V. antibiotic administration as an outpatient with home care support.

LUNG ABSCESS

A lung abscess is a lung infection accompanied by pus accumulation and tissue destruction. The abscess may be putrid (due to anaerobic bacteria) or nonputrid (due to anaerobes or aerobes), and often has a well-defined border. The availability of effective antibiotics has made lung abscesses much less common than they were in the past.

Causes

A lung abscess is a manifestation of necrotizing pneumonia, often the result of aspiration of oropharyngeal contents. Poor oral hygiene with dental or gingival (gum) disease is strongly associated with a putrid lung abscess. Septic pulmonary emboli commonly produce cavitary lesions. Infected cystic lung lesions and cavitating bronchial carcinoma must be distinguished from lung abscesses.

 PREVENTION TIP To prevent a lung abscess in the unconscious patient and the patient with seizures, first prevent aspiration of secretions. Do this by suctioning the patient and by positioning him to promote drainage of secretions.

Signs and symptoms

The clinical effects of lung abscess include a cough that may produce bloody, purulent, or foul-smelling sputum; pleuritic chest pain; dyspnea; excessive sweating; chills; fever; headache; malaise; diaphoresis; and weight loss. Complications include rupture into the pleural space, which results in empyema and, rarely, massive hemorrhage. A chronic lung abscess may cause localized bronchiectasis. Failure of an abscess to improve with antibiotic treatment suggests a possible underlying neoplasm or other causes of obstruction.

Diagnosis

The following tests are used to diagnose a lung abscess:
▶ Auscultation of the chest may reveal crackles and decreased breath sounds.
▶ Chest X-ray shows a localized infiltrate with one or more clear spaces, usually containing air-fluid levels.
▶ Percutaneous aspiration of an abscess or bronchoscopy may be used to obtain cultures to identify the causative organism. Bronchoscopy is only used if abscess resolution is eventful and the patient's condition permits it.
▶ Blood cultures, Gram stain, and culture of sputum are also used to detect the causative organism.
▶ White blood cell count commonly exceeds 10,000/μl.

Treatment

Antibiotic therapy often lasts for months until radiographic resolution or definite stability occurs. Clindamycin is often the drug of choice. Symptoms usually disappear in a few weeks. Postural drainage may facilitate discharge of necrotic material into upper airways, where expectoration is possible; oxygen therapy may relieve hypoxemia. A poor response to therapy may require resection of the lesion or removal of the diseased section of the lung but is not considered routine due to the possibility of infectious spread. All patients need rigorous follow-up and serial chest X-rays.

Special considerations

▶ Provide chest physiotherapy (including coughing and deep breathing).
▶ Increase fluid intake to loosen secretions, and provide a quiet, restful atmosphere.

LYME DISEASE

A multisystem disorder, Lyme disease is caused by the spirochete *Borrelia burgdorferi*, which is carried by the minute tick

Ixodes scapularis or another tick in the Ixodidae family. It often begins in the summer with the classic skin lesion called erythema chronicum migrans (ECM). Weeks or months later, cardiac or neurologic abnormalities sometimes develop, possibly followed by arthritis. Initially, Lyme disease was identified in a group of children in Lyme, Connecticut. Now Lyme disease is known to occur primarily in three parts of the United States:

▶ in the northeast, from Massachusetts to Maryland

▶ in the Midwest, in Wisconsin and Minnesota

▶ in the west, in California and Oregon.

Although Lyme disease is endemic to these areas, cases have been reported in 43 states and 20 other countries, including Germany, Switzerland, France, and Australia.

Causes

Lyme disease occurs when a tick injects spirochete-laden saliva into the bloodstream or deposits fecal matter on the skin. After incubating for 3 to 32 days, the spirochetes migrate out to the skin, causing ECM. Then they disseminate to other skin sites or organs by the bloodstream or lymph system. The spirochetes' life cycle isn't completely clear; they may survive for years in the joints or they may trigger an inflammatory response in the host and then die.

Signs and symptoms

Typically, Lyme disease has three stages.

Stage 1

ECM heralds stage 1 with a red macule or papule, often at the site of a tick bite. This lesion usually feels hot and itchy and may grow to more than 20" (50 cm) in diameter. Within a few days, more lesions may erupt along with a malar rash, conjunctivitis, or diffuse urticaria. In 3 to 4 weeks, lesions are replaced by small red blotches, which persist for several more

> ### DEVELOPING TESTS FOR LYME DISEASE
>
> The National Institute of Allergy and Infectious Diseases (NIAID) is testing an extremely sensitive, rapid enzyme-linked immunosorbent assay test, which could provide for a quicker and more reliable diagnosis of suspected Lyme disease cases. Researchers also hope to develop a procedure that will distinguish among people with active *B. burgdorferi* infection, those who have received the Lymerix vaccine, and those who have recovered from a previous infection.

weeks. Malaise and fatigue are constant, but other findings are intermittent: headache, fever, chills, and regional lymphadenopathy. Less common effects are meningeal irritation, mild encephalopathy, migrating musculoskeletal pain, and hepatitis. A persistent sore throat and dry cough may appear several days before ECM.

Stage 2

Weeks to months later, the second stage begins with neurologic abnormalities — fluctuating meningoencephalitis with peripheral and cranial neuropathy — that usually resolve after days or months. Facial palsy is especially noticeable. Cardiac abnormalities, such as a brief, fluctuating atrioventricular heart block, may also develop.

Stage 3

Characterized by arthritis, stage 3 begins weeks or years later. Migrating musculoskeletal pain leads to frank arthritis with marked swelling, especially in the large joints. Recurrent attacks may precede

LYME DISEASE TREATMENT IN TRIALS

The National Institutes of Health (NIH) is conducting two Phase III trials to determine the efficacy of ceftriaxone and doxycycline in treating chronic Lyme disease. One study involves seropositive patients and the other involves seronegative patients.

chronic arthritis with severe cartilage and bone erosion.

Diagnosis

Because isolation of *B. burgdorferi* is unusual in humans and because indirect immunofluorescent antibody tests are marginally sensitive, diagnosis often rests on the characteristic ECM lesion and related clinical findings, especially in endemic areas. Mild anemia and an elevated erythrocyte sedimentation rate, leukocyte count, serum immunoglobulin M level, and aspartate aminotransferase level support the diagnosis. The National Institute of Allergy and Infectious Diseases (NIAID) is researching a more sensitive diagnostic test for Lyme disease. (See *Developing tests for Lyme disease,* page 161.) Differential diagnoses are chronic fatigue syndrome and fibromyalgia; however, these can also develop in association with, or soon after, contracting Lyme disease.

Treatment

 ALERT Antibiotic therapy should be started early to minimize later complications.

A 28-day course of oral tetracycline is the treatment of choice for adults. Penicillin and erythromycin are alternates. Oral penicillin is usually prescribed for chil-

dren. When given during the late stages, high-dose ceftriaxone I.V. may be a successful treatment. Neurological abnormalities are best treated with I.V. ceftriaxone or I.V. penicillin. (See *Lyme disease treatment in trials.*)

 PREVENTION TIP A vaccine (Lymerix) is available in the U.S. to prevent Lyme disease. For maximal effectiveness, it's given as a series of 3 injections. Lymerix is not likely to be highly effective in Europe and Asia because of the diversity of genospecies that cause Lyme disease in these countries.

Special considerations

▶ Take a detailed patient history, asking about travel to endemic areas and exposure to ticks.

▶ Check for drug allergies, and administer antibiotics carefully.

▶ For a patient with arthritis, help with range-of-motion and strengthening exercises, but avoid overexertion.

▶ Assess the patient's neurologic function and level of consciousness frequently. Watch for signs of increased intracranial pressure and cranial nerve involvement, such as ptosis, strabismus, and diplopia.

▶ Check for cardiac abnormalities, such as dysrhythmias and heart block.

M

MALARIA

Malaria, an acute infectious disease, is caused by protozoa of the genus *Plasmodium: P. falciparum, P. vivax, P. malariae,* and *P. ovale,* all of which are transmitted to humans by mosquito vectors. *P. Falciparum* malaria is the most severe form of the disease. When treated, malaria is rarely fatal; untreated, it's fatal in 10% of victims, usually as a result of complications such as disseminated intravascular coagulation (DIC).

Untreated primary attacks last from a week to a month, or longer. Relapses are common and can recur sporadically for several years. Susceptibility to the disease is universal. Malaria is a tropical and subtropical disease and is most prevalent in Asia, Africa, and Latin America, with highly endemic areas being Southeast Asia and Sub-Sahara Africa. Incidence of malaria in the United States during the last 25 years has ranged from a high of 4,230 cases in 1970 (when the disease occurred mainly among military personnel returning from Vietnam) to a low of 222 cases in 1973. Since 1940, very few cases of malaria have actually been contracted in the United States; most of these were transmitted by blood transfusions or the use of contaminated needles by drug addicts. (See *How to prevent malaria*, page 164.)

Causes

Malaria literally means "bad air" and for centuries was thought to result from the inhalation of swamp vapors. It is now known that malaria is transmitted by the bite of female *Anopheles* mosquitoes, which abound in humid, swampy areas. When an infected mosquito bites, it injects *Plasmodium* sporozoites into the wound. The infective sporozoites migrate by blood circulation to parenchymal cells of the liver; there they form cyst-like structures containing thousands of merozoites. Upon release, each merozoite invades an erythrocyte and feeds on hemoglobin. Eventually, the erythrocyte ruptures, releasing malaria pigment, cell debris, and more merozoites, which, unless destroyed by phagocytes, enter other erythrocytes. At this point, the infected person becomes a reservoir of malaria who infects any mosquito that feeds on him, thus beginning a new cycle of transmission. (See *What happens in malaria*, page 165.) Hepatic parasites (*P. vivax, P. ovale,* and *P. malariae*) may persist for years in the liver. These parasites are responsible for the chronic carrier state. Because blood transfusions and street-drug paraphernalia can also spread malaria, drug addicts have a higher incidence of the disease. Malaria is a worldwide health problem that continues to impede the development of many countries.

Signs and symptoms

After an incubation period of 12 to 30 days, malaria produces chills, fever, headache, and myalgia interspersed with periods of well-being (the hallmark of the benign form of malaria). Acute attacks (paroxysms) occur when erythrocytes rupture and have three stages:

▶ *cold stage,* lasting 1 to 2 hours, ranging from chills to extreme shaking

▶ *hot stage,* lasting 3 to 4 hours, charac-

HOW TO PREVENT MALARIA

▶ Drain, fill, and eliminate breeding areas of the *Anopheles* mosquito.
▶ Install screens in living and sleeping quarters in endemic areas.
▶ Use a residual insecticide on clothing and skin to prevent mosquito bites.
▶ Seek treatment for known cases.
▶ Question blood donors about a history of malaria or possible exposure to malaria. They *may* give blood if: they haven't taken any antimalarial drugs and are asymptomatic after 6 months outside an endemic area; they were asymptomatic after treatment for malaria over 3 years ago; or they were asymptomatic after receiving malaria prophylaxis over 3 years ago.
▶ Seek prophylactic drug therapy before traveling to an endemic area.

terized by a high fever (up to 107° F [41.7° C])
▶ *wet stage,* lasting 2 to 4 hours, characterized by profuse sweating.

Paroxysms occur every 48 to 72 hours when malaria is caused by *P. malariae* and every 42 to 50 hours when malaria is caused by *P. vivax* or *P. ovale.* All three types have low levels of parasitosis and are self-limiting as a result of early acquired immunity. *P. vivax* and *P. ovale* also produce hepatosplenomegaly. Hemolytic anemia occurs in all but the mildest infections. The most severe and only life-threatening form of malaria is caused by *P. falciparum.* This species produces persistent high fever, orthostatic hypotension, and red blood cell (RBC) sludging that leads to capillary obstruction at various sites. Signs and symptoms of obstruction at these sites include the following:

▶ *cerebral* — hemiplegia, seizures, delirium, coma
▶ *pulmonary* — coughing, hemoptysis
▶ *splanchnic* — vomiting, abdominal pain, diarrhea, melena
▶ *renal* — oliguria, anuria, uremia.

During blackwater fever (a complication of *P. falciparum* infection), massive intravascular hemolysis causes jaundice, hemoglobinuria, a tender and enlarged spleen, acute renal failure, and uremia. This dreaded complication is fatal in about 20% of patients.

Diagnosis

A history showing travel to endemic areas, recent blood transfusion, or drug abuse in a person with high fever of unknown origin strongly suggests malaria. But because symptoms of malaria mimic other diseases, unequivocal diagnosis depends on laboratory identification of the parasites in RBCs of peripheral blood smears.

The Centers for Disease Control and Prevention can identify donors responsible for transfusion malaria through indirect fluorescent serum antibody tests. These tests are unreliable in the acute phase because antibodies can be undetectable for 2 weeks after onset.

Supplementary laboratory values that support this diagnosis include decreased hemoglobin levels, normal to decreased leukocyte count (as low as 3,000/µl), and protein and leukocytes in urine sediment. In *falciparum* malaria, serum values reflect DIC: reduced number of platelets (20,000 to 50,000/µl), prolonged prothrombin time (18 to 20 seconds), prolonged partial thromboplastin time (60 to 100 seconds), and decreased plasma fibrinogen.

Treatment

Malaria is best treated with oral chloroquine in all forms except chloroquine-resistant *P. falciparum.* Unfortunately, chloroquine-resistant malaria exists in most parts of the world. Studies are in progress to treat resistance with newer drugs. (See *Artemisinin derivatives to treat*

WHAT HAPPENS IN MALARIA

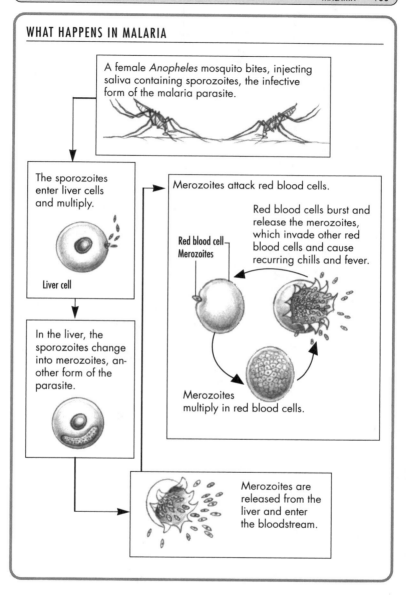

A female *Anopheles* mosquito bites, injecting saliva containing sporozoites, the infective form of the malaria parasite.

The sporozoites enter liver cells and multiply.

Liver cell

In the liver, the sporozoites change into merozoites, another form of the parasite.

Merozoites attack red blood cells.

Red blood cells burst and release the merozoites, which invade other red blood cells and cause recurring chills and fever.

Red blood cell
Merozoites

Merozoites multiply in red blood cells.

Merozoites are released from the liver and enter the bloodstream.

malaria, page 166.) Symptoms and parasitemia decrease within 24 hours after chloroquine therapy begins, and the patient usually recovers within 3 to 4 days. If the patient is comatose or vomiting frequently, chloroquine is given I.M. Toxic reactions, which rarely occur, include GI upset, pruritus, headache, and visual disturbances.

Malaria caused by *P. falciparum,* which is resistant to chloroquine, requires treatment with oral quinine for 10 days, given concurrently with pyrimethamine and a sulfonamide, such as sulfadiazine. Re-

ARTEMISININ DERIVATIVES TO TREAT MALARIA

Quinine-resistant malaria is becoming more problematic, with an increasing number of drug-resistant parasites leading to an increase in mortality. New therapies being considered include the use of artemisinin derivatives. Artemisinin was isolated in 1972 from Artemisia annua, a plant long used in China to treat fever. Studies have demonstrated that artemisinin derivatives are no worse than quinine when used to prevent death from severe or complicated malaria and, therefore, may be a good option for quinine-resistant malaria.

lapses require the same treatment, or quinine alone, followed by tetracycline.

The only drug effective against the hepatic stage of the disease that is available in the United States is primaquine phosphate, given daily for 14 days. This drug can induce hemolytic anemia, especially in patients with glucose-6-phosphate dehydrogenase deficiency.

PREVENTION TIP For travelers spending less than 3 weeks in areas where malaria exists, weekly prophylaxis includes oral chloroquine beginning 2 weeks before the trip and ending 6 weeks after it. Chloroquine and sulfadoxine-pyrimethamine (Fansidar) may be ordered for those staying longer than 3 weeks, although combination treatment can have severe adverse effects. If the traveler is not sensitive to either component of Fansidar, he may be given a single dose to take if he has a febrile episode. (See *Malaria vaccines show promise.*)

ALERT Any traveler who develops an acute febrile illness should seek prompt medical attention, regardless of the prophylaxis taken.

Special considerations

▶ Obtain a detailed patient history, noting any recent travel, foreign residence, blood transfusion, or drug addiction. Record symptom pattern, fever, type of malaria, and any systemic signs.

▶ Assess the patient on admission and daily thereafter for fatigue, fever, orthostatic hypotension, disorientation, myalgia, and arthralgia. Enforce bed rest during periods of acute illness.

▶ Protect the patient from secondary bacterial infection by following proper handwashing and aseptic techniques.

▶ Protect yourself by wearing gloves when handling blood or body fluids containing blood.

▶ Discard needles and syringes in an impervious container designated for incineration.

▶ Double-bag all contaminated linens, and transport them according to hospital policy.

▶ To reduce fever, administer antipyretics, as ordered. Document onset of fever and its duration, and symptoms before and after episodes.

▶ Fluid balance is fragile, so keep a strict record of intake and output. Monitor I.V. fluids closely. Avoid fluid overload (especially with *P. falciparum*) because it can lead to pulmonary edema and aggravate cerebral symptoms. Observe blood chemistry levels for hyponatremia and increased blood urea nitrogen, creatinine, and bilirubin levels. Monitor urine output hourly, and maintain at 40 to 60 ml/hour for an adult and at 15 to 30 ml/hour for a child. Immediately report any decrease in urine output or the onset of hematuria as a possible sign of renal failure; be prepared to do peritoneal dialysis for uremia caused by renal failure. For oliguria, administer furosemide or mannitol I.V., as ordered.

▶ Slowly administer packed RBCs or

whole blood while checking for crackles, tachycardia, and shortness of breath.

▶ If humidified oxygen is ordered because of anemia, note the patient's response, particularly any changes in rate or character of respirations, or improvement in mucous membrane color.

▶ Watch for and immediately report signs of internal bleeding, such as tachycardia, hypotension, and pallor.

▶ Encourage frequent coughing and deep breathing, especially if the patient is on bed rest or has pulmonary complications. Record the amount and color of sputum.

▶ Watch for adverse effects of drug therapy, and take measures to relieve them.

▶ If the patient is comatose, make frequent, gentle changes in his position, and give passive range-of-motion exercises every 3 to 4 hours. If the patient is unconscious or disoriented, use restraints, as needed, and keep an airway or padded tongue blade available.

▶ Provide emotional support and reassurance, especially in critical illness. Explain the procedures and treatment to the patient and his family. Listen sympathetically, and answer questions clearly. Suggest that other family members be tested for malaria. Emphasize the need for follow-up care to check the effectiveness of treatment and to manage residual problems.

▶ Report all cases of malaria to local public health authorities.

MASTITIS AND BREAST ENGORGEMENT

Mastitis (parenchymatous inflammation of the mammary glands) and breast engorgement (congestion) are disorders that may affect lactating females. Mastitis occurs postpartum in about 1%, mainly in primiparas who are breast-feeding. It occurs occasionally in nonlactating females and rarely in males. All breast-feeding mothers develop some degree of engorgement, which is not an infectious

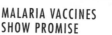

MALARIA VACCINES SHOW PROMISE

Several malaria vaccines recently in trials offer the possibility that effective vaccines for this disease may be on the horizon. One trial involved administering a three-component, blood-stage vaccine against *Plasmodium falciparum* in Papua New Guinean children, and demonstrated efficacy in those who had not received antimalaria pretreatment. Another trial, with Gambian men, involved a pre-erythrocytic malaria vaccine. Efficacy was 65% within the first 2 months, but only 16% overall. Additional studies are under way to improve these vaccines, including DNA vaccines, such as the recombinant RTS, S/SBAS2, developed by the Walter Reed Army Institute of Research.

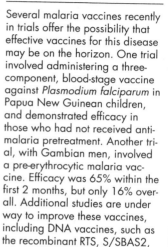

process. The prognosis for both disorders is good.

Causes

Mastitis develops when a pathogen that typically originates in the nursing infant's nose or pharynx invades breast tissue through a fissured or cracked nipple and disrupts normal lactation. The most common pathogen of this type is *Staphylococcus aureus;* less frequently, it's *Staphylococcus epidermidis* or beta-hemolytic streptococci. Rarely, mastitis may result from disseminated tuberculosis or the mumps virus. Predisposing factors include a fissure or abrasion on the nipple; blocked milk ducts; and an incomplete let-down reflex, usually due to emotional trauma. Blocked milk ducts can result from a tight bra or prolonged intervals between breast-feedings. Causes of breast engorgement include venous and lymphatic stasis, and alveolar milk accumulation.

Signs and symptoms

Mastitis may develop anytime during lactation but usually begins 1 to 2 weeks postpartum with fever (101° F [38.3° C] or higher in acute mastitis), malaise, and flu-like symptoms. The breast (or, occasionally, both breasts) becomes tender, hard, swollen, and warm.

 ALERT Unless mastitis is treated adequately, it may progress to breast abscess.

Breast engorgement generally starts with onset of lactation (day 2 to day 5 postpartum). The breasts undergo changes similar to those in mastitis, and body temperature may be elevated. Engorgement may be mild, causing only slight discomfort, or severe, causing considerable pain. A severely engorged breast can interfere with the infant's capacity to feed because of his inability to position his mouth properly on the swollen, rigid breast.

Diagnosis

Diagnosis is usually made early, on clinical grounds. If pus is expressed from a nipple, a culture may be helpful in confirming the impression of mastitis. Differential diagnoses include abscess and inflammatory breast cancer.

Treatment

Antibiotic therapy, the primary treatment for mastitis, generally consists of oral cephalosporins, dicloxacillin or cloxacillin to combat staphylococcus. Azithromycin may be used for penicillin-allergic patients. Although symptoms usually subside 2 to 3 days after treatment begins, antibiotic therapy should continue for 10 days. Other appropriate measures include analgesics for pain and, rarely, when antibiotics fail to control the infection and mastitis progresses to breast abscess, incision and drainage of the abscess.

The goal of treatment for breast engorgement is to relieve discomfort and control swelling, and may include analgesics to alleviate pain, and ice packs and an uplift support bra to minimize edema.

Rarely, oxytocin nasal spray may be necessary to release milk from the alveoli into the ducts. To facilitate breast-feeding, the mother may manually express excess milk before a feeding so the infant can grasp the nipple properly.

Special considerations

If the patient has mastitis:

▶ Isolate the patient and her infant to prevent the spread of infection to other nursing mothers. Explain mastitis to the patient and why isolation is necessary.

▶ Obtain a complete patient history, including a drug history, especially allergy to penicillin.

▶ Assess and record the cause and amount of discomfort. Give analgesics, as needed.

▶ Reassure the mother that breast-feeding during mastitis won't harm her infant because he's the source of the infection. Tell her to offer the infant the affected breast first to promote complete emptying of the breast and prevent clogged ducts. However, if an open abscess develops, she must stop breast-feeding with this breast and use a breast pump until the abscess heals. She should continue to breast-feed on the unaffected side.

▶ Suggest applying a warm, wet towel to the affected breast or taking a warm shower to relax and improve her ability to breast-feed.

▶ Instruct the patient to combat fever by getting plenty of rest, drinking sufficient fluids, and following prescribed antibiotic therapy.

 PREVENTION TIP To prevent mastitis and relieve its symptoms, teach the patient good health care, breast care, and breast-feeding habits. Advise her to always wash her hands before touching her breasts.

If the patient has breast engorgement:

▶ Assess and record the level of discomfort. Give analgesics, and apply ice packs as needed.

▶ Teach the patient how to express excess breast milk manually. She should do this just before nursing to enable the infant to get the swollen areola into his mouth. Caution against excessive expression of milk between feedings because this stimulates milk production and prolongs engorgement.

▶ Explain that because breast engorgement is due to the physiologic processes of lactation, breast-feeding is the best remedy for engorgement. Suggest breast-feeding every 2 to 3 hours and at least once during the night.

▶ Ensure that the mother wears a well-fitted nursing bra and be sure it is not too tight.

MASTOIDITIS

Mastoiditis is a bacterial infection and inflammation of the air cells of the mastoid antrum. Although the prognosis is good with early treatment, possible complications include meningitis, facial paralysis, brain abscess, and suppurative labyrinthitis.

Causes

Bacteria that cause mastoiditis include pneumococci, *Haemophilus influenzae, Moraxella catarrhalis,* beta-hemolytic streptococci, staphylococci, and gram-negative bacteria, the same microbes that cause acute otitis media. Mastoiditis is usually a complication of chronic otitis media; less frequently, it develops after acute otitis media. An accumulation of pus under pressure in the middle ear cavity results in necrosis of adjacent tissue and extension of the infection into the mastoid cells. Chronic systemic diseases or immunosuppression may also lead to mastoiditis. While pneumococcal mastoiditis is usually not symptomatic, it can be very destructive. Coalescence of the mastoid air cells may precede rupture of the tympanic membrane. Streptococcal mastoiditis is generally preceded by early rupture of the tympanic membrane and copious otorrhea.

Signs and symptoms

Symptoms of mastoiditis are usually noticed 2 weeks or more after untreated acute otitis media, due to destruction of one of the mastoid processes. Primary clinical features include persistent and throbbing pain and tenderness in the area of the mastoid process, low-grade fever, headache, and a thick, purulent discharge that gradually becomes more profuse, possibly leading to otitis externa. Postauricular erythema and edema may push the auricle out from the head; pressure within the edematous mastoid antrum may produce swelling and obstruction of the external ear canal, causing conductive hearing loss.

Diagnosis

X-rays of the mastoid area reveal hazy mastoid air cells; the bony walls between the cells appear decalcified due to purulent fluid, swollen mucous membranes, and granulation tissue in the air cells. Audiometric testing may reveal a conductive hearing loss. Physical examination shows a dull, thickened, and edematous tympanic membrane, if the membrane isn't concealed by obstruction. During examination, the external ear canal is cleaned; persistent oozing into the canal indicates perforation of the tympanic membrane. Differential diagnoses include serous otitis media, acute otitis media, petrous apicitis, and sigmoid sinus thrombosis.

Treatment

Treatment of mastoiditis consists of intense parenteral antibiotic therapy. I.V. penicillin is the initial drug of choice for at least a 2-week duration. If bone damage is minimal, myringotomy drains purulent fluid and provides a specimen of discharge for culture and sensitivity testing. Recurrent or persistent infection or signs of intracranial complications necessitate simple mastoidectomy. This procedure involves removal of the diseased bone and cleaning of the affected area, after which a drain is inserted.

A chronically inflamed mastoid requires radical mastoidectomy (excision of the posterior wall of the ear canal, remnants of the tympanic membrane, and the malleus and incus, although these bones are usually destroyed by infection before surgery). The stapes and facial nerve remain intact. Radical mastoidectomy, which is seldom necessary because of antibiotic therapy, does not drastically affect the patient's hearing because significant hearing loss precedes surgery. With either surgical procedure, the patient continues oral antibiotic therapy for several weeks after surgery and hospital discharge.

Special considerations

▶ After simple mastoidectomy, give pain medication, as needed. Check wound drainage, and reinforce dressings. (The surgeon usually changes the dressing daily and removes the drain in 72 hours.) Check the patient's hearing, and watch for signs of complications, especially infection (either localized or extending to the brain); facial nerve paralysis, with unilateral facial drooping; bleeding; and vertigo, especially when the patient stands.

▶ After radical mastoidectomy, the wound is packed with petroleum gauze or gauze treated with an antibiotic ointment. Give pain medication before the packing is removed, on the fourth or fifth postoperative day.

▶ Because of stimulation to the inner ear during surgery, the patient may feel dizzy and nauseated for several days afterward. Keep the side rails up, and assist the patient with ambulation. Also, give antiemetics as needed.

▶ Before discharge, teach the patient and family how to change and care for the dressing. Urge compliance with the prescribed antibiotic treatment, and promote regular follow-up care.

▶ If the patient is diabetic, evaluate him for malignant otitis externa.

MENINGITIS

In meningitis, the brain and the spinal cord meninges become inflamed, usually as a result of viral or bacterial infection. Viral meningitis is more prevalent than a bacterial cause. Such inflammation may involve all three meningeal membranes — the dura mater, arachnoid, and pia mater. The prognosis is good and complications are rare, especially if the disease is recognized early and the infecting organism responds to antibiotics. The prognosis is poorer for infants and older adults. In the case of children, the prognosis is poor for some types of bacterial meningitis, unless antibiotic therapy is started within hours of onset of symptoms.

Causes

Meningitis is almost always a complication of another bacterial infection — bacteremia (especially from pneumonia, empyema, osteomyelitis, and endocarditis), sinusitis, otitis media, encephalitis, myelitis, or brain abscess — usually caused by *Neisseria meningitidis, Haemophilus influenzae, Streptococcus pneumoniae,* and *Escherichia coli.*

Meningitis may also follow skull fracture, a penetrating head wound, lumbar puncture, or ventricular shunting procedures. Aseptic meningitis may result from a virus or other organism. (See *Aseptic meningitis.*) Sometimes no causative organism can be found. Meningitis often begins as an inflammation of the pia-arachnoid, which may progress to congestion of adjacent tissues and destroy some nerve cells.

Signs and symptoms

Typical signs include the following features:

Cardinal signs

Cardinal signs of meningitis include infection (fever, chills, malaise) and increased intracranial pressure (headache, vomiting and, rarely, papilledema).

ASEPTIC MENINGITIS

Aseptic meningitis is a benign syndrome characterized by headache, fever, vomiting, and meningeal symptoms. It results from some form of viral infection, including enteroviruses (most common), arboviruses, herpes simplex virus, mumps virus, and lymphocytic choriomeningitis virus.

Aseptic meningitis begins suddenly with a fever up to 104°F (40.0°C), alterations in consciousness (drowsiness, confusion, stupor), and neck or spine stiffness, which is slight at first. (The patient experiences such stiffness when bending forward.) Other signs and symptoms include headache, nausea, vomiting, abdominal pain, poorly defined chest pain, and sore throat.

Patient history of recent illness and knowledge of seasonal epidemics are essential in differentiating among the many forms of aseptic meningitis. Negative bacteriologic cultures and cerebrospinal fluid (CSF) analysis showing pleocytosis and increased protein levels suggest the diagnosis. Isolation of the virus from CSF confirms it.

Treatment is supportive, including bed rest, maintenance of fluid and electrolyte balance, analgesics for pain, and exercises to combat residual weakness. Isolation is not necessary. Careful handling of excretions and good hand-washing technique prevent spreading the disease.

Meningeal irritation

Signs of meningeal irritation include nuchal rigidity, positive Brudzinski's and Kernig's signs, exaggerated and symmetrical deep tendon reflexes, and opisthotonos (a spasm in which the back and extremities arch backward so that the body rests on the head and heels).

Other manifestations

Other features of meningitis are sinus arrhythmias; irritability; photophobia, diplopia, and other visual problems; delirium, deep stupor, and coma. An infant may show signs of infection but often is simply fretful and refuses to eat. Such an infant may vomit a great deal, leading to dehydration, which prevents a bulging fontanel and thus masks this important sign of increased intracranial pressure (ICP). As the illness progresses, twitching, seizures (in 30% of infants) or coma may develop. Most older children have the same symptoms as adults. In subacute meningitis, onset may be insidious.

Diagnosis

A lumbar puncture showing typical findings in cerebrospinal fluid (CSF) and positive Brudzinski's and Kernig's signs usually establish this diagnosis. (See *Two telltale signs of meningitis,* page 172.) The lumbar puncture usually indicates elevated CSF pressure from obstructed CSF outflow at the arachnoid villi. The fluid may appear cloudy or milky white, depending on the number of white blood cells present. CSF protein levels tend to be high; glucose levels may be low. (In subacute meningitis, CSF findings may vary.) CSF culture and sensitivity tests usually identify the infecting organism, unless it's a virus. Other useful tests include the following:

▶ Cultures of blood, urine, and nose and throat secretions; a chest X-ray; electrocardiography; and a physical examination, with special attention to skin, ears, and sinuses, can uncover the primary infection site.

▶ Blood tests commonly reveal leukocytosis and serum electrolyte abnormalities.

TWO TELLTALE SIGNS OF MENINGITIS

BRUDZINSKI'S SIGN

To test for Brudzinski's sign, place the patient in a dorsal recumbent position; then put your hands behind his neck and bend it forward. Pain and resistance may indicate meningeal inflammation, neck injury, or arthritis. However, if the patient also flexes the hips and knees in response to this manipulation, chances are he has meningitis.

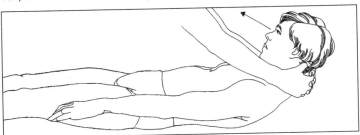

KERNIG'S SIGN

To test for Kernig's sign, place the patient in a supine position. Flex his leg at the hip and knee, then straighten the knee. Pain or resistance points to meningitis.

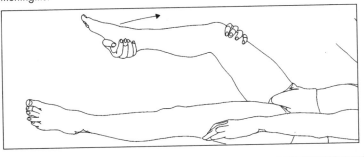

▶ Computed tomography scan can rule out cerebral hematoma, hemorrhage, or tumor.

Differential diagnoses include many diseases that can cause acute meningeal syndrome, such as brain abscess, subdural empyema, epidural abscess, encephalitis, CNS syphilis, bacterial endocarditis, rickettsial infections, sarcoidosis, CNS neoplasms, and neuroleptic malignant syndrome.

Treatment

 ALERT If left untreated, meningitis has a mortality rate of 70% to 100%.

In bacterial meningitis, treatment includes appropriate antibiotic therapy and vigorous supportive care. Usually, I.V. antibiotics are given for at least 2 weeks and are followed by oral antibiotics. Such antibiotics include ampicillin and a third-generation cephalosporin, such as ceftriaxone, or ampicillin and an aminoglycoside. Other drugs include a digitalis glycoside, such as digoxin, to control arrhythmias, mannitol to decrease cerebral edema, an anticonvulsant (usually given I.V.) or a sedative to reduce restlessness, and aspirin or acetaminophen to relieve headache and fever.

PREVENTION TIP Several vaccines are available to protect against certain types of meningitis. There are vaccines against *Haemophilus influenzae,* type B; some strains of *N. meningitidis;* and many types of *Streptococcus pneumoniae.*

Supportive measures include bed rest, fever reduction, and measures to prevent dehydration. Isolation is necessary if nasal cultures are positive. Of course, treatment includes appropriate therapy for any co-existing conditions, such as endocarditis or pneumonia. To prevent meningitis, prophylactic antibiotics are sometimes used after ventricular shunting procedures, skull fracture, or penetrating head wounds, but this use is controversial.

Special considerations

▶ Assess neurologic function often. Observe the patient's level of consciousness, and check for signs of increased ICP (plucking at the bedcovers, vomiting, seizures, change in motor functions and vital signs). Also watch for signs of cranial nerve involvement (ptosis, strabismus, diplopia).

▶ Watch for deterioration in the patient's condition, which may signal an impending crisis.

▶ Monitor fluid balance. Maintain adequate fluid intake to avoid dehydration, but avoid fluid overload because of the danger of cerebral edema. Measure central venous pressure and intake and output accurately.

▶ Watch for adverse reactions to I.V. antibiotics and other drugs. To avoid infiltration and phlebitis, check the I.V. site often, and change the site according to facility policy.

▶ Position the patient carefully to prevent joint stiffness and neck pain. Turn him of-

ten, according to a planned positioning schedule. Assist with range-of-motion exercises.

▶ Maintain adequate nutrition and elimination. It may be necessary to provide small, frequent meals or supplement these meals with nasogastric tube or parenteral feedings.

▶ To prevent constipation and minimize the risk of increased ICP resulting from straining during defecation, give the patient a mild laxative or stool softener.

▶ Ensure the patient's comfort. Provide mouth care regularly. Maintain a quiet environment. Darkening the room may decrease photophobia.

▶ Relieve the patient's headache with a nonnarcotic analgesic, such as aspirin or acetaminophen, as needed. (Narcotics interfere with neurologic assessment.)

▶ Provide reassurance and support. The patient may be frightened by his illness and procedures, such as frequent lumbar punctures. If he is delirious or confused, attempt to reorient him often. Reassure the family that the delirium and behavior changes caused by meningitis usually disappear.

▶ If a severe neurologic deficit appears permanent, refer the patient to a rehabilitation program as soon as the acute phase of this illness has passed.

▶ Follow strict aseptic technique when treating patients with head wounds or skull fractures.

PREVENTION TIP To help prevent development of meningitis, teach patients with chronic sinusitis or other chronic infections the importance of proper medical treatment.

MENINGOCOCCAL INFECTIONS

Two major meningococcal infections (meningitis and meningioma) are caused by the gram-negative bacteria *Neisseria meningitidis,* which also causes primary pneumonia, purulent conjunctivitis, endocarditis, sinusitis, and genital infection. Meningococcemia occurs as simple bacteremia, fulminant meningococcemia and, rarely, chronic meningococcemia. It often accompanies meningitis. (For more information on meningitis, see "Meningitis.") Meningococcal infections may occur sporadically or in epidemics; virulent infections may be fatal within a matter of hours.

Causes

Meningococcal infections occur most often among children (ages 6 months to 1 year) and men, usually military recruits, because of overcrowding. *N. meningitidis* has at least seven serogroups (A, B, C, D, X, Y, Z); group A causes most epidemics.

 PREVENTION TIP There is a vaccine available in the U.S., quadrivalent A/C/Y/W-135. It is not used routinely in the U.S. but is recommended for travelers to endemic areas during the dry season. Duration of immunity is unknown but appears to be at least 3 years in persons over 4 years old.

These bacteria are often present in upper respiratory flora. Transmission takes place through inhalation of an infected droplet from carriers (an estimated 2% to 38% of the population). The bacteria then localize in the nasopharynx. Following an incubation period of approximately 3 or 4 days, the bacteria spread through the bloodstream to the joints, skin, adrenal glands, lungs, and central nervous system. The tissue damage that results (possibly due to the effects of bacterial endotoxins) produces symptoms and, in fulminant meningococcemia and meningococcal bacteremia, progresses to hemorrhage, thrombosis, and necrosis.

Signs and symptoms

Clinical features of meningococcal infection vary. Symptoms of *meningococcal bacteremia* include a sudden, spiking fever; headache; sore throat; cough; chills; myalgia (in the back and legs); arthralgia; tachycardia; tachypnea; mild hypotension;

and a petechial, nodular, or maculopapular rash. In 10% to 20% of patients, this progresses to *fulminant meningococcemia,* with extreme prostration, enlargement of skin lesions, disseminated intravascular coagulation (DIC), and shock.

 ALERT Unless it's treated promptly, fulminant meningococcemia results in death from respiratory or heart failure in 6 to 24 hours.

Characteristics of *chronic meningococcemia* include intermittent fever, maculopapular rash, joint pain, and enlarged spleen.

Diagnosis

Isolation of *N. meningitidis* through a positive blood culture, cerebrospinal fluid (CSF) culture, or lesion scraping confirms the diagnosis, except in nasopharyngeal infections, because *N. meningitidis* exists as part of the normal nasopharyngeal flora. Tests that support the diagnosis include counterimmunoelectrophoresis of the CSF or blood, a low white blood cell count and, in patients with skin or adrenal hemorrhages, decreased platelet and clotting levels. Diagnostic evaluation must rule out Rocky Mountain spotted fever and vascular purpuras.

Treatment

As soon as meningococcal infection is suspected, treatment begins with large doses of aqueous penicillin G, ampicillin, or a cephalosporin, such as cefoxitin, and moxalactam. For the patient who is allergic to penicillin, chloramphenicol I.V is used. Therapy may also include mannitol for cerebral edema, I.V. heparin for disseminated intravascular coagulation (DIC), dopamine for shock, and digoxin and a diuretic if heart failure develops. Supportive measures include fluid and electrolyte maintenance, proper ventilation (patent airway and oxygen if necessary), insertion of an arterial or central venous pressure (CVP) line to monitor cardiovascular status, and bed rest. Chemoprophylaxis with rifampin or minocycline is useful for facility workers who come in close contact with the patient; minocycline can also temporarily eradicate the infection in carriers.

 PREVENTION TIP To prevent the spread of meningococcal infection, impose respiratory isolation until the patient has received antibiotic therapy for 24 hours.

Special considerations

▶ The dosages of I.V. antibiotics should be adjusted as necessary to maintain blood and CSF drug levels.

▶ Enforce bed rest in early stages. Provide a dark, quiet, restful environment.

▶ Maintain adequate ventilation with oxygen or a ventilator if necessary. Suction and turn the patient frequently.

▶ Keep accurate intake and output records to maintain proper fluid and electrolyte levels. Monitor blood pressure, pulse, arterial blood gas levels, and CVP.

▶ Watch for complications, such as DIC, arthritis, endocarditis, and pneumonia.

▶ If the patient is receiving chloramphenicol, monitor his complete blood count.

▶ Check the patient's drug history for allergies before giving antibiotics.

▶ Label all meningococcal specimens. Deliver them to the laboratory quickly because meningococci are very sensitive to changes in humidity and temperature.

▶ Report all meningococcal infections to public health department officials.

METHICILLIN-RESISTANT *STAPHYLOCOCCUS AUREUS* INFECTION

Methicillin-resistant *Staphylococcus aureus* (MRSA) is a mutation of a very common bacterium that is spread easily by direct person-to-person contact. Once limited to large teaching hospitals and tertiary care centers, MRSA is now endemic in nursing homes, long-term care facilities, and even community hospitals. Patients most at risk for MRSA include immunosuppressed patients, burn patients, intubated patients, and those with central venous catheters, surgical wounds, or dermatitis. Others at risk include those with prosthetic devices, heart valves, and postoperative wound infections. Other risk factors include prolonged hospital stays, extended therapy with multiple or broad-spectrum antibiotics, and close proximity to those colonized or infected with MRSA. Also at risk are patients with acute endocarditis, bacteremia, cervicitis, meningitis, pericarditis, and pneumonia.

Causes

MRSA enters health care facilities through an infected or colonized patient or colonized health care worker. Although MRSA has been recovered from environmental surfaces, it's transmitted mainly on health care workers' hands. Many colonized individuals become silent carriers. The most frequent site of colonization is the anterior nares (40% of adults and most children become transient nasal carriers). Other sites include the groin, axilla, and the gut, though these sites aren't as common. Typically, MRSA colonization is diagnosed by isolating bacteria from nasal secretions. In individuals where the natural defense system breaks down, such as after an invasive procedure, trauma, or chemotherapy, the normally benign bacteria can invade tissue, proliferate, and cause infection.

Today up to 90% of *Staphylococcus aureus* isolates or strains are penicillin-resistant, and about 27% of all *S. aureus* isolates are resistant to methicillin, a penicillin derivative. These strains may also resist cephalosporins, aminoglycosides, erythromycin, tetracycline, and clindamycin. MRSA has become prevalent with the overuse of antibiotics. Over the years, overuse has given once-susceptible bacteria the chance to develop defenses against antibiotics. This new capability allows resistant strains to flourish when antibiotics knock out their more sensitive cousins.

Diagnosis

MRSA can be cultured from the suspected site with the appropriate culture method. For example, MRSA in a wound infection can be swabbed for culture. Blood, urine, and sputum cultures will reveal sources of MRSA.

Treatment

To eradicate MRSA colonization in the nares, the doctor may order topical mupirocin applied inside the nostrils. Other protocols involve combining a topical agent and an oral antibiotic. Most facilities keep patients in isolation until surveillance cultures are negative. To attack MRSA infection, vancomycin is the drug of choice. A serious adverse effect (mostly caused by histamine release) is itching, which can progress to anaphylaxis. Some doctors also add rifampin, but whether rifampin acts synergistically or antagonistically when given with vancomycin is controversial. Due to *S. aureus* with reduced or total resistance to vancomycin investigation is ongoing for other effective antibiotics.

 PREVENTION TIP Good hand washing is the most effective way to prevent MRSA from spreading. This includes hand washing between tasks and procedures on the same patient to prevent cross-contamination of different body parts.

Special considerations

▶ Personnel in contact with patients should wash hands before and after patient care.
▶ Use an antiseptic soap, such as chlorhexidine, because bacteria have been cultured from workers' hands after they've washed with milder soap. One study showed that without proper hand washing, MRSA could survive on health care workers' hands for up to 3 hours.
▶ Contact isolation precautions should be used when in contact with the patient. A private room should be used, as well as dedicated equipment and disinfection of the environment.
▶ Change gloves when contaminated or when moving from a "dirty" area of the body to a clean one.
▶ Instruct family and friends to wear protective clothing when they visit the patient and show them how to dispose of it.
▶ Provide teaching and emotional support to the patient and family members.
▶ Consider grouping infected patients together and having the same nursing staff care for them.
▶ Equipment used on the patient should not be laid on the bed or bed stand and should be wiped with appropriate disinfectant before leaving the room.
▶ Ensure careful use of antibiotics. Encourage doctors to limit antibiotic use.
▶ Instruct the patient to take antibiotics for the full prescription period, even if he begins to feel better.

MICROSPORIDIOSIS

Microsporidiosis is present mainly in immunocompromised individuals; it gained momentum as a cause of disease during the onset of the acquired immunodeficiency syndrome (AIDS) epidemic. The prevalence of microsporidiosis in human immunodeficiency virus (HIV)-positive patients is difficult to measure because it is hard to diagnosis and is not usually the first AIDS-defining illness present. Intestinal microsporidiosis is the most common microsporidial disease in people with AIDS. Infections of the eye and other organs may also occur.

Researchers speculate that treatment with antiretroviral therapy, including protease inhibitors, has helped to alleviate microsporidiosis in the HIV population Two small studies in 1997 suggest this possibility. One study treated microsporidial diarrhea with combination antiretroviral therapy, including a protease inhibitor. The diarrhea improved after 12 weeks. The other study evaluated 15 patients with chronic microsporidiosis who had been taking triple antiretroviral therapy, including either indinavir (Crixivan) or ritonavir (Norvir). Four out of six patients revealed no identifiable evidence of parasites in several stool examinations. In 12 of the 15 patients, diarrhea was resolved.

Cause

Microsporidiosis is caused by microsporidia, small intercellular spore-forming protozoan parasites (such as *Enterocytozoon intestinalis, Nosema ocularum,* and *Vittaforma corneae*). When the parasites are present in the lumen of the GI tract, they uncoil and infect a host cell. The resulting intercellular division produces sporoblasts. These sporoblasts mature into spores and pass to other cells, or leave the body via urine, feces, or skin. Not much is known about the routes of transmission. In healthy persons, microsporidia is a common cause of subclinical illness. Fifty percent of healthy persons, especially individuals in tropical environments, present with antibodies to the microsporidium *Enterocytozoon cuniculi.* Only a few cases of infection were reported prior to the AIDS era. These pathogens are opportunistic to people with HIV and the immunocompromised; 30% of AIDS patients with chronic diarrhea have intestinal microsporidiosis. Others develop infections in sites other than the GI tract.

Signs and symptoms

The extent of the clinical disease depends on the parasite species and the patient's immune status. In AIDS patients, the most common presentation is profuse, watery, non-bloody diarrhea. Abdominal pain, cramping, nausea, vomiting, and weight loss may also be present. Microsporidia can also cause cholangitis, or inflammation of the bile ducts, hepatitis, peritonitis, or inflammation of the membrane lining in the abdomen, keratoconjunctivitis, and inflammation of the cornea and conjunctiva. Additional symptoms may include kidney, liver, lung, muscle, and brain infections.

Diagnosis

Microsporidial spores in humans are small (1 to 2μ in diameter) and are difficult to detect. Biopsy or corneal scrapings are necessary to detect organisms present in the infected tissue. Staining with Giemsa, PAS, Gram or acid-fast stains can help identify microsporidia in stools and duodenal fluids. A polymerase chain reaction is also useful for microsporidia detection in stools and in gut biopsies.

Treatment

Currently there is no FDA-approved therapy or standard of care. Albendazole (400 mg P.O. b.i.d.) is given to control the intestinal infection with *Septala intestinalis.* A reduction of *E. bieneusi* may be noted in small bowel biopsies, but this does not indicate elimination of the infection. There is currently no treatment for ocular or disseminated microsporidiosis; however, there has been some success with fumagillin eyedrops and imidazole compounds (fluconazole, itraconazole).

Special considerations

▶ Wash hands between patient contact, after touching infected material, and before touching open wounds or performing invasive procedures.

▶ Dispose of soiled linens appropriately.

▶ Change bed linens regularly.

▶ Dispose of feces and urine appropriately.

▶ Assist patient in maintaining good personal hygiene.

▶ Wear gloves when handling infectious secretions and performing patient care.

▶ Handle bedpans carefully.

▶ Maintain the integrity of the patient's skin.

▶ Promote a healthy diet.

 PREVENTION TIP Patients should practice careful hand-washing techniques. Infected bed linens and other items should be contained in the appropriate receptacles. Reinforce use of universal precaution methods to patients, families, and visitors.

MOLLUSCUM CONTAGIOSUM

Molluscum contagiosum is a benign viral skin infection characterized by skin-colored to pearl-like papules or nodules on the skin. Incidence of infection is higher in males, with the greater incidence occurring in children under age 5 and in young adults. In adults, it occurs as a sexually transmitted disease, appearing in the genitalia. In some cases, molluscum contagiosum is a chronic infection; however, it produces no systemic illness and poses no public health significance.

Causes

Molluscum contagiosum is caused by a virus of the Proxvirus family known as Molluscipoxvirus. It spreads through direct contact and autoinoculation; fomites may also aid in viral spread. The virus spreads in children through direct contact and through sexual contact in adults. It spreads to other parts of the body by autoinoculation; when scratching the infected area, the virus gets under the fingernails and is reinoculated when another area of the body is scratched.

 PREVENTION TIP To prevent transfer of the disorder, teach the patient scrupulous personal and family hygiene measures. Prohibit the sharing of clothing or towels, as well as physical contact with the infected area. Encourage thorough hand washing. Limiting sexual partners and using condoms can prevent the spread of the molluscum virus.

Signs and symptoms

The virus infects the epidermis, with lesions appearing on the face, neck, axilla, arms and hands, or other parts of the body, excluding palms and soles of the feet. In some cases it can also be seen in and around the genitalia. The lesions, usually detected by accident while examining for other sexually transmitted diseases, present as small papules, which become raised and form pearly, flesh-colored nodules. Classically, these papules have been characterized as "umbilicated," in reference to the dimple in the center of the lesion. Nodules are 2 to 5 mm in diameter, appear in lines or crops, and may persist from months to years. In general, spontaneous involution of invisible lesions occurs within 8 weeks. Usually there's no inflammation or redness unless the patient has been scratching the lesions. When the molluscum matures, the nodule can be opened to reveal a white, cheesy, or waxy center.

Complications include secondary bacterial skin infections and the spread and recurrence of the nodules. The initial infection begins in the basal layer with a latent period up to 6 months. Incubation is usually 2 to 7 weeks. New viral particles form when the spindle and granular layers of the epidermis are compromised. These lesions can become inflamed with attendant edema, increased vascularity and infiltration by lymphocytes, neutrophils, and monocytes. This occurs only if there is a secondary bacterial infection and infiltration of the dermis. Since children and HIV-infected patients experience more widespread lesions, cell-mediated immunity is necessary to control the infection. Widespread lesions may also occur in immunocompromised patients, such as those with sarcoidosis or undergoing treatment with prednisone and methotrexate.

Diagnosis

Lesions are usually found in the pubic area. Skin biopsy confirm the virus. Staining with Giemsa, Gram, or Wright's stain should indicate infection. Giemsa staining typically reveals classic molluscum bodies, aiding in diagnosis. Individual virus particles can also be detected by electron microscopy. Differential diagnoses to consider include basal cell carcinoma, folliculitis, furunculosis, keratocanthomas, warts, pyrogenic granuloma, and vesicular skin disorders.

Treatment

Usually the infection disappears within months to a few years in patients with a healthy immune system. In patients with

AIDS or who are otherwise immuno-compromised, the lesions may be more extensive. Surgical removal of individual nodules by scraping, de-coring, and freezing may cause scarring. Needle electro-surgery can be used.

Special considerations

▶ Take necessary precautions to prevent spreading the infection, including washing hands thoroughly before and after patient contact.

▶ Assist the patient with appropriate hygiene practices.

▶ Consider cutting the patient's fingernails to help maintain the integrity of the skin barrier.

MONONUCLEOSIS

Infectious mononucleosis is an acute infectious disease caused by the Epstein-Barr virus (EBV), a member of the herpes group. It primarily affects young adults and children, although in children it's usually so mild that it's often overlooked.

Characteristically, infectious mononucleosis produces fever, sore throat, and cervical lymphadenopathy (the hallmarks of the disease), as well as hepatic dysfunction, increased lymphocytes and monocytes, and development and persistence of heterophil antibodies. The prognosis is excellent, and major complications are uncommon.

Causes

Apparently, the EBV reservoir is limited to humans. Infectious mononucleosis probably spreads by the oropharyngeal route because about 80% of patients carry EBV in their throats during the acute infection and for an indefinite period afterward.

It can also be transmitted by blood transfusion and has been reported after cardiac surgery as the "post-pump perfusion" syndrome. Infectious mononucleosis is probably contagious from before symptoms develop until the fever subsides and oropharyngeal lesions disappear.

Infectious mononucleosis is fairly common in the United States, Canada, and Europe, and both sexes are affected equally. Incidence varies seasonally among college students (most common in the early spring and early fall) but not among the general population.

Signs and symptoms

The symptoms of mononucleosis mimic those of many other infectious diseases, including hepatitis, rubella, and toxoplasmosis. Typically, after an incubation period of about 10 days in children and from 30 to 50 days in adults, infectious mononucleosis produces prodromal symptoms, such as headache, malaise, and fatigue.

After 3 to 5 days, patients typically develop a triad of symptoms: sore throat, cervical lymphadenopathy, and temperature fluctuations, with an evening peak of 101° to 102° F (38.3° to 38.9° C). Splenomegaly, hepatomegaly, stomatitis, exudative tonsillitis, or pharyngitis may also develop. Sometimes, early in the illness, a maculopapular rash that resembles rubella develops; also, jaundice occurs in about 5% of patients. Major complications are rare but may include splenic rupture, aseptic meningitis, encephalitis, hemolytic anemia, and Guillain-Barré syndrome. Symptoms usually subside from 6 to 10 days after onset of the disease but may persist for weeks.

Diagnosis

Physical examination demonstrating the clinical triad suggests infectious mononucleosis. The following abnormal laboratory results confirm it:

▶ White blood cell (WBC) count increases 10,000 to 20,000/µl during the second and third weeks of illness. Lymphocytes and monocytes account for 50% to 70% of the total WBC count; 10% of the lymphocytes are atypical.

▶ Heterophil antibodies (agglutinins for sheep red blood cells) in serum drawn during the acute illness and at 3- to 4-week intervals rise to four times normal.

▶ Indirect immunofluorescence shows antibodies to EBV and cellular antigens. Such testing is usually more definitive than heterophil antibodies.

▶ Liver function studies are abnormal.

Differential diagnoses to consider include other acute infections, such as those caused by cytomegalovirus, toxoplasma, human herpesvirus 6, and hepatitis virus.

Treatment

Infectious mononucleosis resists prevention and antimicrobial treatment. Thus, therapy is essentially supportive: relief of symptoms, bed rest during the acute febrile period, and aspirin or another salicylate for headache and sore throat. If severe throat inflammation causes airway obstruction, steroids can be used to relieve swelling and avoid tracheotomy.

 ALERT Splenic rupture, marked by sudden abdominal pain, requires splenectomy.

About 20% of patients with infectious mononucleosis will also have streptococcal pharyngotonsillitis; these patients should receive antibiotic therapy for at least 10 days.

Special considerations

▶ During the acute illness, stress the need for bed rest. If the patient is a student, tell him that he may continue less demanding school assignments and see friends, but should avoid long, difficult projects until after recovery.

▶ To minimize throat discomfort, encourage the patient to drink milk shakes, fruit juices, and broths, and also to eat cool, bland foods.

▶ Advise the use of saline gargles and aspirin as needed.

▶ Because uncomplicated infectious mononucleosis doesn't require hospitalization, patient teaching is essential. Convalescence may take several weeks, usually until the patient's WBC count returns to normal.

MUCORMYCOSIS

Mucormycosis is a rare and commonly fatal mycotic infection caused by fungi of the order Mucorales; it is among the most acute and fulminant fungal infections known. The mortality rate is high, with an average survival rate of only 36%. The worst prognosis occurs in disseminated disease, with a mortality rate approaching 100%, and the best prognosis occurs with infections limited to skin and subcutaneous tissues of the extremities.

A disease of the immunocompromised, mucormycosis is associated with diabetic ketoacidosis, renal disease, deferoxamine therapy, leukemia, disseminated cancer, organ transplants, human immunodeficiency virus (HIV), extensive burns, and prolonged immunosuppressive therapy. Six forms of infection have been identified and include rhinocerebral, pulmonary, cutaneous, gastrointestinal, central nervous system, and disseminated disease. *Rhinocerebral mucormycosis* is the most common form and is usually associated with diabetic ketoacidosis. Usually associated with leukemia, *pulmonary mucormycosis* is the second most common presentation.

Causes

Mucormycosis is caused by saprophytic fungi, which are usually harmless commensals, but under extraordinary circumstances can cause invasive disease. There are four clinically important fungi in the Mucorales order: *Absida, Mucor, Rhizomucor,* and *Rhizopus.* Usually found in soil, bread and fruit molds, manure, and insects, these fungi derive their energy from breaking down dead organic matter. Infection occurs when the spores become airborne and enter the sinuses or when ingested with foods. In immunocompromised patients, normal body defenses may fail, leading to spore germination and the development of hyphae, which extend into the blood vessels with resultant ischemia and necrosis of adjacent organs.

FORMS OF MUCORMYCOSIS

The chart below lists the forms of mucormycosis and the clinical manifestations that may occur.

TYPES	SIGNS AND SYMPTOMS
Cerebral and rhinocerebral	▸ Nasal obstruction ▸ Dark, blood-tinged nasal discharge ▸ Necrotic crusting of the nasal septum and septal perforation ▸ Proptosis, periorbital edema, lacrimation, and blurred vision ▸ Paresis of cranial nerves III, IV, V, VI, and VII ▸ Changes in level of consciousness
Cutaneous	▸ Superficial: vesicles or pustules of the dermis and subcutaneous tissues ▸ Gangrenous: Ulceration and formation of eschar
Gastrointestinal	▸ Bloody diarrhea ▸ Bowel obstruction or perforation
Pulmonary	▸ Fever ▸ Progressive pulmonary infiltration ▸ Cough, hemoptysis, dyspnea, and pleuritic pain

Signs and symptoms

The pathologic feature most characteristic of mucormycosis is hyphal invasion of the vasculature. Regardless of the area of invasion, a combination of hemorrhage, thrombosis, infarction, and necrosis of the tissue or organ involved is apparent. (See *Forms of mucormycosis*.)

Diagnosis

A definitive diagnosis is established by histological examination of infected tissue. Because much of the necrotic debris does not contain organisms, it is important that the tissue samples be painstakingly examined for large nonseptate hyphae. The hyphae may be visualized on hematoxylin and eosin stain, the periodic acid-Schiff stain, methenamine silver stain, or with direct immunofluorescence conjugate.

For unknown reasons, cultures may test negative, even when hyphae are visible in the tissues. X-rays and computed tomography scans often miss signs of significant bone destruction. There must be a high index of suspicion in order to diagnose mucormycosis in its earliest stages, when clinical symptoms are the most subtle and the disease is most treatable.

Treatment

The initial approach is to reverse the disease state that predisposed the patient to the infection, if at all possible. Immunosuppressive drugs should be reduced or stopped. Antifungal therapy and removal of all necrotic tissue is essential to eradicate the infection. Amphotericin B, most effective, is given I.V. or injected directly into the spinal fluid. Since amphotericin B is unable to penetrate avascular areas, surgical debridement of necrotic tissue is performed to cleanse remaining organisms.

Other therapies include rifampin, tetracycline, and the azole antifungals, in combination with amphotericin B. Lifesaving supportive measures are undertaken according to the patient's condition.

Use of hyperbaric oxygen (HBO) is also recommended. HBO provides fungicidal levels of oxygen to the tissues to slow or inhibit fungal growth and also potentiates amphotericin B.

Special considerations

▶ This is an opportunistic disease of severely immunocompromised patients.
▶ Wash hands before and after patient contact, before and after invasive procedures, dressing changes, and handling food.
▶ Dispose of tissues and dressings in moisture-resistant containers.
▶ Wear mask and gloves when performing patient care.
▶ Dispose of soiled bed linens appropriately.
▶ Maintain blood glucose within prescribed limits.
▶ Monitor for adverse effects of amphotericin B such as nephrogenic diabetes insipidus and agranulocytopenia.
▶ Hemodynamic monitoring and ventilatory assistance may be required.
▶ Patients and significant others may require significant emotional and spiritual support and assistance with end-of-life decisions since the morbidity and mortality rate for this disease remains high.

MUMPS

Also known as infectious or epidemic parotitis, mumps is an acute viral disease caused by a paramyxovirus. It is most prevalent in children older than age 5 but younger than age 9. Infants under age 1 seldom get this disease because of passive immunity from maternal antibodies. Peak incidence occurs during late winter and early spring. The prognosis for complete recovery is good, although mumps sometimes causes complications.

Causes

The mumps paramyxovirus is found in the saliva of an infected person and is transmitted by droplets or by direct contact. The virus is present in the saliva 6 days before to 9 days after onset of parotid gland swelling; the 48-hour period immediately preceding onset of swelling is probably the time of highest communicability. The incubation period ranges from 14 to 25 days (the average is 18 days). One attack of mumps (even if unilateral) almost always confers lifelong immunity.

 PREVENTION TIP Emphasize the importance of routine immunization with live attenuated mumps virus (paramyxovirus) and for susceptible patients (especially males) who are approaching or are past puberty. In the U.S. the mumps vaccine is usually given as part of the MMR at age 15 months, and then again later in childhood; it is over 95% effective in preventing mumps disease. Also, immunization within 24 hours of exposure may prevent or attenuate the actual disease. Immunity against mumps lasts at least 12 years.

Signs and symptoms

The clinical features of mumps vary widely. An estimated 30% of susceptible people have subclinical illness.

Mumps usually begins with prodromal symptoms that last for 24 hours and include myalgia, anorexia, malaise, headache, and low-grade fever. These symptoms are followed by an earache that's aggravated by chewing, parotid gland tenderness and swelling, a temperature of 101° to 104° F (38.3° to 40° C), and pain when chewing or when drinking sour or acidic liquids. Simultaneously with the swelling of the parotid gland, or several days later, one or more of the other salivary glands may become swollen.

Complications can include epididymo-orchitis and mumps meningitis. Epididymo-orchitis, which occurs in approximately 25% of postpubertal males who contract mumps, produces abrupt onset of testicular swelling and tenderness, scrotal erythema, lower abdominal pain, nausea, vomiting, fever, and chills. Swelling and tenderness may last for several weeks; epididymitis may precede or accompany orchitis. In 50% of men with mumps-induced orchitis, the testicles show some atrophy, but sterility is extremely rare.

Mumps meningitis complicates mumps in 10% of patients and affects males three to five times more often than females. Symptoms include fever, meningeal irritation (nuchal rigidity, headache, and irritability), vomiting, drowsiness, and a lymphocyte count in cerebrospinal fluid ranging from 500 to 2,000/μl. Recovery is usually complete. Less common effects are pancreatitis, deafness, arthritis, myocarditis, encephalitis, pericarditis, oophoritis, and nephritis.

Diagnosis

In mumps, a diagnosis is usually made after the characteristic signs and symptoms develop, especially parotid gland enlargement with a history of exposure to mumps. Serologic antibody testing can verify the diagnosis when parotid or other salivary gland enlargement is absent. If comparison between a blood sample obtained during the acute phase of illness and another sample obtained 3 weeks later shows a fourfold rise in antibody titer, the patient most likely had mumps. Differential diagnoses include other infectious viruses (such as those caused by parainfluenza virus type 3, coxsackieviruses, and influenza A virus), sarcoidosis, and Sjögren's syndrome.

Treatment

Effective treatment includes analgesics for pain, antipyretics for fever, and adequate fluid intake to prevent dehydration from fever and anorexia. If the patient can't swallow, I.V. fluid replacement may be necessary.

Special considerations

▶ Stress the need for bed rest during the febrile period.

▶ Give analgesics, and apply warm or cool compresses to the neck to relieve pain.

▶ Give antipyretics and tepid sponge baths for fever.

▶ To prevent dehydration, encourage the patient to drink fluids; to minimize pain and anorexia, advise him to avoid spicy, irritating foods and those that require a lot of chewing.

▶ During the acute phase, observe the patient closely for signs of central nervous system involvement, such as an altered level of consciousness and nuchal rigidity.

▶ Respiratory isolation is advocated for mumps. Precautions should be taken by all personnel in contact with the patient.

▶ Report all cases of mumps to local public health authorities.

▶ The patient should be excluded from school or the workplace for 9 days from the onset of mumps.

MYCOBACTERIUM AVIUM COMPLEX

Mycobacterium avium complex (MAC) is a serious opportunistic bacterial infection which most commonly affects patients in the advanced stages of acquired immunodeficiency syndrome (AIDS). In patients with AIDS, MAC is usually disseminated and affects those with CD4+ T-cell counts below 50/mm^3. Any organ system can be involved, especially those with many mononuclear phagocytes (such as the liver, spleen, and bone marrow). Less commonly, MAC may produce pulmonary disease in nonimmunocompromised people; it may manifest in children as cervical lymphadenitis.

The incidence of MAC is not reportable; however, population-based data available for the Houston and Atlanta metropolitan areas suggest a rate of 1:100,000 cases per year. Incidence is decreasing among those with human immunodeficiency virus (HIV) as a result of chemoprophylaxis and combination antiretroviral therapy.

Causes

The etiologic agents responsible for MAC are *Mycobacterium avium* and *Mycobacterium intracellulare*. MAC is a water and soil saprophyte and enters the body through either the GI or respiratory tracts. It is unclear whether active infection results from recently acquired microbes or from reactivation of latent infection. There are no current recommendations regarding avoidance of exposure.

Signs and symptoms

The signs and symptoms of MAC are generally nonspecific and include fever, night sweats, weight loss, weakness, anorexia, diarrhea, malabsorption, and abdominal pain. Enlargement of the liver and spleen is common. Laboratory findings include anemia, neutropenia, and elevated alkaline phosphatase levels. Respiratory symptoms are uncommon in AIDS-related MAC infection. MAC is usually asymptomatic in patients with CD4+ T-cell counts above 100/mm^3.

 PREVENTION TIP Some practitioners advocate prophylactic treatment for MAC in patients with HIV whose CD4+ T-cell counts are below 100/mm^3. Generally, rifabutin, clarithromycin, or azithromycin are used.

Diagnosis

Blood and bone marrow cultures are the most sensitive diagnostic tests. Disseminated MAC can be diagnosed from one positive blood culture. A positive sputum or stool culture may precede the development of symptomatic disease but may also represent colonization rather than infection. A history of prior opportunistic diseases is usually present.

Other diagnostic tests may include a chest radiograph, dilated eye exam, liver function tests, hepatitis profile, lymph node aspiration, test for cryptococcal antigen, purified protein derivative (PPD) and controls, coccidioidomycosis serologies, and histoplasma antigen.

Treatment

 ALERT Given the morbidity and mortality associated with disseminated MAC, prompt treatment of probable infection is critical.

There is currently no standard therapy for MAC; however, guidelines published by the U.S. Public Health Service and Infectious Diseases Society of America recommend a combination treatment regimen which includes at least two drugs, one of which should be either clarithromycin or azithromycin. Ethambutal is a second-line drug; clofazimine, rifabutin, rifampin, amikacin, and ciprofloxacin are third-line drugs. Clinical and microscopic response is usually evident in 4 to 6 weeks. At this time, treatment is considered to be lifelong. Treatment should also include preventing further infection and reducing the risks of opportunistic infections.

Special considerations

▶ Use proper personal protective gear when obtaining or handling laboratory samples.
▶ Monitor carefully for drug adverse effects; most are minor and include GI symptoms. Be alert for signs of nephro- and ototoxicity (amikacin), pain or tingling of the extremities and yellow skin discoloration (clofazimine), visual disturbances (ethambutol), and anemia (rifabutin).
▶ Monitor nutritional status.

▶ Administer antipyretics and antiemetics as needed.

▶ Frequently monitor CD4+ T-cell counts.

 PREVENTION TIP Stress the importance of compliance with the medication regime to prevent life-threatening MAC infection. Other areas of education should include general lifestyle modifications such as smoking cessation, good nutrition, and regular exercise to enhance quality of life, since so many HIV-infected patients are now living long enough to encounter the chronic diseases found in the general population.

MYELITIS AND ACUTE TRANSVERSE MYELITIS

Myelitis, or inflammation of the spinal cord, can result from several diseases. Poliomyelitis affects the cord's gray matter and produces motor dysfunction; leuko-myelitis affects only the white matter and produces sensory dysfunction. These types of myelitis can attack any level of the spinal cord, causing partial destruction or scattered lesions. Acute transverse myelitis, which affects the entire thickness of the spinal cord, produces both motor and sensory dysfunctions. This form of myelitis, which has a rapid onset, is the most devastating.

Prognosis depends on the severity of cord damage and prevention of complications. If spinal cord necrosis occurs, the prognosis for complete recovery is poor. Even without necrosis, residual neurologic deficits usually persist after recovery. Patients who develop spastic reflexes early in the course of the illness are more likely to recover than those who do not develop spastic reflexes or develop them at a later point in the illness.

Causes

Acute transverse myelitis has a variety of causes. It often follows acute infectious diseases, such as measles or pneumonia (the inflammation occurs after the infection has subsided), and primary infections of the spinal cord itself, such as syphilis or acute disseminated encephalomyelitis. Acute transverse myelitis can accompany demyelinating diseases, such as acute multiple sclerosis, and inflammatory and necrotizing disorders of the spinal cord, such as hematomyelia.

Certain toxic agents (carbon monoxide, lead, and arsenic) can cause a type of myelitis in which acute inflammation (followed by hemorrhage and possible necrosis) destroys the entire circumference (myelin, axis cylinders, and neurons) of the spinal cord. Other forms of myelitis may result from poliovirus, herpes zoster, herpesvirus B, or rabies virus; disorders that cause meningeal inflammation, such as syphilis, abscesses and other suppurative conditions, and tuberculosis; smallpox or polio vaccination; parasitic and fungal infections; and chronic adhesive arachnoiditis.

Signs and symptoms

In acute transverse myelitis, onset is rapid, with motor and sensory dysfunctions below the level of spinal cord damage appearing in 1 to 2 days. Patients with acute transverse myelitis develop flaccid paralysis of the legs (sometimes beginning in just one leg) with loss of sensory and sphincter functions. Such sensory loss may follow pain in the legs or trunk. Reflexes disappear in the early stages but may reappear later. The extent of damage depends on which level of the spinal cord is affected; transverse myelitis rarely involves the arms. If spinal cord damage is severe, it may cause shock (hypotension and hypothermia).

Diagnosis

Paraplegia of rapid onset usually points to acute transverse myelitis. In such patients, neurologic examination confirms paraplegia or neurologic deficit below the level of the spinal cord lesion and absent or, later, hyperactive reflexes. Cerebrospinal fluid may be normal or show increased lymphocyte or protein levels. Diagnostic evaluation must rule out a spinal cord tumor and identify the cause of any underlying infection.

Treatment

No effective treatment exists for acute transverse myelitis. However, this condition requires appropriate treatment of any underlying infection. Some patients with postinfectious or multiple sclerosis-induced myelitis have received steroid therapy, but its benefits aren't clear.

 PREVENTION TIP Prevention of complications is important. Prevent contractures with range-of-motion exercises and proper alignment. Prevent skin infections and pressure ulcers with meticulous skin care. Check pressure points often, keep skin clean and dry, and use a waterbed or another pressure-relieving device.

Special considerations

❱ Assess vital signs frequently. Watch carefully for signs of spinal shock (hypotension and excessive sweating).
❱ Watch for signs of urinary tract infections from indwelling urinary catheters.

 ALERT Initiate rehabilitation immediately. Assist the patient with physical therapy, bowel and bladder training, and any lifestyle changes that his condition requires.

MYOCARDITIS

Myocarditis is focal or diffuse inflammation of the cardiac muscle (myocardium). It may be acute or chronic and can occur at any age. Frequently, myocarditis fails to produce specific cardiovascular symptoms or electrocardiogram (ECG) abnormalities, and recovery is usually spontaneous, without residual defects. Occasionally, myocarditis is complicated by heart failure; rarely, it may lead to cardiomyopathy.

Causes

Myocarditis may result from:
❱ *viral infections* (most common cause in the United States and western Europe): coxsackievirus A and B strains and, possibly, poliomyelitis, influenza, rubeola, rubella, and adenoviruses and echoviruses
❱ *bacterial infections:* diphtheria, tuberculosis, typhoid fever, tetanus, and staphylococcal, pneumococcal, and gonococcal infections
❱ *hypersensitive immune reactions:* acute rheumatic fever and postcardiotomy syndrome
❱ *radiation therapy:* large doses of radiation to the chest in treating lung or breast cancer
❱ *chemical poisons:* such as chronic alcoholism
❱ *parasitic infections:* especially South American trypanosomiasis (Chagas' disease) in infants and immunosuppressed adults; also, toxoplasmosis
❱ *helminthic infections:* such as trichinosis.

Signs and symptoms

Myocarditis usually causes nonspecific symptoms — such as fatigue, dyspnea, palpitations, and fever — that reflect the accompanying systemic infection. Occasionally, it may produce mild, continuous pressure or soreness in the chest (unlike the recurring, stress-related pain of angina pectoris). Although myocarditis is usually self-limiting, it may induce myofibril degeneration that results in right and left heart failure, with cardiomegaly, neck vein distention, dyspnea, persistent fever, with resting or exertional tachycardia disproportionate to the degree of fever, and supraventricular and ventricular arrhythmias. Sometimes myocarditis recurs or produces chronic valvulitis (when it results from rheumatic fever), cardiomyopathy, arrhythmias, and thromboembolism.

Diagnosis

The patient history commonly reveals recent febrile upper respiratory tract infection, viral pharyngitis, or tonsillitis. A physical examination shows supraventricular and ventricular arrhythmias, S_3 and S_4 gallops, a faint S_1, possibly a murmur of mitral insufficiency (from papillary muscle dysfunction) and, if pericarditis is present, a pericardial friction rub.

Electrocardiography typically shows diffuse ST-segment and T-wave abnormalities (as in pericarditis), conduction defects (prolonged PR interval), and other supraventricular arrhythmias. Stool and throat cultures may identify the causative bacteria. An endomyocardial biopsy is used to confirm the diagnosis, but a negative biopsy doesn't exclude the diagnosis. A repeat biopsy may be needed. Laboratory tests can't unequivocally confirm myocarditis, but the following findings support this diagnosis:

▶ Cardiac enzyme levels (creatine kinase [CK], the CK-MB isoenzyme, aspartate aminotransferase, and lactate dehydrogenase) are elevated.

▶ White blood cell count and erythrocyte sedimentation rate are increased.

▶ Antibody titers (such as antistreptolysin O titer in rheumatic fever) are elevated.

Endocardial biopsy remains the gold standard for diagnosis of myocarditis, although results remain controversial and the procedure is invasive and costly.

Treatment

In myocardial infarction, treatment includes antibiotics for bacterial infection, modified bed rest to decrease the cardiac workload, and careful management of complications. Heart failure requires restriction of activity to minimize myocardial oxygen consumption, supplemental oxygen therapy, sodium restriction, diuretics to decrease fluid retention, and digitalis glycosides to increase myocardial contractility. Inotropic support of cardiac function with amrinone, dopamine, or dobutamine may be needed. However, digitalis glycosides must be administered cautiously because some patients with myocarditis show a paradoxical sensitivity to even small doses.

 ALERT Arrhythmias require prompt but cautious administration of antiarrhythmics, such as quinidine or procainamide, because these drugs depress myocardial contractility.

Thromboembolism requires anticoagulation therapy. Treatment with corticosteroids or other immunosuppressants is controversial and therefore limited to combating life-threatening complications such as intractable heart failure.

Special considerations

▶ Assess cardiovascular status frequently, watching for signs of heart failure, such as dyspnea, hypotension, and tachycardia. Check for changes in cardiac rhythm or conduction.

▶ Observe for signs of digitalis toxicity (anorexia, nausea, vomiting, blurred vision, cardiac arrhythmias) and for complicating factors that may potentiate toxicity, such as electrolyte imbalances or hypoxia.

▶ Stress the importance of bed rest. Assist with bathing as necessary; provide a bedside commode, which puts less stress on the heart than using a bedpan. Reassure the patient that activity limitations are temporary.

▶ Offer diversional activities that are physically undemanding.

▶ During recovery, recommend that the patient resume normal activities slowly and avoid competitive sports.

MYRINGITIS

Acute infectious myringitis is characterized by inflammation, hemorrhage, and effusion of fluid into the tissue at the end of the external ear canal and the tympanic membrane. This self-limiting disorder (resolving spontaneously within 3 days to

2 weeks) often follows acute otitis media or upper respiratory tract infection and frequently occurs epidemically in children. Chronic granular myringitis, a rare inflammation of the squamous layer of the tympanic membrane, causes gradual hearing loss.

 ALERT Without specific treatment, chronic granular myringitis can lead to stenosis of the ear canal, as granulation extends from the tympanic membrane to the external ear.

Causes

Acute infectious myringitis usually follows viral infection but may also result from infection with bacteria (pneumococci, *Haemophilus influenzae,* beta-hemolytic streptococci, staphylococci), or any other organism that may cause acute otitis media.

 PREVENTION TIP To help prevent acute infectious myringitis, advise early treatment of acute otitis media.

Myringitis is a rare sequela of atypical pneumonia caused by *Mycoplasma pneumoniae.* The cause of chronic granular myringitis is unknown.

Signs and symptoms

Acute infectious myringitis begins with severe ear pain, commonly accompanied by tenderness over the mastoid process. Small, reddened, inflamed blebs form in the canal, on the tympanic membrane and, with bacterial invasion, in the middle ear. Fever and hearing loss are rare unless fluid accumulates in the middle ear or a large bleb totally obstructs the external auditory meatus. Spontaneous rupture of these blebs may cause bloody discharge. Chronic granular myringitis produces pruritus, purulent discharge, and gradual hearing loss.

Diagnosis

In acute infectious myringitis the diagnosis is based on a physical examination, showing characteristic blebs, and on a typical patient history. Culture and sensitivity testing of exudate identifies secondary infection. In chronic granular myringitis, physical examination may reveal granulation extending from the tympanic membrane to the external ear. Differential diagnosis to consider include teething, tonsilitis, pharyngitis, and temporomandibular joint syndrome.

Treatment

Hospitalization usually isn't required for acute infectious myringitis. Treatment consists of measures to relieve pain. Analgesics, such as aspirin or acetaminophen, and application of heat to the external ear are usually sufficient, but severe pain may necessitate the use of codeine. Since it is difficult to determine viral from bacterial or mycoplasmal otitis, antibiotic therapy as for acute otitis media is also indicated. Systemic or topical antibiotics prevent or treat secondary infection.

Incision of the blebs and evacuation of serum and blood may relieve pressure and help drain exudate, but these measures don't speed recovery. Treatment of chronic granular myringitis consists of systemic antibiotics or local anti-inflammatory antibiotic combination eardrops, and surgical excision and cautery. If stenosis is present, surgical reconstruction is necessary.

Special considerations

▶ Stress the importance of completing the prescribed antibiotic therapy.
▶ Teach the patient how to instill topical antibiotics (eardrops).
▶ When necessary, explain the incision of the blebs to the patient.

N

NECROTIZING ENTEROCOLITIS

Neonatal necrotizing enterocolitis (NEC) is a clinical condition characterized by an initial mucosal intestinal injury that may progress to transmural bowel necrosis. Although NEC occurs frequently, its cause is unknown. NEC is the single most frequent surgical emergency in neonates in North America. With early detection, the survival rate is 60% to 80%. Infectious complications associated with bowel necrosis include bacterial peritonitis, systemic sepsis, and intra-abdominal abscess formation.

Causes

NEC occurs most often in premature infants (less than 34 weeks' gestation) and those of low birth weight (less than 5 lb [2.3 kg]). However, one in ten infants who develop NEC is full-term. NEC is occurring more frequently, possibly because of the higher incidence and survival of premature and low-birth-weight infants. More than 90% of NEC cases occur after initiation of feedings. Among premature and low-birth-weight infants in intensive care nurseries, incidence varies from 1% to 12%. NEC is associated with 2% of all infant deaths.

The exact cause of NEC is unknown. Suggested predisposing factors include birth asphyxia, postnatal hypotension, respiratory failure, hypothermia, sepsis, acidosis, and structural cardiac defects, as well as pharmacological associations, such as cocaine exposure and indomethacin treatment. NEC may also be a response to significant prenatal stress, such as premature rupture of membranes, placenta previa, maternal sepsis, toxemia of pregnancy, or breech or cesarean birth.

According to a current theory, NEC develops when the infant suffers perinatal hypoxemia due to shunting of blood from the gut to more vital organs. Subsequent mucosal ischemia provides an ideal medium for bacterial growth. Hypertonic formula may increase bacterial activity because — unlike maternal breast milk — it doesn't provide protective immunologic activity and because it contributes to the production of hydrogen gas.

 PREVENTION TIP To help prevent NEC, encourage mothers to breast-feed because breast milk contains macrophages that fight infection and has a low pH that inhibits the growth of many microbes. Also, colostrum — fluid secreted before the milk — contains high concentrations of immunoglobulin A, which directly protects the bowel from infection, and which the neonate lacks for several days postpartum.

As the bowel swells and breaks down, gas-forming bacteria invade damaged areas, producing free air in the intestinal wall. This may result in fatal perforation and peritonitis.

Signs and symptoms

Any neonate who has suffered from perinatal hypoxemia has the potential for developing NEC. A distended (especially tense or rigid) abdomen, with gastric retention, is the earliest and most common sign of oncoming NEC, usually appearing from 1 to 10 days after birth. Other clinical features are increasing residual gastric contents (which may contain bile), bilious vomitus, and occult or gross blood in stools. One-fourth of patients have bloody diarrhea. A red or shiny, taut abdomen may indicate peritonitis. Nonspecific signs and symptoms include thermal instability, lethargy, metabolic acidosis, jaundice, and disseminated intravascular coagulation (DIC). The major complication is perforation, which requires surgery. Recurrence of NEC and mechanical and functional abnormalities of the intestine, especially stricture, are the usual cause of residual intestinal malfunction in any infant who survives acute NEC, and may develop as late as 3 months postoperatively.

Diagnosis

Successful treatment of NEC relies on early recognition based on the following diagnostic test results:

▶ Anteroposterior and lateral abdominal X-rays confirm the diagnosis by showing nonspecific intestinal dilation and, in later stages of NEC, pneumatosis cystoides intestinalis (gas or air in the intestinal wall). Portal vein gas and fixed or thickened small bowel loops are also important radiographic findings. Sequential screening films are taken every 6 to 8 hours during the early disease stages.

▶ Platelet count may fall below 50,000/μl.

▶ Serum sodium levels are decreased.

▶ Arterial blood gas (ABG) levels show metabolic acidosis (a result of sepsis).

▶ Bilirubin levels show infection-induced breakdown of red blood cells.

▶ Blood and stool cultures identify the infecting organism.

▶ Guaiac test detects occult blood in stools.

Treatment

Up to 90% of infants with NEC can be managed without surgery. The first signs of NEC necessitate discontinuation of oral intake to rest the injured bowel. I.V. fluids, including hyperalimentation, maintain fluid and electrolyte balance and nutrition during this time; passage of a nasogastric (NG) tube allows bowel decompression. Correction of hypoxemia, hypotension, acidosis, and any other reversible medical problems is needed. Optimizing cardiac performance is necessary. Serial physical examinations, platelet counts, lactate levels, and ABGs are the most useful indications of progressive sepsis. Drug therapy consists of parenteral administration of broad-spectrum antibiotics to suppress bacterial flora and prevent bowel perforation. (These drugs can also be administered through an NG tube if necessary.)

 ALERT Surgery is indicated if the patient shows any signs or symptoms of the following: perforation (free intraperitoneal air on X-ray or symptoms of peritonitis), respiratory insufficiency (caused by severe abdominal distention), progressive and intractable acidosis, or DIC. Surgery removes all necrotic and acutely inflamed bowel and creates a temporary colostomy or ileostomy.

Special considerations

▶ Be alert for signs of gastric distention and perforation.

▶ Do not take any rectal temperatures, to avoid perforating the bowel.

▶ Prevent cross-contamination by disposing of soiled diapers properly and washing hands after diaper changes.

▶ Prepare the parents for a potential deterioration in their infant's condition. Explain all treatments, including why feedings are withheld.

▶ After surgery, the infant needs mechanical ventilation. Gently suction secretions and monitor respirations often.

▶ Replace fluids lost through NG tube and stoma drainage. Include drainage losses in output records. Weigh the infant daily. A daily weight gain of 0.35 to 0.7 oz (10 to 20 g) indicates a good response to therapy.

▶ An infant with a temporary colostomy or ileostomy should be referred to an enterostomal therapy nurse to assist the patient and family in meeting needs.

▶ Encourage the parents to participate in their infant's physical care after his condition is no longer critical.

▶ Because of the infant's small abdomen, the suture line is near the stoma. Maintaining a clean suture line may be problematic. Good skin care is essential because the immature infant's skin is fragile and vulnerable to excoriation and the active enzymes in bowel secretions, which are corrosive.

▶ Improvise infant-sized colostomy bags from urine collection bags, medicine cups, or condoms. Karaya gum is helpful in making a seal.

▶ Watch for wound disruption, infection, dehiscence, and excoriation — potential dangers because of severe catabolism.

▶ Watch for intestinal malfunction from stricture or short-bowel syndrome. Such complications usually develop 1 month after the infant resumes normal feedings.

▶ Encourage parental visits.

▶ Instruct mothers that they may refrigerate their milk for 48 hours but shouldn't freeze or heat it because this destroys antibodies. Tell them to use plastic — not glass — containers because leukocytes adhere to glass.

▶ Breast-feeding mothers should pump milk while the baby is not taking anything by mouth, in order to maintain an adequate milk supply.

NECROTIZING FASCIITIS

Popularly (and inappropriately) referred to as a disease caused by "flesh-eating bacteria," necrotizing fasciitis is a progressive, rapidly spreading inflammatory infection, located in the deep fascia, that destroys fascia and fat with secondary necrosis of subcutaneous tissue. Also referred to as hemolytic streptococcal gangrene, acute dermal gangrene, suppurative fasciitis, and synergistic necrotizing cellulitis, necrotizing fasciitis is most commonly caused by the pathogenic bacteria *Streptococcus pyogenes,* also known as group A *Streptococcus* (GAS), although

other aerobic and anaerobic pathogens may be present.

This severe and potentially fatal infection may begin at the site of a small insignificant wound or a surgical incision, and is characterized by invasive and progressive necrosis of the soft tissue and underlying blood supply. High mortality rates associated with necrotizing fasciitis have been attributed to the emergence of more virulent strains of streptococci caused by changes in the bacteria's DNA, as well as delays in clinical diagnosis. This would account for an increase in frequency and severity of the cases reported since 1985, following a 50- to 60-year span of insignificant clinical disease.

Noted for decades and described in medical literature since the Civil War, necrotizing fasciitis accounts for 8% of reported cases of invasive GAS infections today. Men are 3 times more likely to develop this rare condition than women; the disease rarely occurs in children except in countries with poor hygiene practices. The mean age for contracting the disease is 38 to 44 years of age, with a very high mortality rate at 70% to 80%. Mortality drops significantly and prognosis improves with early intervention and treatment. Cases treated aggressively with surgery, antibiotics, and hyperbaric oxygen therapy have seen mortality rates reduced to as low as 9% to 20%. (See *Hyperbaric oxygen therapy for necrotizing fasciitis,* page 192.)

Causes

More than 80 types of the causative bacteria *S. pyogenes* are in existence, making the epidemiology of GAS infections complex. Wounds as minor as pinpricks, needle punctures, bruises, blisters and abrasions, or as serious as a traumatic injury or surgical incision can provide an opportunity for bacteria to enter the body. In necrotizing fasciitis, group A beta-hemolytic *Streptococcus* and *Staphylococcus aureus,* working alone or together, are most often the primary infecting bacteria, entering the body via local tissue injury or through a breach in the in-

HYPERBARIC OXYGEN THERAPY FOR NECROTIZING FASCIITIS

Reports suggest that the use of hyperbaric oxygen (HBO) therapy decreases mortality rate, significantly improves the tissues' defense against infection, and prevents necrosis from spreading by increasing the normal oxygen saturations of infected wounds by a thousand-fold, thus causing a bactericidal effect. Typical HBO treatment begins aggressively, after the first surgical debridement, and continues for a total of 10 to 15 sessions.

tegrity of a mucous membrane barrier. Other aerobic and anaerobic pathogens, including *Bacteroides, Clostridium, Peptostreptococcus,* Enterobacteriaceae, coliforms, *Proteus, Pseudomonas,* and *Klebsiella,* may be present, proliferating in an environment of tissue hypoxia caused by trauma, recent surgery, and medical compromise. The end product of invasion is necrosis of the surrounding tissue, accelerating the disease process by creating a favorable environment for these microbes.

Signs and symptoms

Pain, out of proportion to the size of the wound or injury it is associated with, is usually the first symptom of necrotizing fasciitis, and is generally present prior to all other physical findings. The infective process usually begins with a mild area of erythema at the site of insult, which quickly progresses within the first 24 hours. During the first 24- to 48-hour period, the erythema changes from red to purple in color and then blue, with the formation of fluid-filled blisters and bullae indicating the rapid progression of the necrotizing

process. By days 4 and 5, multiple patches of this erythema form, producing large areas of gangrenous skin. By days 7 to 10, dead skin begins to separate at the margins of the erythema, revealing extensive necrosis of the subcutaneous tissue. At this stage, fascial necrosis is typically more advanced than appearance would suggest.

Other clinical symptoms include fever and hypovolemia, and in later stages, hypotension, respiratory insufficiency, and signs of overwhelming sepsis requiring supportive care. In the most severe cases, necrosis advances rapidly until several large areas are involved, causing the patient to become mentally cloudy, delirious, or even unresponsive secondary to the intoxication rendered. Other complications include renal failure, septic shock with cardiovascular collapse, and scarring with cosmetic deformities. Without treatment, involvement of deeper muscle layers may occur, resulting in myositis or myonecrosis.

Diagnosis

Tissue biopsy is the best method of diagnosing necrotizing fasciitis. Cultures of microorganisms can be obtained locally from the periphery of the spreading infection, or from deeper tissues during surgical debridement. Gram staining and culturing of biopsied tissue helps establish the type of invasive organisms and the effective treatment against them. Radiographic studies can pinpoint the presence of subcutaneous gases, and computed tomography scans can locate the anatomic site of involvement by locating necrosis. In combination with clinical assessment, magnetic resonance imaging (MRI) is being utilized to determine areas of necrosis and the need for surgical debridement.

Other supportive studies include lab values, such as complete blood count with differential, electrolytes, glucose, blood urea nitrogen and creatinine, urinalysis, and arterial blood gases. Differential diagnoses are cellulitis, Fournier's gangrene, gas gangrene, and toxic shock syndrome.

Treatment

ALERT Most severe cases progress within hours and mortality is high. Early medical treatment is critical. Oral treatment is inappropriate; this is a very deadly infection and requires aggressive treatment, including I.V. antibiotics.

Prompt and aggressive exploration and debridement of suspected necrotizing fasciitis is mandatory to provide early and definitive diagnosis and enhance prognosis. Ninety percent of patients that present with clinical signs and symptoms will need immediate surgical debridement, fasciotomy, or amputation. Ampicillin, clindamycin (Cleocin), metronidazole (Flagyl), ceftriaxone (Rocephin), and gentamicin (Garamycin) are some of the medications used intravenously to treat the organisms that can be involved with necrotizing fasciitis.

The particular drugs are determined by the sensitivity of the organisms in culture, although empiric treatment with multiple broad-spectrum antibiotics is appropriate initially. Drug recommendations continue to change as new antibiotics are developed and new resistance emerges.

Special considerations

▶ Start broad-spectrum antibiotic therapy immediately.

▶ Accurate and frequent assessment of the patient's level of pain, mental status, wound status, and vital signs are essential in recognizing the progression of wound changes or the development of new signs and symptoms. Changes must be reported and documented immediately.

▶ The need for supportive care, such as endotracheal intubation, cardiac monitoring, fluid replacement, and supplemental oxygen should be assessed and provided as warranted.

▶ Care of post-operative patients and those with trauma wounds requires strict aseptic technique, good hand washing, and barriers between health care providers and patients to prevent contamination.

▶ Health care workers with sore throats should see their doctor to determine if they have a streptococcal infection. If diagnosed positive they should stay home from work at least 24 hours after starting antibiotic therapy.

▶ Risk factors for contracting necrotizing fasciitis include alcohol abuse, advanced age, human immunodeficiency virus infection, and varicellar infection. Patients with chronic illnesses such as cancer, diabetes, cardiac and pulmonary disease, kidney disease requiring hemodialysis, and those using steroids are more susceptible to GAS infection due to debilitated immune responsiveness.

ALERT Be alert for signs and symptoms of toxic shock syndrome, which is associated with any streptococcal soft tissue infection, and the development of shock, acute respiratory distress syndrome, renal impairment, and bacteremia, any of which can lead to sudden death.

NOCARDIOSIS

Nocardiosis is an acute, subacute, or chronic bacterial infection caused by a weakly gram-positive species of the genus *Nocardia* — usually *N. asteroides*. It is most common in men, especially those with a compromised immune system. In patients with brain infection, mortality exceeds 80%; in other forms, mortality is 50%, even with appropriate therapy.

Causes

Nocardia are aerobic gram-positive bacteria with branching filaments similar in appearance to fungi. Normally found in soil, these microbes cause occasional sporadic disease in humans and animals throughout the world. Their incubation period is unknown but is probably several weeks. The usual mode of transmission is inhalation of organisms suspended in dust. Transmission by direct inoculation through puncture wounds or abrasions is less common.

Signs and symptoms

Nocardiosis originates as a pulmonary infection with a cough that produces thick, tenacious, purulent, mucopurulent, and possibly blood-tinged sputum. It may also cause a fever as high as 105° F (40.6° C), chills, night sweats, anorexia, malaise, and weight loss. This infection may lead to pleurisy, intrapleural effusions, and empyema. Other effects include tracheitis, bronchitis, pericarditis, endocarditis, peritonitis, mediastinitis, septic arthritis, and keratoconjunctivitis. If the infection spreads through the blood to the brain, abscesses form, causing confusion, disorientation, dizziness, headache, nausea, and seizures. Rupture of a brain abscess can cause purulent meningitis. Extrapulmonary, hematogenous spread may cause endocarditis and lesions in the kidneys, liver, subcutaneous tissue, and bone.

Diagnosis

Identifying *Nocardia* by culture of sputum or discharge is difficult. In many cases, special staining techniques must be used to make the diagnosis, in conjunction with a typical clinical picture (usually progressive pneumonia, despite antibiotic therapy). Occasionally, diagnosis requires biopsy of lung or other tissue. Chest X-rays vary and may show fluffy or interstitial infiltrates, nodules, or abscesses. Unfortunately, up to 40% of nocardial infections elude diagnosis until postmortem examination.

In brain infection with meningitis, lumbar puncture shows nonspecific changes, such as increased opening pressure; cerebrospinal fluid with increased white blood cell and protein levels; and decreased glucose levels compared to serum glucose.

Treatment

Nocardiosis requires 12 to 18 months of treatment, preferably with co-trimoxazole or high doses of sulfonamides. In patients who do not respond to sulfonamide treatment, other drugs, such as ampicillin, erythromycin, or minocycline, may be added. Treatment also includes surgical drainage of abscesses and excision of necrotic tissue. The acute phase requires complete bed rest; as the patient improves, activity can increase.

Special considerations

Because it is not transmitted from person to person, nocardiosis requires no isolation.

◗ Provide adequate nourishment through total parenteral nutrition, nasogastric tube feedings, or a balanced diet.

◗ Give the patient tepid sponge baths and antipyretics, as ordered, to reduce his fever.

◗ Monitor for allergic reactions to antibiotics.

◗ High-dose sulfonamide therapy (especially sulfadiazine) predisposes the patient to crystalluria and oliguria, so assess him frequently, force fluids, and alkalinize the urine with sodium bicarbonate, as ordered, to prevent these complications.

◗ In patients with pulmonary infection, administer chest physiotherapy. Auscultate the lungs daily, checking for increased crackles or consolidation. Note and record the amount, color, and thickness of sputum.

◗ In brain infection, regularly assess neurologic function. Watch for signs of increased intracranial pressure, such as decreased level of consciousness, and respiratory abnormalities.

◗ In long-term hospitalization, turn the patient often, and assist with range-of-motion exercises.

◗ Before the patient is discharged, stress the need to follow a regular medication schedule to maintain therapeutic blood levels, and to continue drugs even after symptoms subside. Explain the importance of frequent follow-up examinations.

◗ Provide support and encouragement to help the patient and his family cope with this long-term illness.

O

ORBITAL CELLULITIS

Orbital cellulitis is an acute infection of the orbital tissues and eyelids that doesn't involve the eyeball. With treatment, the prognosis is good; if cellulitis is not treated, however, infection may spread to the cavernous sinus or the meninges, where it can be life-threatening. Orbital cellulitis in young children is spread from adjacent sinuses (especially the ethmoid air cell) and accounts for the majority of postseptal cellulitis cases. Immunosuppressed patients and people with poor dental hygiene are also at risk.

Causes

Orbital cellulitis may result from bacterial, fungal, or parasitic infections. The most common bacterial pathogens in children are *Haemophilus influenzae, Streptococcus pneumoniae,* and *Staphylococcus aureus.* The organisms invade the orbit, frequently by direct extension through the sinuses, the bloodstream, or the lymphatic ducts. The periorbital tissues may be inoculated as a result of surgery, foreign body trauma, or animal or insect bites.

Signs and symptoms

Orbital cellulitis generally produces unilateral eyelid edema, hyperemia of the orbital tissues, reddened eyelids, and matted lashes. Although the eyeball is initially unaffected, proptosis develops later due to edematous tissues within the bony confines of the orbit. Other indications include extreme orbital pain, impaired eye movement, chemosis, and purulent discharge from indurated areas. The severity of associated systemic symptoms (chills, fever, and malaise) varies with the cause.

Complications include posterior extension, causing cavernous sinus thrombosis, meningitis, or brain abscess and, rarely, atrophy and subsequent loss of vision secondary to optic neuritis.

Diagnosis

Typical clinical features establish the diagnosis. Wound culture and sensitivity testing determines the causative organism and specific antibiotic therapy. Other tests include white blood cell count, ophthalmologic examination, and a computed tomography (CT) scan of orbit tissues. A CT scan will rule out cellulitis due to preseptal or deeper structural causes, and will determine if a tumor is the cause of the swelling.

Treatment

Prompt treatment is necessary to prevent complications. Primary treatment consists of antibiotic therapy. Systemic antibiotics (I.V. or oral) and eyedrops or ointment will be ordered. Supportive therapy consists of fluids; warm, moist compresses; and bed rest. The patient should be followed closely. If there's no improvement during the first 48 to 72 hours of treatment, antibiotic adjustment guided by drug sensitivity should be considered. An orbital abscess may necessitate surgical incision and drainage.

Special considerations

▶ Monitor vital signs, assess visual acuity, and maintain fluid and electrolyte balance.

❯ Have the patient instill antibiotic eye-drops during the day and use antibiotic ointment at night as prescribed.

❯ Apply compresses every 3 to 4 hours to localize inflammation and relieve discomfort. Teach the patient to apply these compresses. Give pain medication, as ordered, after assessing pain level.

❯ Before discharge, stress the importance of completing the prescribed antibiotic therapy.

 PREVENTION TIP To prevent orbital cellulitis, tell the patient to maintain good general hygiene and to carefully clean abrasions and cuts that occur near the orbit. Urge early treatment of orbital cellulitis to prevent infection from spreading.

ORNITHOSIS

Ornithosis (also called psittacosis or parrot fever) is caused by the gram-negative intracellular parasite *Chlamydia psittaci* and is transmitted by infected birds. This disease occurs worldwide and is mainly associated with occupational exposure to birds (such as poultry farming). Incidence is higher in women and in people ages 20 to 50. With adequate antimicrobial therapy, ornithosis is fatal in fewer than 4% of patients.

Causes

Psittacine birds (parrots, parakeets, cockatoos), pigeons, and turkeys may harbor *C. psittaci* in their blood, feathers, tissues, nasal secretions, liver, spleen, and feces. Transmission to humans occurs primarily through inhalation of dust containing *C. psittaci* from bird droppings; less often, transmission occurs through direct contact with infected secretions or body tissues, as in laboratory personnel who work with birds. Person-to-person transmission seldom occurs but usually causes severe ornithosis.

Signs and symptoms

After an incubation period of 4 to 15 days, onset of symptoms may be insidious or sudden. Clinical effects include chills and a low-grade fever that increases to 103° to 105° F (39.4° to 40.6° C) for 7 to 10 days, then, with treatment, declines during the 2nd or 3rd week. Other signs and symptoms include headache, myalgia, sore throat, cough (may be dry, hacking, and nonproductive, or may produce blood-tinged sputum), abdominal distention and tenderness, nausea, vomiting, photophobia, decreased pulse rate, slightly increased respiratory rate, secondary purulent lung infection, and a faint macular rash. Severe infection also produces delirium, stupor and, in extensive pulmonary infiltration, cyanosis. Ornithosis may recur, but is usually milder.

Diagnosis

Characteristic symptoms and a recent history of exposure to birds suggest ornithosis. Firm diagnosis requires recovery of *C. psittaci* from mice, eggs, or tissue culture that has been inoculated with the patient's blood or sputum.

Comparison of acute and convalescent serum shows a fourfold rise in *Chlamydia* antibody titers. In addition, a patchy lobar infiltrate appears on chest X-rays during the 1st week of illness.

Treatment

Ornithosis calls for treatment with tetracycline. If the infection is severe, tetracycline may be given I.V. until the fever subsides. Fever and other symptoms should begin to subside 48 to 72 hours after antibiotic treatment begins, but treatment must continue for 2 weeks after temperature returns to normal. If the patient can't tolerate tetracycline, penicillin G procaine or chloramphenicol is an alternative.

Special considerations

❯ Monitor fluid and electrolyte balance. Give I.V. fluids as needed.

▶ Carefully monitor vital signs. Watch for signs of overwhelming infection.

▶ Reduce fever with tepid alcohol or sponge baths and a hypothermia blanket.

▶ Reposition the patient often.

▶ Observe secretion precautions. During the acute, febrile stage, if the patient has a cough, wear a face mask and wash your hands carefully. Instruct him to use tissues when he coughs and to dispose of them in a closed plastic bag.

▶ Report all cases of ornithosis to public health authorities.

 PREVENTION TIP To prevent ornithosis, those who raise birds for sale should feed them tetracycline-treated birdseed and follow regulations on bird importation. They should also segregate infected or possibly infected birds from healthy birds, and disinfect structures that housed infected ones.

OSTEOMYELITIS

A pyogenic bone infection, osteomyelitis may be chronic or acute. It commonly results from a combination of local trauma — usually quite trivial but resulting in hematoma formation — and an acute infection originating elsewhere in the body. Although osteomyelitis often remains localized, it can spread through the bone to the marrow, cortex, and periosteum.

Acute osteomyelitis is usually a bloodborne disease, which most often affects rapidly growing children. Chronic osteomyelitis (rare) is characterized by multiple draining sinus tracts and metastatic lesions.

Osteomyelitis occurs more often in children than in adults — and particularly in boys — usually as a complication of an acute localized infection. The most common sites in children are the lower end of the femur and the upper end of the tibia, humerus, and radius. In adults, the most common sites are the pelvis and vertebrae,

generally the result of contamination associated with surgery or trauma.

The incidence of both chronic and acute osteomyelitis is declining, except in drug abusers. With prompt treatment, the prognosis for acute osteomyelitis is very good; for chronic osteomyelitis, which is more prevalent in adults, the prognosis remains poor.

Causes

The most common pyogenic organism in osteomyelitis is *Staphylococcus aureus;* others include *Streptococcus pyogenes, Pneumococcus, Pseudomonas aeruginosa, Escherichia coli,* and *Proteus vulgaris.* Typically, these microbes find a culture site in a hematoma from recent trauma or in a weakened area, such as the site of local infection (for example, furunculosis), and spread directly to bone.

As the microbes grow and form pus within the bone, tension builds within the rigid medullary cavity, forcing pus through the haversian canals. This forms a subperiosteal abscess that deprives the bone of its blood supply and eventually may cause necrosis. In turn, necrosis stimulates the periosteum to create new bone (involucrum); the old bone (sequestrum) detaches and works its way out through an abscess or the sinuses. By the time sequestrum forms, osteomyelitis is chronic.

Signs and symptoms

Onset of *acute* osteomyelitis is usually rapid, with sudden pain in the affected bone, and tenderness, heat, swelling, and restricted movement over it. Associated systemic symptoms may include tachycardia, sudden fever, nausea, and malaise. Generally, the clinical features of both chronic and acute osteomyelitis are the same, except that chronic infection can persist intermittently for years, flaring up spontaneously after minor trauma. Sometimes, however, the only symptom of chronic infection is the persistent drainage of pus from an old pocket in a sinus tract.

Diagnosis

Patient history, physical examination, and laboratory tests help to confirm osteomyelitis.

▶ White blood cell count shows leukocytosis.

▶ Erythrocyte sedimentation rate and C-reactive protein (CRP) are elevated; however, CRP appears to be a better diagnostic tool.

▶ Blood cultures identify the causative organism.

X-rays may not show bone involvement until the disease has been active for some time, usually 2 to 3 weeks. Bone scans can detect early infection. Computed tomography scan and magnetic resonance imaging may be necessary to delineate the extent of infection. Diagnosis must rule out poliomyelitis, rheumatic fever, myositis, and bone fractures.

Treatment

Treatment varies for acute and chronic osteomyelitis. Acute osteomyelitis should be treated before a definitive diagnosis. Treatment includes administration of large doses of I.V. antibiotics (usually a penicillinase-resistant penicillin, such as nafcillin or oxacillin, or a cephalosporin) after blood cultures are taken; early surgical drainage to relieve pressure buildup and sequestrum formation; immobilization of the affected bone by plaster cast, traction, or bed rest; and supportive measures, such as administration of analgesics and I.V. fluids.

If an abscess forms, treatment includes incision and drainage, followed by a culture of the drainage. Antibiotic therapy to control infection may include administration of systemic antibiotics; intracavitary instillation of antibiotics through closed-system continuous irrigation with low intermittent suction; limited irrigation with blood drainage system with suction (Hemovac); or local application of packed, wet, antibiotic-soaked dressings.

In chronic osteomyelitis, surgery is usually required to remove dead bone (sequestrectomy) and to promote drainage (saucerization). The prognosis is poor even after surgery. Patients are often in great pain and require prolonged hospitalization. Resistant chronic osteomyelitis in an arm or leg may necessitate amputation.

Some facilities also use hyperbaric oxygen to increase the activity of naturally occurring leukocytes.

Free tissue transfers and local muscle flaps are also used to fill in dead space and increase blood supply.

Special considerations

The caregiver's major concerns are to control infection, protect the bone from injury, and offer meticulous supportive care.

▶ Use strict aseptic technique when changing dressings and irrigating wounds.

▶ If the patient is in skeletal traction for compound fractures, cover insertion points of pin tracks with small, dry dressings, and tell him not to touch the skin around the pins and wires.

▶ Administer I.V. fluids to maintain adequate hydration as necessary.

▶ Provide a diet high in protein and vitamin C.

▶ Assess vital signs and wound appearance daily, and monitor daily for new pain, which may indicate secondary infection.

▶ Carefully monitor suctioning equipment. Keep containers filled of solution being instilled. Monitor the amount of solution instilled and suctioned.

▶ Support the affected limb with firm pillows. Keep the limb level with the body; don't let it sag.

▶ Provide good skin care. Turn the patient gently every 2 hours and watch for signs of developing pressure ulcers.

▶ Provide good cast care. Support the cast with firm pillows and "petal" the edges with pieces of adhesive tape or moleskin to smooth rough edges.

▶ Check circulation and drainage. If a wet spot appears on the cast, circle it with a marking pen and note the time of appearance (on the cast). Be aware of how much drainage is expected. Check the circled spot at least every 4 hours. Watch for any enlargement.

▶ Protect the patient from mishaps, such as jerky movements and falls, which may threaten bone integrity.

▶ Be alert for sudden pain, crepitus, or deformity. Watch for any sudden malposition of the limb, which may indicate fracture.

▶ Provide emotional support and appropriate diversions.

▶ Stress the need for follow-up examinations.

▶ Instruct the patient to seek prompt treatment for possible sources of recurrence — blisters, boils, styes, and impetigo.

 PREVENTION TIP Before discharge, teach the patient how to protect and clean the wound and, most importantly, how to recognize signs of recurring infection (increased temperature, redness, localized heat, and swelling).

OTITIS EXTERNA

Also known as external otitis and swimmer's ear, otitis externa is an inflammation of the skin of the external ear canal and auricle. It may be acute, chronic, or invasive and it is most common in the summer among children and young adults. With treatment, acute otitis externa usually subsides within 7 days (although it may become chronic) and tends to recur. Malignant otitis externa is potentially life-threatening and most commonly occurs in controlled diabetic patients. It is caused by *Pseudomonas aeruginosa* and slowly invades from the external canal into adjacent soft tissues, mastoid, and temporal bone. It may spread across the base of the skull.

Causes

Otitis externa usually results from bacterial infection with an organism, such as *Pseudomonas, Proteus vulgaris,* streptococci, or *Staphylococcus aureus;* sometimes it stems from a fungus, such as *As-*

pergillus niger or *Candida albicans* (fungal otitis externa is most common in the tropics). Occasionally, chronic otitis externa results from dermatologic conditions, such as seborrhea or psoriasis. Predisposing factors include swimming in contaminated water; cleaning the ear canal with a cotton swab, bobby pin, finger, or other foreign object; exposure to dust, hair care products, or other irritants; regular use of earphones, earplugs, or earmuffs; and chronic drainage from a perforated tympanic membrane.

Signs and symptoms

Acute otitis externa characteristically produces moderate to severe pain that is exacerbated by manipulation of the auricle or tragus, clenching the teeth, opening the mouth, or chewing. The canal appears red and swollen. Its other clinical effects may include fever, foul-smelling aural discharge, regional cellulitis, and partial hearing loss.

Fungal otitis externa may be asymptomatic, although *A. niger* produces a black or gray blotting paper-like growth in the ear canal. In chronic otitis externa, pruritus replaces pain, which may lead to scaling and skin thickening with a resultant narrowing of the lumen. An aural discharge may also occur. Asteatosis (lack of cerumen) is common.

Diagnosis

Physical examination confirms otitis externa. In acute otitis externa, otoscopy reveals a swollen external ear canal (sometimes to the point of complete closure), periauricular lymphadenopathy (tender nodes in front of the tragus, behind the ear, or in the upper neck) and, occasionally, regional cellulitis.

In fungal otitis externa, removal of growth shows thick red epithelium. Microscopic examination or culture and sensitivity tests can identify the causative organism and determine antibiotic treatment. Pain on palpation of the tragus or auricle distinguishes acute otitis externa from oti-

DIFFERENTIATING ACUTE OTITIS TYPES

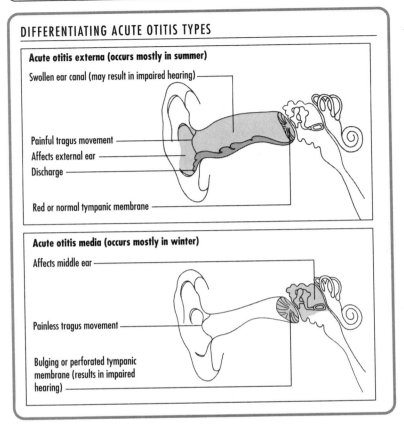

Acute otitis externa (occurs mostly in summer)

Swollen ear canal (may result in impaired hearing)

Painful tragus movement

Affects external ear

Discharge

Red or normal tympanic membrane

Acute otitis media (occurs mostly in winter)

Affects middle ear

Painless tragus movement

Bulging or perforated tympanic membrane (results in impaired hearing)

tis media. (See *Differentiating acute otitis types*.)

In chronic otitis externa, physical examination shows thick red epithelium in the ear canal. Severe chronic otitis externa may reflect underlying diabetes mellitus, hypothyroidism, or nephritis. Other conditions to consider are the presence of a foreign body in the ear canal, pruritus, malignant otitis externa, and squamous cell carcinoma of the external ear.

Treatment

Treatment varies, depending on the type of otitis externa. To relieve the pain of acute otitis externa, treatment includes heat therapy to the periauricular region (heat lamp; hot, damp compresses; heating pad), aspirin or acetaminophen, and codeine. Instillation of antibiotic eardrops such as polymyxin (with or without hydrocortisone) follows cleaning of the ear with alcohol-acetic acid mixtures and removal of debris. If fever persists or regional cellulitis develops, a systemic antibiotic is necessary.

As with other forms of this disorder, fungal otitis externa necessitates careful cleaning of the ear. Application of a keratolytic or 2% salicylic acid in cream containing nystatin may help treat otitis externa resulting from candidal organisms.

Instillation of slightly acidic eardrops creates an unfavorable environment in the ear canal for most fungi as well as *Pseudomonas*.

Primary treatment of chronic otitis externa consists of cleaning the ear and removing debris. Supplemental therapy includes instillation of antibiotic eardrops or application of antibiotic ointment or cream (neomycin, bacitracin, or polymyxin, possibly combined with hydrocortisone). Another ointment contains phenol, salicylic acid, precipitated sulfur, and petrolatum, and produces exfoliative and antipruritic effects.

For mild chronic otitis externa, treatment may include instilling antibiotic eardrops once or twice weekly and wearing specially fitted earplugs while showering, shampooing, or swimming.

Special considerations

If the patient has acute otitis externa:

▶ Monitor vital signs, particularly temperature. Watch for and record the type and amount of aural drainage.

▶ Remove debris and gently clean the ear canal with mild Burow's solution (aluminum acetate). Place a wisp of cotton soaked with solution into the ear, and apply a saturated compress directly to the auricle. Afterward, dry the ear gently but thoroughly. (In severe otitis externa, cleaning may be delayed until after initial treatment with antibiotic eardrops.)

▶ To instill eardrops in an adult, pull the pinna upward and backward to straighten the canal. For children, pull the pinna downward and backward. To ensure that the drops reach the epithelium, insert a wisp of cotton moistened with eardrops.

▶ If the patient has chronic otitis externa, clean the ear thoroughly. Use wet soaks intermittently on oozing or infected skin. If the patient has a chronic fungal infection, clean the ear canal well, then apply an exfoliative ointment.

 PREVENTION TIP To prevent otitis externa, suggest using lamb's wool earplugs coated with petrolatum to keep water out of the ears when showering or shampooing. Also, tell the patient to wear earplugs or to keep his head above water when swimming and to instill two or three drops of 3% boric acid solution in 70% alcohol before and after swimming to toughen the skin of the external ear canal. Warn the patient against cleaning the ears with cotton swabs or other objects and urge prompt treatment of otitis media to prevent perforation of the tympanic membrane. If the patient is diabetic, evaluate him for malignant otitis externa. Hearing aid users who are prone to otitis externa should consider having the device vented to improve aeration of the external ear canal.

OTITIS MEDIA

An inflammation of the middle ear, otitis media may be suppurative or secretory, acute or chronic. Acute otitis media is common in children; its incidence rises during the winter months, paralleling the seasonal rise in nonbacterial respiratory tract infections. It occurs most commonly between ages 6 months and 24 months due to developmental changes involving the eustachian tube.

With prompt treatment, the prognosis for acute otitis media is excellent; however, prolonged accumulation of fluid within the middle ear cavity causes chronic otitis media, with possible perforation of the tympanic membrane.

Chronic suppurative otitis media may lead to scarring, adhesions, and severe structural or functional ear damage; chronic secretory otitis media, with its persistent inflammation and pressure, may cause conductive hearing loss.

Causes

Otitis media results from disruption of eustachian tube patency. (See *Locating otitis media*, page 202.)

In the suppurative form, respiratory tract infection, allergic reaction, nasotracheal intubation, or positional changes allow nasopharyngeal flora to reflux through the eustachian tube and colonize the middle ear. Suppurative otitis media usually re-

LOCATING OTITIS MEDIA

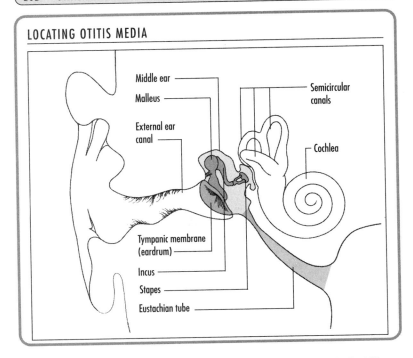

Middle ear

Malleus

External ear canal

Semicircular canals

Cochlea

Tympanic membrane (eardrum)

Incus

Stapes

Eustachian tube

sults from bacterial infection with pneumococci, *Haemophilus influenzae* (the most common cause in children under age 6), *Moraxella catarrhalis,* beta-hemolytic streptococci, staphylococci (most common cause in children age 6 or older), or gram-negative bacteria.

Predisposing factors include the normally wider, shorter, more horizontal eustachian tubes and increased lymphoid tissue in children as well as anatomic anomalies. Chronic suppurative otitis media results from inadequate treatment of acute otitis episodes or from infection by resistant strains of bacteria or, rarely, tuberculosis.

Secretory otitis media results from obstruction of the eustachian tube. This causes a buildup of negative pressure in the middle ear that promotes transudation of sterile serous fluid from blood vessels in the membrane of the middle ear. Such effusion may be secondary to eustachian tube dysfunction from viral infection or allergy. It may also follow barotrauma

(pressure injury caused by inability to equalize pressures between the environment and the middle ear), as can occur during rapid aircraft descent in a person with an upper respiratory tract infection or during rapid underwater ascent in scuba diving (barotitis media).

Chronic secretory otitis media follows persistent eustachian tube dysfunction from mechanical obstruction (adenoidal tissue overgrowth, tumors), edema (allergic rhinitis, chronic sinus infection), or inadequate treatment of acute suppurative otitis media.

Generally, risk factors include male sex; genetic factors; adenoid hypertrophy; bottle feeding, especially in the supine position; exposure to upper respiratory tract infections (such as in day-care settings or during the winter season); history of allergies; exposure to cigarette smoke; craniofacial abnormalities (such as cleft palate); and previous episodes of acute otitis media.

Signs and symptoms

Clinical features vary with the specific type of the disorder. Symptoms of acute suppurative otitis media include severe, deep, throbbing pain (from pressure behind the tympanic membrane); signs of upper respiratory tract infection (sneezing, coughing); mild to very high fever; hearing loss (usually mild and conductive); dizziness; nausea; and vomiting. Other possible effects include bulging of the tympanic membrane, with concomitant erythema and purulent drainage in the ear canal from tympanic membrane rupture. However, many patients are asymptomatic.

In acute secretory otitis media, a severe conductive hearing loss varies from 15 to 35 decibels, depending on the thickness and amount of fluid in the middle ear cavity and, possibly, a sensation of fullness in the ear, and popping, crackling, or clicking sounds on swallowing or with jaw movement. Accumulation of fluid may also cause the patient to hear an echo when he speaks and to experience a vague feeling of top-heaviness.

The cumulative effects of chronic otitis media include thickening and scarring of the tympanic membrane, decreased or absent tympanic membrane mobility, cholesteatoma (a cyst-like mass in the middle ear) and, in chronic suppurative otitis media, a painless, purulent discharge. The extent of associated conductive hearing loss varies with the size and type of tympanic membrane perforation and ossicular destruction.

If the tympanic membrane has ruptured, the patient may state that the pain has suddenly stopped. Complications may include abscesses (brain, subperiosteal, and epidural), sigmoid sinus or jugular vein thrombosis, septicemia, meningitis, suppurative labyrinthitis, facial paralysis, and otitis externa.

Diagnosis

Diagnostic tests vary with the specific type of otitis media. In acute suppurative otitis media, otoscopy reveals obscured or distorted bony landmarks of the tympanic membrane. Pneumatoscopy can show decreased tympanic membrane mobility, but this procedure is painful with an obviously bulging, erythematous tympanic membrane. The pain pattern is diagnostically significant: In acute suppurative otitis media, for example, pulling the auricle doesn't exacerbate the pain.

In acute secretory otitis media, otoscopic examination reveals tympanic membrane retraction, which causes the bony landmarks to appear more prominent.

Examination also detects clear or amber fluid behind the tympanic membrane. If hemorrhage into the middle ear has occurred, as in barotrauma, the tympanic membrane appears blue-black.

In patients with chronic otitis media, the history discloses recurrent or unresolved otitis media. Otoscopy shows thickening and sometimes scarring, and decreased mobility of the tympanic membrane; pneumatoscopy shows decreased or absent tympanic membrane movement. History of recent air travel or scuba diving suggests barotitis media.

Other conditions to consider are infectious myringitis, pharyngitis, tonsillitis, teething, and temporomandibular joint syndrome.

Treatment

The type of otitis media dictates the treatment guidelines. In acute suppurative otitis media, antibiotic therapy includes ampicillin or amoxicillin for 10 days. In areas with a high incidence of beta lactamase-producing *H. influenzae* and in patients who are not responding to ampicillin or amoxicillin, amoxicillin/clavulanate potassium may be used.

For those who are allergic to penicillin derivatives, therapy may include cefaclor, cefuroxime axetil, cefprozil, cefixime, erythromycin, sulfisoxazole, or cotrimoxazole. Severe, painful bulging of the tympanic membrane usually necessitates myringotomy. Broad-spectrum antibiotics can help prevent acute suppurative otitis media in high-risk patients. In patients with recurring otitis, antibiotics must be used with discretion to prevent development of resistant strains of bacteria. Acetaminophen may be used for pain. Systemic decongestants and expectorants may also be of benefit. However, antihistamines should not be used.

For patients with acute secretory otitis media, inflation of the eustachian tube by performing Valsalva's maneuver several times a day may be the only treatment required. Otherwise, nasopharyngeal decongestant therapy may be helpful. It should continue for at least 2 weeks and sometimes indefinitely, with periodic evaluation.

If decongestant therapy fails, myringotomy and aspiration of middle ear fluid are necessary, followed by insertion of a polyethylene tube into the tympanic membrane, for immediate and prolonged equalization of pressure. The tube falls out spontaneously after 9 to 12 months. Concomitant treatment of the underlying cause (such as elimination of allergens, or adenoidectomy for hypertrophied adenoids) may also be helpful in correcting this disorder.

Treatment of chronic otitis media includes broad-spectrum antibiotics, such as amoxicillin/clavulanate potassium or cefuroxime, for exacerbations of acute otitis media; elimination of eustachian tube obstruction; treatment of otitis externa; myringoplasty and tympanoplasty to reconstruct middle ear structures when thickening and scarring are present; and, possibly, mastoidectomy. Cholesteatoma requires excision.

Special considerations

▶ Explain all diagnostic tests and procedures.

▶ After myringotomy, maintain drainage flow. Don't place cotton or plugs deep in the ear canal; however, sterile cotton may be placed loosely in the external ear to absorb drainage.

▶ To prevent infection, change the cotton whenever it gets damp, and wash hands before and after giving ear care. Watch for headache, fever, severe pain, or disorientation.

▶ After tympanoplasty, reinforce dressings, and observe for excessive bleeding from the ear canal. Administer analgesics as needed. Warn the patient against blowing his nose or getting the ear wet when bathing.

▶ Encourage the patient to complete the prescribed course of antibiotic treatment. If nasopharyngeal decongestants are ordered, teach correct instillation.

▶ Suggest application of heat to the ear to relieve pain.

▶ Advise the patient with acute secretory otitis media to watch for and immediately report pain and fever — signs of secondary infection.

 PREVENTION TIP To prevent otitis media, teach recognition of upper respiratory tract infections and encourage early treatment. Instruct parents not to feed their infant in a supine position or put him to bed with a bottle. This prevents reflux of nasopharyngeal flora. To promote eustachian tube patency, instruct the patient to perform Valsalva's maneuver several times daily. Parents should be advised that tobacco smoke increases the risk of middle ear infections in children. Allergens in the home, such as pets, house dust, and mold, should be eliminated as much as possible.

PQ

PANCREATITIS

Pancreatitis, inflammation of the pancreas, occurs in acute and chronic forms. In this disease, the enzymes normally excreted by the pancreas digest pancreatic tissue (autodigestion). Acute pancreatitis can range from mild self-limiting episodes of abdominal discomfort to severe systemic illness associated with fluid sequestration, metabolic disorder, hypotension, sepsis, and death. In 85% to 90% of patients with pancreatitis, the disease subsides with conventional treatment. Chronic pancreatitis is persistent inflammation that produces irreversible changes in the structure and function of the pancreas. It sometimes follows accute pancreatitis. Two sets of criteria are used to determine the patient's prognosis. These are the Ranson/Imrie criteria and Acute Physiology and Chronic Health Evaluation (APACHE$_{II}$). Patients with any two criteria have a mortality rate of 20% to 30%. Life-threatening illness is associated with pancreatic hemorrhage or necrosis in about 10% of patients.

Causes

The most common causes of pancreatitis are biliary tract disease and alcoholism, but it can also result from pancreatic carcinoma, trauma, or certain drugs, such as glucocorticoids, sulfonamides, chlorothiazide, and azathioprine.

This disease also may develop as a complication of peptic ulcer, mumps, or hypothermia. Rarer causes are stenosis or obstruction of the sphincter of Oddi, hypercalcemia, duodenal obstruction, hyperlipemia, ischemia from vasculitis or vascular disease, viral infections, mycoplasmal pneumonia, scorpion venom, and pregnancy. It may also be familial or idiopathic.

Pancreatitis may also develop in a patient after surgery. This occurrence has the highest morbidity and mortality. Whatever the cause, complications from acute pancreatitis are possible.

Signs and symptoms

In many patients, the first and only symptom of mild pancreatitis is steady epigastric pain centered close to the umbilicus. The pain usually begins as a gradually increasing mid-epigastric pain reaching its maximum intensity several hours after the beginning of the illness. In pancreatitis resulting from alcohol ingestion, the pain commences 12 to 48 hours after an episode of binge drinking. Nausea and vomiting generally accompany the abdominal pain. However, a severe attack causes extreme pain, persistent vomiting, abdominal rigidity, diminished bowel activity (suggesting peritonitis), right or left pleural effusion, or left hemidiaphragm elevation.

Severe pancreatitis may produce extreme malaise and restlessness, mottled skin, tachycardia, and diaphoresis. Hypotension, hypovolemia, hypoperfusion, sepsis, and shock may ensue. Pulmonary complications and secondary pancreatic infections such as pancreatic abscess or infected pancreatic necrosis, and later, pancreatic pseudocyst, may also occur. Proximity of the inflamed pancreas to the bowel may cause ileus. Renal failure may occur as a result of severe hypovolemia.

CHRONIC PANCREATITIS

Usually associated with alcoholism (in over half of all patients), chronic pancreatitis can also follow hyperparathyroidism, hyperlipemia or, infrequently, gallstones, trauma, peptic ulcer, posttraumatic stricture, pancreas division, and hereditary or familial pancreatitis. Inflammation and fibrosis cause progressive pancreatic insufficiency and eventually destroy the pancreas.

SYMPTOMS

Chronic pancreatitis is usually associated with constant dull pain with occasional exacerbations, malabsorption, severe weight loss, and hyperglycemia (leading to diabetic symptoms). Relevant diagnostic measures include patient history, abdominal X-rays or computed tomography scans showing pancreatic calcification, elevated erythrocyte sedimentation rate, and examination of stools for steatorrhea.

TREATMENT

The severe pain of chronic pancreatitis often requires large doses of analgesics or narcotics. Addiction may be common. Treatment also includes a low-fat diet and oral administration of pancreatic enzymes, such as pancreatin or pancrelipase to control steatorrhea; insulin or oral antidiabetic agents to curb hyperglycemia; and, occasionally, surgical repair of biliary or pancreatic ducts or the sphincter of Oddi to reduce pressure and promote the flow of pancreatic juice. The prognosis is good if the patient can avoid alcohol but poor if he can't.

If pancreatitis damages the islets of Langerhans, complications may include diabetes mellitus and enzyme deficiency. (See *Chronic pancreatitis*.) Fulminant pancreatitis causes massive hemorrhage and total destruction of the pancreas, resulting in diabetic acidosis, shock, or coma.

Diagnosis

Clinical presentation along with combined laboratory and radiographic findings form the basis for diagnosis. A careful patient history (especially for alcoholism) and physical examination are the first steps in diagnosis, but the retroperitoneal position of the pancreas makes physical assessment difficult.

Dramatically elevated serum amylase levels — frequently over 500 U/L — confirm pancreatitis and rule out perforated peptic ulcer, acute cholecystitis, appendicitis, and bowel infarction or obstruction. Persistent elevation of serum amylase levels may indicate pancreatic necrosis, pseudocyst, or abscess.

Similarly dramatic elevations of amylase are also found in urine, ascites, or pleural fluid. Characteristically, amylase levels return to normal 48 hours after onset of pancreatitis, despite continuing symptoms. Supportive laboratory values include:
- increased serum lipase levels — which rise more slowly than serum amylase
- white blood cell counts — ranging from 8,000 to 20,000/µl, with increased polymorphonuclear leukocytes
- elevated glucose levels — as high as 500 to 900 mg/dl, indicating hyperglycemia.

Other tests that may be used to diagnose pancreatitis include:
- abdominal X-rays — show dilation of the small or large bowel or calcification of the pancreas
- chest X-rays — show left-sided pleural effusion
- abdominal computed tomography scan with contrast — most sensitive noninvasive test used to confirm the diagnosis of pancreatitis.

Treatment

The goal of therapy is to maintain circulation and fluid volume. Treatment measures must also relieve pain and decrease pancreatic secretions. In 90% of patients with acute pancreatitis, the disease occurs as a mild self-limiting illness and requires simple supportive care alone. In the remaining 10% of patients, the disease can evolve into a severe form of acute pancreatitis with significant complications, a lengthy duration of illness, and a significant mortality rate.

 ALERT Emergency treatment for shock (the most common cause of death in early-stage pancreatitis) consists of vigorous I.V. replacement of electrolytes and proteins.

Metabolic acidosis that develops secondary to hypovolemia and impaired cellular perfusion requires vigorous fluid volume replacement.

Drug treatment choices may include morphine sulfate for pain; diazepam for restlessness and agitation; and antibiotics for documented bacterial infections.

Specific metabolic complications, such as hypokalemia, hypocalcemia, hemorrhage, and coagulopathy, must be treated with appropriate replacement products, such as potassium chloride, I.V. calcium gluconate or chloride, red blood cells, and fresh frozen plasma. Hyperglycemia and glycosuria signal altered carbohydrate metabolism. Treatment consists of careful titration of glucose and insulin to maintain a euglycemic state.

After the emergency phase, continuing I.V. therapy should provide adequate electrolytes and protein solutions. If the patient is unable to resume oral feedings, hyperalimentation may be necessary. Nonstimulating enteral feedings may be safer because of the decreased risk of infection and maintenance of normal physiology.

Surgery for acute pancreatitis is reserved for specific complications and to correct an anatomic problem. Surgery is usually required for patients with necrotizing pancreatitis in order to debride devitalized tissue and to provide external drainage. Debridement is often required frequently, usually at 24-to 48-hour intervals, until the necrotic tissue is replaced by a granulating wound.

Special considerations

Acute pancreatitis is a life-threatening emergency. Provide meticulous supportive care and continuous monitoring of vital systems.

❚ Monitor vital signs and pulmonary artery pressure closely.

❚ Monitor fluid intake and output, and electrolyte levels.

❚ Assess for crackles, rhonchi, decreased breath sounds, or respiratory failure.

❚ Observe for signs of calcium deficiency — tetany, cramps, carpopedal spasm, and seizures.

❚ Administer analgesics, as needed, to relieve the patient's pain and anxiety.

❚ Observe for adverse reactions to antibiotics: nephrotoxicity with aminoglycosides; pseudomembranous enterocolitis with clindamycin; and blood dyscrasias with chloramphenicol.

❚ Monitor for complications due to hyperalimentation, such as sepsis, hypokalemia, overhydration, and metabolic acidosis.

❚ Observe for fever, cardiac irregularities, changes in arterial blood gas measurements, and deep respirations (signs of sepsis).

PARAINFLUENZA

Human parainfluenza virus (HPIV) infections are a leading cause of upper and lower respiratory tract illness throughout the world. About 40% of acute respiratory infections in children are attributed to HPIVs. HPIVs affect all age groups, but serious infections tend to occur among elderly patients and those who are immunocompromised. The viruses can cause repeated infections throughout the life span, but they are usually mild and short-lived.

There are four serotypes of HPIV, and each has different clinical and epidemiological features. HPIV-1 is the leading cause of croup in children, but both HPIV-1 and HPIV-2 can cause upper and lower tract respiratory illness. HPIV-3 is usually associated with bronchiolitis and pneumonia, whereas HPIV-4 is infrequently detected. Serological studies have shown that 90% to 100% of children aged 5 years and older have antibodies to HPIV-3, 75% have antibodies to HPIV-1 and 58% have antibodies to HPIV-2. HPIV-1 tends to occur biennially in the fall; HPIV-2 causes annual or biennial fall outbreaks; and HPIV-3 occurs annually during the spring and early summer months. All of the HPIVs can be infectious throughout the year.

Causes

HPIVs are single-stranded RNA virions. Transmission occurs through direct contact and by inhalation of droplets. The incubation period depends upon the infecting virus — for HPIV-3 it's generally 24 to 48 hours; for HPIV-1 it's 4 to 5 days.

Signs and symptoms

Parainfluenza symptoms at onset include fever, moderate inflammation of the nasal mucous membrane with profuse nasal discharge, moderate sore throat, and dry cough. Malaise is directly related to the intensity of the fever, which usually does not exceed 101°F (38.3° C). In many cases, a characteristic barking cough (usually occurring at night) and hoarseness are prominent. Acute laryngotracheobronchitis, the most severe form of croup in children, can cause life-threatening respiratory distress and often requires hospitalization.

Shortness of breath and rigors usually accompany pneumonia, and auscultation of the lung fields may reveal moist rales, bronchophony, egophony, or whispered pectoriloquy. Tactile fremitus and tubular breath sounds may indicate acute bronchitis. Exacerbations of chronic bronchitis and asthma symptoms may also occur.

Diagnosis

Most cases of HPIV are diagnosed clinically based on presenting symptoms. When absolutely necessary to distinguish between the four serotypes, the virus can be confirmed by isolation and identification of the virus in cell culture or by direct detection of the virus in respiratory secretions using immunofluorescence, enzyme immunoassay, or polymerase chain reaction assay. A significant rise in specific IgG or IgM antibodies in a serum specimen is also diagnostic.

A chest X-ray is the most effective method for detecting pneumonia. The differential diagnosis includes pertussis, respiratory syncytial virus, adenovirus, Group A or B streptococcal infection, mycoplasma pneumonia, and *Chlamydia trachomatis, Staphylococcus aureus, Pseudomonas aeruginosa,* and *Haemophilus influenzae* infection.

Treatment

Currently no specific therapy exists beyond supportive measures such as rest and adequate fluid intake for mild cases. Acetaminophen may be given to relieve fever and other symptoms to allow for proper rest. To avoid the risk of Reye's syndrome with influenza, acetaminophen is preferable to aspirin if children require analgesics or antipyretics. Antitussives may be prescribed to suppress cough. Mild croup symptoms can often be alleviated with steam. Treatment of severe infection emphasizes airway maintenance.

Special considerations

▶ Wash hands thoroughly before and after patient contact, performing invasive procedures, and dressing changes. Dispose of tissues and dressings in a moisture-resistant container for proper disposal.
▶ Pediatric patients may require a mist tent; adult patients may require supplementary oxygen.
▶ Monitor proper diet and fluids.
▶ Encourage the patient to move, cough and deep breathe every 2 hours.

▶ Assess the patient's breath sounds frequently. Observe for the development of secondary bacterial infections.

▶ Dispose of bed linens appropriately.

▶ Promote regular bathing and proper hygiene.

 PREVENTION TIP Instruct the patient to cover the mouth when coughing or sneezing, and to appropriately dispose of infected tissues. Encourage children to maintain good personal hygiene, to wash hands thoroughly with soap and water, and to avoid sharing items such as cups, glasses, and utensils. Breast feeding during the first few months of life should also be encouraged, as passively acquired maternal antibodies play a role in the protection against HPIV types 1 and 2. Teach patients and parents how to monitor for signs of impending respiratory failure and the importance of seeking immediate medical care.

PEDICULOSIS

Pediculosis is caused by parasitic forms of lice: *Pediculus humanus* var. *capitis* causes pediculosis capitis (head lice); *Pediculus humanus* var. *corporis* causes pediculosis corporis (body lice); and *Phthirus pubis* causes pediculosis pubis (crab lice). These lice feed on human blood and lay their eggs (nits) in body hairs or clothing fibers.

After the nits hatch, the lice must feed within 24 hours or die; they mature in about 2 to 3 weeks. When a louse bites, it injects a toxin into the skin that produces mild irritation and a purpuric spot. Repeated bites cause sensitization to the toxin, leading to more serious inflammation. Treatment can effectively eliminate lice.

Causes

P. humanus var. *capitis* (most common species) feeds on the scalp and, rarely, in the eyebrows, eyelashes, and beard. This form of pediculosis is caused by overcrowded conditions and poor personal hygiene, and commonly affects children, especially girls. It spreads through shared clothing, hats, combs, and hairbrushes.

P. humanus var. *corporis* lives in the seams of clothing, next to the skin, leaving only to feed on blood. Common causes include prolonged wearing of the same clothing (which might occur in cold climates), overcrowding, and poor personal hygiene. It spreads through shared clothing and bedsheets.

P. pubis is primarily found in pubic hairs, but this species may extend to the eyebrows, eyelashes, and axillary or body hair. Pediculosis pubis is transmitted through sexual intercourse or by contact with clothes, bedsheets, or towels harboring lice.

Signs and symptoms

Clinical features vary with the cause. Signs and symptoms of pediculosis capitis include itching; excoriation (with severe itching); matted, foul-smelling, lusterless hair (in severe cases); occipital and cervical lymphadenopathy; and a rash on the trunk probably due to sensitization. Adult lice migrate from the scalp and deposit oval gray-white nits on hair shafts.

Pediculosis corporis initially produces small red papules (usually on the shoulders, trunk, or buttocks). Later wheals (probably a sensitivity reaction) may develop. Untreated pediculosis corporis may lead to vertical excoriations and ultimately to dry, discolored, thickly encrusted, scaly skin, with bacterial infection and scarring. In severe cases, headache, fever, and malaise may accompany cutaneous symptoms.

Pediculosis pubis causes skin irritation from scratching, which is usually more obvious than the bites. Small gray-blue spots (maculae caeruleae) may appear on the thighs or upper body.

Diagnosis

Pediculosis is visible on physical examination as follows:

▶ in *pediculosis capitis* there are oval grayish nits that can't be shaken loose like dandruff (the closer the nits are to the end of the hair shaft, the longer the infection has been present, because the ova are laid close to the scalp)

▶ in *pediculosis corporis* there are characteristic skin lesions with nits found on clothing

▶ in *pediculosis pubis* nits are attached to pubic hairs, which feel coarse and grainy to the touch. Other conditions to consider are dandruff, impetigo, and scabies.

Treatment

For pediculosis capitis, treatment consists of permethrin cream rinse rubbed into the hair and rinsed after 10 minutes. A single treatment should be sufficient. Use of lindane has been questioned because of a significant failure rate and concerns regarding neurotoxicity. Removing nits with a fine-tooth comb dipped in vinegar is vital; washing hair with ordinary shampoo removes encrustations.

Pediculosis corporis requires bathing with soap and water to remove lice from the body. Lice may be removed from clothes by washing them in hot water, ironing, or dry-cleaning. Storing clothes for more than 30 days or placing them in dry heat of 140° F (60° C) kills lice. If clothes can't be washed or changed, application of 10% lindane powder is effective.

Treatment of pediculosis pubis includes application of a topical pediculocide. Various agents such as 0.5% malathion emulsion, permethrin cream, and lindane ointment have been used according to the patient's status and health care provider's preference. Clothes and bedsheets must be laundered to prevent reinfestation.

Special considerations

▶ Instruct patients how to use the creams, ointments, powders, and shampoos that can eliminate lice. To prevent self-infestation, avoid prolonged contact with the patient's hair, clothing, and bedsheets.

▶ Ask the patient with pediculosis pubis for a history of recent sexual contacts, so that they can be examined and treated.

▶ To prevent the spread of pediculosis to other hospitalized persons, examine all high-risk patients on admission, especially the elderly who depend on others for care, those admitted from nursing homes, or persons living in crowded conditions.

PELVIC INFLAMMATORY DISEASE

Pelvic inflammatory disease (PID) is any acute, subacute, recurrent, or chronic infection of the oviducts and ovaries, with adjacent tissue involvement. It includes inflammation of the cervix (cervicitis), uterus (endometritis), fallopian tubes (salpingitis), and ovaries (oophoritis), which can extend to the connective tissue lying between the broad ligaments (parametritis).

Early diagnosis and treatment prevents damage to the reproductive system. Untreated PID may cause infertility and may lead to potentially fatal septicemia, pulmonary emboli, and shock.

Causes

PID can result from infection with aerobic or anaerobic microbes. The aerobe, *Neisseria gonorrhoeae,* is its most common cause because it most readily penetrates the bacteriostatic barrier of cervical mucus.

Normally, cervical secretions have a protective and defensive function. Conditions or procedures that alter or destroy cervical mucus impair this bacteriostatic mechanism and allow bacteria present in the cervix or vagina to ascend into the uterine cavity; such procedures include conization or cauterization of the cervix.

Uterine infection can also follow the transfer of contaminated cervical mucus into the endometrial cavity by instrumentation. Consequently, PID can follow insertion of an intrauterine device (IUD), use of a biopsy curet or of an irrigation catheter, or tubal insufflation. Other predisposing factors include abortion, pelvic surgery, and infection during or after pregnancy.

Bacteria may also enter the uterine cavity through the bloodstream or from drainage from a chronically infected fallopian tube, a pelvic abscess, a ruptured appendix, diverticulitis of the sigmoid colon, or other infectious foci.

Common bacteria found in cervical mucus are staphylococci, streptococci, diphtheroids, chlamydiae, and coliforms, including *Pseudomonas* and *Escherichia coli.*

Uterine infection can result from any one or several of these organisms or may follow the multiplication of normally nonpathogenic bacteria in an altered endometrial environment. Bacterial multiplication is most common during parturition, because the endometrium is atrophic, quiescent, and not stimulated by estrogen.

Signs and symptoms

Clinical features of PID vary with the affected area but generally include a profuse, purulent vaginal discharge, sometimes accompanied by low-grade fever and malaise (particularly if gonorrhea is the cause). The patient experiences lower abdomen pain; movement of the cervix or palpation of the adnexa may be extremely painful. (See *Forms of pelvic inflammatory disease,* pages 212 and 213.)

Diagnosis

Diagnostic tests generally include Gram stain of secretions from the endocervix or cul de sac. Culture and sensitivity testing aids selection of the appropriate antibiotic. Urethral and rectal secretions may also be cultured. Ultrasonography is used to identify an adnexal or uterine mass. (X-rays seldom identify pelvic masses.) Culdocentesis is performed to obtain peritoneal fluid or pus for culture and sensitivity testing. Complete blood count and pregnancy test should also be completed.

In addition, patient history is significant. In general, PID is associated with recent sexual intercourse, IUD insertion, childbirth, or abortion.

Other conditions to consider are appendicitis, ectopic pregnancy, ovarian cyst rupture, endometritis, ovarian torsion, inflammatory bowel disease, and diverticulitis.

Treatment

To prevent progression of PID, antibiotic therapy begins immediately after culture specimens are obtained. Such therapy can be reevaluated as soon as laboratory results are available (usually after 24 to 48 hours). Infection may become chronic if treated inadequately.

The guidelines of the Centers for Disease Control and Prevention (CDC) for outpatient treatment include ofloxacin and metronidazole for 14 days or ceftriaxone (or another third-generation cephalosporin) with doxycycline for 14 days. The CDC guidelines for inpatient treatment include doxycycline with a combination of clindamycin and gentamicin or cefotetan.

Development of a pelvic abscess necessitates adequate drainage. A ruptured abscess is life-threatening. If this complication develops, the patient may need a total abdominal hysterectomy with bilateral salpingo-oophorectomy, although laparoscopic drainage with preservation of the ovaries and uterus appears promising.

Special considerations

▶ After establishing that the patient has no drug allergies, administer antibiotics and analgesics as necessary.

▶ Check for fever. If it persists, carefully monitor fluid intake and output for signs of dehydration.

▶ Watch for abdominal rigidity and distention — possible signs of developing peritonitis. Provide frequent perineal care if vaginal drainage occurs.

▶ To prevent a recurrence, explain the nature and seriousness of PID, and encourage the patient to comply with the treatment regimen.

FORMS OF PELVIC INFLAMMATORY DISEASE

The Centers for Disease Control and Prevention (CDC) defines pelvic inflammatory disease (PID) as an infection of the upper genital tract. Endometriosis is not considered PID by itself but may accompany PID.

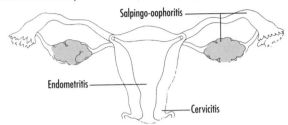

CLINICAL FEATURES	DIAGNOSTIC FINDINGS
Salpingo-oophoritis ▶ *Acute:* sudden onset of lower abdominal and pelvic pain, usually following menses; increased vaginal discharge; fever; malaise; lower abdominal pressure and tenderness; tachycardia; pelvic peritonitis ▶ *Chronic:* adhesions, chronic pelvic pain, infertility	▶ Laparoscopy reveals intratubal pus. ▶ Blood studies show leukocytosis or normal white blood cell (WBC) count. ▶ X-ray may show ileus with severe peritonitis. ▶ Pelvic exam reveals extreme tenderness. ▶ Smear of cervical or periurethral gland exudate shows gram-negative intracellular diplococci if gonorrhea is the causative agent.
Cervicitis ▶ *Acute:* purulent, foul-smelling vaginal discharge; vulvovaginitis, with itching or burning; red, edematous cervix; pelvic discomfort; sexual dysfunction; metrorrhagia; infertility; spontaneous abortion ▶ *Chronic:* cervical dystocia, laceration or eversion of the cervix, ulcerative vesicular lesion (when cervicitis results from herpes simplex virus II)	▶ Cultures for *Neisseria gonorrhoeae* are positive (more than 90% of patients). ▶ Cytologic smears may reveal severe inflammation. ▶ If cervicitis isn't complicated by salpingitis, WBC count is normal or slightly elevated; erythrocyte sedimentation rate (ESR) is elevated. ▶ In *acute cervicitis,* cervical palpation reveals tenderness. ▶ In *chronic cervicitis,* causative organisms are usually staphylococci or streptococci.

FORMS OF PELVIC INFLAMMATORY DISEASE *(continued)*

CLINICAL FEATURES	DIAGNOSTIC FINDINGS
Endometritis **(generally postpartum or postabortion)** ▶ *Acute:* mucopurulent or purulent vaginal discharge oozing from the cervix; edematous, hyperemic endometrium, possibly leading to ulceration and necrosis (with virulent organisms); lower abdominal pain and tenderness; fever; rebound pain; abdominal muscle spasm; thrombophlebitis of uterine and pelvic vessels (in severe forms) ▶ *Chronic:* recurring acute episodes (increasingly common because of widespread use of intrauterine devices)	▶ In severe infection, palpation may reveal boggy uterus. ▶ Uterine and blood samples are positive for causative organism, usually staphylococcus. ▶ WBC count and ESR are elevated.

▶ Stress the need for the patient's sexual partner to be examined and, if necessary, treated for infection.

▶ Because PID may cause painful intercourse, advise the patient to consult with her health care provider about sexual activity.

 PREVENTION TIP To prevent infection after minor gynecologic procedures, such as dilatation and curettage, tell the patient to immediately report any fever, increased vaginal discharge, or pain. After such procedures, instruct her to avoid douching and intercourse for at least 7 days.

PERICARDITIS

Pericarditis is an inflammation of the pericardium, the fibroserous sac that envelops, supports, and protects the heart. It occurs in both acute and chronic forms. Acute pericarditis can be fibrinous or effusive, with purulent, serous, or hemorrhagic exudate; chronic constrictive pericarditis is characterized by dense fibrous pericardial thickening. The prognosis depends on the underlying cause but is generally good in acute pericarditis, unless constriction occurs.

Causes

Common causes of this disease include bacterial, fungal, or viral infection (infectious pericarditis); neoplasms (primary, or metastases from lungs, breasts, or other organs); high-dose radiation to the chest; uremia; hypersensitivity or autoimmune disease, (such as acute rheumatic fever, systemic lupus erythematosus, and rheumatoid arthritis); postcardiac injury, such as myocardial infarction (MI), which later causes an autoimmune reaction (Dressler's syndrome) in the pericardium; trauma, or surgery that causes pericardial effusion; drugs, such as hydralazine or procainamide; and idiopathic factors (most common in acute pericarditis).

Less common causes include aortic aneurysm with pericardial leakage and myxedema with cholesterol deposits in the pericardium.

Signs and symptoms

In acute pericarditis, a sharp and often sudden pain usually starts over the sternum

PATTERNS OF CARDIAC PAIN

PERICARDITIS	ANGINA	MYOCARDIAL INFARCTION
Onset and duration ▶ Sudden onset; continuous pain lasting for days; residual soreness	▶ Gradual or sudden onset; pain usually lasting less than 15 minutes and not more than 30 minutes (average: 3 minutes)	▶ Sudden onset; pain lasting 30 minutes to 2 hours; waxing and waning; residual soreness 1 to 3 days
Location and radiation ▶ Substernal pain to left of midline; radiation to back or subclavicular area	▶ Substernal or anterior chest pain, not sharply localized; radiation to back, neck, arms, jaws, even upper abdomen or fingers	▶ Substernal, midline, or anterior chest pain; radiation to jaws, neck, back, shoulders, or one or both arms
Quality and intensity ▶ Mild ache to severe pain, deep or superficial; stabbing, knife-like	▶ Mild-to-moderate pressure; deep sensation; varied pattern of attacks; tightness, squeezing, crushing, pressure	▶ Persistent, severe pressure; deep sensation; crushing, squeezing, heavy, oppressive
Signs and symptoms ▶ Precordial friction rub; increased pain with movement, inspiration, laughing, coughing; decreased pain with sitting or leaning forward (sitting up pulls the heart away from the diaphragm)	▶ Dyspnea, diaphoresis, nausea, desire to void, belching, apprehension	▶ Nausea, vomiting, apprehension, dyspnea, diaphoresis, increased or decreased blood pressure, gallop heart sound, sensation of impending doom
Precipitating factors ▶ Myocardial infarction or upper respiratory tract infection; invasive cardiac trauma	▶ Exertion, stress, eating, cold or hot and humid weather	▶ Occurring at rest or during physical exertion or emotional stress

and radiates to the neck, shoulders, back, and arms. However, unlike the pain of MI, pericardial pain is often pleuritic, increasing with deep inspiration and decreasing when the patient sits up and leans forward, pulling the heart away from the diaphragmatic pleurae of the lungs. (See *Patterns of cardiac pain*.)

Pericardial effusion, the major complication, may produce effects of heart failure (dyspnea, orthopnea, and tachycardia) as well as ill-defined substernal chest pain and a feeling of fullness in the chest.

 ALERT If the fluid accumulates rapidly, cardiac tamponade may occur, resulting in pallor, clammy skin, hypotension, pulsus paradoxus (a decrease in systolic blood pressure of more than 10 mm Hg during slow inspiration), neck vein distention and, eventually, cardiovascular collapse and death.

Chronic constrictive pericarditis causes a gradual increase in systemic venous pressure and produces symptoms similar to those of chronic right-sided heart failure (fluid retention, ascites, hepatomegaly).

Diagnosis

Because pericarditis often coexists with other conditions, diagnosis of the acute form depends on typical clinical features and elimination of other possible causes.

A classic symptom, the pericardial friction rub, is a grating sound heard as the heart moves. It can usually be auscultated best during forced expiration, while the patient leans forward or is on his hands and knees in bed.

Pericardial friction rub may have up to three components, corresponding to the timing of atrial systole, ventricular systole, and the rapid filling phase of ventricular diastole. Occasionally, it's heard only briefly or not at all. However, its presence, along with other characteristic features, is diagnostic of acute pericarditis.

In addition, if acute pericarditis has caused very large pericardial effusions, the physical examination reveals increased cardiac dullness and diminished or absent apical impulse and distant heart sounds. In patients with chronic pericarditis, acute inflammation or effusions do not occur— only restricted cardiac filling.

Laboratory results reflect inflammation and may identify its cause. There is a normal or elevated white blood cell count, especially in infectious pericarditis, an elevated erythrocyte sedimentation rate, and

slightly elevated cardiac enzyme levels with associated myocarditis. Cultures of pericardial fluid obtained by open surgical drainage or cardiocentesis sometimes identifies a causative organism in bacterial or fungal pericarditis.

Electrocardiography shows the following changes in acute pericarditis: elevation of ST segments in the standard limb leads and most precordial leads without significant changes in QRS morphology that occur with MI, atrial ectopic rhythms such as atrial fibrillation, and diminished QRS complex in pericardial effusion.

Other pertinent laboratory studies include blood urea nitrogen level to check for uremia, antistreptolysin-O titers to detect rheumatic fever, and a purified protein derivative skin test to check for tuberculosis. In pericardial effusion, echocardiography is diagnostic when it shows an echo-free space between the ventricular wall and the pericardium.

Differential diagnoses include pulmonary emboli, angina, MI, pneumonia, and heart failure.

Treatment

The treatment goal is to relieve symptoms and manage underlying systemic disease.

In acute idiopathic pericarditis and postthoracotomy pericarditis, treatment consists of bed rest as long as fever and pain persist, and nonsteroidal anti-inflammatory drugs (NSAIDS), such as aspirin and indomethacin, to relieve pain and reduce inflammation. If these drugs fail to relieve symptoms, corticosteroids may be used. Although corticosteroids produce rapid and effective relief, they must be used cautiously because episodes may recur when therapy is discontinued. In post-MI pericarditis, aspirin, NSAIDS, and steroids should be avoided because they may interfere with myocardial scar formation.

Infectious pericarditis that results from disease of the left pleural space, mediastinal abscesses, or septicemia requires antibiotics (possibly by direct pericardial injection), surgical drainage, or both. Cardiac tamponade may require pericardiocentesis. Signs of tamponade include pulsus paradoxus, neck vein distention, dyspnea, and shock.

Recurrent pericarditis may necessitate partial pericardectomy, which creates a window that allows fluid to drain into the pleural space. In constrictive pericarditis, total pericardectomy to permit adequate filling and contraction of the heart may be necessary. Treatment must also include management of rheumatic fever, uremia, tuberculosis, and other underlying disorders

Special considerations
▶ Provide complete bed rest.
▶ Assess pain in relation to respiration and body position to distinguish pericardial pain from myocardial ischemic pain.
▶ Place the patient in an upright position to relieve dyspnea and chest pain. Provide analgesics and oxygen, and reassure the patient with acute pericarditis that his condition is temporary and treatable.
▶ Monitor the patient for signs of cardiac compression or cardiac tamponade, possible complications of pericardial effusion. Signs include decreased blood pressure, increased central venous pressure, and pulsus paradoxus. Because cardiac tamponade requires immediate treatment, keep a pericardiocentesis set handy whenever pericardial effusion is suspected.
▶ Explain tests and treatments to the patient. If surgery is necessary, he should learn deep breathing and coughing exercises beforehand. Postoperative care is similar to that given after cardiothoracic surgery.

PERIRECTAL ABSCESS AND FISTULA

A perirectal abscess is a localized collection of pus caused by inflammation of the soft tissue outside the anal verge. Such inflammation may produce an anal fistula — an abnormal opening in the anal skin — that may communicate with the rectum. Men are affected by this disease three times as often as women.

Causes
The inflammatory process that leads to abscess may begin with an abrasion or tear in the lining of the anal canal, rectum, or perianal skin, and subsequent infection by *Escherichia coli,* staphylococci, or streptococci. Such trauma may result from injections for treatment of internal hemorrhoids, enema-tip abrasions, puncture wounds from ingested eggshells or fish bones, or insertion of foreign objects.

Other preexisting lesions include infected anal fissure, infections from the anal crypt through the anal gland, ruptured anal hematoma, prolapsed thrombotic internal hemorrhoids, and septic lesions in the pelvis, such as acute appendicitis, acute salpingitis, and diverticulitis. Systemic illnesses that may cause abscesses include ulcerative colitis and Crohn's disease. However, many abscesses develop without preexisting lesions. Other causes include trauma, malignancy, radiation, infectious dermatitis, and an immunocompromised state.

As the abscess produces more pus, a fistula may form in the soft tissue beneath the muscle fibers of the sphincters (especially the external sphincter), usually extending into the perianal skin. The internal (primary) opening of the abscess or fistula is usually near the anal glands and crypts; the external (secondary) opening, in the perianal skin.

Signs and symptoms
Characteristics are throbbing pain and tenderness at the site of the abscess and painful swelling that is exacerbated by defecation. A hard, painful lump develops on one side, preventing comfortable sitting.

Diagnosis
Perianal abscess is a red, tender, localized, oval swelling close to the anus. Sitting or coughing increases pain, and pus may

drain from the abscess. Digital examination reveals no abnormalities. Ischiorectal abscess involves the entire perianal region on the affected side of the anus. The only symptom of this large erythematous, indurated, tender mass at the buttock may be pain. It's tender but may not produce drainage. Digital rectal examination reveals a tender induration bulging into the anal canal. A flexible sigmoidoscopy should be performed at a later date on these patients to rule out carcinoma or inflammatory bowel disease.

Submucous or high intermuscular abscess (5% of patients) may produce a dull, aching pain in the rectum, tenderness and, occasionally, induration. Digital examination reveals a smooth swelling of the upper part of the anal canal or lower rectum.

Pelvirectal abscess (rare) produces fever, malaise, and myalgia but no local anal or external rectal signs or pain. Digital examination reveals a tender mass high in the pelvis, perhaps extending into one of the ischiorectal fossae.

If the abscess drains by forming a fistula, the pain usually subsides and the major signs become pruritic drainage and subsequent perianal irritation.

Pain and discharge are symptoms of fistula development and when the external or secondary opening has closed.

The external opening of a fistula generally appears as a pink or red, elevated, discharging sinus or ulcer on the skin near the anus. Depending on the infection's severity, the patient may have chills, fever, nausea, vomiting, and malaise. Digital rectal examination may reveal a palpable indurated tract and a drop or two of pus on palpation. The internal opening may be palpated as a depression or ulcer in the midline anteriorly or at the dentate line posteriorly. To identify an internal opening, an examination under anesthesia should be performed.

Flexible sigmoidoscopy, barium studies, and colonoscopy should be performed to rule out underlying conditions.

Treatment

Perirectal abscesses require surgical incision and drainage. The area may be explored to identify a fistula tract, and a fistulotomy may be performed at a later date. Fistulas require a fistulotomy — removal of the fistula tract and associated granulation tissue — under general, spinal, or caudal anesthesia. If the fistula tract is epithelialized, treatment requires fistulectomy — removal of the fistulous tract — followed by insertion of drains, which are gradually removed over time.

Special considerations

After incision and drainage:
◗ Provide adequate medication for pain relief.
◗ Examine the wound frequently to assess proper healing, which should progress from the inside out. Healing should be complete in 4 to 5 weeks for perianal fistulas; in 12 to 16 weeks for deeper wounds.
◗ Inform the patient that complete recovery takes time. Offer encouragement.
◗ Stress the importance of perianal cleanliness.
◗ Dispose of soiled dressings properly.
◗ Be alert for the first postoperative bowel movement. The patient may suppress the urge to defecate because of anticipated pain; the resulting constipation increases pressure at the wound site. Such a patient may benefit from a stool-softening laxative.

PERITONITIS

Peritonitis is an acute or chronic inflammation of the peritoneum, the membrane that lines the abdominal cavity and covers the visceral organs. Inflammation may extend throughout the peritoneum or may be localized as an abscess.

Peritonitis commonly decreases intestinal motility and causes intestinal distention with gas. Mortality is 10%, with death usually resulting from bowel obstruction; the mortality rate was much higher before the introduction of antibiotics.

Causes

Although the GI tract normally contains bacteria, the peritoneum is sterile. In peritonitis, however, bacteria invade the peritoneum. Generally, such infection results from inflammation and perforation of the GI tract, allowing bacterial invasion. Usually, this results from appendicitis, diverticulitis, peptic ulcer, ulcerative colitis, volvulus, strangulated obstruction, abdominal neoplasm, or a penetrating wound.

Peritonitis may also result from chemical inflammation, as in rupture of the fallopian tube or the bladder; perforation of a gastric ulcer; or released pancreatic enzymes.

In both chemical and bacterial inflammation, accumulated fluids containing protein and electrolytes make the transparent peritoneum opaque, red, inflamed, and edematous. Because the peritoneal cavity is so resistant to contamination, such infection is often localized as an abscess instead of disseminated as a generalized infection.

Signs and symptoms

The key symptom of peritonitis is sudden, severe, and diffuse abdominal pain that tends to intensify and localize in the area of the underlying disorder. Direct or rebound tenderness may be elicited over an area affected by diverticulitis.

Pain may be accompanied by anorexia, nausea, vomiting, and altered bowel habits (particularly constipation). For instance, if appendicitis causes the rupture, pain eventually localizes in the lower right quadrant. The patient often displays weakness, pallor, excessive sweating, and cold skin as a result of excessive loss of fluid, electrolytes, and protein into the abdominal cavity.

Decreased intestinal motility and paralytic ileus result from the effect of bacterial toxins on the intestinal muscles. Intestinal obstruction causes nausea, vomiting, and abdominal rigidity.

Other typical clinical features include hypotension, tachycardia, signs of dehydration (oliguria, thirst, dry swollen tongue, pinched skin), acutely tender abdomen associated with rebound tenderness, temperature of 103° F (39.4° C) or higher, and hypokalemia. Inflammation of the diaphragmatic peritoneum may cause shoulder pain and hiccups.

Abdominal distention and resulting upward displacement of the diaphragm may decrease respiratory capacity. Typically, the patient with peritonitis tends to breathe shallowly and move as little as possible to minimize pain.

Diagnosis

Severe abdominal pain in a patient with direct or rebound tenderness suggests peritonitis. Abdominal X-rays showing edematous and gaseous distention of the small and large bowel support the diagnosis. In the case of perforation of a visceral organ, the X-ray shows air in the abdominal cavity. Other appropriate tests include:
◗ chest X-ray — may show elevation of the diaphragm
◗ blood studies — shows leukocytosis (more than 20,000/µl)
◗ paracentesis — reveals bacteria, exudate, blood, pus, or urine
◗ laparotomy — may be necessary to identify the underlying cause.

Other conditions to consider are acute appendicitis, pancreatitis, cholecystitis, and pelvic inflammatory disease.

Treatment

Early treatment of GI inflammatory conditions and preoperative and postoperative antibiotic therapy help prevent peritonitis. After peritonitis develops, emergency treatment must combat infection, restore intestinal motility, and replace fluids and electrolytes.

Empiric antibiotic therapy usually includes administration of cefoxitin with an aminoglycoside or penicillin G and clindamycin with an aminoglycoside, depending on the infecting organisms. To decrease peristalsis and prevent perforation, the patient should receive nothing by mouth; I.V. fluids are administered. Other supportive measures include preoperative and postoperative administration of analgesia and nasogastric (NG) decompression.

When peritonitis results from perforation, surgery is necessary. The aim of surgery is to eliminate the source of infection by evacuating the spilled contents and repairing any organ perforation.

Special considerations

▶ Monitor vital signs, fluid intake and output, and the amount of NG drainage or vomitus.

▶ Place the patient in semi-Fowler's position to facilitate pulmonary toileting.

▶ Encourage the patient to deep-breathe, cough effectively, and use an incentive spirometer.

▶ Teach splinting of the incision to facilitate pulmonary toileting.

▶ Counteract mouth and nose dryness due to fever and NG intubation with regular cleaning and lubrication.

▶ Maintain parenteral fluid and electrolyte administration as ordered. Accurately record fluid intake and output, including NG and incisional drainage.

▶ Place the patient in Fowler's position to promote drainage (through drainage tube) by gravity.

▶ Encourage and assist ambulation as ordered, usually on the first postoperative day.

▶ Observe for signs of dehiscence (the patient may complain that "something gave way") and abscess formation (persistent abdominal tenderness and fever).

▶ Frequently assess for peristaltic activity by listening for bowel sounds and evaluating for passage of flatus, bowel movements, and soft abdomen.

▶ When peristalsis returns and temperature and pulse rate are normal or when NG output diminishes (less than 200 cc/24 hrs), the NG tube is removed.

▶ Gradually decrease parenteral fluids and increase oral intake.

PERTUSSIS

Also known as whooping cough, pertussis is a highly contagious respiratory infection usually caused by the nonmotile, gram-negative coccobacillus *Bordetella pertussis* and, occasionally, by the related similar bacteria *B. parapertussis* and *B. bronchiseptica*. Characteristically, whooping cough produces an irritating cough that becomes paroxysmal and commonly ends in a high-pitched inspiratory whoop.

Since the 1940s, immunization and aggressive diagnosis and treatment have significantly reduced mortality from whooping cough in the United States. Mortality in children under age 1 is usually a result of pneumonia and other complications. The disease is also dangerous in the elderly but tends to be less severe in older children and adults. Since the 1980s reported cases of pertussis in the U.S. has increased.

Causes

Whooping cough is usually transmitted by the direct inhalation of contaminated droplets from a patient in the acute stage; it may also be spread indirectly through soiled linen and other articles contaminated by respiratory secretions.

Whooping cough is endemic throughout the world, usually occurring in late winter and early spring. In about 50% of cases, it strikes unimmunized children under age 1, probably because women of childbearing age don't usually have high serum levels of *B. pertussis* antibodies to transmit to their offspring.

Signs and symptoms

After an incubation period of about 7 to 10 days, *B. pertussis* enters the tracheobronchial mucosa, where it produces progressively tenacious mucus. Whooping cough follows a classic 6-week course that includes three stages, each of which lasts about 2 weeks.

First, the *catarrhal stage* characteristically produces an irritating hacking, nocturnal cough; anorexia; sneezing; listlessness; infected conjunctiva and, occasionally, a low-grade fever. This stage is highly communicable.

After 7 to 14 days, the *paroxysmal stage* produces spasmodic and recurrent coughing that may expel tenacious mucus. Each cough characteristically ends in a loud, crowing inspiratory whoop, and choking on mucus causes vomiting. (Very young infants, however, may not develop the typical whoop.) Paroxysmal coughing may induce such complications as nosebleed, increased venous pressure, periorbital edema, conjunctival hemorrhage, hemorrhage of the anterior chamber of the eye, detached retina (and blindness), rectal prolapse, inguinal or umbilical hernia, seizures, atelectasis, and pneumonitis. In infants, choking spells may cause apnea, anoxia, and disturbed acid-base balance. During this stage, patients are highly vulnerable to fatal secondary bacterial or viral infections. Suspect such secondary infection (usually otitis media or pneumonia) in any whooping cough patient with a fever during this stage, because whooping cough itself seldom causes fever.

During the *convalescent stage,* paroxysmal coughing and vomiting gradually subside. However, for months afterward, even a mild upper respiratory tract infection may trigger paroxysmal coughing.

Central nervous system complications are uncommon but one should be aware of these. Seizures and encephalopathy may be seen. The mechanisms may include hypoxia or a toxin.

Diagnosis

Classic clinical findings, especially during the paroxysmal stage, suggest this diagnosis; laboratory studies confirm it. Nasopharyngeal swabs and sputum cultures show *B. pertussis* only in the early stages of this disease; fluorescent antibody screening of nasopharyngeal smears provides quicker results than cultures but is less reliable. In addition, the white blood cell (WBC) count is usually increased, especially in children older than 6 months and early in the paroxysmal stage. Sometimes, the WBC count may reach 175,000 to 200,000/μl, with 60% to 90% lymphocytes.

Other conditions to rule out are adenovirus infections, tuberculosis, bronchitis, and influenza.

Treatment

Vigorous supportive therapy requires hospitalization of infants (commonly in the intensive care unit), and fluid and electrolyte replacement. Other measures include adequate nutrition, codeine and mild sedation to decrease coughing, and oxygen therapy in apnea. Antibiotics, such as erythromycin and, possibly, ampicillin, must be initiated during the catarrhal phase of the illness to be effective in eliminating the infection. Antibiotics are also helpful in shortening the period of communicability and preventing secondary infections. Corticosteroids, especially in infants, may reduce the severity and course of illness.

Because very young infants are particularly susceptible to whooping cough, immunization — most commonly with the diphtheria-tetanus acellular-pertussis (DTaP) vaccine — begins at 2, 4, and 6 months. Boosters follow at 18 months and at 4 to 6 years. The risk of pertussis is greater than the risk of vaccine complications such as neurologic damage. However, seizures or unusual and persistent crying may be a sign of a severe neurologic reaction and the doctor may not order the other doses. The vaccine is contraindicated in children over age 6 because it can cause a severe fever.

Special considerations

▶ Whooping cough calls for aggressive, supportive care and respiratory isolation (masks only) for 5 to 7 days after initiation of antibiotic therapy.

▶ Monitor acid-base, fluid, and electrolyte balances.

▶ Carefully suction secretions, and monitor oxygen therapy. *Remember:* Suctioning removes oxygen as well as secretions.

▶ Create a quiet environment to decrease coughing stimulation. Provide small, frequent meals, and treat constipation or nausea caused by codeine.

▶ Offer emotional support to parents of children with whooping cough.

▶ To decrease exposure to organisms, change soiled linen, empty the suction bottle, and change the trash bag at least once each shift.

 PREVENTION TIP Stress to parents the importance of correct immunization of infants, toddlers, and older children to increase protection against infection.

PHARYNGITIS

The most common throat disorder, pharyngitis is an acute or chronic inflammation of the pharynx. It is widespread among adults who live or work in dusty or very dry environments, use their voices excessively, habitually use tobacco or alcohol, or suffer from chronic sinusitis, persistent coughs, or allergies.

Causes

Pharyngitis is usually caused by respiratory viruses such as rhinovirus, coronavirus, adenovirus, influenza, and parainfluenza viruses. The most common concern is infection due to group A beta-hemolytic streptococci, because of the associated, preventable risk of rheumatic fever. Other common causes include *Mycoplasma* and *Chlamydia*. A host of other bacteria, viruses, fungi, and spirochetes have also been identified as etiologic agents. *Mycobacterium tuberculosis* is a rare cause of pharyngitis.

Signs and symptoms

Pharyngitis produces a sore throat and slight difficulty in swallowing. Swallowing saliva is usually more painful than swallowing food. Pharyngitis may also cause the sensation of a lump in the throat as well as a constant, aggravating urge to swallow. Associated features may include fever, headache, muscle and joint pain, coryza, and rhinorrhea. Inquire about drooling, any preferred neck position, and pain on extension of the neck. Uncomplicated pharyngitis usually subsides in 3 to 10 days.

Diagnosis

Physical examination of the pharynx reveals generalized redness and inflammation of the posterior wall and red, edematous mucous membranes studded with white or yellow exudate. Exudate is usually confined to the lymphoid areas of the throat, sparing the tonsillar pillars. Bacterial pharyngitis usually produces a large amount of exudate. Assess for anterior vs. posterior cervical adenopathy, gingivitis or necrotic tonsillar ulcers. Associated physical findings, such as viral exanthem, conjunctivitis, petechiae, generalized lymphadenopathy, splenomegaly, or hepatic tenderness, may provide important clues to etiology.

 ALERT Patients with severe dysphagia or dyspnea require urgent evaluation to exclude airway obstruction. If epiglottitis is suspected, the airway should not be instrumented.

A throat culture may be performed to identify bacterial organisms that may be the cause of the inflammation. Rapid screening for streptococci can be performed from a throat swab with antigen agglutination kits. It should be performed in patients with an intermediate likelihood of strep throat as well as those patients at high risk for complications. Because there is a 5% to 10% false negative rate, some clinicians suggest routine backup of all negatives with blood agar culture.

Special tests should be performed only if the history warrants. Such tests include screening for gonococcal infection (requires warm Thayer-Martin plate) and Monospot test for Epstein-Barr virus. Gram stain can be suggestive, and streptococcal isolates can be immunologically typed.

Obtain a lateral neck radiograph if drooling is present and look for epiglottitis.

Other conditions to consider are acute epiglottitis, peritonsillar abscess, Ludwig's angina, influenza, rhinovirus, adenovirus, parainfluenza virus, Epstein-Barr virus, and coxsackievirus.

Treatment

There are several approaches to the management of pharyngitis. Deciding factors include the reliability of cultures and rapid tests for streptococci, the incidence of pharyngitis not due to group A beta-hemolytic streptococci, patient follow-up, medical compliance, and costs.

In acute viral pharyngitis, treatment is usually symptomatic, and consists mainly of rest, warm saline gargles, throat lozenges containing a mild anesthetic, plenty of fluids, and analgesics as needed. If the patient can't swallow fluids, hospitalization may be required for I.V. hydration.

Suspected bacterial pharyngitis requires rigorous treatment with penicillin or another broad-spectrum antibiotic because *Streptococcus* is the chief infecting microbe. Antibiotic therapy should continue for 48 hours until culture results are known.

If the culture (or a rapid strep test) is positive for group A beta-hemolytic streptococci, or if bacterial infection is suspected despite negative culture results, penicillin therapy should be continued for 10 days. This is to prevent the sequelae of acute rheumatic fever. Erythromycin, amoxicillin, or penicillin are effective. Patients suspected of noncompliance may be given a long-acting parenteral penicillin such as benzathine penicillin. The macrolide antibiotics have also been reported to be successful in shorter-duration regimens. Azithromycin need only be taken for 3 days.

Chronic pharyngitis requires the same supportive measures as acute pharyngitis but with greater emphasis on eliminating the underlying cause, such as an allergen. Preventive measures include adequate humidification and avoiding excessive exposure to air conditioning. In addition, the patient should be urged to stop smoking.

Antibiotic choices for treatment failures are controversial. Alternatives to penicillin include cefuroxime and certain other cephalosporins, dicloxacillin, and amoxicillin with clavulanate. In cases of prior severe penicillin reaction, cephalosporins should probably be avoided. The cross-reaction is believed to be higher than the overall 8% rate.

Special considerations

▶ Administer analgesics and warm saline gargles as appropriate.
▶ Encourage the patient to drink plenty of fluids. Monitor intake and output scrupulously, and watch for signs of dehydration. Assess skin turgor, mucous membranes and, in young children, tearing.
▶ Provide meticulous mouth care to prevent dry lips and oral pyoderma, and maintain a restful environment.
▶ Elevate the patient's head with three or four pillows.
▶ Obtain throat cultures, and administer antibiotics as required if the patient has acute bacterial pharyngitis.
▶ Teach the patient with chronic pharyngitis how to minimize sources of throat irritation in the environment, such as using a bedside humidifier.
▶ Refer the patient to a self-help group to stop smoking, if appropriate.
▶ In severe cases, anesthetic gargles and lozenges (such as benzocaine) may provide additional symptomatic relief.

 PREVENTION TIP Stress to patients the importance of completing the 10-day course of antibiotics regardless of symptom response. Patients are presumed to be noninfectious after 24 hours of antibiotic coverage.

PLAGUE

Plague, also known as the Black Death, is an acute infection that occurs in several forms. *Bubonic plague,* the most common, causes the characteristic swollen, and sometimes suppurating, lymph glands (buboes) that give this infection its name. Other forms include *septicemic plague,* a severe, rapid systemic form, and *pneumonic plague,* which can be primary or secondary to the other two forms. *Primary pneumonic plague* is an acutely fulminant, highly contagious form that causes acute prostration, respiratory distress, and death— in many cases within 2 to 3 days after onset.

Without treatment, mortality is about 60% in bubonic plague and approaches 100% in both septicemic and pneumonic plagues. With treatment, mortality is approximately 18%, largely due to the delay between onset and treatment and the patient's age and physical condition.

Bubonic plague is notorious for the historic pandemics in Europe and Asia during the Middle Ages, which in some areas killed up to two-thirds of the population. This form is rarely transmitted from person to person. However, the untreated bubonic form may progress to a secondary pneumonic form, which is transmitted by contaminated respiratory droplets (coughing) and is highly contagious. In the United States, the primary pneumonic form usually occurs after inhalation of *Y. pestis* in a laboratory.

Sylvatic (wild rodent) plague remains endemic in South America, the Near East, central and Southeast Asia, north central and southern Africa, Mexico, and western United States and Canada. In the United States, its incidence has been rising, a possible reflection of different bacterial strains or environmental changes that favor rodent growth in certain areas. Plague tends to occur between May and September; between October and February it usually occurs in hunters who skin wild ani-

BUBONIC PLAGUE CARRIER

Bubonic plague is usually transmitted to humans through the bite of a flea *(Xenopsylla cheopis)* shown here.

mals. One attack confers permanent immunity.

Causes

Plague is caused by the gram-negative, nonmotile, nonsporulating bacillus *Yersinia pestis* (formerly called *Pasteurella pestis*). It's usually transmitted to humans through the bite of a flea from an infected rodent host, such as a rat, squirrel, prairie dog, or hare. Occasionally, transmission occurs from handling infected animals or their tissues. (See *Bubonic plague carrier.*)

Signs and symptoms

The incubation period, early symptoms, severity at onset, and clinical course vary in the three forms of plague. In *bubonic plague,* the incubation period is 2 to 6 days. The milder form begins with malaise, fever, and pain or tenderness in regional lymph nodes, possibly associated with swelling. Lymph node damage (usually axillary or inguinal) eventually produces painful, inflamed, and possibly suppurative buboes. The classic sign of plague is an excruciatingly painful bubo. Hemorrhagic areas may become necrotic; in the skin, such areas appear dark— hence the name "Black Death."

This infection can progress extremely rapidly: A seemingly mildly ill person with only fever and adenitis may become moribund within hours. Plague may also begin dramatically, with a sudden high fever of 103° to 106° F (39.5° to 41.1° C), chills, myalgia, headache, prostration, restlessness, disorientation, delirium, toxemia, and staggering gait. Occasionally, it causes abdominal pain, nausea, vomiting, and constipation, followed by diarrhea (frequently bloody), skin mottling, petechiae, and circulatory collapse.

In *primary pneumonic plague,* the incubation period is 2 to 3 days, followed by a typically acute onset, with high fever, chills, severe headache, tachycardia, tachypnea, dyspnea, and a productive cough (first mucoid sputum, later frothy pink or red).

Secondary pneumonic plague, the pulmonary extension of the bubonic form, complicates about 5% of cases of untreated plague. A cough producing bloody sputum signals this complication. Both the primary and secondary forms of pneumonic plague rapidly cause severe prostration, respiratory distress and, usually, death.

Septicemic plague usually develops without overt lymph node enlargement. In this form, the patient shows toxicity, hyperpyrexia, seizures, prostration, shock, and disseminated intravascular coagulation (DIC). Septicemic plague causes widespread nonspecific tissue damage — such as peritoneal or pleural effusions, pericarditis, and meningitis — and is rapidly fatal unless promptly and correctly treated.

Diagnosis

Because plague is rare in the United States, it's commonly overlooked until after the patient dies or multiple cases develop. Characteristic buboes and a history of exposure to rodents strongly suggest bubonic plague.

Stained smears and cultures of *Y. pestis* obtained from a needle aspirate of a small amount of fluid from skin lesions confirm this diagnosis.

Postmortem examination of a guinea pig inoculated with a sample of blood or purulent drainage allows isolation of the organism. Other laboratory findings include a white blood cell count of over 20,000/μl with increased polymorphonuclear leukocytes, and hemoagglutination reaction (antibody titer) studies. Diagnosis should rule out tularemia, typhus, and typhoid.

In pneumonic plague, diagnosis requires a chest X-ray to show fulminating pneumonia, and stained smear and culture of sputum to identify *Y. pestis.* Other bacterial pneumonias and psittacosis must be ruled out. Stained smear and blood culture containing *Y. pestis* are diagnostic in septicemic plague. However, cultures of *Y. pestis* grow slowly; so, in suspected plague (especially pneumonic and septicemic plagues), treatment should begin without waiting for laboratory confirmation. For a presumptive diagnosis of plague, a fluorescent antibody test may be ordered.

Treatment

Antimicrobial treatment of suspected plague must begin immediately after blood specimens have been taken for culture and shouldn't be delayed for laboratory confirmation. Generally, treatment consists of large doses of streptomycin, the drug proven most effective against *Y. pestis.* Other effective drugs include gentamicin, doxycycline, and chloramphenicol. Penicillins are ineffective against plague.

In both septicemic and pneumonic plagues, life-saving antimicrobial treatment must begin within 18 hours of onset. Supportive management aims to control fever, shock, and seizures, and to maintain fluid balance.

After antimicrobial therapy has begun, glucocorticoids can combat life-threatening toxemia and shock; diazepam relieves restlessness; and if the patient develops DIC, treatment may include heparin.

Special considerations

Patients with plague require strict isolation, which may be discontinued 48 hours after antimicrobial therapy begins unless respiratory symptoms develop.

▶ Use an approved insecticide to rid the patient and his clothing of fleas. Carefully dispose of soiled dressings and linens, feces, and sputum. If the patient has pneumonic plague, wear a gown, mask, and gloves. Handle all exudates, purulent discharge, and laboratory specimens with rubber gloves. For more information, consult your infection control officer.

▶ Give medications and treat complications, as ordered.

▶ Treat buboes with hot, moist compresses. Never excise or drain them because this could spread the infection.

▶ When septicemic plague causes peripheral tissue necrosis, prevent further injury to necrotic tissue. Avoid using restraints or armboards, and pad the bed's side rails.

▶ Obtain a history of patient contacts so that they can be quarantined for 6 days of observation. Administer prophylactic tetracycline as ordered.

▶ Report suspected cases of plague to local public health department officials so they can identify the source of infection.

 PREVENTION TIP To help prevent plague, discourage contact with wild animals (especially those that are sick or dead), and support programs aimed at reducing insect and rodent populations. Recommend immunization with plague vaccine to travelers to or residents of endemic areas, even though the effect of immunization is transient.

PLEURISY

Pleurisy, also known as pleuritis, is an inflammation of the visceral and parietal pleurae that line the inside of the thoracic cage and envelop the lungs.

Causes

Pleurisy develops as a complication of pneumonia, tuberculosis, viruses, systemic lupus erythematosus, rheumatoid arthritis, uremia, Dressler's syndrome, cancer, pulmonary infarction, and chest trauma.

Pleuritic pain is caused by the inflammation or irritation of sensory nerve endings in the parietal pleura. As the lungs inflate and deflate, the visceral pleura covering the lungs moves against the fixed parietal pleura lining the pleural space, causing pain. This disorder usually begins suddenly.

Signs and symptoms

Sharp, stabbing pain that increases with respiration may be so severe that it limits movement on the affected side during breathing. Dyspnea also occurs. Other symptoms vary according to the underlying pathologic process.

Diagnosis

Auscultation of the chest reveals a characteristic pleural friction rub — a coarse, creaky sound heard during late inspiration and early expiration, directly over the area of pleural inflammation. Palpation over the affected area may reveal coarse vibration. Other conditions to consider are myocardial infarction, pericarditis, and pulmonary embolus.

Treatment

Generally, symptomatic treatment includes anti-inflammatory agents, analgesics, and bed rest. Severe pain may require an intercostal nerve block of two or three intercostal nerves. Pleurisy with pleural effusion calls for thoracentesis as both a therapeutic and a diagnostic measure.

Special considerations

▶ Stress the importance of bed rest and plan your care to allow the patient as much uninterrupted rest as possible.

▶ Administer antitussives and pain medication as necessary, but be careful not to overmedicate.

▶ If the pain requires a narcotic analgesic, warn the patient about to be discharged to avoid overuse because such medication depresses coughing and respiration.
▶ Encourage the patient to cough. Tell him to apply firm pressure at the site of pain during coughing exercises to minimize pain.

PNEUMOCYSTIS CARINII PNEUMONIA

Because of its association with human immunodeficiency virus (HIV) infection, *Pneumocystis carinii* pneumonia (PCP), an opportunistic infection, has increased in incidence since the 1980s. Before the advent of PCP prophylaxis, this disease was the first clue in about 60% of patients that HIV infection was present.

PCP occurs in up to 90% of HIV-infected patients in the United States at some point during their lifetime. It is the leading cause of death in these patients. Disseminated infection doesn't occur. PCP also is associated with other immunocompromised conditions, including organ transplantation, leukemia, and lymphoma.

Causes
P. carinii, the cause of PCP, usually is classified as a protozoan, although some investigators consider it more closely related to fungi. The organism exists as a saprophyte in the lungs of humans and various animals.

Part of the normal flora in most healthy people, *P. carinii* becomes an aggressive pathogen in the immunocompromised patient. Impaired cell-mediated (T-cell) immunity is thought to be more important than impaired humoral (B-cell) immunity in predisposing the patient to PCP, but the immune defects involved are poorly understood.

The organism invades the lungs bilaterally and multiplies extracellularly. As the infestation grows, alveoli fill with organisms and exudate, impairing gas exchange. The alveoli hypertrophy and thicken progressively, eventually leading to extensive consolidation.

The primary transmission route seems to be air, although the organism is already present in most people. The incubation period probably lasts for 4 to 8 weeks.

Signs and symptoms
The patient typically has a history of an immunocompromising condition (such as HIV infection, leukemia, or lymphoma) or procedure (such as organ transplantation).

PCP begins insidiously with increasing shortness of breath and a nonproductive cough. Anorexia, generalized fatigue, and weight loss may follow. Although the patient may have hypoxemia and hypercapnia, he may not exhibit significant symptoms. He may, however, have a low-grade, intermittent fever.

Other signs and symptoms include tachypnea, dyspnea, accessory muscle use for breathing, crackles (in about one-third of patients), and decreased breath sounds (in advanced pneumonia). Cyanosis may appear with acute illness; pulmonary consolidation develops later.

Diagnosis
Histologic studies confirm *P. carinii*. In patients with HIV infection, initial examination of a first morning sputum specimen (induced by inhaling an ultrasonically dispersed saline mist) may be sufficient; however, this technique usually is ineffective in patients without HIV infection.

Fiberoptic bronchoscopy remains the most commonly used study to confirm PCP. Invasive procedures, such as transbronchial biopsy and open lung biopsy, are performed less commonly.

Chest X-ray may show slowly progressing, fluffy infiltrates and occasionally nodular lesions or a spontaneous pneumothorax. Gallium scan may show increased uptake over the lungs even when the chest X-ray appears relatively normal. Arterial blood gas (ABG) studies detect hypoxia and an increased alveolar-arterial gradient.

These findings must be differentiated from findings in other types of pneumonia, adult respiratory distress syndrome, asthma, heart failure, and lung cancer.

Treatment

PCP may respond to drug therapy with cotrimoxazole or pentamidine isethionate. Because of immune system impairment, many patients who also have HIV experience severe adverse reactions to drug therapy. These reactions include bone marrow suppression, thrush, fever, hepatotoxicity, and anaphylaxis. Nausea, vomiting, and rashes are common. Diphenhydramine may be prescribed to treat the latter effects and leucovorin may reduce bone marrow suppression (and may be used prophylactically in patients with HIV infection).

Pentamidine may be administered I.V. or in aerosol form. I.V. pentamidine is associated with a high incidence of severe toxic effects. The inhaled form usually is well tolerated. However, inhaled pentamidine may not effectively reach the lung apices. Adverse reactions associated with inhalation include metallic taste, pharyngitis, cough, bronchospasm, shortness of breath, rhinitis, and laryngitis.

Supportive measures, such as oxygen therapy, mechanical ventilation, adequate nutrition, and fluid balance, are important adjunctive therapies.

Oral or I.V. morphine sulfate solution may reduce the respiratory rate and the patient's anxiety, thereby enhancing oxygenation.

Special considerations

▶ Implement universal precautions to prevent contagion.
▶ Frequently assess the patient's respiratory status, and monitor ABG levels every 4 hours.

▶ Administer oxygen therapy as necessary. Encourage the patient to ambulate and to perform deep-breathing exercises and incentive spirometry to facilitate effective gas exchange.
▶ Administer antipyretics, as required, to relieve fever.
▶ Monitor intake and output and daily weight to evaluate fluid balance. Replace fluids as necessary.
▶ Give antimicrobial drugs as required. Never give pentamidine I.M. because it can cause pain and sterile abscesses. Administer the I.V. drug form slowly over 60 minutes to reduce the risk of hypotension.
▶ Monitor the patient for adverse reactions to antimicrobial drugs. If he's receiving cotrimoxazole, watch for nausea, vomiting, rash, bone marrow suppression, thrush, fever, hepatotoxicity, and anaphylaxis. If he's receiving pentamidine, watch for cardiac arrhythmias, hypotension, dizziness, azotemia, hypocalcemia, and hepatic disturbances.
▶ Provide diversional activities and coordinate health care team activities to allow adequate rest periods between procedures.
▶ Teach the patient energy conservation techniques as well.
▶ Supply nutritional supplements as needed. Encourage the patient to eat a high-calorie, protein-rich diet. Offer small, frequent meals if the patient cannot tolerate large amounts of food.
▶ Reduce anxiety by providing a relaxing environment, eliminating excessive environmental stimuli, and allowing ample time for meals.
▶ Give emotional support and help the patient identify and use meaningful support systems.
▶ Instruct the patient about the medication regimen, especially about possible adverse effects.
▶ If the patient will require oxygen therapy at home, explain that an oxygen concentrator may be most effective.

PNEUMONIA

An acute infection of the lung parenchyma, pneumonia often impairs gas exchange. The prognosis is generally good for people who have normal lungs and adequate host defenses before the onset of pneumonia; however, pneumonia is the sixth leading cause of death in the United States.

Causes

Pneumonia can be classified in several ways:

▶ *Microbiologic etiology* — Pneumonia can be viral, bacterial, fungal, protozoal, mycobacterial, mycoplasmal, or rickettsial in origin.

▶ *Location* — Bronchopneumonia involves distal airways and alveoli; lobular pneumonia, part of a lobe; and lobar pneumonia, an entire lobe.

▶ *Type* — Primary pneumonia results from inhalation or aspiration of a pathogen; it includes pneumococcal and viral pneumonia. Secondary pneumonia may follow initial lung damage from a noxious chemical or other insult (superinfection), or may result from hematogenous spread of bacteria from a distant focus (See *Types of pneumonia*, pages 230 to 233.)

Predisposing factors to bacterial and viral pneumonia include chronic illness and debilitation; cancer (particularly lung cancer); abdominal and thoracic surgery; atelectasis; common colds or other viral respiratory infections; chronic respiratory disease (chronic obstructive pulmonary disease [COPD], asthma, bronchiectasis, cystic fibrosis); influenza; smoking; malnutrition; alcoholism; sickle cell disease; tracheostomy; exposure to noxious gases; aspiration; and immunosuppressant therapy.

Predisposing factors to aspiration pneumonia include old age, debilitation, nasogastric tube feedings, impaired gag reflex, poor oral hygiene, and decreased level of consciousness.

Signs and symptoms

The five cardinal symptoms of early bacterial pneumonia are coughing, sputum production, pleuritic chest pain, shaking chills, and fever. Physical signs vary widely, ranging from diffuse, fine rales to signs of localized or extensive consolidation and pleural effusion.

Complications include hypoxemia, respiratory failure, pleural effusion, empyema, lung abscess, and bacteremia, with spread of infection to other parts of the body resulting in meningitis, endocarditis, and pericarditis.

Diagnosis

Clinical features, chest X-ray showing infiltrates, and sputum smear demonstrating acute inflammatory cells support this diagnosis. Positive blood cultures in patients with pulmonary infiltrates strongly suggest pneumonia produced by the organisms isolated from the blood cultures.

Pleural effusions, if present, should be tapped and fluid analyzed for evidence of infection in the pleural space. Occasionally, a transtracheal aspirate of tracheobronchial secretions or bronchoscopy with brushings or washings may be done to obtain material for smear and culture. The patient's response to antimicrobial therapy also provides important evidence of the presence of pneumonia.

Other conditions to consider are lung cancer, heart failure, Wegener's granulomatosis, and tuberculosis.

Treatment

Antimicrobial therapy varies with the causative agent. Therapy should be reevaluated early in the course of treatment.

Supportive measures include humidified oxygen therapy for hypoxia, mechanical ventilation for respiratory failure, a high-calorie diet and adequate fluid intake, bed rest, and an analgesic to relieve pleuritic chest pain. Patients with severe pneumonia on mechanical ventilation may require positive end-expiratory pressure to facilitate adequate oxygenation.

Special considerations

▶ Maintain a patent airway and adequate oxygenation. Measure arterial blood gas levels, especially in hypoxic patients. Administer supplemental oxygen if partial pressure of arterial oxygen is less than 60 mm Hg. Patients with underlying chronic lung disease should be given oxygen cautiously.

▶ Teach the patient how to cough and perform deep-breathing exercises to clear secretions, and encourage him to do so often.

▶ In severe pneumonia that requires endotracheal intubation or tracheostomy with or without mechanical ventilation, provide thorough respiratory care and suction often, using sterile technique, to remove secretions.

▶ Obtain sputum specimens as needed, by suction if the patient can't produce specimens independently. Collect specimens in a sterile container and deliver them promptly to the microbiology laboratory.

▶ Administer antibiotics as necessary, and pain medication as needed; record the patient's response to medications. Fever and dehydration may require I.V. fluids and electrolyte replacement.

▶ Maintain adequate nutrition to offset high caloric utilization secondary to infection. Ask the dietary department to provide a high-calorie, high-protein diet consisting of soft, easy-to-eat foods. Encourage the patient to eat.

▶ As necessary, supplement oral feedings with nasogastric tube feedings or parenteral nutrition. Monitor fluid intake and output.

▶ Provide a quiet, calm environment for the patient, with frequent rest periods.

▶ To control the spread of infection, dispose of secretions properly. Tell the patient to sneeze and cough into a disposable tissue; tape a waxed bag to the side of the bed for used tissues.

▶ To prevent aspiration during nasogastric tube feedings, elevate the patient's head, check the tube's position, and administer the formula slowly. Don't give large volumes at one time; this could cause vomiting. If the patient has an endotracheal tube, inflate the tube cuff. Keep the patient's head elevated for at least 30 minutes after the feeding. Check for residual formula at 4- to 6-hour intervals.

 PREVENTION TIP Advise the patient to avoid using antibiotics indiscriminately during minor viral infections because this may result in upper airway colonization with antibiotic-resistant bacteria. If the patient then develops pneumonia, the organisms producing the pneumonia may require treatment with more toxic antibiotics.

Encourage annual influenza vaccination and Pneumovax for high-risk patients, such as those with COPD, chronic heart disease, or sickle cell disease.

Urge all bedridden and postoperative patients to perform deep-breathing and coughing exercises frequently. Position such patients properly to promote full aeration and drainage of secretions.

POLIOMYELITIS

Poliomyelitis, also called polio or infantile paralysis, is an acute communicable disease caused by the poliovirus and ranges in severity from inapparent infection to fatal paralytic illness. First recognized in 1840, poliomyelitis became epidemic in Norway and Sweden in 1905. Outbreaks reached pandemic proportions in Europe, North America, Australia, and New Zealand during the first half of this century. Incidence peaked during the 1940s and early 1950s, and led to the development of the Salk vaccine. (See *Polio protection,* page 234.)

Minor polio outbreaks still occur, usually among nonimmunized groups such as the Amish of Pennsylvania. The disease usually strikes during the summer and fall.

Once confined mainly to infants and children, poliomyelitis mostly occurs today in people over age 15. Adults and girls

TYPES OF PNEUMONIA

TYPE	SIGNS AND SYMPTOMS
Viral	
Influenza (prognosis poor even with treatment; 50% mortality)	▶ Cough (initially nonproductive; later, purulent sputum), marked cyanosis, dyspnea, high fever, chills, substernal pain and discomfort, moist crackles, frontal headache, myalgia ▶ Death resulting from cardiopulmonary collapse
Adenovirus (insidious onset; generally affects young adults)	▶ Sore throat, fever, cough, chills, malaise, small amounts of mucoid sputum, retrosternal chest pain, anorexia, rhinitis, adenopathy, scattered crackles, and rhonchi
Respiratory syncytial virus (most prevalent in infants and children)	▶ Listlessness, irritability, tachypnea with retraction of intercostal muscles, wheezing, slight sputum production, fine moist crackles, fever, severe malaise and, possibly, cough or croup
Measles (rubeola)	▶ Fever, dyspnea, cough, small amounts of sputum, coryza, skin rash, and cervical adenopathy
Chickenpox (varicella) (uncommon in children, but present in 30% of adults with varicella)	▶ Cough, dyspnea, cyanosis, tachypnea, pleuritic chest pain, hemoptysis, and rhonchi 1 to 6 days after onset of rash
Cytomegalovirus	▶ Difficult to distinguish from other nonbacterial pneumonias ▶ Fever, cough, shaking chills, dyspnea, cyanosis, weakness, and diffuse crackles ▶ Occurs in neonates as devastating multisystemic infection; in normal adults resembles mononucleosis; in immunocompromised hosts, varies from clinically inapparent to devastating infection

DIAGNOSIS	TREATMENT
▶ *Chest X-ray:* diffuse bilateral bronchopneumonia from hilus ▶ *White blood cell (WBC) count:* normal to slightly elevated; lymphocytic predominance ▶ *Sputum smears:* no specific organisms	▶ *Supportive:* for respiratory failure, endotracheal intubation and ventilator assistance; for fever, hypothermia blanket or antipyretics; for influenza A, amantadine or rimantadine
▶ *Chest X-ray:* patchy distribution of pneumonia, more severe than indicated by physical examination ▶ *WBC count:* normal to slightly elevated	▶ Symptomatic treatment only ▶ Mortality low, usually clears with no residual effects
▶ *Chest X-ray:* patchy bilateral consolidation ▶ *WBC count:* normal to slightly elevated	▶ *Supportive:* humidified air, oxygen, antimicrobials often given until viral etiology confirmed, aerosolized ribavirin ▶ Complete recovery in 1 to 3 weeks
▶ *Chest X-ray:* reticular infiltrates, sometimes with hilar lymph node enlargement ▶ *Lung tissue specimen:* characteristic giant cells	▶ *Supportive:* bed rest, adequate hydration, antimicrobials; assisted ventilation, if necessary
▶ *Chest X-ray:* shows more extensive pneumonia than indicated by physical examination, and bilateral, patchy, diffuse, nodular infiltrates ▶ *Sputum analysis:* predominant mononuclear cells and characteristic intranuclear inclusion bodies with skin rash confirm diagnosis	▶ *Supportive:* adequate hydration, oxygen therapy in critically ill patients ▶ Therapy with I.V. acyclovir
▶ *Chest X-ray:* in early stages, variable patchy infiltrates; later, bilateral, nodular, and more predominant in lower lobes ▶ *Percutaneous aspiration of lung tissue, transbronchial biopsy or open lung biopsy:* microscopic examination shows intranuclear and cytoplasmic inclusions, virus can be cultured from lung tissue	▶ Generally, benign and self-limiting in mononucleosis-like form ▶ *Supportive:* adequate hydration and nutrition, oxygen therapy, bed rest ▶ In immunosuppressed patients, disease more severe and possibly fatal, ganciclovir or foscarnet treatment warranted

(continued)

TYPES OF PNEUMONIA *(continued)*

TYPE	SIGNS AND SYMPTOMS
Bacterial	
Streptococcus (Diplococcus pneumoniae)	▶ Sudden onset of a single, shaking chill, and sustained temperature of 102° to 104° F (38.9° to 40° C), often preceded by upper respiratory tract infection
Klebsiella	▶ Fever and recurrent chills; cough producing rusty, bloody, viscous sputum (currant jelly); cyanosis of lips and nail beds due to hypoxemia; shallow, grunting respirations ▶ Common in patients with chronic alcoholism, pulmonary disease, diabetes, and those at risk for aspiration
Staphylococcus	▶ Temperature of 102° to 104° F (38.9° to 40° C), recurrent shaking chills, bloody sputum, dyspnea, tachypnea, and hypoxemia ▶ Should be suspected with viral illness, such as influenza or measles, and in patients with cystic fibrosis
Protozoan	
Pneumocystis carinii	▶ Occurs in immunocompromised persons ▶ Dyspnea and nonproductive cough ▶ Anorexia, weight loss, and fatigue ▶ Low-grade fever
Aspiration	
Results from vomiting and aspiration of gastric or oropharyngeal contents into trachea and lungs	▶ Noncardiogenic pulmonary edema may follow damage to respiratory epithelium from contact with stomach acid ▶ Crackles, dyspnea, cyanosis, hypotension, and tachycardia ▶ Possibly subacute pneumonia with cavity formation, or lung abscess if foreign body is present

are at greater risk for infection; boys, for paralysis.

If the central nervous system (CNS) is spared, the prognosis is excellent. However, CNS infection can cause paralysis and death. The mortality for all types of poliomyelitis is 5% to 10%.

DIAGNOSIS	TREATMENT
▶ *Chest X-ray:* areas of consolidation, often lobar ▶ *WBC count:* elevated ▶ *Sputum culture:* may show gram-positive *S. pneumoniae;* this organism not always recovered	▶ *Antimicrobial therapy:* macrolide for 7 to 10 days; begun after obtaining culture specimen but without waiting for results
▶ *Chest X-ray:* typically, but not always, consolidation in the upper lobe that causes bulging of fissures ▶ *WBC count:* elevated ▶ *Sputum culture and Gram stain:* may show gram-negative cocci *(Klebsiella)*	▶ *Antimicrobial therapy:* an aminoglycoside and a cephalosporin
▶ *Chest X-ray:* multiple abscesses and infiltrates; high incidence of empyema ▶ *WBC count:* elevated ▶ *Sputum culture and Gram stain:* may show gram-positive staphylococci	▶ *Antimicrobial therapy:* nafcillin or oxacillin for 14 days if staphylococci are penicillinase producing ▶ *Supportive:* Chest tube drainage of empyema
▶ *Fiber-optic bronchoscopy:* obtains specimens for histologic studies ▶ *Chest X-ray:* nonspecific infiltrates, nodular lesions, or spontaneous pneumothorax	▶ *Antimicrobial therapy:* co-trimoxazole or pentamidine by I.V. or inhalation ▶ *Supportive:* oxygen, improved nutrition, mechanical ventilation
▶ *Chest X-ray:* locates areas of infiltrates, which suggest diagnosis	▶ *Antimicrobial therapy:* penicillin G or clindamycin ▶ *Supportive:* oxygen therapy, suctioning, coughing, deep breathing, adequate hydration

Causes

The poliovirus has three antigenically distinct serotypes — types I, II, and III — all of which cause poliomyelitis. These viruses are found worldwide and are transmitted from person to person by direct contact with infected oropharyngeal secretions or feces. The incubation period ranges from 5 to 35 days — 7 to 14 days on average.

POLIO PROTECTION

Dr. Jonas Salk's poliomyelitis vaccine, which became available in 1955, has been rightly called one of the miracle drugs of modern medicine. The vaccine contains dead (formalin-inactivated) polioviruses that stimulate production of circulating antibodies in the human body. This vaccine so effectively eliminated poliomyelitis that today it's hard to appreciate how feared the disease once was.

However, even miracle drugs can be improved. Today, the Sabin vaccine, which can be taken orally and is more than 90% effective, is the vaccine of choice in preventing poliomyelitis. The Sabin vaccine is available in trivalent and monovalent forms. The trivalent form (TOPV) contains live but weakened organisms of all three poliovirus serotypes in one solution. TOPV is generally preferred to the monovalent form, which contains only one viral type and is useful only when the particular serotype is known.

All infants should be immunized with the Sabin vaccine; pregnant women may be vaccinated without risk. However, because of the risk of contracting poliomyelitis from the vaccine, it's contraindicated in patients with immunodeficiency diseases, leukemia, or lymphoma, and in those receiving corticosteroids, antimetabolites, other immunosuppressants, or radiation therapy. These patients are usually immunized with the Salk vaccine. When possible, immunodeficient patients should avoid contact with family members who are receiving the Sabin vaccine for at least 2 weeks after vaccination. The Sabin vaccine is no longer routinely advised for adults unless they're apt to be exposed to polio or plan to travel to endemic areas.

The virus usually enters the body through the alimentary tract, multiplies in the oropharynx and lower intestinal tract, then spreads to regional lymph nodes and the blood. Factors that increase the risk of paralysis include pregnancy; old age; localized trauma, such as a recent tonsillectomy, tooth extraction, or inoculation; and unusual physical exertion at or just before the clinical onset of poliomyelitis.

Signs and symptoms

Manifestations of poliomyelitis follow three basic patterns. Inapparent (subclinical) infections constitute 95% of all poliovirus infections. Abortive poliomyelitis (minor illness), which accounts for 4% to 8% of all cases, causes slight fever, malaise, headache, sore throat, inflamed pharynx, and vomiting. The patient usually recovers within 72 hours. Most cases of inapparent or abortive poliomyelitis go unnoticed.

Major poliomyelitis, however, involves the CNS and takes two forms: nonparalytic and paralytic. Children commonly show a biphasic course, in which the onset of major illness occurs after recovery from the minor illness stage. *Nonparalytic poliomyelitis* produces moderate fever, headache, vomiting, lethargy, irritability, and pains in the neck, back, arms, legs, and abdomen. It also causes muscle tenderness, weakness, and spasms in the extensors of the neck and back, and sometimes in the hamstring and other muscles. (These spasms may be observed during maximum range-of-motion exercises.) Nonparalytic polio usually lasts about a week, with meningeal irritation persisting for about 2 weeks.

Paralytic poliomyelitis usually develops within 5 to 7 days of the onset of fever. The patient displays symptoms similar to those of nonparalytic poliomyelitis, with asymmetrical weakness of various muscles, loss of superficial and deep reflexes, paresthesia, hypersensitivity to touch, urine retention, constipation, and abdominal distention. The extent of paralysis depends on the level of the spinal cord lesions, which may be cervical, thoracic, or lumbar.

Resistance to neck flexion is characteristic in nonparalytic and paralytic poliomyelitis. The patient will "tripod"—extend his arms behind him for support—when he sits up. He'll display Hoyne's sign—his head will fall back when he is supine and his shoulders are elevated. From a supine position, he won't be able to raise his legs a full 90 degrees. Paralytic poliomyelitis also causes positive Kernig's and Brudzinski's signs.

When the disease affects the medulla of the brain, it's called *bulbar paralytic poliomyelitis,* which is the most perilous type. This form affects the respiratory muscle nerves, which leads to respiratory paralysis, and weakens the muscles supplied by the cranial nerves (particularly the IX and X), producing symptoms of encephalitis. Other signs and symptoms include facial weakness, diplopia, dysphasia, difficulty in chewing, inability to swallow or expel saliva, regurgitation of food through the nasal passages, and dyspnea as well as abnormal respiratory rate, depth, and rhythm, which may lead to respiratory arrest. Fatal pulmonary edema and shock are possible.

Complications—many of which result from prolonged immobility and respiratory muscle failure—include hypertension, urinary tract infection, urolithiasis, atelectasis, pneumonia, myocarditis, cor pulmonale, skeletal and soft-tissue deformities, and paralytic ileus.

Diagnosis

Diagnosis requires isolation of the poliovirus from throat washings early in the disease, from stools throughout the disease, and from cerebrospinal fluid (CSF) cultures in CNS infection.

Coxsackievirus and echovirus infections must be ruled out. Convalescent serum antibody titers four times greater than acute titers support a diagnosis of poliomyelitis. Routine laboratory tests are usually within normal limits; however, CSF pressure and protein levels may be slightly increased and white blood cell count elevated initially, mostly due to polymorphonuclear leukocytes, which constitute 50% to 90% of the total count. Thereafter, mononuclear cells constitute most of the diminished number of cells.

Rarely, certain group A and B coxsackieviruses (especially A7), several echoviruses, and enterovirus type 71 may produce muscle weakness or paralysis that cannot be clinically differentiated from paralytic poliomyelitis. Guillain-Barré syndrome is often confused with paralytic poliomyelitis. CNS involvement due to mumps or herpesviruses, meningoencephalitis due to arboviruses in certain geographic areas, tuberculous meningitis, or brain abscess should also be considered.

Treatment

Treatment is supportive and includes analgesics to ease headache, back pain, and leg spasms; morphine is contraindicated because of the danger of additional respiratory suppression. Moist heat applications may also reduce muscle spasm and pain.

Bed rest is necessary only until extreme discomfort subsides; in paralytic polio, this may take a long time. Paralytic polio also requires long-term rehabilitation using physical therapy, braces, corrective shoes and, in some cases, orthopedic surgery.

Special considerations

▶ Observe the patient carefully for signs of paralysis and other neurologic damage, which can occur rapidly. Maintain a patent airway, and watch for respiratory weakness and difficulty in swallowing. A tracheotomy is commonly done at the first sign of respiratory distress, after which the patient is placed on a mechanical ventilator. Remember to reassure the patient that his breathing is being supported. Practice strict aseptic technique during suctioning, and use only sterile solutions to nebulize medications.

▶ Perform a brief neurologic assessment at least once a day, but don't demand any vigorous muscle activity. Encourage a return to mild activity as soon as the patient is able.

▶ Check blood pressure frequently, especially in bulbar poliomyelitis, which can cause hypertension or shock because of its effect on the brain stem.

▶ Watch for signs of fecal impaction (due to dehydration and intestinal inactivity). To prevent this, give sufficient fluids to ensure an adequate daily output of low-specific-gravity urine (1.5 to 2 L/day for adults).

▶ Monitor the bedridden patient's food intake for an adequate, well-balanced diet. If tube feedings are required, give liquid baby foods, juices, lactose, and vitamins.

▶ To prevent pressure ulcers, provide good skin care, reposition the patient often, and keep the bed dry. Remember, muscle paralysis may cause bladder weakness or transient bladder paralysis.

▶ Apply high-top sneakers or use a footboard to prevent footdrop. To alleviate discomfort, use foam rubber pads and sandbags, as needed, and light splints, as ordered.

▶ To control the spread of poliomyelitis, wash your hands thoroughly after contact with the patient, especially after contact with excretions. Instruct the ambulatory patient to do the same. (Only hospital personnel who have been vaccinated against poliomyelitis may have direct contact with the patient.)

▶ Provide emotional support to the patient and his family. Reassure the nonparalytic patient that his chances for recovery are good. Long-term support and encouragement are essential for maximum rehabilitation.

▶ When caring for a paralytic patient, help set up an interdisciplinary rehabilitation program. Such a program should include physical and occupational therapists, physicians and, if necessary, a psychiatrist to help manage the emotional problems that develop in a patient suddenly facing severe physical disabilities.

PROGRESSIVE MULTIFOCAL LEUKOENCEPHALOPATHY

Progressive multifocal leukoencephalopathy (PML) is a rare disorder of the nervous system that primarily affects individuals with suppressed immune systems (such as those with cancers such as leukemia or lymphoma, or acquired immunodeficiency syndrome [AIDS]). The disorder, which is caused by a virus, is characterized by demyelination or destruction of the myelin sheath that covers nerve cells, specifically oligodendrocytes. The myelin sheath is the fatty covering — which acts as an insulator — of nerve fibers in the brain.

Though rare, PML occurs more frequently in people whose immunity is compromised by HIV, usually in those with CD4+ counts of less than 100 cells/μl of blood, and is rapidly progressive. The interval between first neurologic symptoms and death may be as short as 3 to 4 months; in rare cases, remission has occurred and patients have survived for several years. In general, however, PML is an incurable, fatal disease.

Causes

PML is caused by the opportunistic JC virus (JCV), a member of the papovavirus family. (The name JC comes from the initials of a patient with the disorder.) PML is believed to be caused by reactivation of latent JCV infection, resulting in demyelination of the central nervous system. Initial brain lesions occur around blood vessels, suggesting dissemination via the blood.

Signs and symptoms

Symptoms include mental status changes followed by speech or language deficits, visual deficits, and generalized or focal weakness. Neurologic signs include lack of coordination (weakness of one limb or one side of the body), cranial nerve palsies, loss of vision on one side, sensory loss in one limb or one side of the body, language disturbance, and unsteadiness.

Diagnosis

Definitive diagnosis of PML requires a brain biopsy. Clinically, detecting focal lesions and abnormalities of the white matter on computed tomography scan or magnetic resonance imaging suggests the diagnosis. Recently, DNA of the JC virus has been detected in the cerebral spinal fluid, and used as a diagnostic tool.

Because of the neurological symptoms that occur with PML, differential diagnosis should include toxoplasmosis, central nervous system (CNS) lymphoma, cerebral vascular disease, HIV encephalopathy, HIV dementia, CNS infection, lymphoma, and tuberculosis.

Treatment

There is no accepted treatment regimen for PML, other than highly aggressive antiretroviral therapy. Corticosteroids may be utilized if the patient is having difficulty with edema. Supportive care for the patient's activities of daily living, nutrition, safety and prevention of further neurologic accident or head injury are important.

Special considerations

▶ Observe the patient with PML closely for antiretroviral therapy response.
▶ Family members and care providers should be included in the evaluation of the therapy. Depending on the patient's memory and mentation, they may need a great deal of support.
▶ Stress the importance of taking the medications on schedule.

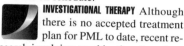 **INVESTIGATIONAL THERAPY** Although there is no accepted treatment plan for PML to date, recent research involving combination drug therapies such as cidofovir and cytosine arabinoside (ARA-C) has shown some favorable results.

 PREVENTION TIP When a diagnosis of PML has been established or suggested due to a clinical picture of neurologic deterioration, the nurse must initiate a discussion of plans for terminal care (including wills, advance directives, and supportive care and services) with the patient and caregiver. Supportive treatment will be necessary for an undetermined period of time, and hospice referral should be considered if the patient doesn't respond to a highly aggressive antiretroviral regimen.

PROSTATITIS

Prostatitis, inflammation of the prostate gland, may be acute or chronic. Acute prostatitis most often results from gram-negative bacteria and is easy to recognize and treat. However, chronic prostatitis, the most common cause of recurrent urinary tract infections (UTIs) in men, is less easy to recognize. As many as 35% of men over age 50 have chronic prostatitis.

Causes

About 80% of bacterial prostatitis cases result from infection by *Escherichia coli;* the rest, from infection by *Klebsiella, Enterobacter, Proteus, Pseudomonas, Streptococcus,* or *Staphylococcus.* These organisms probably spread to the prostate by the bloodstream or from ascending urethral infection, invasion of rectal bacteria via lymphatics, reflux of infected bladder urine into prostate ducts or, less commonly, infrequent or excessive sexual intercourse or such procedures as cystoscopy or catheterization. Chronic prostatitis usually results from bacterial invasion from the urethra.

Signs and symptoms

Acute prostatitis begins with fever, chills, low back pain, myalgia, malaise, nausea, vomiting, perineal fullness, and arthralgia. Urination is frequent and urgent. Dysuria, nocturia, urinary obstruction, and decreased sex drive may also occur. The urine may appear cloudy. When palpated rectally, the prostate is tender, indurated, swollen, firm, and warm.

Chronic bacterial prostatitis sometimes produces no symptoms but usually elicits the same urinary symptoms as the acute form but to a lesser degree. UTI is a common complication. Other possible signs include painful ejaculation, hemospermia, persistent urethral discharge, and sexual dysfunction.

Diagnosis

Characteristic rectal examination findings suggest prostatitis. In many cases, a urine culture can identify the causative infectious organism.

However, firm diagnosis depends on a comparison of urine cultures of specimens obtained by the Meares and Stamey technique. This test requires four specimens: one collected when the patient starts voiding (voided bladder one — VB1); another midstream (VB2); another after the patient stops voiding and the doctor massages the prostate to produce secretions (expressed prostate secretions — EPS); and a final voided specimen (VB3). A significant increase in colony count in the prostatic specimens confirms prostatitis.

Other conditions to consider are benign prostatic hypertrophy, prostate cancer, and epididymitis.

Treatment

Systemic antibiotic therapy is the treatment of choice for acute prostatitis. Septra, Bactrim, or a fluoroquinolone is given orally and, if clinical response is satisfactory, continued for 30 days. If sepsis is likely, I.V. gentamicin plus ampicillin may be given until sensitivity test results are known. If test results and clinical response are favorable, parenteral therapy continues for 48 hours to 1 week; then an oral agent is substituted for 30 more days. In chronic prostatitis due to *E. coli,* fluoroquinolones are given for 3 months.

Supportive therapy includes bed rest, adequate hydration, and administration of analgesics, antipyretics, sitz baths, and stool softeners as necessary. In symptomatic chronic prostatitis, regular massage of the prostate is most effective. Regular ejaculation may help promote drainage of prostatic secretions. Anticholinergics and analgesics may help relieve nonbacterial prostatitis symptoms. Alpha-adrenergic blockers and muscle relaxants may relieve prostatodynia.

If drug therapy is unsuccessful, treatment may include transurethral resection of the prostate, which requires removal of all infected tissue. However, this procedure is usually not performed on young adults because it may cause retrograde ejaculation and sterility. Total prostatectomy is curative but may cause impotence and incontinence.

Special considerations

▶ Ensure bed rest and adequate hydration. Provide stool softeners and administer sitz baths, as ordered.
▶ As necessary, prepare to assist with suprapubic needle aspiration of the bladder or a suprapubic cystostomy.
▶ Emphasize the need for strict adherence to the prescribed drug regimen. Instruct the patient to drink at least 8 glasses of water a day. Have him report adverse drug reactions (rash, nausea, vomiting, fever, chills, and GI irritation).

PSEUDOMEMBRANOUS ENTEROCOLITIS

Pseudomembranous enterocolitis is an acute inflammation and necrosis of the small and large intestines, which usually affects the mucosa but may extend into submucosa and, rarely, other layers. Marked by severe diarrhea, this rare condition is generally fatal in 1 to 7 days from severe dehydration and from toxicity, peritonitis, or perforation.

Causes

The exact cause of pseudomembranous enterocolitis is unknown; however, *Clostridium difficile* is thought to produce a toxin that may play a role in its development. Pseudomembranous enterocolitis has occurred postoperatively in debilitated patients who undergo abdominal surgery and in patients treated with broad-spectrum antibiotics. Whatever the cause, necrotic mucosa is replaced by a pseudomembrane filled with staphylococci, leukocytes, mucus, fibrin, and inflammatory cells.

Signs and symptoms

Pseudomembranous enterocolitis begins suddenly with copious watery or bloody diarrhea, abdominal pain, and fever. Serious complications, including severe dehydration, electrolyte imbalance, hypotension, shock, and colonic perforation, may occur in this disorder.

Diagnosis

Diagnosis is difficult in many cases because of the abrupt onset of enterocolitis and the emergency situation it creates, so consideration of patient history is essential. A rectal biopsy through sigmoidoscopy confirms pseudomembranous enterocolitis. Stool cultures can identify *C. difficile*. Other conditions to consider are ulcerative colitis and Crohn's disease.

Treatment

A patient receiving broad-spectrum antibiotic therapy must discontinue antibiotics at once. Effective treatment usually includes oral metronidazole. Oral vancomycin is usually given for severe or resistant cases. A patient with mild pseudomembranous enterocolitis may receive anion exchange resins, such as cholestyramine, to bind the toxin produced by *C. difficile*. Supportive treatment must maintain fluid and electrolyte balance and combat hypotension and shock with pressors, such as dopamine and levarterenol. The value of systemic corticosteroids is not established. In extreme cases, subtotal colectomy has been required as a life-saving measure.

Special considerations

▶ Monitor vital signs, skin color, and level of consciousness. Report signs of shock immediately.
▶ Record fluid intake and output, including fluid lost in stools. Watch for dehydration (poor skin turgor, sunken eyes, and decreased urine output).
▶ Check serum electrolytes daily, and watch for clinical signs of hypokalemia, especially malaise, and weak, rapid, irregular pulse.

PSEUDOMONAS INFECTIONS

Pseudomonas is a small gram-negative aerobic bacillus that produces nosocomial infections, superinfections of various parts of the body, and a rare disease called melioidosis. (See *Melioidosis*, page 240.) This bacillus is also associated with bacteremia, endocarditis, and osteomyelitis in drug addicts. In local *Pseudomonas* infections, treatment is usually successful and complications are rare; however, in patients with poor immunologic resistance — premature infants, the elderly, or those with debilitating disease, burns, or wounds — septicemic *Pseudomonas* infections are serious and sometimes fatal.

Causes

The most common species of *Pseudomonas* is *P. aeruginosa*. Other species that

MELIOIDOSIS

Melioidosis results from wound penetration by, or inhalation or ingestion of, the gram-negative bacteria *Pseudomonas pseudomallei*. Although it was once confined to southeast Asia, Central America, South America, Madagascar, and Guam, incidence in the United States is rising as a result of the recent influx of Southeast Asians.

Melioidosis occurs in two forms: chronic melioidosis, which causes osteomyelitis and lung abscesses; and the rare acute melioidosis, which causes pneumonia, bacteremia, and prostration. Acute melioidosis is commonly fatal; however, most infections are chronic and asymptomatic, producing clinical symptoms only with accompanying malnutrition, major surgery, or severe burns.

Diagnostic measures consist of isolation of *P. pseudomallei* in a culture of exudate, blood, or sputum; serology tests (complement fixation, passive hemagglutination); and chest X-ray (findings resemble tuberculosis). Treatment includes oral tetracycline — and co-trimoxazole, abscess drainage and, in severe cases, chloramphenicol — until X-rays show resolution of primary abscesses.

The prognosis is good because most patients have a mild infection and acquire permanent immunity; aggressive use of antibiotics and sulfonamides has improved the prognosis in acute melioidosis.

benzalkonium chloride, hexachlorophene soap, saline solution, penicillin, water in flower vases, and fluids in incubators, humidifiers, and inhalation therapy equipment. *P. aeruginosa* is associated with chronic obstructive pulmonary disease and cystic fibrosis. In elderly patients, *Pseudomonas* infection usually enters through the genitourinary tract; in infants, through the umbilical cord, skin, and GI tract.

Signs and symptoms

The most common infections associated with *Pseudomonas* include skin infections (such as burns and pressure ulcers), urinary tract infections (UTIs), infant epidemic diarrhea and other diarrheal illnesses, bronchitis, pneumonia, bronchiectasis, meningitis, corneal ulcers, mastoiditis, otitis externa, otitis media, endocarditis, and bacteremia.

Drainage in *Pseudomonas* infections has a distinct, sickly sweet odor and a greenish blue pus that forms a crust on wounds. Other symptoms depend on the site of infection. For example, when it invades the lungs, *Pseudomonas* causes pneumonia with fever, chills, and a productive cough.

Diagnosis

Diagnosis requires isolation of the *Pseudomonas* organism in blood, spinal fluid, urine, exudate, or sputum culture.

Treatment

In the debilitated or otherwise vulnerable patient with clinical evidence of *Pseudomonas* infection, treatment should begin immediately, without waiting for results of laboratory tests. Antibiotic treatment includes aminoglycosides, such as gentamicin or tobramycin, combined with a *Pseudomonas*-sensitive penicillin, such as carbenicillin disodium or ticarcillin. An alternative combination is amikacin and a similar penicillin. Two newer drugs, imipenem and the anti-pseudomonal fluoroquinolones, in combination with an aminoglycoside, are also effective. Such

typically cause disease in humans include *P. maltophilia, P. cepacia, P. fluorescens, P. testosteroni, P. acidovorans, P. alcaligenes, P. stutzeri, P. putrefaciens,* and *P. putida.* These organisms are commonly found in hospital liquids that have been allowed to stand for a long time, such as

combination therapy is necessary because *Pseudomonas* quickly becomes resistant to carbenicillin alone. However, in UTIs, carbenicillin indanyl sodium can be used alone if the organism is susceptible and the infection doesn't have systemic effects; the drug is excreted in the urine and builds up high urine levels that prevent resistance.

Local *Pseudomonas* infections or septicemia secondary to wound infection requires 1% acetic acid irrigations, topical applications of colistimethate sodium and polymyxin B, and debridement or drainage of the infected wound.

Special considerations

▶ Observe and record the character of wound exudate and sputum.

▶ Before administering antibiotics, ask the patient about a history of drug allergies, especially to penicillin. If combinations of carbenicillin or ticarcillin and an aminoglycoside are ordered, schedule the doses 1 hour apart (carbenicillin and ticarcillin may decrease the antibiotic effect of the aminoglycoside). Don't give both antibiotics through the same administration set.

▶ Monitor the patient's renal function (output, blood urea nitrogen level, specific gravity, urinalysis, creatinine level) during treatment with aminoglycosides.

 PREVENTION TIP Protect immunocompromised patients from exposure to this infection. Proper hand washing and aseptic techniques prevent further spread. To prevent *Pseudomonas* infection, maintain proper endotracheal and tracheostomy suctioning technique: Use strict sterile technique when caring for I.V. lines, catheters, and other tubes; dispose of suction bottle contents properly; and label and date solution bottles and change them frequently, according to policy.

PUERPERAL INFECTION

A common cause of childbirth-related death, puerperal infection is an infection of the birth canal and other structures during the postpartum period.

It can result in endometritis, parametritis, pelvic and femoral thrombophlebitis, and peritonitis. In the United States, puerperal infection develops in about 6% of maternity patients. The prognosis is good with treatment.

Causes

Microbes that commonly cause puerperal infection include streptococci, coagulase-negative staphylococci, *Clostridium perfringens, Bacteroides fragilis,* and *Escherichia coli.* Most of these microbes are considered normal vaginal flora. But they may cause puerperal infection in the presence of certain predisposing factors, such as prolonged and premature rupture of the membranes, prolonged (more than 24 hours) or traumatic labor, cesarean section, frequent or unsanitary vaginal examinations or unsanitary delivery, retained products of conception, hemorrhage, and maternal conditions, such as anemia or debilitation from malnutrition.

Signs and symptoms

A characteristic sign of puerperal infection is fever (at least 100.4° F [38° C]) that occurs on any 2 consecutive days up to the 11th day postpartum (excluding the first 24 hours). This fever can spike as high as 105° F (40.6° C) and is commonly associated with chills, headache, malaise, restlessness, and anxiety.

Accompanying signs and symptoms depend on the extent and site of infection. With endometritis there is heavy, sometimes foul-smelling lochia; tender, enlarged uterus; backache; severe uterine contractions persisting after childbirth. Parametritis (pelvic cellulitis) symptoms are vaginal tenderness and abdominal pain and tenderness (pain may become more intense as infection spreads).

The inflammation may remain localized, may lead to abscess formation, or may spread through the blood or lymphatic system. Widespread inflammation may cause pelvic thrombophlebitis with severe, repeated chills and dramatic swings in body temperature; lower abdominal or flank pain; and, possibly, a palpable tender mass over the affected area, which usually develops near the second postpartum week. Also, femoral thrombophlebitis may develop with pain, stiffness, or swelling in a leg or the groin; inflammation or shiny, white appearance of the affected leg; malaise; fever; and chills, usually beginning 10 to 20 days postpartum (these signs may precipitate pulmonary embolism). Finally, peritonitis is possible with its associated symptoms of fever with tachycardia (greater than 140 beats per minute), weak pulse, hiccups, nausea, vomiting, and diarrhea, and constant and possibly excruciating abdominal pain.

Diagnosis

Development of the typical clinical features, especially fever within 48 hours after delivery, suggests a diagnosis of puerperal infection.

A culture of lochia, blood, incisional exudate (from cesarean incision or episiotomy), uterine tissue, or material collected from the vaginal cuff that reveals the causative organism may confirm the diagnosis.

Within 36 to 48 hours, white blood cell count usually demonstrates leukocytosis (15,000 to 30,000/μl).

Typical clinical features usually suffice for diagnosis of endometritis and peritonitis. In parametritis, pelvic examination shows induration without purulent discharge; culdoscopy shows pelvic adnexal induration and thickening. Red, swollen abscesses on the broad ligaments are even more serious indications because rupture leads to peritonitis.

Diagnosis of pelvic or femoral thrombophlebitis is suggested by characteristic clinical signs, venography, Doppler ultrasonography, Rielander's sign (palpable veins inside the thigh and calf), Payr's sign (pain in the calf when pressure is applied on the inside of the foot), and Homans' sign (pain on dorsiflexion of the foot with the knee extended). Homan's sign should be elicited passively by asking the patient to dorsiflex her foot because active dorsiflexion could, in theory, lead to embolization of a clot.

Other conditions to consider are pelvic abscess, deep venous thrombophlebitis, pyelonephritis, cystitis, mastitis, atelectasis, and wound infection.

Treatment

Treatment of puerperal infection usually begins with I.V. infusion of broad-spectrum antibiotics and is continued for 48 hours after fever is resolved.

Ancillary measures include analgesics for pain; antiseptics for local lesions; and antiemetics for nausea and vomiting from peritonitis. Supportive care includes bed rest, adequate fluid intake, I.V. fluids when necessary, and measures to reduce fever. Sitz baths and heat lamps may relieve discomfort from local lesions.

Surgery may be necessary to remove any remaining products of conception or to drain local lesions, such as an abscess in parametritis.

Management of septic pelvic thrombophlebitis consists of heparinization for approximately 10 days in conjunction with broad-spectrum antibiotic therapy.

Special considerations

▶ Monitor vital signs every 4 hours (more frequently if peritonitis has developed), intake, and output. Enforce strict bed rest.
▶ Frequently inspect the perineum. Assess the fundus, and palpate for tenderness (subinvolution may indicate endometritis). Note the amount, color, and odor of vaginal drainage, and document your observations.

▶ Administer antibiotics and analgesics, as ordered. Assess and document the type, degree, and location of pain as well as the patient's response to analgesics. Give the patient an antiemetic to relieve nausea and vomiting, as necessary.

▶ Provide sitz baths and a heat lamp for local lesions. Change bed linen, perineal pads, and under pads frequently. Keep the patient warm.

▶ Elevate the thrombophlebitic leg about 30 degrees. Don't rub or manipulate it or compress it with bed linen. Provide warm soaks for the leg. Watch for signs of pulmonary embolism, such as cyanosis, dyspnea, and chest pain.

▶ Offer reassurance and emotional support. Thoroughly explain all procedures to the patient and family.

▶ If the mother is separated from her infant, provide her with frequent reassurance about his progress. Encourage the father to reassure the mother about the infant's condition as well.

▶ Maintain aseptic technique when performing a vaginal examination. Limit the number of vaginal examinations performed during labor. Take care to wash your hands thoroughly after each patient contact.

▶ Keep the episiotomy site clean.

▶ Screen personnel and visitors to keep persons with active infections away from maternity patients.

 PREVENTION TIP Instruct all pregnant patients to call the health care provider immediately when their membranes rupture. Warn them to avoid intercourse after rupture or leak of the amniotic sac. Teach the patient how to maintain good perineal hygiene following delivery.

PYELONEPHRITIS, ACUTE

One of the most common renal diseases, acute pyelonephritis (also known as acute infective tubulointerstitial nephritis) is a sudden inflammation caused by bacteria that primarily affects the interstitial area and the renal pelvis or, less often, the renal tubules. With treatment and continued follow-up care, the prognosis is good, and extensive permanent damage is rare.

Pyelonephritis occurs more often in females, probably because of a shorter urethra and the proximity of the urinary meatus to the vagina and the rectum — both conditions allow bacteria to reach the bladder more easily — and a lack of the antibacterial prostatic secretions produced in the male.

Incidence increases with age and is higher in certain groups. Sexually active women are more prone to pyelonephritis because intercourse increases the risk of bacterial contamination. About 5% of pregnant women develop asymptomatic bacteriuria; if untreated, about 40% develop pyelonephritis. In diabetics neurogenic bladder causes incomplete emptying and urinary stasis and glycosuria may support bacterial growth in the urine. Persons with other renal diseases have compromised renal function that aggravates susceptibility.

Causes

Acute pyelonephritis results from bacterial infection of the kidneys. The infecting bacteria usually are normal intestinal and fecal flora that grow readily in urine. The most common causative microbe is *Escherichia coli,* but *Proteus, Pseudomonas, Staphylococcus aureus,* and *Enterococcus faecalis* (formerly *Streptococcus faecalis*) may also cause such infections.

Typically, the infection spreads from the bladder to the ureters, then to the kidneys, as in vesicoureteral reflux. Vesicoureteral reflux may result from congenital weakness at the junction of the ureter and the bladder. Bacteria refluxed to intrarenal tissues may create colonies of infection within 24 to 48 hours. Infection may also result from instrumentation (such as catheterization, cystoscopy, or urologic surgery), from a hematogenic infection (as in septicemia or endocarditis), or possibly from lymphatic infection.

Pyelonephritis may also result from an inability to empty the bladder (for example, in patients with neurogenic bladder), urinary stasis, or urinary obstruction due to tumors, strictures, or benign prostatic hyperplasia.

Signs and symptoms

Typical clinical features include urgency, frequency, burning during urination, dysuria, nocturia, and hematuria (usually microscopic but may be gross). Urine may appear cloudy and have an ammonia-like or fishy odor. Other common symptoms include a temperature of 102° F (38.9° C) or higher, shaking chills, unilateral or bilateral flank pain, anorexia, and general fatigue.

These symptoms characteristically develop rapidly over a few hours or a few days. Although the symptoms may disappear within days, even without treatment, residual bacterial infection is likely and may cause symptoms to recur later.

 AGE ALERT Elderly patients may exhibit decreased alertness or GI symptoms, such as nausea and vomiting, rather than the usual febrile responses to pyelonephritis.

Diagnosis

Diagnosis requires urinalysis and culture. Typical findings include:

▶ Pyuria (pus in urine): Urine sediment reveals the presence of leukocytes singly, in clumps, and in casts; and, possibly, a few red blood cells.

▶ Significant bacteriuria: urine culture reveals more than 100,000 organisms/µl of urine.

▶ Low specific gravity and osmolality: These findings result from a temporarily decreased ability to concentrate urine.

▶ Slightly alkaline urine pH.

▶ Proteinuria, glycosuria, and ketonuria: These conditions are less common.

X-rays also help in the evaluation of acute pyelonephritis. A plain film of the kidneys-ureters-bladder may reveal calculi, tumors, or cysts in the kidneys and the urinary tract. Excretory urography may show asymmetrical kidneys.

Other conditions to consider are acute glomerulonephritis, acute renal artery dissection, acute renal vein thrombosis, renal infarct, obstructive uropathy, hepatitis, pancreatitis, cholecystitis, appendicitis, perforated viscus, splenic infarct, aortic dissection, and pelvic inflammatory disease.

Treatment

Treatment centers on antibiotic therapy appropriate to the specific infecting microbe after identification by urine culture and sensitivity studies. For example, *Enterococcus* requires treatment with ampicillin, penicillin G, or vancomycin. *Staphylococcus* requires penicillin G or, if resistance develops, a semisynthetic penicillin, such as nafcillin, or a cephalosporin. *Escherichia coli* may be treated with sulfisoxazole, nalidixic acid, and nitrofurantoin; *Proteus,* with ampicillin, sulfisoxazole, nalidixic acid, and a cephalosporin; and *Pseudomonas,* with gentamicin, tobramycin, and carbenicillin.

When the infecting microbe cannot be identified, therapy usually consists of a broad-spectrum antibiotic, such as ampicillin or cephalexin. If the patient is pregnant, antibiotics must be prescribed cautiously. Urinary analgesics such as phenazopyridine are also appropriate.

Symptoms may disappear after several days of antibiotic therapy. Although urine usually becomes sterile within 48 to 72 hours, the course of such therapy is 10 to 14 days. Follow-up treatment includes reculturing urine 1 week after drug therapy stops, then periodically for the next year to detect residual or recurring infection. Most patients with uncomplicated infections respond well to therapy and don't suffer reinfection.

In infection from obstruction or vesicoureteral reflux, antibiotics may be less effective; treatment may then necessitate surgery to relieve the obstruction or correct the anomaly. Patients at high risk of recurring urinary tract and kidney infections, such as those with prolonged use of an indwelling catheter or maintenance antibiotic therapy, require long-term follow-up.

Recurrent episodes of acute pyelonephritis can eventually result in chronic pyelonephritis. (See *Chronic pyelonephritis.*)

Special considerations

▶ Administer antipyretics for fever.

▶ Force fluids to achieve urine output of more than 2,000 ml/day. This helps to empty the bladder of contaminated urine. Don't encourage intake of more than 2 to 3 qt (2 to 3 L) because this may decrease the effectiveness of the antibiotics.

▶ Provide an acid-ash diet to prevent stone formation.

▶ Teach proper technique for collecting a clean-catch urine specimen. Be sure to refrigerate or culture a urine specimen within 30 minutes of collection to prevent overgrowth of bacteria.

▶ Stress the need to complete prescribed antibiotic therapy, even after symptoms subside. Encourage long-term follow-up care for high-risk patients.

▶ Observe strict sterile technique during catheter insertion and care.

 PREVENTION TIP Instruct female patients to avoid bacterial contamination by wiping the perineum from front to back after defecation. Advise routine checkups for patients with a history of urinary tract infections. Teach them to recognize signs of infection, such as cloudy urine, burning on urination, urgency, and frequency, especially when accompanied by a low-grade fever.

CHRONIC PYELONEPHRITIS

Chronic pyelonephritis is a persistent kidney inflammation that can scar the kidneys and may lead to chronic renal failure. Its etiology may be bacterial, metastatic, or urogenous. This disease is most common in patients who are predisposed to recurrent acute pyelonephritis, such as those with urinary obstructions or vesicoureteral reflux.

CLINICAL FEATURES

Patients with chronic pyelonephritis may have a childhood history of unexplained fevers or bed-wetting. Clinical effects may include flank pain, anemia, low urine specific gravity, proteinuria, leukocytes in urine and, especially in late stages, hypertension. Uremia rarely develops from chronic pyelonephritis unless structural abnormalities exist in the excretory system. Bacteriuria may be intermittent. When no bacteria are found in the urine, diagnosis depends on excretory urography (renal pelvis may appear small and flattened) and renal biopsy.

TREATMENT

Effective treatment of chronic pyelonephritis requires control of hypertension, elimination of the existing obstruction (when possible), and long-term antimicrobial therapy.

R

RABIES

Usually transmitted by an animal bite, rabies (hydrophobia) is an acute central nervous system (CNS) infection caused by a ribonucleic acid virus.

If the bite is on the face, the risk of developing rabies is about 60%; on the upper extremities, 15% to 40%; and on the lower extremities, about 10%. In the United States, dog vaccinations have reduced rabies transmission to humans. Wild animals, such as skunks, foxes, and bats, account for 70% of rabies cases.

If symptoms occur, rabies is almost always fatal. Treatment soon after a bite, however, may prevent fatal CNS invasion.

Causes

Generally, the rabies virus is transmitted to a human through the bite of an infected animal that introduces the virus through the skin or mucous membrane. The virus begins to replicate in the striated muscle cells at the bite site.

It next spreads up the nerve to the CNS and replicates in the brain. Finally, it moves through the nerves into other tissues, including the salivary glands. Occasionally, airborne droplets and infected tissue transplants can transmit the virus.

Signs and symptoms

Clinical features are progressive. Typically, after an incubation period of 1 to 3 months, rabies produces local or radiating pain or burning, a sensation of cold, pruritus, and tingling at the bite site. It also produces prodromal symptoms, such as malaise, a slight fever (100° to 102° F

[37.8° to 38.9° C]), headache, anorexia, nausea, sore throat, and persistent loose cough. After this, the patient begins to show nervousness, anxiety, irritability, hyperesthesia, photophobia, sensitivity to loud noises, pupillary dilation, tachycardia, shallow respirations, and excessive salivation, lacrimation, and perspiration.

About 2 to 10 days after onset of prodromal symptoms, a phase of excitation begins. It's characterized by agitation, marked restlessness, anxiety and apprehension, and cranial nerve dysfunction that causes ocular palsies, strabismus, asymmetrical pupillary dilation or constriction, absence of corneal reflexes, weakness of facial muscles, and hoarseness. Severe systemic symptoms include tachycardia or bradycardia, cyclic respirations, urinary retention, and a temperature of about 103° F (39.4° C).

About 50% of affected patients exhibit hydrophobia (literally, "fear of water"), during which forceful, painful pharyngeal muscle spasms expel liquids from the mouth and cause dehydration, and possibly apnea, cyanosis, and death. Difficulty swallowing causes frothy saliva to drool from the patient's mouth. Eventually, even the sight, mention, or thought of water causes uncontrollable pharyngeal muscle spasms and excessive salivation. Between episodes of excitation and hydrophobia, the patient commonly is cooperative and lucid.

After about 3 days, excitation and hydrophobia subside and the progressively paralytic, terminal phase of this illness begins.

The patient experiences gradual, generalized, flaccid paralysis that ultimately leads to peripheral vascular collapse, coma, and death.

Diagnosis

Because rabies is fatal unless treated promptly, always suspect rabies in any person who suffers an unprovoked animal bite until you can prove otherwise.

Virus isolation from the patient's saliva or throat and examination of his blood for fluorescent rabies antibody (FRA) are considered the tests that provide the most definitive diagnosis. Other results typically include an elevated white blood cell count, with increased polymorphonuclear and large mononuclear cells, and elevated urinary glucose, acetone, and protein levels.

Confinement of the suspected animal for 10 days of observation by a veterinarian also helps support this diagnosis. If the animal appears rabid, it should be killed and its brain tissue tested for FRA and Negri bodies (oval or round masses that conclusively confirm rabies). (See *Evidence of rabies.*)

EVIDENCE OF RABIES

Negri bodies (outlined below) in the brain tissue of an animal suspected of being rabid confirm rabies. This electron micrograph also shows the rabies virus; Negri bodies are the areas of viral inclusion.

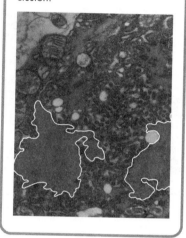

Treatment

The patient requires wound treatment and immunization as soon as possible after exposure. Thoroughly wash all bite wounds and scratches with soap and water. (See *First aid in animal bites,* page 248.)

Check the patient's immunization status, and administer tetanus-diphtheria prophylaxis, if needed. Take measures to control bacterial infection. If the wound requires suturing, special treatment and suturing techniques must be used to allow proper wound drainage. Antiserum is infiltrated locally if the wound is sutured.

After rabies exposure, a patient who hasn't been immunized before must receive passive immunization with rabies immune globulin (RIg) and active immunization with human diploid cell vaccine (HDCV) as soon as possible. If the patient has received HDCV before and has an adequate rabies antibody titer, he doesn't need RIg immunization, just an HDCV booster.

Special considerations

▶ When injecting rabies vaccine, rotate injection sites on the upper arm or thigh. Watch for and treat symptoms of redness, itching, pain, and tenderness at the injection site.

▶ Cooperate with public health authorities to determine the vaccination status of the animal. If the animal is proven rabid, help identify others at risk.

▶ If rabies develops, provide aggressive supportive care (even after onset of coma) to make probable death less agonizing.

▶ Monitor cardiac and pulmonary function continuously.

▶ Isolate the patient.

▶ Keep the room dark and quiet.

FIRST AID IN ANIMAL BITES

▶ Immediately wash the bite vigorously with soap and water for at least 10 minutes to remove the animal's saliva.
▶ Flush the wound with a viricidal agent, followed by a clear-water rinse.
▶ Apply a sterile dressing.
▶ If possible, don't suture the wound and don't immediately stop the bleeding (unless it's massive), because blood flow helps to clean the wound.
▶ Question the patient about the bite. Ask if he provoked the animal (if so, chances are it's not rabid) and if he can identify it or its owner (the animal may be confined for observation).
▶ Consult local health authorities for treatment information.

▶ Establish communication with the patient and his family. Provide psychological support to help them cope with the patient's symptoms and probable death.

 ALERT Wear a gown, gloves, and protection for the eyes and mouth when handling saliva and articles contaminated with saliva. Take precautions to avoid being bitten by the patient during the excitation phase.

 PREVENTION TIP To help prevent this dreaded disease, stress the need for vaccination of household pets that may be exposed to rabid wild animals. Warn people not to try to touch wild animals, especially if they appear ill or overly docile (a possible sign of rabies). Recommend prophylactic rabies vaccine to high-risk people, such as farm workers, forest rangers, spelunkers (cave explorers), and veterinarians.

REITER'S SYNDROME

A self-limiting syndrome associated with polyarthritis (dominant feature), urethritis, balanitis, conjunctivitis, and mucocutaneous lesions, Reiter's syndrome appears to be related to infection, either venereal or enteric. This disease, also called reactive arthritis, usually affects young men (ages 20 to 40) but can be seen in women and children.

Causes

The cause of Reiter's syndrome is unknown, but most cases follow venereal or enteric infection. Because 75% to 85% of patients with Reiter's syndrome test positive for the human leukocyte antigen B27, genetic susceptibility is likely. Reiter's syndrome has followed infections caused by *Mycoplasma, Shigella, Salmonella, Yersinia,* and *Chlamydia* organisms. More common in patients who are infected with the human immunodeficiency virus (HIV), it may precede or follow acquired immunodeficiency syndrome.

Signs and symptoms

The patient with Reiter's syndrome may complain of dysuria, hematuria, urgent and frequent urination, and mucopurulent penile discharge, with swelling and reddening of the urethral meatus. Small painless ulcers may erupt on the glans penis (balanitis) and coalesce to form irregular patches that cover the penis and scrotum. He may also experience suprapubic pain, fever, anorexia with weight loss, and other genitourinary (GU) complications, such as prostatitis and hemorrhagic cystitis. Female patients may complain of suprapubic pain, dysuria, and vaginal discharge. Enteric infections may manifest as fever, abdominal cramps, and loose stools.

Arthritic symptoms usually follow GU or enteric symptoms and last from 2 to 4 months, although some patients may go on to have chronic monoarthritis or oligoarthritis. Asymmetrical and extremely variable polyarticular arthritis is most common and tends to develop in weight-bearing joints of the legs and sometimes in the low back or sacroiliac joints. The arthritis is usually acute, with warm, erythematous, and painful joints, but it may be mild, with minimal synovitis. Muscle wasting is common near affected joints. Fingers and toes may swell and appear sausagelike.

Ocular symptoms include mild bilateral conjunctivitis, possibly complicated by keratitis, iritis, retinitis, or optic neuritis. In severe cases, burning, itching, and profuse mucopurulent discharge are possible.

In 30% of patients, skin lesions (keratoderma blennorrhagicum) develop 4 to 6 weeks after onset of other symptoms and may last for several weeks. These macular to hyperkeratotic lesions commonly resemble those of psoriasis. They usually occur on the palms and soles but can develop anywhere on the trunk, extremities, or scalp. Nails become thick, opaque, and brittle; keratic debris accumulates under the nails. In many patients, painless, transient ulcerations erupt on the buccal mucosa, palate, and tongue.

Diagnosis

Many patients with Reiter's syndrome test positive for the HLA-B27 antigen and have an elevated white blood cell (WBC) count and erythrocyte sedimentation rate. Mild anemia may develop. Urethral discharge and synovial fluid contain many WBCs, mostly polymorphonuclear leukocytes; synovial fluid is high in complement and protein and is grossly purulent. Cultures or smears of discharge and synovial fluid rule out other causes, such as gonococci or chlamydia.

Examination of urethral, cervical, or nasopharyngeal swabs may have proved helpful in the diagnosis of new-onset Reiter's syndrome because they provide a way to identify early-stage infections with *Chlamydia trachomatis,* which are often subtle and may go unnoticed.

During the first few weeks, X-rays are normal and may remain so, but some patients may show osteoporosis in inflamed areas. If inflammation persists, X-rays may show erosions of the small joints, periosteal proliferation (new bone formation) of involved joints, and calcaneal spurs.

Treatment

No specific treatment exists for Reiter's syndrome. Most patients recover in 2 to 16 weeks. About 50% of patients have recurring acute attacks, while the rest follow a chronic course, experiencing continued synovitis and sacroiliitis. In acute stages, limited weight bearing may be necessary.

Anti-inflammatory agents, the primary treatment, can be given to relieve discomfort and fever. Steroids may be used for persistent skin lesions; gold therapy, sulfasalazine, methotrexate, or azathioprine, for bony erosion. Testing for HIV is also indicated. Physical therapy includes range-of-motion and strengthening exercises and the use of padded or supportive shoes to prevent contractures and foot deformities.

Special considerations

▶ Explain Reiter's syndrome. Discuss the medications and their possible adverse effects. Warn the patient to take medications with meals or milk to prevent GI bleeding.

▶ Encourage normal daily activity and moderate exercise. Suggest a firm mattress and encourage good posture and body mechanics.

▶ Arrange for occupational counseling if the patient has severe or chronic joint impairment.

RELAPSING FEVER

An acute infectious disease caused by spirochetes of the genus *Borrelia,* relapsing fever (also called tick, fowl-nest, cabin, or vagabond fever, or bilious typhoid) is transmitted to humans by lice or ticks and is characterized by relapses and remissions. Rodents and other wild animals serve as the primary reservoirs for the *Borrelia* spirochetes. Humans can become secondary reservoirs but cannot transmit this infection by ordinary contagion; however, congenital infection and transmission by contaminated blood are possible.

Untreated louse-borne relapsing fever normally carries a mortality rate of more than 10%, but during an epidemic, the mortality rate may rise to as high as 50%. The victims are usually indigent people who are already suffering from other infections and malnutrition. With treatment, however, the prognosis for both louse- and tick-borne relapsing fevers is excellent.

Louse-borne relapsing fever is most common in North and Central Africa, Europe, Asia, and South America. No cases of louse-borne relapsing fever have been reported in the United States since 1900. Tick-borne relapsing fever, however, is found in the United States. This form of the disease is most prevalent in Texas and other western states, usually during the summer, when ticks and their hosts (chipmunks, goats, prairie dogs) are most active; however, cold-weather outbreaks sometimes afflict people, such as campers, who sleep in tick-infested cabins.

Causes

The body louse (*Pediculus humanus* var. *corporis*) carries louse-borne relapsing fever, which typically occurs in epidemics during wars, famines, and mass migrations. Cold weather and crowded living conditions also favor the spread of body lice. Inoculation takes place when the victim crushes the louse, causing its infected blood or body fluid to soak into the victim's bitten or abraded skin, or mucous membranes.

Tick-borne relapsing fever is caused by three species of *Borrelia* most closely identified with tick carriers: *B. hermsii* (associated with *Ornithodoros hermsii*), *B. turicatae* (associated with *Ornithodoros turicata*), and *B. parkeri* (associated with *Ornithodoros parkeri*). Because tick bites are virtually painless, and most *Ornithodoros* ticks feed at night but do not imbed themselves in the victim's skin, many people are bitten unknowingly.

Signs and symptoms

The incubation period for relapsing fever is 5 to 15 days (the average is 7 days). Clinically, tick- and louse-borne diseases are similar. Both begin suddenly, with a temperature approaching 105° F (40.5° C), prostration, headache, severe myalgia, arthralgia, diarrhea, vomiting, coughing, and eye or chest pains. Splenomegaly is common; hepatomegaly and lymphadenopathy may occur. During febrile periods, the victim's pulse and respiratory rates rise, and a transient macular rash may develop over his torso.

The first attack usually lasts from 3 to 6 days; then the patient's temperature drops quickly and is accompanied by profuse sweating. About 5 to 10 days later, a second febrile, symptomatic period begins. In louse-borne infection, additional relapses are unusual; but in tick-borne cases, a second or third relapse is common. As the afebrile intervals become longer, relapses become shorter and milder because of antibody accumulation. Relapses are possibly due to antigenic changes in the *Borrelia* organism.

Complications from relapsing fever include nephritis, bronchitis, pneumonia, endocarditis, seizures, cranial nerve lesions, paralysis, and coma. Death may occur from hyperpyrexia, massive bleeding, circulatory failure, splenic rupture, or a secondary infection.

Diagnosis

Diagnosis requires demonstration of the spirochetes in blood smears during febrile periods, using Wright's or Giemsa stain.

Borrelia spirochetes may be harder to detect in later relapses because their number in the blood declines. In such cases, injecting the patient's blood or tissue into a young rat and incubating the microbe in the rat's blood for 1 to 10 days commonly allows spirochete identification.

In severe infection, spirochetes are found in the urine and cerebrospinal fluid. Other abnormal laboratory results usually include a white blood cell (WBC) count as high as 25,000/μl, with increases in lymphocytes and erythrocyte sedimentation rate; however, the WBC count may be normal. Because *Borrelia* is a spirochete, relapsing fever may cause a false-positive test for syphilis.

Differential diagnoses include malaria, Lyme arthritis, dengue, influenza, typhus, yellow fever, leptospirosis, and the enteric fevers.

Treatment
Doxycycline or erythromycin is the treatment of choice and should continue for 4 to 5 days. In cases of drug allergy or resistance, penicillin G may be administered as an alternative. However, neither drug should be given at the height of a severe febrile attack because it may cause Jarisch-Herxheimer reaction, resulting in malaise, rigors, leukopenia, flushing, fever, tachycardia, rising respiration rate, and hypotension. This reaction, which is caused by toxic by-products from massive spirochete destruction, can mimic septic shock and may prove fatal. Antimicrobial therapy should be postponed until the fever subsides. Until then, supportive therapy (consisting of parenteral fluids and electrolytes) should be given instead.

Special considerations
▶ During the initial evaluation period, obtain a complete history of the patient's travels.
▶ Throughout febrile periods, monitor vital signs, level of consciousness (LOC), and temperature every 4 hours. Watch for and immediately report any signs of neurologic complications, such as decreasing LOC or seizures. To reduce fever, give

tepid sponge baths and antipyretics, as ordered.
▶ Maintain adequate fluid intake to prevent dehydration. Provide I.V. fluids as ordered. Measure intake and output accurately, especially if the patient is vomiting and has diarrhea.
▶ Administer antibiotics carefully. Document and report any hypersensitive reactions (rash, fever, anaphylaxis), especially a Jarisch-Herxheimer reaction.
▶ Treat flushing, hypotension, or tachycardia with vasopressors or fluids, as ordered.
▶ Look for symptoms of relapsing fever in family members and in others who may have been exposed to ticks or lice along with the victim.
▶ Use proper hand-washing technique, and teach it to the patient. Isolation is unnecessary because the disease isn't transmitted from person to person.
▶ Report all cases of louse- or tickborne relapsing fever to the local public health department, as required by law.

 PREVENTION TIP To prevent relapsing fever, advise anyone traveling to tick-infested areas (Asia, North and Central Africa, South America) to wear clothing that covers as much skin as possible and to tuck pant legs into boots or socks.

RESPIRATORY SYNCYTIAL VIRUS INFECTION

A subgroup of the myxoviruses resembling paramyxovirus causes respiratory syncytial virus (RSV) infection. RSV is the leading cause of lower respiratory tract infections in infants and young children; it's the major cause of pneumonia, tracheobronchitis, and bronchiolitis in this age-group and a suspected cause of the fatal respiratory diseases of infancy. It has been linked to apnea in cases of acute infection in infants. Antibody titers seem to indicate that few children under age 4 escape contracting some form of RSV infection, even if it's mild. In fact, RSV infection is the only viral disease that has its maximum impact during the first few months of life. (Incidence of RSV bronchiolitis peaks at age 2 months.)

This virus creates annual epidemics that occur during the late winter and early spring in temperate climates, and during the rainy season in the tropics.

Causes

The organism is transmitted from person to person by respiratory secretions and has an incubation period of 4 to 5 days.

Reinfection is common, producing milder symptoms than the primary infection. School-age children, adolescents, and young adults with mild reinfections are probably the source of infection for infants and young children.

Signs and symptoms

Clinical features of RSV infection vary in severity, ranging from mild coldlike symptoms to bronchiolitis or bronchopneumonia and, in a few patients, severe, life-threatening lower respiratory tract infections. Generally, symptoms include coughing, wheezing, malaise, pharyngitis, dyspnea, and inflamed mucous membranes in the nose and throat.

Otitis media is a common complication of RSV in infants. RSV has also been identified in patients with a variety of central nervous system disorders, such as meningitis and myelitis.

Diagnosis

Diagnosis is usually based on clinical findings and epidemiologic information.

Cultures of nasal and pharyngeal secretions may show RSV; however, the virus is very labile, so cultures aren't always reliable. Serum antibody titers may be elevated, but before age 6 months, maternal antibodies may impair test results. Two serologic techniques that aid in diagnosis are the indirect immunofluorescence and the enzyme-linked immunosorbent assay (ELISA) methods. These tests are sensitive and will give results in less than one hour. Chest X-rays help detect pneumonia.

Other conditions to consider are pneumonia, croup, asthma, influenza, and the common cold.

Treatment

Among the goals of treatment are support of respiratory function, maintenance of fluid balance, and relief of symptoms. Mild and even moderated cases do not require specific therapy. Treating the symptoms with nebulized beta-agonists (albuterol) or racemic epinephrine have been shown to be effective. Short courses of oral steroids may also help decrease inflammation of the bronchioles.

Special considerations

▶ Monitor respiratory status. Observe the rate and pattern; watch for nasal flaring or retraction, cyanosis, pallor, and dyspnea; and auscultate for wheezing, rhonchi, or other signs of respiratory distress. Monitor arterial blood gas values.

▶ Maintain a patent airway, and be especially watchful when the patient has periods of acute dyspnea. Perform percussion and provide drainage and suction when necessary. Provide a high-humidity atmosphere. Semi-Fowler's position may help prevent aspiration of secretions.

▶ The head of the bed or crib may be elevated to help prevent aspiration of secretions.

▶ Monitor intake and output carefully. Observe for signs of dehydration such as decreased skin turgor. Encourage the patient to drink plenty of high-calorie fluids. Administer I.V. fluids as needed.

▶ Promote bed rest, allowing for as much uninterrupted rest as possible.

▶ Hold and cuddle infants; talk to and play with toddlers. Offer diversional activities suitable to the child's condition and age. Foster parental visits and cuddling. Restrain a child only as necessary.

▶ Impose contact isolation. Enforce strict hand washing, because RSV may be transmitted from fomites.

▶ Staff members with respiratory illnesses shouldn't care for infants.

RHEUMATIC FEVER AND RHEUMATIC HEART DISEASE

Often recurrent, acute rheumatic fever is a systemic inflammatory disease of childhood that follows a group A beta-hemolytic streptococcal infection. Rheumatic heart disease refers to the cardiac manifestations of rheumatic fever, and includes pancarditis (myocarditis, pericarditis, and endocarditis) during the early acute phase, and chronic valvular disease later.

Long-term antibiotic therapy can minimize recurrence of rheumatic fever, reducing the risk of permanent cardiac damage and eventual valvular deformity. However, severe pancarditis occasionally produces fatal heart failure during the acute phase. Of the patients who survive this complication, about 20% die within 10 years. Although rheumatic fever tends to run in families, this may merely reflect contributing environmental factors. For example, in lower socioeconomic groups, incidence is highest in children between ages 5 and 15, probably as a result of malnutrition and crowded living conditions.

This disease strikes most often during cool, damp weather in the winter and early spring. In the United States, it's most common in the northern states.

Causes

Rheumatic fever appears to be a hypersensitivity reaction to a group A beta-hemolytic streptococcal infection, in which antibodies manufactured to combat streptococci react and produce characteristic lesions at specific tissue sites, especially in the heart and joints. Because very few people (about 0.3%) with streptococcal infections ever contract rheumatic fever, altered host resistance must be involved in its development or recurrence.

Signs and symptoms

In 95% of patients, rheumatic fever characteristically follows a streptococcal infection that appeared a few days to 6 weeks earlier. A temperature of at least 100.4° F (38° C) occurs.

Most patients complain of migratory joint pain or polyarthritis. Swelling, redness, and signs of effusion usually accompany such pain, which most commonly affects the knees, ankles, elbows, or hips.

In 5% of patients (generally those with carditis), rheumatic fever causes skin lesions such as erythema marginatum. This nonpruritic, macular, transient rash gives rise to red lesions with blanched centers.

Rheumatic fever may also produce firm, movable, nontender, subcutaneous nodules about 3 mm to 2 cm in diameter, usually near tendons or bony prominences of joints (especially the elbows, knuckles, wrists, and knees) and less often on the scalp and backs of the hands. These nodules persist for a few days to several weeks and, like erythema marginatum, often accompany carditis.

Later, rheumatic fever may cause transient chorea, which develops up to 6 months after the original streptococcal infection.

Mild chorea may produce hyperirritability, a deterioration in handwriting, or an inability to concentrate. Severe chorea causes purposeless, nonrepetitive, involuntary muscle spasms; poor muscle coordination; and weakness. Chorea always resolves without residual neurologic damage.

The most destructive effect of rheumatic fever is carditis, which develops in up to 50% of patients. It may affect the endocardium, myocardium, pericardium, or the heart valves.

Pericarditis causes a pericardial friction rub and, occasionally, pain and effusion. Myocarditis produces characteristic lesions called Aschoff's bodies (in the acute stages) and cellular swelling and fragmentation of interstitial collagen, leading to formation of a progressively fibrotic nodule and interstitial scars.

Endocarditis causes valve leaflet swelling, erosion along the lines of leaflet closure, and blood, platelet, and fibrin deposits, which form beadlike vegetations. Endocarditis affects the mitral valve most often in females; the aortic valve most often in males. In both sexes, endocarditis affects the tricuspid valves occasionally and the pulmonic valve only rarely.

Severe rheumatic carditis may cause heart failure with dyspnea, upper right quadrant pain, tachycardia, tachypnea, significant mitral and aortic murmurs, and a hacking, nonproductive cough.

The most common of such murmurs include a systolic murmur of mitral insufficiency (high-pitched, blowing, holosystolic, loudest at apex, possibly radiating to the anterior axillary line); a midsystolic murmur caused by stiffening and swelling of the mitral leaflet; and, occasionally, a diastolic murmur of aortic insufficiency. Valvular disease may eventually result in chronic valvular stenosis and insufficiency, including mitral stenosis and insufficiency and aortic insufficiency. In children, mitral insufficiency remains the major sequela of rheumatic heart disease.

Diagnosis

Recognition of one or more of the classic symptoms (carditis, polyarthritis, chorea, erythema marginatum, or subcutaneous nodules) and a detailed patient history allow diagnosis.

Supportive laboratory data include the following:

▶ White blood cell count and erythrocyte sedimentation rate may be elevated (during the acute phase) and blood studies show slight anemia from suppressed erythropoiesis during inflammation.

▶ C-reactive protein is positive (especially during the acute phase).

▶ Cardiac enzyme levels may be increased in severe carditis.

▶ Antistreptolysin-O titer is elevated in 95% of patients within 2 months of onset.

▶ Electrocardiography changes aren't diagnostic, but the PR interval is prolonged in 20% of patients.

▶ Chest X-rays show normal heart size (except with myocarditis, heart failure, or pericardial effusion).

▶ Echocardiography helps evaluate valvular damage, chamber size, and ventricular function.

▶ Cardiac catheterization evaluates valvular damage and left ventricular function in severe cardiac dysfunction.

Several other conditions may have similar signs and symptoms and need to be considered, including systemic lupus erythematosus, sickle cell anemia, leukemia, serum sickness, traumatic arthritis, gonococcal arthritis, systemic juvenile rheumatoid arthritis, and congenital heart disease.

Treatment

Effective management eradicates the streptococcal infection, relieves symptoms, and prevents recurrence, reducing the chance of permanent cardiac damage.

During the acute phase, treatment includes penicillin or (for patients with penicillin hypersensitivity) erythromycin. Salicylates such as aspirin relieve fever and minimize joint swelling and pain; if carditis is present or salicylates fail to relieve pain and inflammation, corticosteroids may be used.

Supportive treatment requires strict bed rest for about 5 weeks during the acute phase with active carditis, followed by a progressive increase in physical activity, depending on clinical and laboratory findings and the response to treatment.

After the acute phase subsides, a monthly I.M. injection of penicillin G benzathine or daily doses of oral sulfadiazine or penicillin G may be used to prevent recurrence. Such preventive treatment usually continues for 5 to 10 years.

Heart failure necessitates continued bed rest and diuretics. Severe mitral or aortic valvular dysfunction causing persistent heart failure requires corrective valvular surgery, including commissurotomy (separation of the adherent, thickened leaflets of the mitral valve), valvuloplasty (inflation of a balloon within a valve), or valve replacement (with a prosthetic valve). Corrective valvular surgery is rarely necessary before late adolescence.

Special considerations
▶ Teach the patient and family about this disease and its treatment.
▶ Before giving penicillin, ask the parents if the child has ever had a hypersensitivity reaction to it. Even if the patient has never had a reaction to penicillin, warn that such a reaction is possible. Tell the child's parents to stop the drug and immediately report the development of a rash, fever, chills, or other signs of allergy at any time during penicillin therapy.
▶ Instruct the parents to watch for and report early signs of heart failure, such as dyspnea and a hacking, nonproductive cough.
▶ Stress the need for bed rest during the acute phase and suggest appropriate, physically undemanding diversions.
▶ After the acute phase, encourage family and friends to spend as much time as possible with the child to minimize boredom. Advise the parents to secure a tutor to help the child keep up with schoolwork during his long convalescence.
▶ Help the parents overcome any guilt they may feel about their child's illness. Tell them that failure to seek treatment for streptococcal infection is common, because this illness often seems no worse than a cold.
▶ If the child has severe carditis, help parents prepare for permanent changes in the child's lifestyle.
▶ Warn the parents to watch for and immediately report signs of recurrent streptococcal infection — sudden sore throat,

diffuse throat redness and oropharyngeal exudate, swollen and tender cervical lymph glands, pain on swallowing, a temperature of 101° to 104° F (38.3° to 40° C), headache, and nausea. Urge them to keep the child away from people with respiratory tract infections.
▶ Arrange for a visiting nurse to oversee home care if necessary.

 PREVENTION TIP Explain the importance of good dental hygiene in preventing gingival infection, which can make the gums prone to bleeding, thus putting the patient at risk for infection. Make sure the child and his family understand the need to comply with prolonged antibiotic therapy and follow-up care and the need for additional antibiotics for dental or oral surgical procedures likely to cause gingival bleeding, for upper respiratory tract surgery, and for surgery or instrumentation of the GU and lower GI tracts.

ROCKY MOUNTAIN SPOTTED FEVER

Rocky Mountain spotted fever (RMSF) is a febrile, rash-producing illness caused by *Rickettsia rickettsii*. The disease is transmitted to humans by a tick bite. Endemic throughout the continental United States, RMSF is particularly prevalent in the southeast and southwest. Because RMSF is associated with outdoor activities, such as camping and backpacking, the incidence of this illness is usually higher in the spring and summer. Epidemiologic surveillance reports for RMSF indicate that the incidence is also higher in children ages 5 to 9, men and boys, and whites.

RMSF is fatal in about 5% of patients. Mortality rises when treatment is delayed and in older patients.

Causes
R. rickettsii is transmitted to a human or small animal by a prolonged bite (4 to 6

TICK CLOSEUP

Rocky Mountain spotted fever is transmitted by the prolonged bite of an adult tick.

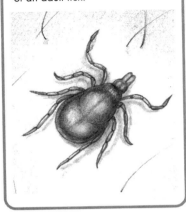

hours) of an adult tick — the wood tick (*Dermacentor andersoni*) in the west and by the dog tick (*Dermacentor variabilis*) in the east. Occasionally, it's acquired through inhalation or through contact of abraded skin with tick excreta or tissue juices. (This explains why people should not crush ticks between their fingers when removing them from other people and animals.) In most tick-infested areas, 1% to 5% of the ticks harbor *R. rickettsii.* (See *Tick closeup.*)

Signs and symptoms

The incubation period is usually about 7 days, but it can range from 2 to 14 days. Generally, the shorter the incubation time, the more severe the infection. Signs and symptoms, which usually begin abruptly, include a persistent temperature of 102° to 104° F (38.9° to 40° C); a generalized, excruciating headache; nausea and vomiting; and aching in the bones, muscles, joints, and back. In addition, the tongue is covered with a thick white coating that gradually turns brown as the fever persists and rises.

Initially, the skin may simply appear flushed. Between days 2 and 5, eruptions begin around the wrists, ankles, or forehead; within 2 days, they cover the entire body, including the scalp, palms, and soles. The rash consists of erythematous macules 1 to 5 mm in diameter that blanch on pressure; if untreated, the rash may become petechial and maculopapular. By the 3rd week, the skin peels off and may become gangrenous over the elbows, fingers, and toes.

The pulse is strong initially, but it gradually becomes rapid (possibly reaching 150 beats/minute) and thready.

 ALERT A rapid pulse rate and hypotension (systolic pressure less than 90 mm Hg) herald imminent death from complete vascular collapse.

Other signs and symptoms include a bronchial cough, a rapid respiratory rate (as high as 60 breaths/minute), anorexia, constipation, abdominal pain, hepatomegaly, splenomegaly, insomnia, restlessness and, in extreme cases, delirium. Urine output falls to half of the normal level or less, and the urine is dark and contains albumin. Complications, although uncommon, include lobar pneumonia, otitis media, parotitis, disseminated intravascular coagulation (DIC) and, possibly, renal failure. In rare cases, RMSF leads to death.

Diagnosis

Diagnosis is usually based on a history of a tick bite or travel to a tick-infested area and a positive complement fixation test (which shows a fourfold increase in convalescent antibody titer compared with acute titers). Blood cultures should be performed to isolate the organism and confirm the diagnosis.

Another common but less reliable antibody test is the Weil-Felix reaction, which also shows a fourfold increase between the acute and convalescent sera titer levels. Increased titers usually develop after

10 to 14 days and persist for several months.

Additional recommended laboratory tests consist of a platelet count for thrombocytopenia (12,000 to 150,000/µl) and a white blood cell count (elevated to 11,000 to 33,000/µl) during the 2nd week of illness.

Other conditions to consider are meningococcemia, rubeola, typhus, Lyme disease, and Q fever.

Treatment

Treatment requires careful removal of the tick and administration of antibiotics, such as chloramphenicol or tetracycline, until 3 days after the fever subsides. Treatment also includes symptomatic measures and, in DIC, heparin and platelet transfusion.

Special considerations

▶ Carefully monitor intake and output. Watch closely for decreased urine output — a possible indicator of renal failure.

▶ Be alert for signs of dehydration, such as poor skin turgor and dry mouth.

▶ Administer antipyretics, as ordered, and provide tepid sponge baths to reduce fever.

▶ Monitor vital signs, and watch for profound hypotension and shock.

▶ Locate the necessary equipment and be prepared to administer oxygen therapy and assisted ventilation if pulmonary complications develop.

▶ Turn the patient frequently to prevent such complications of immobility as pressure ulcers and pneumonia.

▶ Pay attention to the patient's nutritional needs because vomiting may necessitate parenteral nutrition or frequent small meals.

▶ Provide meticulous mouth care and other oral hygiene measures.

 PREVENTION TIP When the patient recovers sufficiently, initiate patient teaching about disease prevention. Instruct the patient to report any recurrent symptoms to the doctor at once so that treatment measures may resume

immediately. Advise the patient to avoid tick-infested areas (woods, meadows, streams, and canyons) if possible. If he can't avoid tick-infested areas, tell him how to protect himself from a prolonged tick bite. Advise him to inspect his entire body (including his scalp) every 3 to 4 hours for attached ticks, to wear protective clothing, such as a long-sleeved shirt, pants securely tucked into laced boots, and a protective head covering, such as a cap, and to apply insect repellant to exposed skin and even to his clothing. Offer printed and illustrated instructions, if available, that teach the patient and his family members or other caregivers how to correctly and safely remove a tick. Or show them how to use tweezers or forceps and how to apply steady traction to release the whole tick without leaving its mouth parts still in the skin. After the patient removes the tick, caution him not to handle it or its fragments. Finally, instruct him to clean his skin with alcohol at the point of attachment.

ROSEOLA INFANTUM

Also called exanthema subitum, roseola infantum is an acute, benign, presumably viral infection. It usually affects infants and young children (ages 6 months to 3 years).

Roseola affects boys and girls alike. It occurs year-round but is most prevalent in the spring and fall. Overt roseola, the most common exanthem in infants under age 2, affects 30% of all children; inapparent roseola (febrile illness without a rash) may affect the rest.

Characteristically, roseola first causes a high fever and then a rash that accompanies an abrupt drop to normal temperature. (See *Survey of common rash-producing infections,* page 258.)

SURVEY OF COMMON RASH-PRODUCING INFECTIONS

INFECTION	INCUBATION (DAYS)	DURATION (DAYS)
Herpes simplex	2 to 12	7 to 21
Roseola	10 to 15	3 to 6
Rubella	14 to 21	3
Rubeola	8 to 14	5
Varicella	14 to 17	7 to 14

Causes

The mode of transmission isn't known. Only rarely does an infected child transmit roseola to a sibling.

Signs and symptoms

After a 10- to 15-day incubation period, the infant with roseola develops an abruptly rising, unexplainable fever and, sometimes, seizures. Temperature peaks at 103° to 105° F (39.4° to 40.6° C) for 3 to 5 days, then drops suddenly. In the early febrile period, the infant may be anorexic, irritable, and listless but doesn't seem particularly ill.

Simultaneously with an abrupt drop in temperature, a maculopapular, nonpruritic rash develops, which blanches on pressure. The rash is profuse on the infant's trunk, arms, and neck, and is mild on the face and legs. It fades within 24 hours. Although possible, complications are extremely rare.

Diagnosis

Diagnosis requires observation of the typical rash that appears about 48 hours after fever subsides. Other conditions to consider are varicella, rubeola, rubella, and herpes simplex.

Treatment

Because roseola is self-limiting, treatment is supportive and symptomatic: antipyretics to lower fever and, if necessary, anticonvulsants to relieve seizures.

 PREVENTION TIP Teach parents how to lower their infant's fever by giving tepid baths, keeping him in lightweight clothes, and maintaining normal room temperature. Stress the need for adequate fluid intake. Strict bed rest and isolation are unnecessary. Tell parents that a short febrile convulsion will not cause brain damage. Explain that convulsions will cease after fever subsides and that phenobarbital is likely to cause drowsiness; parents should call immediately if it causes stupor.

ROTAVIRUS

Rotavirus is the most common cause of severe diarrhea among children, resulting in the hospitalization of approximately 55,000 children each year in the United States and the death of over 600,000 children annually worldwide, as reported by the Centers for Disease Control and Prevention. The highest rates of illness occur among infants and young children, and most children in the United States are infected by 2 years of age. The incubation period for rotavirus disease is approximately 2 days. The disease is characterized by vomiting and watery diarrhea for 3 to 8 days, and fever and abdominal pain occur frequently. Immunity after infection is incomplete, but repeat infections tend to be less severe than the original infection. About one in 40 children with rotavirus gastroenteritis will require hospitalization for intravenous fluids. In the United States and other countries with a temperate climate, the disease has a winter seasonal pattern, with annual epidemics occurring from November to April.

Causes

The primary mode of transmission is fecal-oral, although some have reported low titers of virus in respiratory tract secretions and other bodily fluids. Due to the stability of the virus within the environment, transmission can occur through ingestion of contaminated water or food and contact with contaminated surfaces. Billions of rotavirus particles are passed in the stool of the infected individual. Tiny amounts of the rotavirus can lead to infection if a baby puts fingers or other objects contaminated with the virus into the mouth. Young children may pass it on to siblings and parents.

Signs and symptoms

Rotavirus gastroenteritis frequently starts with a fever, nausea and vomiting followed by diarrhea. The illness can range from mild to severe and last from 3 to 9 days. Diarrhea and vomiting may result in dehydration.

Diagnosis

Diagnosis is determined by rapid antigen detection of rotavirus in stool specimens.

Rotavirus is the most common diagnosis for young children with acute diarrhea, but other causes that require differential diagnosis include bacteria (*Salmonella, Shigella, Campylobacter* most common), parasites (*Giardia* and *Cryptosporidium* most common), localized infection elsewhere, antibiotic-associated (antibiotic side effect as well as *Clostridium difficile*), and food poisoning. Noninfectious causes may include overfeeding, (particularly of fruit juices), irritable bowel syndrome, celiac disease, milk protein intolerance,
lactose intolerance, cystic fibrosis, and inflammatory bowel syndrome.

Treatment

For individuals with healthy immune systems, rotavirus gastroenteritis is a self-limited illness, lasting for only days. Treatment is nonspecific and consists of oral rehydration therapy to prevent dehydration.

Special considerations

▶ Strict hand washing and careful cleaning of all equipment, including any toys the child may have, is most important in the prevention of spreading the rotavirus.
▶ Help the patient maintain adequate hydration. Remember that dehydration occurs rapidly within infants and young children. Ice pops, Jell-O, and ice chips may be included in the diet to maintain hydration.
▶ Breast-fed infants should continue to nurse without restrictions. Lactose-free soybean formulas may be used for those who are bottle-fed.
▶ Carefully monitor intake and output (including stools).
▶ Cleanse the perineum thoroughly to prevent skin breakdown.

 PREVENTION TIP Instruct the patient's parents on proper hand-washing technique for themselves and the infant, diaper changing, and cleansing of all affected surfaces. Include the parents and caregivers in the measurement of intake and output as it relates to the infants' diapers, and instruct them to notify their doctor with any increased diarrhea, or dehydration. Warn travelers that rotavirus is pandemic and can be contracted via contaminated food or water so that appropriate precautions may be undertaken.

RUBELLA

Commonly called German measles, rubella is an acute, mildly contagious viral disease that produces a distinctive 3-day rash and lymphadenopathy. It occurs most often among children ages 5 to 9, adolescents, and young adults.

Worldwide in distribution, rubella flourishes during the spring (particularly in big cities), and epidemics occur sporadically. This disease is self-limiting, and the prognosis is excellent.

Causes

The rubella virus is transmitted through contact with the blood, urine, stools, or nasopharyngeal secretions of infected persons and, possibly, by contact with contaminated articles of clothing. Transplacental transmission, especially in the first trimester of pregnancy, can cause serious birth defects.

Humans are the only known hosts for the rubella virus. The period of communicability lasts from about 10 days before the rash appears until 5 days later.

Signs and symptoms

In children, after an incubation period of from 14 to 21 days, an exanthematous, maculopapular rash erupts abruptly. In adolescents and adults, prodromal symptoms — headache, anorexia, malaise, low-grade fever, coryza, lymphadenopathy and, sometimes, conjunctivitis — appear first. Suboccipital, postauricular, and postcervical lymph node enlargement is a hallmark of rubella.

Typically, the rubella rash begins on the face. This maculopapular eruption spreads rapidly, often covering the trunk and extremities within hours. Small, red, petechial macules on the soft palate (Forschheimer spots) may precede or accompany the rash.

By the end of the second day, the facial rash begins to fade, but the rash on the trunk may be confluent and may be mistaken for scarlet fever. The rash continues to fade in the downward order in which it appeared. The rash generally disappears on the third day, but it may persist for 4 or 5 days — sometimes accompanied by mild coryza and conjunctivitis.

The rapid appearance and disappearance of the rubella rash distinguishes it from rubeola. Rubella can occur without a rash, but this is rare. Low-grade fever (99° to 101° F [37.2° to 38.3° C]) may accompany the rash, but it usually doesn't persist after the first day of the rash; rarely, temperature may reach 104° F (40° C).

Complications seldom occur in children with rubella, but when they do, they often appear as hemorrhagic problems such as thrombocytopenia. Young women, however, often experience transient joint pain or arthritis, usually just as the rash is fading. Fever may then recur. These complications usually subside spontaneously within 5 to 30 days.

Diagnosis

The rubella rash, lymphadenopathy, other characteristic signs, and a history of exposure to infected people usually permit clinical diagnosis without laboratory tests. However, cell cultures of the throat, blood, urine, and cerebrospinal fluid can confirm the virus's presence. Convalescent serum that shows a fourfold rise in antibody titers confirms the diagnosis.

Differential diagnosis includes measles, scarlet fever, secondary syphilis, drug rashes, erythema infectiosum, and infectious mononucleosis as well as echovirus, coxsackievirus, and adenovirus infections.

Treatment

Because the rubella rash is self-limiting and only mildly pruritic, it doesn't require topical or systemic medication. Treatment consists of aspirin for fever and joint pain. Bed rest isn't necessary, but the patient should be isolated until the rash disappears.

Immunization with live-virus vaccine RA27/3, the only rubella vaccine available in the United States, is necessary for prevention and appears to be more immunogenic than previous vaccines. The rubella vaccine should be given with measles and mumps vaccines at age 15 months to decrease the cost and the number of injections needed.

Special considerations

▶ Make the patient with active rubella as comfortable as possible. Give children books to read or games to play to keep them occupied.

▶ Explain why respiratory isolation is necessary. Make sure the patient understands how important it is to avoid exposing pregnant women to this disease.

▶ Report confirmed cases of rubella to local public health officials.

▶ Obtain a history of allergies, especially to neomycin. If the patient has this allergy or has had a reaction to immunization in the past, check with the doctor before giving the rubella vaccine.

▶ Ask women of childbearing age if they're pregnant. If they are or think they may be, don't give the vaccine.

▶ Warn women who receive rubella vaccine to use an effective means of birth control for at least 3 months after immunization.

▶ Give the vaccine at least 3 months after any administration of immune globulin or blood, which could have antibodies that neutralize the vaccine.

▶ Don't vaccinate any immunocompromised patients, patients with immunodeficiency diseases, or those receiving immunosuppressive, radiation, or corticosteroid therapy. Instead, administer immune serum globulin to prevent or reduce infection in susceptible patients.

▶ After giving the vaccine, observe for signs of anaphylaxis for at least 30 minutes. Keep epinephrine 1:1,000 handy.

▶ Warn about possible mild fever, slight rash, transient arthralgia (in adolescents), and arthritis (in elderly patients). Suggest aspirin or acetaminophen for fever.

▶ Advise the patient to apply warmth to the injection site for 24 hours after immunization (to help the body absorb the vaccine). If swelling persists after the initial 24 hours, suggest a cold compress to promote vasoconstriction and prevent antigenic cyst formation.

RUBEOLA

Also known as measles or morbilli, rubeola is an acute, highly contagious paramyxovirus infection. It is one of the most common and the most serious of all communicable childhood diseases.

In temperate zones, incidence is highest in late winter and early spring. Before the availability of measles vaccine, epidemics occurred every 2 to 5 years in large urban areas. Use of the vaccine has reduced the occurrence of measles during childhood; as a result, measles is becoming more prevalent in adolescents and adults. (See *Administering measles vaccine,* page 262.)

In the United States, the prognosis is usually excellent. However, measles is a major cause of death in children in developing countries.

Causes

Measles is spread by direct contact or by contaminated airborne respiratory droplets. The portal of entry is the upper respiratory tract.

Signs and symptoms

Incubation is from 8 to 14 days. Initial symptoms begin and greatest communicability occurs during a prodromal phase beginning about 11 days after exposure to the virus. This phase lasts from 4 to 5 days; symptoms include fever, photophobia, malaise, anorexia, conjunctivitis, coryza, hoarseness, and hacking cough.

At the end of the prodrome, Koplik's spots, the hallmark of the disease, appear.

ADMINISTERING MEASLES VACCINE

Generally one bout of measles renders immunity. (A second infection is extremely rare and may represent misdiagnosis.) Infants under age 4 months may be immune because of circulating maternal antibodies.

Under normal conditions, measles vaccine isn't administered to children younger than age 15 months. However, during an epidemic, infants as young as 6 months may receive the vaccine and they must be reimmunized at age 15 months.

An alternative approach calls for administration of gamma globulin to infants between ages 6 and 15 months who are likely to be exposed to measles.

SPECIAL CONSIDERATIONS

▶ Warn the patient or his parents that possible adverse effects of the vaccine include anorexia, malaise, rash, mild thrombocytopenia or leukopenia, and fever. Explain that the vaccine may produce slight reactions, usually within 7 to 10 days.
▶ Ask the patient about known allergies, especially to neomycin (each dose contains a small amount). However, a patient who's allergic to eggs may receive the vaccine because it contains only minimal amounts of albumin and yolk components.
▶ Avoid giving the vaccine to a pregnant woman (ask for the date of her last menstrual period). Warn women receiving the vaccine to avoid pregnancy for at least 3 months after vaccination
▶ Don't vaccinate children with untreated tuberculosis, immunodeficiencies, leukemia, or lymphoma or those receiving immunosuppressives. If such children are exposed to the virus, recommend that they receive gamma globulin. (Gamma globulin won't prevent measles but will lessen its severity.)
▶ Older unimmunized children who have been exposed to measles for more than 5 days may also require gamma globulin. Be sure to immunize them 3 months later.
▶ Delay vaccination for 8 to 12 weeks after administration of whole blood, plasma, or gamma globulin because measles antibodies in these components may neutralize the vaccine.
▶ Watch for signs of anaphylaxis for 30 minutes after vaccination. Keep epinephrine 1:1,000 handy.
▶ Advise application of a warm compress to the vaccination site to facilitate absorption of the vaccine. If swelling occurs within 24 hours after vaccination, tell the patient to apply cold compresses to promote vasoconstriction and to prevent antigenic cyst formation.

These spots look like tiny, bluish gray specks surrounded by a red halo. They appear on the oral mucosa opposite the molars and occasionally bleed.

About 5 days after Koplik's spots appear, temperature rises sharply, spots slough off, and a slightly pruritic rash appears. This characteristic rash starts as faint macules behind the ears and on the neck and cheeks.

These macules become papular and erythematous, rapidly spreading over the entire face, neck, eyelids, arms, chest, back, abdomen, and thighs. When the rash reaches the feet (2 to 3 days later), it begins to fade in the same sequence it appeared, leaving a brownish discoloration that disappears in 7 to 10 days.

The disease climax occurs 2 to 3 days after the rash appears and is marked by a temperature of 103° to 105° F (39.4° to 40.6° C), severe cough, rhinorrhea, and puffy, red eyes. About 5 days after the rash appears, other symptoms disappear and communicability ends.

Symptoms are usually mild in patients with partial immunity (conferred by administration of gamma globulin) or infants with transplacental antibodies. More severe symptoms and complications are more likely to develop in young infants, adolescents, adults, and immunocompromised patients than in young children.

Atypical measles may appear in patients who received the killed measles vaccine. These patients are acutely ill with a fever and maculopapular rash that's most obvious in the arms and legs, or with pulmonary involvement and no skin lesions.

Severe infection may lead to secondary bacterial infection and to autoimmune reaction or organ invasion by the virus, resulting in otitis media, pneumonia, and encephalitis. Subacute sclerosing panencephalitis (SSPE), a rare and invariably fatal complication, may develop several years after measles. SSPE is less common in patients who have received the measles vaccine.

Diagnosis

Measles results in distinctive clinical features, especially the pathognomonic Koplik's spots. Mild measles may resemble rubella, roseola infantum, enterovirus infection, toxoplasmosis, and drug eruptions; laboratory tests are required for a differential diagnosis.

If necessary, measles virus may be isolated from the blood, nasopharyngeal secretions, and urine during the febrile period. Serum antibodies appear within 3 days after onset of the rash and reach peak titers 2 to 4 weeks later.

Treatment

Therapy consists of bed rest, relief of symptoms, and respiratory isolation throughout the communicable period. Vaporizers and a warm environment help reduce respiratory irritation, but cough preparations and antibiotics are generally ineffective; antipyretics can reduce fever. Treatment must also combat complications.

 PREVENTION TIP Teach parents supportive measures, and stress the need for isolation, plenty of rest, and increased fluid intake. Advise them to cope with photophobia by darkening the room or providing sunglasses and to reduce fever with antipyretics and tepid sponge baths. Warn parents to watch for and report the early signs and symptoms of complications, such as encephalitis, otitis media, and pneumonia. Children at home should be kept out of school for at least 4 days after the rash appears. Teach parents the importance of immunizing their children against measles, and follow appropriate procedures when giving the vaccine.

S

SALMONELLOSIS

A common infection in the United States, salmonellosis is caused by gram-negative bacilli of the genus *Salmonella*, a member of the Enterobacteriaceae family. It occurs as enterocolitis, bacteremia, localized infection, typhoid, or paratyphoid fever. (See *Types of salmonellosis*.) Nontyphoidal forms usually produce mild to moderate illness with low mortality.

Typhoid, the most severe form of salmonellosis, usually lasts from 1 to 4 weeks. Mortality is about 3% in persons who are treated and 10% in those untreated, usually as a result of intestinal perforation or hemorrhage, cerebral thrombosis, toxemia, pneumonia, or acute circulatory failure.

An attack of typhoid confers lifelong immunity, although the patient may become a carrier. Most typhoid patients are under age 30; most carriers are women over age 50. Incidence of typhoid in the United States is increasing as a result of travelers returning from endemic areas.

Enterocolitis and bacteremia are common (and more virulent) among infants, elderly people, and people already weakened by other infections; paratyphoid fever is rare in the United States.

Salmonellosis occurs 20 times more often in patients with acquired immunodeficiency syndrome. Features are increased incidence of bacteremia, inability to identify the infection source, and tendency of the infection to recur after therapy is stopped.

Causes

Of an estimated 1,700 serotypes of *Salmonella,* 10 cause the diseases most common in the United States, and all 10 can survive for weeks in water, ice, sewage, or food. Nontyphoidal salmonellosis generally follows the ingestion of contaminated or inadequately processed foods, especially eggs, chicken, turkey, and duck. Proper cooking reduces the risk of contracting salmonellosis.

Other causes include contact with infected people or animals or ingestion of contaminated dry milk, chocolate bars, or drugs of animal origin. Salmonellosis may occur in children under age 5 from fecaloral spread.

Typhoid results most frequently from drinking water contaminated by excretions of a carrier.

Signs and symptoms

Clinical manifestations of salmonellosis vary but usually include fever, abdominal pain, and severe diarrhea with enterocolitis. Headache, increasing fever, and constipation are more common with typhoidal infection.

Diagnosis

Generally, diagnosis depends on isolation of the microbe in a culture, particularly blood (in typhoid, paratyphoid, and bacteremia) or feces (in enterocolitis, paratyphoid, and typhoid). Other appropriate culture specimens include urine, bone marrow, pus, and vomitus.

In endemic areas, clinical symptoms of enterocolitis allow a working diagnosis before cultures are positive. Presence of

TYPES OF SALMONELLOSIS

TYPE	CAUSE	CLINICAL FEATURES
Bacteremia	Any *Salmonella* species, but most commonly *S. choleraesuis* *Incubation period*: varied	Fever, chills, anorexia, weight loss (without GI symptoms), joint pain
Enterocolitis	Any species of nontyphoidal *Salmonella*, but usually *S. enteritidis* *Incubation period*: 6 to 48 hours	Mild to severe abdominal pain, diarrhea, sudden fever up to 102°F (38.8°C), nausea, vomiting; usually self-limiting, but may progress to enteric fever (resembling typhoid), local abscesses (usually abdominal), dehydration, septicemia
Localized infections	Usually follows bacteremia caused by *Salmonella* species	Symptoms determined by site of localization: possible osteomyelitis, endocarditis, bronchopneumonia, pyelonephritis, and arthritis
Paratyphoid	*S. paratyphi* and *S. schottmuelleri* (formerly *S. paratyphi* B) *Incubation period*:3 weeks or more	Fever and transient diarrhea; generally resembles typhoid but less severe
Typhoid fever	*S. typhi* entering GI tract, invading bloodstream via the lymphatics, and setting up intracellular sites; during this phase, infection of biliary tract leading to intestinal seeding with millions of bacilli; involved lymphoid tissues (especially Peyer's patches in ilium) that enlarge, ulcerate, and necrose, resulting in hemorrhage *Incubation period*: usually 1 to 2 weeks	Symptoms of enterocolitis possibly developing within hours of ingestion of *S. typhi;* usually subside before onset of typhoid fever symptoms *First week:* gradually increasing fever, anorexia, myalgia, malaise, headache, slow pulse *Second week:* remittent fever up to 104°F (40°C) usually in the evening, chills, diaphoresis, weakness, delirium, increasing abdominal pain and distention, diarrhea or constipation, cough, moist crackles, tender abdomen with enlarged spleen, maculopapular rash (especially on abdomen) *Third week:* persistent fever, increasing fatigue and weakness; usually subsides end of third week, although relapses may occur *Complications:* intestinal perforation, hemorrhage, abscesses, thrombophlebitis, cerebral thrombosis, pneumonia, osteomyelitis, myocarditis, acute circulatory failure, chronic carrier state

S. typhi in stools 1 or more years after treatment indicates that the patient is a carrier, which is true of 3% of patients.

Widal's test, an agglutination reaction against somatic and flagellar antigens, may suggest typhoid with a fourfold rise in titer. However, drug use or hepatic disease can also increase these titers and invalidate test results.

Other supportive laboratory values may include transient leukocytosis during the first week of typhoidal salmonellosis, leukopenia during the third week, and leukocytosis in local infection.

Treatment

Antimicrobial therapy for typhoid, paratyphoid, and bacteremia depends on the microbe's sensitivity. It may include amoxicillin, chloramphenicol and, in severely toxemic patients, cotrimoxazole, ciprofloxacin, or ceftriaxone. Localized abscesses may also need surgical drainage.

Enterocolitis requires a short course of antibiotics only if it causes septicemia or prolonged fever. Other treatments include bed rest and replacement of fluids and electrolytes. Camphorated opium tincture, kaolin with pectin, diphenoxylate hydrochloride, codeine, or small doses of morphine may be necessary to relieve diarrhea and control cramps in patients who must remain active.

Special considerations

▶ Follow standard precautions. Always wash your hands thoroughly before and after any contact with the patient, and advise other hospital personnel to do the same. Teach the patient to use proper handwashing technique, especially after defecating and before eating or handling food. Wear gloves and a gown when disposing of feces or fecally contaminated objects.

▶ Continue standard precautions until three consecutive stool cultures are negative — the first one 48 hours after antibiotic treatment ends, followed by two more at 24-hour intervals.

▶ Observe the patient closely for indications of bowel perforation: sudden pain in the lower right abdomen, possibly after one or more rectal bleeding episodes; sudden fall in temperature or blood pressure; and rising pulse rate.

▶ During acute infection, allow the patient as much rest as possible. Raise the side rails and use other safety measures because the patient may become delirious.

▶ The patient should have a room close to the nurses' station so he can be checked on often. Use a room deodorizer (preferably electric) to minimize odor from diarrhea and to provide a comfortable atmosphere for rest.

▶ Accurately record intake and output. Maintain adequate I.V. hydration. When the patient can tolerate oral feedings, encourage high-calorie fluids such as milk shakes. Watch for constipation.

▶ Provide good skin and mouth care. Turn the patient frequently, and perform mild passive exercises as indicated. Apply mild heat to the abdomen to relieve cramps.

▶ Don't administer antipyretics. These mask fever and lead to possible hypothermia. Instead, to promote heat loss through the skin without causing shivering (which keeps fever high by vasoconstriction), apply tepid, wet towels (don't use alcohol or ice) to the patient's groin and axillae. To promote heat loss by vasodilation of peripheral blood vessels, use additional wet towels on the arms and legs, wiping with long, vigorous strokes.

▶ After draining the abscesses of a joint, provide heat, elevation, and passive range-of-motion exercises to decrease swelling and maintain mobility.

▶ If the patient has positive stool cultures on discharge, tell him to use a different bathroom than other family members if possible (while he's on antibiotics); to wash his hands afterwards; and to avoid preparing uncooked foods, such as salads, for family members.

 PREVENTION TIP To prevent salmonellosis, advise prompt refrigeration of meat and cooked foods (avoid keeping them at room temperature for any prolonged period), and teach the importance of proper hand washing. Advise those at high risk of contracting typhoid (laboratory workers, travelers) to seek vaccination.

SCABIES

An age-old skin infection, scabies results from infestation with *Sarcoptes scabiei* var. *hominis* (itch mite), which provokes a sensitivity reaction. It occurs worldwide, is predisposed by overcrowding and poor hygiene, and can be endemic.

Causes
Mites can live their entire life cycles in the skin of humans, causing chronic infection. The female mite burrows into the skin to lay her eggs, from which larvae emerge to copulate and then reburrow under the skin. (See *Scabies: Cause and effect,* page 268.)

Transmission of scabies occurs through skin or sexual contact. The adult mite can survive without a human host for only 2 or 3 days.

Signs and symptoms
Typically, scabies causes itching that intensifies at night. Characteristic lesions take many forms but are usually excoriated and may appear as erythematous nodules.

Burrows are threadlike lesions approximately 3/8" long and generally occur between fingers, on flexor surfaces of the wrists, on elbows, in axillary folds, at the waistline, on nipples in females, and on genitalia in males. In infants, the burrows may appear on the head and neck.

Intense scratching can lead to severe excoriation and secondary bacterial infection. Itching may become generalized secondary to sensitization.

Diagnosis
A drop of mineral oil placed over the burrow, followed by superficial scraping and examination of expressed material under a low-power microscope, may reveal the mite, ova, or mite feces. However, excoriation or inflammation of the burrow often makes such identification difficult.

If diagnostic tests offer no positive identification of the mite and if scabies is still suspected (for example, if close contacts of the patient also report itching), skin clearing that occurs after a therapeutic trial of a pediculicide confirms the diagnosis. Other conditions to consider include eczema, pruritus, and insect bites.

Treatment
Generally, treatment of scabies consists of application of a pediculicide — permethrin cream or lindane lotion — in a thin layer over the entire skin surface. The pediculicide is left on for 8 to 12 hours. To make certain that all areas have been treated, this application should be repeated in approximately 1 week. Another pediculicide, crotamiton cream, may be applied on 5 consecutive nights but is not as effective. Widespread bacterial infections require systemic antibiotics.

Persistent pruritus (from mite sensitization or contact dermatitis) may develop from repeated use of pediculicides rather than from continued infection. An antipruritic emollient or topical steroid can reduce itching; intralesional steroids may resolve erythematous nodules.

Special considerations
▶ Instruct the adult patient to apply permethrin cream or lindane lotion at bedtime from the neck down, covering the entire body. The cream or lotion should be washed off in 8 to 12 hours. Contaminated clothing and linens must be washed in hot water or dry-cleaned.
▶ Tell the patient not to apply lindane lotion if skin is raw or inflamed. Advise the patient to report any skin irritation or hypersensitivity reaction immediately, to dis-

SCABIES: CAUSE AND EFFECT

Infestation with *Sarcoptes scabiei* (the itch mite) causes scabies. This mite (shown enlarged below) has a hard shell and measures a microscopic 0.1 mm. The second illustration shows the erythematous nodules with excoriation that appear in patients with scabies. These lesions are highly pruritic.

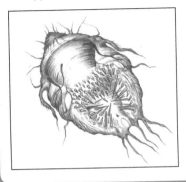 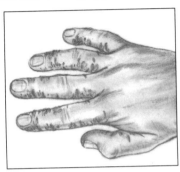

continue using the drug, and to wash it off thoroughly.

▶ Suggest that family members and other close contacts of the patient be checked for possible symptoms and be treated if necessary.

▶ If a hospitalized patient has scabies, prevent transmission to other patients: Practice good hand-washing technique or wear gloves when touching the patient, observe wound and skin precautions for 24 hours after treatment with a pediculicide, gas autoclave blood pressure cuffs before using them on other patients, isolate linens until the patient is noninfectious, and thoroughly disinfect the patient's room after discharge.

SCARLET FEVER

Scarlet fever is an infectious disease caused by Group A beta-hemolytic streptococcal bacteria (GAS). The disease most commonly arises from tonsillar and pharyngeal infections, although it may follow streptococcal infections of the skin and soft tissue, surgical wounds (surgical scarlet fever), or the uterus (puerperal scarlet fever), making definitive diagnosis of scarlet fever difficult in these cases.

Considered a childhood disease, and formerly known as scarlatina, scarlet fever is a syndrome caused by exotoxins produced by GAS, and is characterized by a scarlatiniform rash. Over the past century, the number of cases of reported scarlet fever has remained high. Scarlet fever occurs predominately in children ages 5 to 15. The disease tends to be rare in children under age 2, likely because of acquired immunity from maternal anti-exotoxin antibodies and lack of prior sensitization. By age 10, 80% of all children have developed life-long protective antibodies against streptococcal pyrogenic exotoxins.

Scarlet fever occurs year round, but the incidence of pharyngeal disease is highest in the winter and spring months. Up to 10% of GAS pharyngitis cases contract scarlet fever. Acquisition of the disease is high in over-crowded situations such as schools, childcare settings, hospitals, and areas of lower socioeconomic status. Today, due to the widespread use of antibiotics, scarlet fever runs a benign course with a death rate of less than 2%. Suppurative complications are the most common cause of death. Prognosis is excellent, with most patients having a full recovery.

Causes

Most cases of scarlet fever are associated with GAS replication in the tonsillar and pharyngeal regions. GAS secretes a number of toxins, enzymes, and erythrogenic toxins. These erythrogenic toxins cause the rash of scarlet fever. The epidemiology of GAS is complex. Five separate and distinct streptococcal pyrogenic exotoxins (SPEs) have been described. Hypersensitivity to the exotoxins of GAS contributes to the susceptibility of contracting the disease. It is proposed that minor changes in the structure of the bacteria's DNA over time has caused GAS to become more invasive and severe, allowing it to mimic a virus. Transmission of the bacteria is most common via airborne respiratory particles. The incubation period for scarlet fever is 12 hours to 7 days, but persons infected are contagious during the acute illness and before the appearance of clinical signs and symptoms. Isolation of infected individuals is essential. Children should not return to school or day care settings until 24 hours of antibiotic therapy has been completed.

Signs and symptoms

Most people who have contracted scarlet fever initially appear moderately well — presenting with raw, red tonsils and pharynx with or without exudates. Other symptoms include fever, headache, abdominal pain, and vomiting.

The characteristic rash of scarlet fever appears 12 to 24 hours after the onset of the illness, first on the trunk then extending rapidly over the entire body to finally involve the extremities. It then becomes especially prominent in the skin folds of the axilla, groin, and buttocks, producing Patia's lines, which are lines of petechiae

caused by increased capillary fragility. The rash consists of scarlet macules overlying generalized erythema. The erythema blanches with pressure. Between days 1 and 5, the rash eruptions become more palpable than visible, having the texture of coarse sandpaper or goose bumps. By day 3 to 4 after the onset of the rash, it will begin to fade and a desquamation period begins, with peeling of the face, palms, and fingers occurring between days 7 and 10. This phase can continue for up to 6 weeks, the extension and duration being directly related to the initial intensity of the rash.

The tongue also exhibits specific and characteristic signs and symptoms of scarlet fever infection. During the first 2 days, it will have a white coating through which red and edematous papillae project. This is called "white strawberry tongue". After 2 days, the tongue desquamates, resulting in a red tongue with prominent papillae, called "red strawberry tongue".

Although rare, complications may arise from scarlet fever infection, such as arthritis, bronchopneumonia, pericarditis, peritonsillar abscess, sinusitis, jaundice, otitis media, meningitis, cervical lymphadenitis, brain abscess, and septicemia. Rare — but potentially fatal — complications include early toxin-related diagnoses, such as myocarditis and toxic shock syndrome. Late complications, such as rheumatic fever and glomerulonephritis, are associated with immune deficiency and may appear weeks to months after illness.

Diagnosis

Throat culture remains the definitive diagnostic tool for confirming a GAS upper respiratory infection. Throat cultures are about 90% sensitive for the presence of GAS in the pharynx. Direct antigen detection kits, also known as Rapid Antigen Tests (RATs), have been found to be sensitive only 50% to 90% of the time, and if the results are negative, a throat culture must be performed. With positive results, however, these RATs allow immediate di-

TYPES OF SCHISTOSOMES

SPECIES AND INCIDENCE	SIGNS AND SYMPTOMS	TREATMENT
Schistosoma mansoni Western hemisphere, particularly Puerto Rico, Lesser Antilles, Brazil, and Venezuela; also Nile delta, Sudan, and central Africa	Irregular fever, malaise, weakness, abdominal distress, weight loss, diarrhea, ascites, hepatosplenomegaly, portal hypertension, fistulas, intestinal stricture	Praziquantel: 60 mg/kg in three equally divided doses at 4- to 6-hour intervals on the same day
Schistosoma japonicum Affects men more than women; particularly prevalent among farmers in Japan, China, and the Philippines	Irregular fever, malaise, weakness, abdominal distress, weight loss, diarrhea, ascites, hepatosplenomegaly, portal hypertension, fistulas, intestinal stricture	Praziquantel: 60 mg/kg in three equally divided doses at 4- to 6-hour intervals on the same day
Schistosoma haematobium Africa, Cyprus, Greece, India	Terminal hematuria, dysuria, ureteral colic; with secondary infection — colicky pain, intermittent flank pain, vague GI complaints, total renal failure	Praziquantel: 60 mg/kg in three equally divided doses at 4- to 6-hour intervals on the same day

agnosis and prompt administration of antibiotics.

Serologic tests include streptococcal antibody tests to confirm recent GAS infection, but are not useful as a diagnostic tool during the acute phase of the illness. These tests include the Antistreptolysin O Titer (ASO) and the Streptozyme test.

Other conditions to consider include erythema multiforme, pediatric Kawasaki disease, pediatric measles, rubella, Rocky Mountain spotted fever, infectious mononucleosis, roseola, secondary syphilis, staphylococcal scalded skin syndrome, viral exanthema, Mycoplasma pneumoniae, exfoliative dermatitis, pediatric pharyngitis and pneumonia, scabies, toxic epidermal necrolysis, toxic shock syndrome, severe sunburn, and drug hypersensitivities.

Treatment

Treatment of scarlet fever involves a standard 10-day course of penicillin or erythromycin. Treatment of streptococcal infections is primarily focused on the prevention of acute renal failure from poststreptococcal glomerulonephritis. Acute renal failure is prevented even if antibiotic treatment is initiated 1 week after onset of acute pharyngitis. Supportive care would include hospitalization and I.V. therapy for those with difficulty swallowing secondary to throat pain and swelling.

Special considerations

▶ Stress the importance of prompt and complete antibiotic therapy.
▶ Teach the signs and symptoms of complications related to scarlet fever.
▶ To maximize sensitivity of test results, throat cultures must be properly obtained.

ADVERSE EFFECTS

Abdominal discomfort, dizziness, drowsiness, fever, headache, malaise, minimal increase in liver enzyme levels, nausea, urticaria

Abdominal discomfort, dizziness, drowsiness, fever, headache, malaise, minimal increase in liver enzyme levels, nausea, urticaria

Abdominal discomfort, dizziness, drowsiness, fever, headache, malaise, minimal increase in liver enzyme levels, nausea, urticaria

The posterior pharynx and tonsils and any exudates present should be swabbed vigorously with a cotton or Dacron swab under strong lighting to allow for maximum visualization. Caution should be maintained to avoid touching the swab to the lips, tongue, or buccal membranes to prevent contamination of the specimen.

▶ Be aware that prior antibiotic therapy will alter tests, causing negative throat cultures and a delayed or negative ASO titer.

▶ Care should be taken in disposing of all purulent drainage.

▶ Offer comfort measures, such as acetaminophen or ibuprofen to relieve pain and reduce fever. Soothing gargles for adults and children who can gargle safely will help relieve sore throat pain. Cool mist humidifiers soothe breathing passages and throat discomfort. A liquid diet can be incorporated including warm soups and cool fluids for patients who are having difficulty swallowing.

▶ Patients must be instructed on the importance of completing their entire course of antibiotic therapy, even if their symptoms have resolved. Patients should be warned that they will have generalized exfoliation over the course of the next 2 to 6 weeks.

▶ Review the warning signs and symptoms for complications secondary to scarlet fever, such as persistent fever, increased throat or sinus pain, and generalized swelling (possible renal impairment) and the need for prompt reporting of these to a physician.

SCHISTOSOMIASIS

Schistosomiasis, also known as bilharzia, is a slowly progressive disease caused by blood flukes of the class Trematoda. There are three major types: *Schistosoma mansoni* and *S. japonicum* infect the intestinal tract; *S. haematobium* infects the urinary tract. (See *Types of schistosomes.*) The degree of infection determines the intensity of illness. Complications — such as portal hypertension, pulmonary hypertension, heart failure, ascites, hematemesis from ruptured esophageal varices, and renal failure — can be fatal.

Causes

The mode of transmission is bathing, swimming, wading, or working in water contaminated with Schistosoma larvae. These larvae penetrate the skin or mucous membranes and eventually work their way to the liver's venous portal circulation. There, they mature in 1 to 3 months. The adults then migrate to other parts of the body.

The female cercariae lay spiny eggs in blood vessels surrounding the large intestine or bladder. After penetrating the mucosa of these organs, the eggs are excreted in feces or urine. If the eggs hatch in fresh water, the first-stage larvae (miracidia) penetrate freshwater snails, which act as passive intermediate hosts. Cercariae produced in snails escape into water and begin a new life cycle.

Signs and symptoms

Initial signs and symptoms of schistosomiasis depend on the site of infection and the stage of the disease. Initially, a transient, pruritic rash develops at the site of cercariae penetration, along with fever, myalgia, and cough. Later signs and symptoms may include hepatomegaly, splenomegaly, and lymphadenopathy. Worm migration and egg deposition may cause such complications as flaccid paralysis, seizures, and skin abscesses.

Diagnosis

Typical symptoms and a history of travel to endemic areas suggest the diagnosis; ova in the urine or stool or a mucosal lesion biopsy confirms it. The white blood cell count shows eosinophilia.

Treatment

The treatment of choice is the anthelmintic drug praziquantel. Between 3 and 6 months after treatment, the patient will need to be examined again. If this checkup detects any living eggs, treatment may be resumed.

 PREVENTION TIP To help prevent schistosomiasis, teach those in endemic areas the importance of a pure water supply and to avoid contaminated water. If they must enter this water, tell them to wear protective clothing and to dry themselves afterward.

SEPTIC ARTHRITIS

A medical emergency, septic (infectious) arthritis is caused by bacterial invasion of a joint, resulting in inflammation of the synovial lining. If the microbes enter the joint cavity, effusion and pyogenesis follow, with eventual destruction of bone and cartilage.

Septic arthritis can lead to ankylosis and even fatal septicemia. However, prompt antibiotic therapy and joint aspiration or drainage cures most patients.

Causes

In most cases of septic arthritis, bacteria spread from a primary site of infection, usually in adjacent bone or soft tissue, through the bloodstream to the joint.

Common infecting microbes include four strains of gram-positive cocci — *Staphylococcus aureus, Streptococcus pyogenes, Streptococcus pneumoniae,* and *Streptococcus viridans* — and two strains of gram-negative cocci — *Neisseria gonorrhoeae* and *Haemophilus influenzae.* Various gram-negative bacilli — *Escherichia coli, Salmonella,* and *Pseudomonas,* for example — also cause infection.

Anaerobic microbes such as gram-positive cocci usually infect adults and children over age 2. *H. influenzae* most often infects children under age 2.

Various factors can predispose a person to septic arthritis. Any concurrent bacterial infection (of the genitourinary or the upper respiratory tract, for example) or serious chronic illness (such as cancer, renal failure, rheumatoid arthritis, systemic lupus erythematosus, diabetes, or cirrhosis) heightens susceptibility. Consequently, alcoholics and elderly people run a higher risk of developing septic arthritis.

Of course, susceptibility increases with diseases that depress the autoimmune system or with prior immunosuppressive therapy. I.V. drug abuse (by heroin addicts, for example) can also cause septic arthritis.

Other predisposing factors include recent articular trauma, joint surgery, intra-articular injections, and local joint abnormalities.

Signs and symptoms

Acute septic arthritis begins abruptly, causing intense pain, inflammation, and swelling of the affected joint, with low-grade fever. It usually affects a single joint.

It most often develops in the large joints but can strike any joint, including the spine and small peripheral joints.

Systemic signs of inflammation may not appear in some patients. Migratory polyarthritis sometimes precedes localization of the infection. If the bacteria invade the hip, pain may occur in the groin, upper thigh, or buttock, or may be referred to the knee.

Diagnosis

Two sets of positive culture and Gram stain smears of skin exudates, sputum, urethral discharge, stools, urine, or nasopharyngeal smear confirm septic arthritis. Joint fluid analysis shows gross pus or watery, cloudy fluid of decreased viscosity, usually with 50,000/µl or more white blood cells (WBCs), primarily neutrophils.

When synovial fluid culture is negative, a positive blood culture may confirm the diagnosis. Synovial fluid glucose is often low compared with a simultaneous 6-hour postprandial blood glucose test.

Other diagnostic measures include the following:

▶ X-rays can show typical changes as early as 1 week after initial infection — distention of joint capsules, for example, followed by narrowing of joint space (indicating cartilage damage) and erosions of bone (joint destruction).

▶ Radioisotope joint scan for less accessible joints (such as spinal articulations) may help detect infection or inflammation but isn't itself diagnostic.

▶ C-reactive protein may be elevated, as well as WBC count, with many polymorphonuclear cells; erythrocyte sedimentation rate is increased.

▶ Lactic assay can distinguish septic from nonseptic arthritis.

Treatment

Antibiotic therapy should begin promptly; it may be modified when sensitivity results become available. Penicillin G is effective against infections caused by *S. aureus, S. pyogenes, S. pneumoniae,* *S. viridans,* and *N. gonorrhoeae.* A penicillinase-resistant penicillin, such as nafcillin, is recommended for penicillin G-resistant strains of *S. aureus;* ampicillin, for *H. influenzae;* gentamicin, for gram-negative bacilli.

Medication selection requires drug sensitivity studies of the infecting organism. Bioassays or bactericidal assays of synovial fluid and bioassays of blood may confirm clearing of the infection.

Treatment of septic arthritis requires monitoring of progress through frequent analysis of joint fluid cultures, synovial fluid WBC counts, and glucose determinations.

Codeine or propoxyphene can be given for pain if needed. (Aspirin causes a misleading reduction in swelling, hindering accurate monitoring of progress.) The affected joint can be immobilized with a splint or traction until movement can be tolerated.

Needle aspiration (arthrocentesis) to remove grossly purulent joint fluid should be repeated daily until fluid appears normal. If excessive fluid is aspirated or the WBC count remains elevated, open surgical drainage (usually arthrotomy with lavage of the joint) may be necessary for resistant infection or chronic septic arthritis.

Late reconstructive surgery is warranted only for severe joint damage and only after all signs of active infection have disappeared, which usually takes several months. In some cases, the recommended procedure may be arthroplasty or joint fusion.

Prosthetic replacement remains controversial; it may exacerbate the infection. However, it has helped patients with damaged femoral heads or acetabula.

Special considerations

▶ Practice strict aseptic technique with all procedures. Prevent contact between immunosuppressed patients and infected patients.

▶ Watch for signs of joint inflammation: heat, redness, swelling, pain, or drainage. Monitor vital signs and fever pattern. Remember that corticosteroids mask signs of infection.

▶ Check splints or traction regularly. Keep the joint in proper alignment, but avoid prolonged immobilization. Start passive range-of-motion exercises immediately, and progress to active exercises as soon as the patient can move the affected joint and put weight on it.

▶ Monitor pain levels and medicate accordingly, especially before exercise (remember that the pain of septic arthritis is easy to underestimate). Administer analgesics and narcotics for acute pain and heat or ice packs for moderate pain.

▶ Carefully evaluate the patient's condition after joint aspiration. Provide emotional support throughout the diagnostic tests and procedures, which should be previously explained to the patient. Warn the patient before the first aspiration that it will be extremely painful.

SEPTIC SHOCK

Second only to cardiogenic shock as the leading cause of shock death, septic shock (usually a result of bacterial infection) causes inadequate blood perfusion and circulatory collapse. It occurs most often among hospitalized patients, especially men over age 40 and women ages 25 to 45.

About 25% of patients who develop gram-negative bacteremia go into shock. Unless vigorous treatment begins promptly, preferably before symptoms fully develop, septic shock rapidly progresses to death (often within a few hours) in up to 80% of these patients.

Causes

In two-thirds of patients, septic shock results from infection with gram-negative bacteria: *Escherichia coli, Klebsiella, Enterobacter, Proteus, Pseudomonas,* and *Bacteroides;* in others, from gram-positive bacteria: *Streptococcus pneumoniae, Streptococcus pyogenes,* and *Actinomyces.* Infections with viruses, rickettsiae, chlamydiae, and protozoa may be complicated by shock.

These microbes produce septicemia in persons whose resistance is already compromised by an existing condition. Infection also results from translocation of bacteria from other areas of the body through surgery, I.V. therapy, and catheters.

Septic shock often occurs in patients hospitalized for primary infection of the genitourinary, biliary, GI, and gynecologic tracts. Other predisposing factors include immunodeficiency, advanced age, trauma, burns, diabetes mellitus, cirrhosis, and disseminated cancer.

Signs and symptoms

Indications of septic shock vary according to the stage of the shock, the microbe causing it, and the age of the patient.

▶ *Early stage:* oliguria, sudden fever (over 101° F [38.3° C]), chills, nausea, vomiting, diarrhea, and prostration.

▶ *Late stage:* restlessness, apprehension, irritability, thirst from decreased cerebral tissue perfusion, tachycardia, and tachypnea. Hypotension, altered level of consciousness, and hyperventilation may be the *only* signs among infants and elderly people.

Hypothermia and anuria are common late signs. Complications of septic shock include disseminated intravascular coagulation (DIC), renal failure, heart failure, GI ulcers, and abnormal hepatic function.

Diagnosis

Observation of one or more typical signs (fever, confusion, nausea, vomiting, hyperventilation) in a patient suspected of having an infection suggests septic shock and necessitates immediate treatment.

In the early stages, arterial blood gas (ABG) analysis indicates respiratory alkalosis (low partial pressure of carbon dioxide [$PaCO_2$], low or normal bicarbonate [HCO_3^-] level, and high pH). As shock progresses, metabolic acidosis develops, with hypoxemia indicated by decreasing PCO_2 (which may increase as respiratory failure ensues), as well as decreasing partial pressure of oxygen, HCO_3^-, and pH levels.

The following laboratory tests support the diagnosis and determine the treatment:

◗ blood cultures to isolate the microbe
◗ decreased platelet count and leukocytosis (15,000 to 30,000/μl)
◗ increased blood urea nitrogen and creatinine levels and decreased creatinine clearance
◗ abnormal prothrombin and partial thromboplastin time
◗ simultaneous measurement of urine and plasma osmolalities for renal failure (urine osmolality below 400 milliosmoles, with a ratio of urine to plasma below 1.5)
◗ decreased central venous pressure (CVP), pulmonary artery wedge pressure (PAWP), and cardiac output (in early septic shock, cardiac output increases)
◗ electrocardiogram demonstrating ST-segment depression, inverted T waves, and arrhythmias resembling myocardial infarction.

Treatment

The first goal of treatment is to monitor and reverse shock through volume expansion. I.V. fluids are administered, and a pulmonary artery catheter is inserted to check pulmonary circulation and PAWP. Administration of whole blood or plasma can then raise the PAWP to a satisfactory level of 14 to 18 mm Hg. A ventilator may be necessary for proper ventilation to overcome hypoxia. A urinary catheter allows accurate measurement of hourly urine output.

Treatment also requires immediate administration of I.V. antibiotics to control the infection. Depending on the organism, the antibiotic combination usually includes an aminoglycoside, such as gentamicin or tobramycin for gram-negative bacteria, combined with a penicillin, such as piperacillin or ticarcillin.

Sometimes treatment includes a cephalosporin, such as cefazolin, and nafcillin for suspected staphylococcal infection instead of ticarcillin. Therapy may also include metronidazole for nonsporulating anaerobes (*Bacteroides*), although it may cause bone marrow depression, and clindamycin, which may produce pseudomembranous enterocolitis.

Appropriate anti-infectives for other causes of septic shock depend on the suspected organism. Other measures to combat infections include surgery to drain and excise abscesses, and debridement.

If shock persists after fluid infusion, treatment with vasopressors, such as dopamine, maintains adequate blood perfusion in the brain, liver, GI tract, kidneys, and skin. Other treatment includes I.V. bicarbonate to correct acidosis and I.V. corticosteroids, which may improve blood perfusion and increase cardiac output.

Special considerations

◗ Determine which of your patients are at high risk for developing septic shock. Know the signs of impending septic shock, but don't rely solely on technical aids to judge the patient's status. Consider any change in mental status and urine output as significant as a change in CVP.
◗ Carefully maintain the pulmonary artery catheter. Check ABG values for adequate oxygenation or gas exchange, watching for any changes.
◗ Keep accurate intake and output records. Maintain adequate urine output (0.5 to 1 ml/kg/hour) and systolic pressure. Be careful to avoid fluid overload.
◗ Monitor serum gentamicin level, and administer drugs.
◗ Watch closely for complications of septic shock: DIC (abnormal bleeding); renal failure (oliguria, increased specific gravity); heart failure (dyspnea, edema, tachycardia, distended neck veins); GI ulcers (hematemesis, melena); and hepatic

abnormalities (jaundice, hypoprothrombinemia, and hypoalbuminemia).

SHIGELLOSIS

Shigellosis, also known as bacillary dysentery, is an acute intestinal infection caused by the bacteria *Shigella,* a short, nonmotile, gram-negative rod. *Shigella* can be classified into four groups, all of which may cause shigellosis: group A (*Shigella dysenteriae*), which is most common in Central America and causes particularly severe infection and septicemia; group B (*Shigella flexneri*); group C (*Shigella boydii*); and group D (*Shigella sonnei*). Typically, shigellosis causes a high fever (especially in children), acute self-limiting diarrhea with tenesmus (ineffectual straining at stool) and, possibly, electrolyte imbalance and dehydration. It's most common in children ages 1 to 4; however, many adults acquire the illness from children.

Shigellosis is endemic in North America, Europe, and the tropics. In the United States, about 23,000 cases appear annually, usually in children or in elderly, debilitated, or malnourished people. Shigellosis commonly occurs among confined populations such as those in mental institutions; it's also common in hospitals.

The prognosis is good. Mild infections usually subside within 10 days; severe infections may persist for 2 to 6 weeks. With prompt treatment, shigellosis is fatal in only 1% of cases, although in severe *Shigella dysenteriae* epidemics, mortality may reach 8%.

Causes

Transmission occurs through the fecal-oral route, by direct contact with contaminated objects, or through ingestion of contaminated food or water. Occasionally, the housefly is a vector.

Signs and symptoms

After an incubation period of 1 to 4 days, *Shigella* bacteria invade the intestinal mucosa and cause inflammation. In children, shigellosis usually produces high fever, diarrhea with tenesmus, nausea, vomiting, irritability, drowsiness, and abdominal pain and distention. Within a few days, the child's stool may contain pus, mucus, and — from the superficial intestinal ulceration typical of this infection — blood. Without treatment, dehydration and weight loss are rapid and overwhelming.

In adults, shigellosis produces sporadic, intense abdominal pain, which may be relieved at first by passing formed stools. Eventually, however, it causes rectal irritability, tenesmus and, in severe infection, headache and prostration. Stools may contain pus, mucus, and blood. In adults, shigellosis doesn't usually cause fever.

Complications of shigellosis, such as electrolyte imbalance (especially hypokalemia), metabolic acidosis, and shock, are not common but may be fatal in children and debilitated patients. Less common complications include conjunctivitis, iritis, arthritis, rectal prolapse, secondary bacterial infection, acute blood loss from mucosal ulcers, and toxic neuritis.

Diagnosis

Fever (in children) and diarrhea with stools containing blood, pus, and mucus point to this diagnosis; microscopic bacteriologic studies and culture help confirm it.

Microscopic examination of a fresh stool may reveal mucus, red blood cells, and polymorphonuclear leukocytes; direct immunofluorescence with specific antisera may reveal *Shigella*. Severe infection increases hemagglutinating antibodies. Sigmoidoscopy or proctoscopy may reveal typical superficial ulcerations.

Diagnosis must rule out other causes of diarrhea, such as enteropathogenic *Escherichia coli* infection, malabsorption diseases, and amebic or viral diseases.

Treatment

Treatment of shigellosis includes enteric precautions, low-residue diet and, most important, replacement of fluids and electrolytes with I.V. infusions of normal saline solution (with electrolytes) in sufficient quantities to maintain a urine output of 40 to 50 ml/hour. Antibiotics are of questionable value but may be used in an attempt to eliminate the microbe and thereby prevent further spread. Ampicillin, tetracycline, or co-trimoxazole may be useful in severe cases, especially in children with overwhelming fluid and electrolyte loss.

Antidiarrheals that slow intestinal motility are contraindicated in shigellosis because they delay fecal excretion of *Shigella* and prolong fever and diarrhea. An investigational vaccine containing attenuated strains of *Shigella* appears promising in preventing shigellosis.

Special considerations
Supportive care can minimize complications and increase patient comfort.
▶ To prevent dehydration, administer I.V. fluids, as ordered. Measure intake and output (including stools) carefully.
▶ Correct identification of *Shigella* requires examination and culture of fresh stool specimens. Therefore, hand-carry specimens directly to the laboratory. Because shigellosis is suspected, include this information on the laboratory slip.
▶ Use a disposable hot-water bottle to relieve abdominal discomfort, and schedule care to conserve patient strength.

 PREVENTION TIP To help prevent spread of this disease, maintain enteric precautions until microscopic bacteriologic studies confirm that the stool specimen is negative. If a risk of exposure to the patient's stool exists, put on a gown and gloves before entering the room. Keep the patient's (and your own) nails short to avoid harboring microbes. Change soiled linen promptly and store in an isolation container.
▶ During shigellosis outbreaks, obtain stool specimens from all potentially infected staff, and instruct those infected to remain away from work until two stool specimens are negative.

SINUSITIS

Inflammation of the paranasal sinuses is a common problem. The most common type, maxillary sinusitis, is followed in frequency by ethmoid, frontal, and sphenoid sinusitis. Sinusitis may be acute, subacute, chronic, allergic, or hyperplastic.

Acute sinusitis usually results from the common cold and lingers in subacute form in only about 10% of patients. Chronic sinusitis follows persistent bacterial infection; allergic sinusitis accompanies allergic rhinitis; hyperplastic sinusitis is a combination of purulent acute sinusitis and allergic sinusitis or rhinitis. The prognosis is good for all types.

Causes
Sinusitis may result from viral, bacterial, or fungal infection. The bacteria responsible for acute sinusitis are usually pneumococci, other streptococci, *Haemophilus influenzae,* and *Moraxella catarrhalis.* Staphylococci and gram-negative bacteria are more likely to occur in chronic cases or in patients in intensive care.

On rare occasions, fungi can also be an etiologic factor. *Aspergillus fumigatus* is the fungus most frequently associated with sinus disease.

Predisposing factors include any condition that interferes with drainage and ventilation of the sinuses, such as chronic nasal edema, deviated septum, viscous mucus, nasal polyps, allergic rhinitis, nasal intubation, nasogastric tubes, or debilitation related to chemotherapy; malnutrition, diabetes, blood dyscrasias, chronic use of steroids, or immunodeficiency.

Bacterial invasion commonly occurs from the conditions listed above or after a viral infection. It may also result from swimming in contaminated water.

Signs and symptoms
The primary symptom of *acute sinusitis* is nasal congestion, followed by a gradual buildup of pressure in the affected sinus. For 24 to 48 hours after onset, nasal dis-

charge may be present and later may become purulent. Associated symptoms include malaise, sore throat, headache, low-grade fever (temperature of 99° to 99.5° F [37.2° to 37.5° C]), malodorous breath, painless morning periorbital swelling, and a sense of facial fullness.

Characteristic pain depends on the affected sinus: maxillary sinusitis causes pain over the cheeks and upper teeth; ethmoid sinusitis, pain over the eyes or retroorbital; frontal sinusitis, pain over the eyebrows; and sphenoid sinusitis (rare), pain behind the eyes with radiation to the occiput or to the upper half of the face.

Purulent nasal drainage that continues for longer than 3 weeks after an acute infection subsides suggests *subacute sinusitis*. Other clinical features of the subacute form include a stuffy nose, vague facial discomfort, fatigue, and a nonproductive cough.

The effects of *chronic sinusitis* are similar to those of acute sinusitis, but the chronic form causes continuous mucopurulent discharge.

The effects of *allergic sinusitis* are the same as those of allergic rhinitis. In both conditions, the prominent symptoms are sneezing, frontal headache, watery nasal discharge, and a stuffy, burning, itchy nose.

In *hyperplastic sinusitis,* bacterial growth on the diseased tissue causes pronounced tissue edema. Thickening of the mucosal lining, as well as the development of mucosal polyps, combine to produce chronic stuffiness of the nose in addition to headaches.

Diagnosis

The following measures are useful:
◗ Nasal examination reveals inflammation and pus.
◗ Four view sinus X-rays reveal cloudiness in the affected sinus, air and fluid, and any thickening of the mucosal lining.
◗ Antral puncture promotes drainage of purulent material. It may also be used to provide a specimen for culture and sensitivity testing of the infecting microbe, but is rarely done.
◗ Ultrasonography and computed tomography (CT) scan aid in diagnosing suspected complications. CT scans are more sensitive than routine X-rays in detecting sinusitis.

The common cold and allergic or vasomotor rhinitis are the most common causes of sinus symptoms. Other conditions that produce symptoms resembling sinusitis include polyps, tumors, cysts, foreign bodies, and vasculitides such as Wegener's granulomatosis.

Treatment

In acute sinusitis, local decongestants usually are tried before systemic decongestants; steam inhalation may also be helpful. Local application of heat may help to relieve pain and congestion.

Antibiotics are necessary to combat purulent or persistent infection. (The patient should be aware that allergic reactions to penicillin can occur.) Amoxicillin, ampicillin, and trimethoprim-sulfamethoxazole are usually the antibiotics of choice; question the patient about any known allergy to penicillin. Sinusitis is a deep-seated infection, so antibiotics should be given for 2 to 3 weeks. Surgery to widen the ostia and drain thick secretions may be necessary in severe acute sinusitis, especially when the disease fails to respond to initial intravenous therapy.

In subacute sinusitis, antibiotics and decongestants may be helpful. Treatment of allergic sinusitis must include treatment of allergic rhinitis — administration of antihistamines, identification of allergens by skin testing, and desensitization by immunotherapy. Severe allergic symptoms may require treatment with corticosteroids and epinephrine.

In both chronic sinusitis and hyperplastic sinusitis, antihistamines, antibiotics, and a steroid nasal spray may relieve pain and congestion. If irrigation fails to relieve symptoms, one or more sinuses may require surgery.

Special considerations

▶ Enforce bed rest, and encourage the patient to drink plenty of fluids to promote drainage. Don't elevate the head of the bed more than 30 degrees.

▶ To relieve pain and promote drainage, apply warm compresses continuously, or four times daily for 2-hour intervals. In addition, give analgesics and antihistamines as needed.

▶ Watch for complications, such as vomiting, chills, fever, edema of the forehead or eyelids, blurred or double vision, and personality changes.

▶ If surgery is necessary, tell the patient what to expect postoperatively: A nasal packing will be in place for 12 to 24 hours after surgery; he'll have to breathe through his mouth and he won't be able to blow his nose. After surgery, monitor for excessive drainage or bleeding and watch for complications.

▶ To prevent edema and promote drainage, place the patient in semi-Fowler's position. To relieve edema and pain and to minimize bleeding, apply ice compresses or a rubber glove filled with ice chips over the nose and iced saline gauze over the eyes. Continue these measures for 24 hours.

▶ Frequently change the mustache dressing or drip pad, and record the consistency, amount, and color of drainage (expect scant, bright red, and clotty drainage).

▶ Because the patient will be breathing through his mouth, provide meticulous mouth care.

▶ Tell the patient that even after the packing is removed, nose blowing may cause bleeding and swelling. If the patient is a smoker, instruct him not to smoke for at least 2 or 3 days after surgery.

▶ Instruct the patient to finish the prescribed antibiotics, even if his symptoms disappear.

▶ Vasoconstrictive nose drops and spray are associated with rebound edema if used for more than 5 to 7 days.

SPOROTRICHOSIS

Sporotrichosis is a chronic disease caused by the fungus *Sporothrix schenckii*. It occurs in three forms: *cutaneous lymphatic,* which produces nodular erythematous primary lesions and secondary lesions along lymphatic channels; *pulmonary,* a rare form that produces a productive cough and pulmonary lesions; and *disseminated,* another rare form that may cause arthritis or osteomyelitis. The course of sporotrichosis is slow, the prognosis is good, and fatalities are rare. However, untreated skin lesions may cause secondary bacterial infection.

Causes

S. schenckii is found in soil, wood, sphagnum moss, and decaying vegetation throughout the world. Because this fungus usually enters through broken skin (the pulmonary form through inhalation), sporotrichosis is more common in horticulturists, agricultural workers, and home gardeners. Perhaps because of occupational exposure, it's more prevalent in adult men than in women and children.

Signs and symptoms

After an incubation period that lasts from 1 week to 3 months, cutaneous lymphatic sporotrichosis produces characteristic skin lesions, usually on the hands or fingers. Each lesion begins as a small, painless, movable subcutaneous nodule, but grows progressively larger, discolors, and eventually ulcerates. Later, additional lesions form along the adjacent lymph node chain. (See *Recognizing sporotrichosis,* page 280.)

Pulmonary sporotrichosis causes a productive cough, lung cavities and nodules, hilar adenopathy, pleural effusion, fibrosis, and the formation of a fungus ball. It's often associated with sarcoidosis and tuberculosis.

Disseminated sporotrichosis produces multifocal lesions that spread from the primary lesion in the skin or lungs. The dis-

RECOGNIZING SPOROTRICHOSIS

Ulceration, swelling, and crusting of nodules on fingers is characteristic of cutaneous lymphatic sporotrichosis.

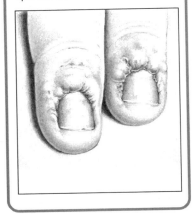

ease begins insidiously, typically causing weight loss, anorexia, synovial or bony lesions and, possibly, arthritis or osteomyelitis.

Diagnosis

Typical clinical findings and a culture of *S. schenckii* in sputum, pus, or bone drainage confirm this diagnosis.

Histologic identification is difficult. Diagnosis must rule out tuberculosis, sarcoidosis and, in patients with the disseminated form, bacterial osteomyelitis and neoplasm.

Treatment

Sporotrichosis doesn't require isolation. The cutaneous lymphatic form usually responds to application of a saturated solution of potassium iodide, generally continued for 1 to 2 months after lesions heal. Occasionally, cutaneous lesions must be excised or drained. The disseminated form responds to itraconazole but may require several weeks of treatment. Local heat ap-

plication relieves pain. Cavitary pulmonary lesions may require surgery.

Special considerations

▶ Keep lesions clean, make the patient as comfortable as possible, and carefully dispose of contaminated dressings.

▶ Warn patients about possible adverse effects of drugs. Because amphotericin B may cause fever, chills, nausea, and vomiting, give antipyretics and antiemetics, as ordered.

▶ To help prevent sporotrichosis, advise horticulturists and home gardeners to wear gloves while working.

STAPHYLOCOCCAL INFECTIONS

Staphylococci are coagulase-negative (*Staphylococcus epidermidis*) or coagulase-positive (*Staphylococcus aureus*) gram-positive bacteria. Coagulase-negative staphylococci grow abundantly as normal flora on skin, but they can also cause boils, abscesses, and carbuncles. In the upper respiratory tract, they are usually nonpathogenic but can cause serious infections. Pathogenic strains of staphylococci are found in many adult carriers — usually on the nasal mucosa, axilla, or groin. Sometimes, carriers shed staphylococci, infecting themselves or other susceptible people. Coagulase-positive staphylococci tend to form pus; they cause many types of infections. (See *Comparing staphylococcal infections,* pages 282 to 287.)

STAPHYLOCOCCAL SCALDED SKIN SYNDROME

A severe skin disorder, staphylococcal scalded skin syndrome (SSSS) is marked by epidermal erythema, peeling, and superficial necrosis that give the skin a scalded appearance. SSSS is most prevalent in

IDENTIFYING STAPHYLOCOCCAL SCALDED SKIN SYNDROME

Staphylococcal scalded skin syndrome is a severe skin disorder that commonly affects infants and children. The illustration below shows the typical scalded skin appearance, with areas of denuded skin found in an infant.

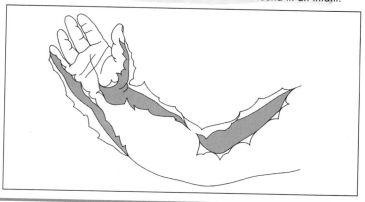

infants ages 1 to 3 months but may develop in children; it's rare in adults.

This disease follows a consistent pattern of progression, and most patients recover fully. Mortality is 2% to 3%, with death usually resulting from complications of fluid and electrolyte loss, sepsis, and involvement of other body systems.

Causes

The causative microbe in SSSS is Group 2 *Staphylococcus aureus,* primarily phage type 71. Predisposing factors may include impaired immunity and renal insufficiency — present to some extent in the normal neonate because of immature development of these systems.

Signs and symptoms

SSSS can often be traced to a prodromal upper respiratory tract infection, possibly with concomitant purulent conjunctivitis. Cutaneous changes progress through three stages.

▶ *Erythema:* In the first stage, erythema becomes visible, usually around the mouth and other orifices, as well as body fold areas, and may spread in widening circles over the entire body surface. The skin becomes tender; Nikolsky's sign (sloughing of the skin when friction is applied) may appear.

▶ *Exfoliation:* About 24 to 48 hours later, exfoliation occurs. In the more common, localized form of this disease, superficial erosions and minimal crusting develop, generally around body orifices, and may spread to exposed areas of the skin. In the more severe forms of this disease, large, flaccid bullae erupt and may spread to cover extensive areas of the body. These bullae eventually rupture, revealing denuded skin.

▶ *Desquamation:* In this final stage, affected areas dry up and powdery scales form. Normal skin replaces these scales in 5 to 7 days. (See *Identifying staphylococcal scalded skin syndrome.*)

Diagnosis

Careful observation of the three-stage progression of this disease allows diagnosis. Results of exfoliative cytology and a biopsy aid in the differential diagnosis, ruling out erythema multiforme and drug-induced

COMPARING STAPHYLOCOCCAL INFECTIONS

PREDISPOSING FACTORS	SIGNS AND SYMPTOMS	DIAGNOSIS
Bacteremia ▶ Infected surgical wounds ▶ Abscesses ▶ Infected I.V. or intra-arterial catheter sites or catheter tips ▶ Infected vascular grafts or prostheses ▶ Infected pressure ulcers ▶ Osteomyelitis ▶ Parenteral drug abuse ▶ Source unknown (primary bacteremia) ▶ Cellulitis ▶ Burns ▶ Immunosuppression ▶ Debilitating diseases, such as chronic renal insufficiency and diabetes ▶ Infective endocarditis (coagulase-positive staphylococci) and subacute bacterial endocarditis (coagulase-negative staphylococci) ▶ Cancer (leukemia) or neutrophil nadir after chemotherapy or radiation	▶ Fever (high fever with no obvious source in children under age 1), shaking chills, tachycardia ▶ Cyanosis or pallor ▶ Confusion, agitation, stupor ▶ Skin microabscesses ▶ Joint pain ▶ Complications: shock; acute bacterial endocarditis (in prolonged infection; indicated by new or changing systolic murmur); retinal hemorrhages; splinter hemorrhages under nails and small, tender red nodes on pads of fingers and toes (Osler's nodes); abscess formation in skin, bones, lungs, brain, and kidneys; pulmonary emboli if tricuspid valve is infected ▶ Prognosis poor in patients over age 60 or with chronic illness	▶ Blood cultures (two to four samples from different sites at different times): growing staphylococci and leukocytosis (usually 12,000 white blood cells [WBCs]/µl), with shift to the left of polymorphonuclear leukocytes (70% to 90% neutrophils) ▶ Urinalysis: microscopic hematuria. ▶ Erythrocyte sedimentation rate (ESR): elevated, especially in chronic or subacute bacterial endocarditis ▶ Severe anemia or thrombocytopenia (possible) ▶ Prolonged partial thromboplastin time and prothrombin time; low fibrinogen and platelet counts, and low factor assays; possible disseminated intravascular coagulation ▶ Cultures of urine, sputum, and draining skin lesions; chest X-rays; scans of lungs, liver, abdomen, and brain: may identify primary infection site ▶ Echocardiogram: may show heart valve vegetation

toxic epidermal necrolysis, both of which are similar to SSSS.

A blood culture is necessary to rule out sepsis.

Treatment
Systemic antibiotics, usually penicillinase-resistant penicillin, treat the underlying infection. Replacement measures maintain fluid and electrolyte balance.

Special considerations
▶ Provide special care for the neonate if required, including placement in a warming infant incubator to maintain body temperature and provide isolation.
▶ Carefully monitor intake and output to assess fluid and electrolyte balance. In severe cases, I.V. fluid replacement may be necessary.

TREATMENT

▶ Semisynthetic penicillins (oxacillin, nafcillin) or cephalosporins (cefazolin) given I.V.
▶ Vancomycin I.V. for those with penicillin allergy or suspected methicillin-resistant organism
▶ Possibly, probenecid given to partially prevent urinary excretion of penicillin and to prolong blood levels
▶ I.V. fluids to reverse shock
▶ Removal of infected catheter or foreign body
▶ Surgery

SPECIAL CONSIDERATIONS

▶ *S. aureus* bacteremia can be fatal within 12 hours. Be especially alert for it in debilitated patients with I.V. catheters or in those with a history of drug abuse.
▶ Administer antibiotics on time to maintain adequate blood levels, but give them slowly, using the prescribed amount of diluent, to prevent thrombophlebitis.
▶ Watch for signs of penicillin allergy, especially pruritic rash (possible anaphylaxis). Keep epinephrine 1:1,000 and resuscitation equipment handy. Monitor vital signs, urine output, and mental state for signs of shock.
▶ Obtain cultures carefully, and observe for clues to the primary site of infection. Never refrigerate blood cultures; it delays identification of organisms by slowing their growth.
▶ Impose wound and skin precautions if the primary site of infection is draining. Special blood precautions are not necessary because the number of organisms present, even in fulminant bacteremia, is minimal.
▶ Obtain peak and trough levels of vancomycin to determine the adequacy of treatment.

(continued)

▶ Check vital signs. Be especially alert for a sudden rise in temperature, indicating sepsis, which requires prompt, aggressive treatment.
▶ Maintain skin integrity. Remember to use strict aseptic technique to preclude secondary infection, especially during the exfoliative stage, because of open lesions.
▶ To prevent friction and sloughing of the patient's skin, leave affected areas un-covered or loosely covered. Place cotton between fingers and toes that are severely affected to prevent webbing.
▶ Administer warm baths and soaks during the recovery period. Gently debride exfoliated areas.
▶ Reassure parents that complications are rare and residual scars are unlikely.

(Text continues on page 289.)

COMPARING STAPHYLOCOCCAL INFECTIONS (continued)

PREDISPOSING FACTORS	SIGNS AND SYMPTOMS	DIAGNOSIS

Pneumonia

▶ Immune deficiencies, especially in elderly people and in children under age 2
▶ Chronic lung diseases and cystic fibrosis
▶ Malignant tumors
▶ Antibiotics that kill normal respiratory flora but spare *S. aureus*
▶ Viral respiratory infections, especially influenza
▶ Hematogenous (blood-borne) bacteria spread to the lungs from primary sites of infections (such as heart valves, abscesses, and pulmonary emboli)
▶ Recent bronchial or endotracheal suctioning or intubation

▶ High temperature: adults, 103° to 105° F (39.4° to 40.6° C); children, 101° F (38.3° C)
▶ Cough, with purulent, yellow, or bloody sputum
▶ Dyspnea, crackles, and decreased breath sounds
▶ Pleuritic pain
▶ In infants: mild respiratory infection that suddenly worsens: irritability, anxiety, dyspnea, anorexia, vomiting, diarrhea, spasms of dry coughing, marked tachypnea, expiratory grunting, sternal retractions, and cyanosis
▶ Complications: necrosis, lung abscess, pyopneumothorax; empyema; pneumatocele; shock, hypotension, oliguria or anuria, cyanosis, loss of consciousness

▶ WBC count elevated (15,000 to 40,000/µl in adults; 15,000 to 20,000/µl in children), with predominance of polymorphonuclear leukocytes
▶ Sputum Gram stain: mostly gram-positive cocci in clusters, with many polymorphonuclear leukocytes
▶ Sputum culture: mostly coagulase-positive staphylococci
▶ Chest X-rays: usually patchy infiltrates
▶ Arterial blood gas analysis: hypoxia and respiratory acidosis

Enterocolitis

▶ Broad-spectrum antibiotics (tetracycline, chloramphenicol, or neomycin) or aminoglycosides (tobramycin, streptomycin, or kanamycin) as prophylaxis for bowel surgery or treatment of hepatic coma
▶ Usually occurs in elderly people but also in neonates (associated with staphylococcal skin lesions)

▶ Sudden onset of profuse, watery diarrhea usually 2 days to several weeks after start of antibiotic therapy, I.V. or P.O.
▶ Nausea, vomiting, abdominal pain and distention
▶ Hypovolemia and dehydration (decreased skin turgor, hypotension, fever)

▶ Stool Gram stain: many gram-positive cocci and polymorphonuclear leukocytes, with few gram-negative rods
▶ Stool culture: *S. aureus*
▶ Sigmoidoscopy: mucosal ulcerations
▶ Blood studies: leukocytosis, moderately increased blood urea nitrogen level, and decreased serum albumin level

TREATMENT	SPECIAL CONSIDERATIONS

▶ Semisynthetic penicillins (oxacillin, nafcillin) or cephalosporins given I.V.
▶ Vancomycin I.V. for those with penicillin allergy or methicillin-resistant organisms
▶ Isolation until sputum shows minimal numbers of *S. aureus* (about 24 to 72 hours after starting antibiotics)

▶ Use masks with isolated patient because staphylococci from lungs spread by air as well as direct contact. Use gown and gloves only when handling contaminated respiratory secretions. Use respiratory isolation precautions.
▶ Keep the door to the patient's room closed. Don't store extra supplies in the room. Empty suction bottles carefully. Place any articles containing sputum (such as tissues and clothing) in a sealed plastic bag. Mark them "contaminated," and dispose of them promptly by incineration.
▶ When obtaining sputum specimens, make sure you're collecting thick sputum, not saliva. The presence of epithelial cells (found in the mouth, not lungs) indicates a poor specimen.
▶ Administer antibiotics strictly on time, but slowly. Watch for signs of penicillin allergy and for signs of infection at I.V. sites. Change the I.V. site at least every third day.
▶ Perform frequent chest physical therapy. Do chest percussion and postural drainage after intermittent positive pressure breathing treatments. Concentrate on consolidated areas (revealed by X-rays or auscultation).

▶ Broad-spectrum antibiotics discontinued
▶ Possibly, antistaphylococcal agents such as vancomycin P.O.
▶ Normal flora replenished with yogurt

▶ Monitor vital signs frequently to prevent shock. Force fluids to correct dehydration.
▶ Know serum electrolyte levels. Measure and record bowel movements when possible. Check serum chloride level for alkalosis (hypochloremia).
▶ Collect serial stool specimens for Gram stain, and culture for diagnosis and for evaluating effectiveness of treatment.
▶ Observe enteric precautions.
▶ Consider reporting requirements, especially in a group situation such as a nursing home.

(continued)

COMPARING STAPHYLOCOCCAL INFECTIONS *(continued)*

PREDISPOSING FACTORS	SIGNS AND SYMPTOMS	DIAGNOSIS
Osteomyelitis ▶ Hematogenous organisms ▶ Skin trauma ▶ Infection spreading from adjacent joint or other infected tissues ▶ *S. aureus* bacteremia ▶ Orthopedic surgery or trauma ▶ Cardiothoracic surgery ▶ Occurs in growing bones of children under age 12	▶ Abrupt onset of fever — usually 101° F (38.3° C); shaking chills; pain and swelling over infected area; restlessness; headache ▶ Chronic infection in about 20% of children, if not properly treated	▶ Positive bone and pus cultures (and blood cultures in about 50% of patients) ▶ X-ray changes apparent after 2nd or 3rd week ▶ ESR elevated with leukocyte shift to the left
Food poisoning ▶ Enterotoxin produced by toxigenic strains of *S. aureus* in contaminated food (second most common cause of food poisoning in U.S.)	▶ Nausea, vomiting, diarrhea, and abdominal cramps 1 to 6 hours after ingestion of contaminated food ▶ Usually subside within 18 hours	▶ Clinical findings sufficient ▶ Stool cultures usually negative for *S. aureus*
Skin infections ▶ Decreased resistance ▶ Burns or pressure ulcers ▶ Decreased blood flow ▶ Possibly skin contamination from nasal discharge ▶ Foreign bodies ▶ Underlying skin diseases, such as eczema and acne ▶ Common in persons with poor hygiene living in crowded quarters	▶ Cellulitis — diffuse, acute inflammation of soft tissue (no drainage) ▶ Pus-producing lesions in and around hair follicles ▶ Boil-like lesions (painful, red, and indurated, 1 to 2 cm, with a purulent yellow discharge) extending from hair follicles to subcutaneous tissues ▶ Small macule or skin bleb that may develop into vesicle containing pus (bullous impetigo); common in school-age children ▶ Mild or spiking fever ▶ Malaise	▶ Clinical findings and analysis of pus cultures if sites are draining ▶ Cultures of nondraining cellulitis taken from the margin of the reddened area by infiltration with 1 ml sterile saline solution and immediate fluid aspiration

TREATMENT	SPECIAL CONSIDERATIONS
▶ Surgical debridement ▶ Prolonged antibiotic therapy (4 to 8 weeks) ▶ Vancomycin I.V. for patients with penicillin allergy or methicillin-resistant organisms	▶ Identify the infected area, and mark it on the care plan. Check the penetration wound from which the organism originated for evidence of present infection. ▶ Severe pain may render the patient immobile. If so, perform passive range-of-motion exercises. Apply heat as needed, and elevate the affected part. (Extensive involvement may require casting until the infection subsides.) ▶ Before such procedures as surgical debridement, warn the patient to expect some pain. Explain that drainage is essential for healing, and that he will continue to receive analgesics and antibiotics after surgery.
▶ No treatment necessary unless dehydration becomes a problem (usually in infants and elderly); then, possible I.V. therapy to replace fluids	▶ Obtain a complete history of symptoms, recent meals, and other episodes of food poisoning. ▶ Monitor vital signs, fluid balance, and serum electrolyte levels. ▶ Check for dehydration if vomiting is severe or prolonged, and for decreased blood pressure. ▶ Observe and report the number and color of stools.
▶ Topical ointments; bacitracin-neomycin-polymyxin or gentamicin ▶ P.O. cloxacillin, dicloxacillin, or erythromycin; I.V. oxacillin or nafcillin for severe infection; I.V. vancomycin for oxacillin-resistant organisms ▶ Application of heat to reduce pain ▶ Surgical drainage ▶ Identification and treatment of sources of reinfection (nostrils, perineum) ▶ Cleaning and covering the area with moist, sterile dressings	▶ Identify the site and extent of infection. ▶ Keep lesions clean with saline solution and peroxide irrigations as ordered. Cover infections near wounds or genitourinary tract with gauze pads. Keep pressure off the site to facilitate healing. ▶ Be alert for the extension of skin infections. ▶ Severe infection or abscess may require surgical drainage. Explain the procedure to the patient. Determine if cultures will be taken, and be ready to collect a specimen. ▶ Impetigo is contagious. Isolate the patient and alert the family. Use secretion precautions for all draining lesions.

TYPES OF ORAL INFECTIONS

DISEASE AND CAUSE	SIGNS AND SYMPTOMS	TREATMENT
Gingivitis (inflammation of the gingiva) ▶ Early sign of hypovitaminosis, diabetes, blood dyscrasias ▶ Occasionally related to use of oral contraceptives	▶ Inflammation with painless swelling, redness, change of normal contours, bleeding, and periodontal pocket (gum detachment from teeth)	▶ Removal of irritating factors (calculus, faulty dentures) ▶ Good oral hygiene; regular dental checkups; vigorous chewing ▶ Oral or topical corticosteroids
Periodontitis (progression of gingivitis; inflammation of the oral mucosa) ▶ Early sign of hypovitaminosis, diabetes, blood dyscrasias ▶ Occasionally related to use of oral contraceptives ▶ Dental factors: calculus, poor oral hygiene, and malocclusion ▶ Major cause of tooth loss after middle-age	▶ Acute onset of bright red gum inflammation, painless swelling of interdental papillae, easy bleeding ▶ Loosening of teeth, typically without inflammatory symptoms, progressing to loss of teeth and alveolar bone ▶ Acute systemic infection (fever, chills)	▶ Scaling, root planing, and curettage for infection control ▶ Periodontal surgery to prevent recurrence ▶ Good oral hygiene, regular dental checkups, vigorous chewing
Vincent's angina (trench mouth, necrotizing ulcerative gingivitis) ▶ Fusiform bacillus or spirochete infection ▶ Predisposing factors: stress, poor oral hygiene, insufficient rest, nutritional deficiency, smoking	▶ Sudden onset: painful, superficial bleeding gingival ulcers (rarely, on buccal mucosa) covered with a gray-white membrane ▶ Ulcers that become punched-out lesions after slight pressure or irritation ▶ Malaise, mild fever, excessive salivation, bad breath, pain on swallowing or talking, enlarged submaxillary lymph nodes	▶ Removal of devitalized tissue with ultrasonic cavitron ▶ Antibiotics (penicillin or erythromycin P.O.) for infection ▶ Analgesics, as needed ▶ Hourly mouth rinses (with equal amounts of hydrogen peroxide and warm water) ▶ Soft, nonirritating diet; rest; no smoking ▶ With treatment, improvement common within 24 hours

TYPES OF ORAL INFECTIONS *(continued)*

DISEASE AND CAUSE	SIGNS AND SYMPTOMS	TREATMENT
Glossitis (inflammation of the tongue) ▶ Streptococcal infection ▶ Irritation or injury; jagged teeth; ill-fitting dentures; biting during convulsions; alcohol; spicy foods; smoking; sensitivity to toothpaste or mouthwash ▶ Vitamin B deficiency; anemia ▶ Skin conditions: lichen planus, erythema multiforme, pemphigus vulgaris	▶ Reddened, ulcerated, or swollen tongue (may obstruct airway) ▶ Painful chewing and swallowing ▶ Speech difficulty ▶ Painful tongue without inflammation	▶ Treatment of underlying cause ▶ Topical anesthetic mouthwash or systemic analgesics (aspirin and acetaminophen) for painful lesions ▶ Good oral hygiene; regular dental checkups; vigorous chewing ▶ Avoidance of hot, cold, or spicy foods, and alcohol

STOMATITIS AND OTHER ORAL INFECTIONS

A common infection, stomatitis — inflammation of the oral mucosa — may extend to the buccal mucosa, lips, and palate. It may occur alone or as part of a systemic disease.

There are two main types: *acute herpetic stomatitis* and *aphthous stomatitis.* Acute herpetic stomatitis is common and mild. Aphthous stomatitis is common in young girls and female adolescents.

Acute herpetic stomatitis is usually short-lived and easily recognized; however, it may be severe and, in neonates, may be generalized and potentially fatal. Aphthous stomatitis usually heals spontaneously, without a scar, in 10 to 14 days.

Other oral infections include gingivitis, periodontitis, Vincent's angina, and glossitis. (See *Types of oral infections.*)

Causes

Acute herpetic stomatitis results from herpes simplex virus. The cause of aphthous stomatitis is unclear.

Signs and symptoms

Acute herpetic stomatitis begins with burning mouth pain. In immunocompromised individuals, reactivation of the herpes simplex virus infection may be frequent and severe. Gums are swollen and bleed easily, and the mucous membranes are extremely tender. Papulovesicular ulcers appear in the mouth and throat and eventually become punched-out lesions with reddened areolae. The small vesicles rupture and form scales. Another common finding is submaxillary lymphadenitis.

Pain usually disappears from 2 to 4 days before healing of ulcers is complete.

A patient with aphthous stomatitis will typically report burning, tingling, and slight swelling of the mucous membrane. Single or multiple small, round ulcers with whitish centers and red borders appear and heal at one site but then appear at another. The painful stage lasts 7 to 10 days, with healing complete in 1 to 3 weeks.

Diagnosis

Physical examination allows diagnosis. In Vincent's angina, a smear of ulcer exudate allows identification of the causative microbe.

Treatment

For acute herpetic stomatitis, treatment is conservative. For local symptoms, management includes warm-water mouth rinses (antiseptic mouthwashes are contraindicated because they're irritating) and a topical anesthetic to relieve mouth ulcer pain.

A course of acyclovir (200 to 800 mg, 5 times daily for 7 to 14 days) may shorten the course and reduce postherpetic pain.

Supplementary treatment includes bland or liquid diet and, in severe cases, I.V. fluids to maintain hydration, and bed rest.

For aphthous stomatitis, primary treatment is application of a topical anesthetic.

Special considerations

▶ Effective long-term treatment requires alleviation or prevention of precipitating factors.

STREPTOCOCCAL INFECTIONS

Streptococci are small gram-positive bacteria, spherical to ovoid in shape and linked together in pairs of chains. Several species occur as part of normal human flora in the respiratory, GI, and genitourinary tracts. Although researchers have identified 21 species of streptococci, three classes — groups A, B, and D — cause most of the infections. Microbes belonging to groups A and B beta-hemolytic streptococci are associated with a characteristic pattern of human infections. Most disorders due to

group D streptococcus are caused by *Enterococcus faecalis,* formerly called *Streptococcus faecalis,* or *Streptococcus bovis.*

Clinically, there are three states of streptococcal infection: carrier, acute, and delayed nonsuppurative complications. In the carrier state, the patient is infected with a disease-causing species of streptococci without evidence of infection. In the acute form, streptococci invade the tissues and cause physical symptoms. In the delayed nonsuppurative complications state, specific complications associated with streptococcal infection occur. These include the inflammatory state of acute rheumatic fever, chorea, and glomerulonephritis. If complications occur, they usually appear about 2 weeks after the acute illness, but they may be evident after a nonsymptomatic illness. (See *Comparing streptococcal infections,* pages 292 through 297.)

STRONGYLOIDIASIS

Strongyloidiasis, also called threadworm infection, is a parasitic intestinal infection caused by the helminth *Strongyloides stercoralis.* This worldwide infection is endemic in the tropics and subtropics. Susceptibility to strongyloidiasis is universal. Infection doesn't confer immunity, and immunocompromised people may suffer overwhelming disseminated infection. Because the threadworm's reproductive cycle may continue in an untreated individual for up to 45 years, autoinfection is highly probable. Most patients with strongyloidiasis recover, but debilitation from protein loss may result in death.

Causes

Transmission to humans usually occurs through contact with soil that contains infective *S. stercoralis* filariform larvae; such larvae develop from noninfective rhabdoid (rod-shaped) larvae in human feces. The filariform larvae penetrate the human skin, usually at the feet, then migrate by way of the lymphatic system to the bloodstream and the lungs.

Once they enter into pulmonary circulation, the filariform larvae break through the alveoli and migrate upward to the pharynx, where they are swallowed. Then, they lodge in the small intestine, where they deposit eggs that mature into noninfectious rhabdoid larvae. Next, these larvae migrate into the large intestine and are excreted in feces, starting the cycle again. The threadworm life cycle — which begins with penetration of the skin and ends with excretion of rhabdoid larvae — takes 17 days.

In autoinfection, rhabdoid larvae mature within the intestine to become infective filariform larvae.

Signs and symptoms

The patient's resistance and the extent of infection determine the severity of symptoms. Some patients have no symptoms, but many develop an erythematous maculopapular rash at the site of penetration that produces swelling and pruritus and that may be confused with an insect bite. As the larvae migrate to the lungs, pulmonary signs develop, including minor hemorrhage, pneumonitis, and pneumonia; later, intestinal infection produces frequent, watery, and bloody diarrhea, accompanied by intermittent abdominal pain.

Severe infection can cause malnutrition from substantial fat and protein loss, anemia, and lesions resembling ulcerative colitis, all of which invite secondary bacterial infection. Ulcerated intestinal mucosa may lead to perforation and, possibly, potentially fatal dissemination, especially in patients with malignancy or immunodeficiency diseases or in those who receive immunosuppressants.

Diagnosis

Diagnosis requires observation of *S. stercoralis* larvae in a fresh stool specimen (2 hours after excretion, rhabdoid larvae look

like hookworm larvae). During the pulmonary phase, sputum may show many eosinophils and larvae; marked eosinophilia also occurs in disseminated strongyloidiasis.

Other helpful tests include:
◗ chest X-ray — positive during pulmonary phase of infection
◗ hemoglobin — as low as 6 to 10 g
◗ white blood cell count with differential (eosinophil count 450 to 700/µl).

Treatment

Because of potential autoinfection, treatment with thiabendazole is required for 2 to 3 days (total dose not to exceed 3 g). Other drugs available for treatment are albendazole and ivermectin. Patients also need protein replacement, blood transfusions, and I.V. fluids. Retreatment is necessary if *S. stercoralis* remains in stools after therapy. Glucocorticoids are contraindicated because they increase the risk of autoinfection and dissemination.

Special considerations

◗ Keep accurate intake and output records, especially if treatment includes blood transfusions and I.V. fluids. Ask the dietary department to provide a high-protein diet. The patient may need tube feedings to increase caloric intake.
◗ Wear gloves when handling bedpans or giving perineal care, and dispose of feces promptly.
◗ Because direct person-to-person transmission doesn't occur, isolation is not required. Label stool specimens for laboratory as contaminated.
◗ Warn the patient that thiabendazole may cause mild nausea, vomiting, drowsiness, and giddiness.
◗ In pulmonary infection, reposition the patient frequently, encourage coughing and deep breathing, and administer oxygen, as ordered.
◗ Check the patient's family and close contacts for signs of infection. Emphasize the

COMPARING STREPTOCOCCAL INFECTIONS

CAUSES AND INCIDENCE	SIGNS AND SYMPTOMS

Streptococcus pyrogenes (Group A streptococcus)

Streptococcal pharyngitis (strep throat)

▶ Accounts for 95% of all cases of bacterial pharyngitis
▶ Most common in children ages 5 to 10 from October to April
▶ Spread by direct person-to-person contact via droplets of saliva or nasal secretions
▶ Usually colonizes throats of persons with no symptoms; up to 20% of school children possible carriers; pets also possible carriers

▶ After 1- to 5-day incubation period: temperature of 101° to 104° F (38.3° to 40° C), sore throat with severe pain on swallowing, beefy red pharynx, tonsillar exudate, edematous tonsils and uvula, swollen glands along the jaw line, generalized malaise and weakness, occasional abdominal discomfort
▶ In up to 40% of small children, symptoms too mild for diagnosis
▶ Fever abating in 3 to 5 days; nearly all symptoms subsiding within a week

Scarlet fever (scarlatina)

▶ Usually follows streptococcal pharyngitis; may follow wound infections or puerperal sepsis
▶ Caused by streptococcal strain that releases an erythrogenic toxin
▶ Most common in children ages 2 to 10
▶ Spread by inhalation or direct contact

▶ Streptococcal sore throat, fever, strawberry tongue, fine erythematous rash that blanches on pressure and resembles sunburn with goosebumps
▶ Rash usually appearing first on upper chest, then spreading to neck, abdomen, legs, and arms, sparing soles and palms; flushed cheeks; pallor around mouth
▶ Skin shedding during convalescence

Erysipelas

▶ Occurs primarily in infants and adults over age 30
▶ Usually follows strep throat
▶ Exact mode of spread to skin unknown

▶ Sudden onset, with reddened, swollen, raised lesions that sting and itch (skin resembles orange peel), usually on face and scalp, bordered by areas that often contain easily ruptured blebs filled with yellow-tinged fluid (Lesions on the trunk, arms, or legs usually affect incision or wound sites.)
▶ Other symptoms: vomiting, fever, headache, cervical lymphadenopathy, sore throat

---

need for follow-up stool examination, continuing for several weeks after treatment.

 PREVENTION TIP To prevent reinfection, teach the patient proper hand-washing technique.

Stress the importance of washing hands before eating and after defecating, and of wearing shoes when in endemic areas.

DIAGNOSIS	COMPLICATIONS	TREATMENT AND SPECIAL CONSIDERATIONS
▶ Clinically indistinguishable from viral pharyngitis ▶ Throat culture showing group A beta-hemolytic streptococci (carriers have positive throat culture) ▶ Elevated white blood cell (WBC) count ▶ Serology shows a four-fold rise in streptozyme titers during convalescence	▶ Most frequently, acute otitis media or acute sinusitis ▶ Rarely, bacteremic spread may cause arthritis, endocarditis, meningitis, osteomyelitis, or liver abscess ▶ Poststreptococcal sequelae: acute rheumatic fever or acute glomerulonephritis ▶ Reye's syndrome	▶ Penicillin or erythromycin, analgesics, and antipyretics ▶ Bed rest and isolation from other children for 24 hours after antibiotic therapy begins ▶ Full compliance with antibiotic treatment with no skipped doses, even if symptoms subside, to avoid abscess, glomerulonephritis, and rheumatic fever ▶ Proper disposal of soiled tissues.
▶ Characteristic rash and strawberry tongue ▶ Culture and Gram stain showing *S. pyogenes* from nasopharynx ▶ Granulocytosis	▶ Rarely, high fever, arthritis, jaundice, pneumonia, pericarditis, and peritonsillar abscess	▶ Penicillin or erythromycin ▶ Isolation for first 24 hours ▶ Careful disposal of purulent discharge ▶ Prompt and complete antibiotic treatment
▶ Typical reddened lesions ▶ Culture taken from edge of lesions showing group A beta-hemolytic streptococci ▶ Throat culture almost always positive for group A beta-hemolytic streptococci	▶ Untreated lesions on trunk, arms, or legs possibly involving large body areas and leading to death	▶ Penicillin or erythromycin I.V. or P.O. ▶ Cold packs, analgesics (aspirin and codeine for local discomfort), topical anesthetics ▶ Prevention: prompt treatment of streptococcal infections, and drainage and secretion precautions

(continued)

STYE

A localized, purulent staphylococcal infection, a stye (or hordeolum) can occur externally (in the lumen of the smaller glands of Zeis or in Moll's glands) or internally (in the larger meibomian gland). A stye can occur at any age. Generally,

(Text continues on page 298.)

COMPARING STREPTOCOCCAL INFECTIONS (continued)

CAUSES AND INCIDENCE	SIGNS AND SYMPTOMS

Streptococcus pyogenes (Group A streptococcus) (continued)

Impetigo (streptococcal pyoderma)

▶ Common in poor children ages 2 to 5 in hot, humid weather; high rate of familial spread
▶ Predisposing factors: close contact in schools, overcrowded living quarters, poor skin hygiene, minor skin trauma
▶ May spread by direct contact, environmental contamination, or arthropod vector

▶ Small macules that rapidly develop into vesicles, then become pustular and encrusted, causing pain, surrounding erythema, regional adenitis, cellulitis, and itching; infection spread by scratching
▶ Lesions that commonly affect the face, heal slowly, and leave depigmented areas

Streptococcal gangrene (necrotizing fasciitis)

▶ More common in elderly patients with arteriosclerotic vascular disease or diabetes
▶ Predisposing factors: surgery, wounds, skin ulcers, diabetes, peripheral vascular disease
▶ Spread by direct contact

▶ Mimics gas gangrene; within 72 hours of onset, red-streaked, painful skin lesions with dusky red surrounding tissue; then, development and rupture of bullae with yellow or reddish black fluid
▶ Other signs and symptoms: fever, tachycardia, lethargy, prostration, disorientation, hypotension, jaundice, hypovolemia, severe pain followed by anesthesia (due to nerve destruction)

Streptococcus agalactiae (Group B streptococcus)

Neonatal streptococcal infections

▶ Incidence of early-onset infection (age 5 days or less): 2/1,000 live births
▶ Incidence of late-onset infection (age 7 days to 3 months): 1/1,000 live births
▶ Predisposing factors: maternal genital tract colonization, membrane rupture over 24 hours before delivery, vaginal delivery, crowded nursery

▶ Early onset: bacteremia, pneumonia, and meningitis; mortality from 14% for infants over 1,500 g at birth to 61% for infants under 1,500 g at birth
▶ Late onset: bacteremia with meningitis, fever, and bone and joint involvement; mortality 15% to 20%
▶ Other signs and symptoms, such as skin lesions, depending on site affected

Adult group B streptococcal infection

▶ Most adult infections occur in postpartum women, usually in the form of endometritis or wound infection following cesarean section
▶ Incidence of group B streptococcal endometritis: 1.3/1,000 live births

▶ Fever, malaise, uterine tenderness
▶ Change in lochia

DIAGNOSIS	COMPLICATIONS	TREATMENT AND SPECIAL CONSIDERATIONS
▶ Characteristic lesions with honey-colored crust ▶ Culture and Gram stain of swabbed lesions showing *S. pyogenes*	▶ Septicemia (rare) ▶ Ecthyma, a form of impetigo with deep ulcers	▶ Penicillin I.V. or P.O., or erythromycin, or antibiotic ointments ▶ Frequent washing of lesions with antiseptics, followed by thorough drying ▶ Isolation of patient with draining wounds ▶ Good hygiene and proper wound care
▶ Culture and Gram stain usually showing *S. pyogenes* from early bullous lesions and commonly from blood	▶ Extensive necrotic sloughing ▶ Bacteremia, metastatic abscesses, and death ▶ Thrombophlebitis, when lower extremities are involved	▶ Immediate, wide, deep surgery of all necrotic tissues ▶ High-dose penicillin I.V. ▶ Good preoperative skin preparation, aseptic surgical and suturing technique
▶ Isolation of group B streptococcus from blood, cerebrospinal fluid (CSF), or skin ▶ Chest X-ray showing massive infiltrate similar to that of respiratory distress syndrome or pneumonia	▶ Overwhelming pneumonia, sepsis, and death	▶ Penicillin or ampicillin and an aminoglycoside I.V. ▶ Patient isolation if open draining lesion is present ▶ Careful hand washing; drainage and secretion precautions, if draining lesion is present ▶ Vaccine in development
▶ Isolation of group B streptococcus from blood or infection site	▶ Bacteremia followed by meningitis or endocarditis	▶ Ampicillin or penicillin I.V. ▶ Observe for symptoms of infection after delivery ▶ Drainage and secretion precautions

(continued)

COMPARING STREPTOCOCCAL INFECTIONS (continued)

CAUSES AND INCIDENCE	SIGNS AND SYMPTOMS

Streptococcus pneumoniae (Group D streptococcus) (continued)

Pneumococcal pneumonia
▶ Accounts for 70% of all cases of bacterial pneumonia
▶ More common in men, elderly people, Blacks, and Native Americans, in winter and early spring
▶ Spread by air and contact with infective secretions
▶ Predisposing factors: trauma, viral infection, underlying pulmonary disease, overcrowded living quarters, chronic diseases, immunodeficiency
▶ Among the 10 leading causes of death in the United States

▶ Sudden onset with severe shaking chills, temperature of 102° to 105° F (38.9° to 40.6° C), bacteremia, cough (with thick, scanty, blood-tinged sputum) accompanied by pleuritic pain
▶ Malaise, weakness, and prostration common
▶ Tachypnea, anorexia, nausea, and vomiting less common
▶ Severity of pneumonia usually due to host's cellular defenses, not bacterial virulence

Otitis media
▶ Occurring at least once in about 76% to 95% of all children, with *S. pneumoniae* causing half of these cases

▶ Ear pain, ear drainage, hearing loss, fever, lethargy, irritability
▶ Other possible symptoms: vertigo, nystagmus, tinnitus

Meningitis
▶ Can follow bacteremic pneumonia, mastoiditis, sinusitis, skull fracture, or endocarditis
▶ Mortality (30% to 60%) highest in infants and in elderly patients

▶ Fever, headache, nuchal rigidity, vomiting, photophobia, lethargy, coma, wide pulse pressure, bradycardia

Endocarditis
▶ Group D streptococcus (enterococcus) causes 10% to 20% of all bacterial endocarditis
▶ Most common in elderly patients and in those who abuse I.V. substances
▶ Often follows bacteremia from an obvious source, such as a wound infection, urinary tract infection, or I.V. insertion site infection
▶ Most cases subacute

▶ Weakness, fatigability, weight loss, fever, night sweats, anorexia, arthralgia, splenomegaly, new systolic murmur

DIAGNOSIS	COMPLICATIONS	TREATMENT AND SPECIAL CONSIDERATIONS
▶ Gram stain of sputum showing gram-positive diplococci; culture showing *S. pneumoniae* ▶ Chest X-ray showing lobular consolidation in adults; bronchopneumonia in children and in elderly patients ▶ Elevated WBC count ▶ Blood cultures often positive for *S. pneumoniae*	▶ Pleural effusion occurs in 25% of patients ▶ Pericarditis (rare) ▶ Lung abscess (rare) ▶ Bacteremia followed by meningitis or endocarditis ▶ Disseminated intravascular coagulation ▶ Death possible if bacteremia is present	▶ Penicillin or erythromycin I.V. or I.M. ▶ Respiratory monitoring and support as needed; recording of sputum color and amount ▶ Fluids to prevent dehydration ▶ Avoidance of sedatives and narcotics to preserve cough reflex ▶ Careful disposal of all purulent drainage (respiratory isolation unnecessary) ▶ For high-risk patients, vaccine and avoidance of infected persons
▶ Fluid in middle ear ▶ Isolation of *S. pneumoniae* from aspirated fluid if necessary	▶ Possible hearing loss from recurrent attacks	▶ Amoxicillin or ampicillin and analgesics ▶ Patient to report lack of response to therapy after 72 hours
▶ Isolation of *S. pneumoniae* from CSF or blood culture ▶ Increased CSF cell count and protein level; decreased CSF glucose level ▶ Computed tomography scan of head ▶ EEG	▶ Persistent hearing deficits, seizures, hemiparesis, or other nerve deficits ▶ Encephalitis	▶ Penicillin I.V. or chloramphenicol ▶ Close monitoring for neurologic changes and symptoms of septic shock, such as acidosis and tissue hypoxia
▶ Anemia, increased erythrocyte sedimentation rate and serum immunoglobulin level, and positive blood culture for group D streptococcus ▶ Echocardiogram showing vegetation on valves	▶ Embolization ▶ Pulmonary infarction ▶ Osteomyelitis	▶ Penicillin for *Streptococcus bovis* (non-enterococcal group D streptococcus) ▶ Penicillin or ampicillin and an aminoglycoside for enterococcal group D streptococcus

RECOGNIZING A STYE

A stye is a localized red, swollen, and tender abscess of the lid margin.

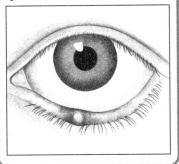

this infection responds well to treatment but tends to recur. If untreated, a stye can eventually lead to cellulitis of the eyelid.

Signs and symptoms

Typically, a stye produces redness, swelling, and pain. An abscess frequently forms at the lid margin, with an eyelash pointing outward from its center. (See *Recognizing a stye*.)

Diagnosis

Visual examination generally confirms this infection. Culture of purulent material from the abscess usually reveals a staphylococcal microbe.

Treatment

Treatment consists of warm compresses applied for 10 to 15 minutes, four times a day for 3 to 4 days, to facilitate drainage of the abscess, to relieve pain and inflammation, and to promote suppuration. Drug therapy includes a topical sulfonamide or antibiotic eyedrops or ointment and, occasionally, a systemic antibiotic for secondary eyelid cellulitis. If conservative treatment fails, incision and drainage may be necessary.

Special considerations

▶ Instruct the patient to use a clean cloth for each application of warm compresses and to dispose of it or launder it separately.
▶ Warn against squeezing the stye; this spreads the infection and may cause cellulitis.
▶ Teach the patient or family members the proper technique for instilling eyedrops or ointments into the cul-de-sac of the lower eyelid.

SYPHILIS

A chronic, infectious, sexually transmitted disease, syphilis begins in the mucous membranes and quickly becomes systemic, spreading to nearby lymph nodes and the bloodstream. This disease, when untreated, is characterized by progressive stages: primary, secondary, latent, and late (formerly called tertiary).

About 34,000 cases of syphilis, in primary and secondary stages, are reported annually in the United States. Incidence is highest among urban populations, especially in persons between ages 15 and 39, drug users, and those infected with the human immunodeficiency virus (HIV).

Untreated syphilis leads to crippling or death, but the prognosis is excellent with early treatment.

Causes

Infection from the spirochete *Treponema pallidum* causes syphilis. Transmission occurs primarily through sexual contact during the primary, secondary, and early latent stages of infection. Prenatal transmission from an infected mother to her fetus is also possible. (See *Prenatal syphilis*.)

Signs and symptoms

Each stage produces distinctive signs and symptoms.

PRENATAL SYPHILIS

A woman can transmit syphilis transplacentally to her unborn child throughout pregnancy. This type of syphilis is often called congenital, but prenatal is a more accurate term. Approximately 50% of infected fetuses die before or shortly after birth. The prognosis is better for infants who develop overt infection after age 2.

SIGNS AND SYMPTOMS

The infant with prenatal syphilis may appear healthy at birth, but usually develops characteristic lesions — vesicular, bullous eruptions, often on the palms and soles — 3 weeks later. Shortly afterward, a maculopapular rash similar to that in secondary syphilis may erupt on the face, mouth, genitalia, palms, or soles. Condylomata lata often occur around the anus. Lesions may erupt on the mucous membranes of the mouth, pharynx, and nose. When the infant's larynx is affected, his cry becomes weak and forced. If nasal mucous membranes are involved, he may also develop nasal discharge, which can be slight and mucopurulent or copious with blood-tinged pus. Visceral and bone lesions, liver or spleen enlargement with ascites, and nephrotic syndrome may also occur.

Late prenatal syphilis becomes apparent after age 2; it may be identifiable only through blood studies or may cause unmistakable syphilitic changes: screwdriver-shaped central incisors, deformed molars or cusps, thick clavicles, saber shins, bowed tibias, nasal septum perforation, eighth nerve deafness, and neurosyphilis.

DIAGNOSIS AND TREATMENT

In the infant with prenatal syphilis, the Venereal Disease Research Laboratory (VDRL) titer, if reactive at birth, stays the same or rises, indicating active disease. The infant's titer drops in 3 months if the mother has received effective prenatal treatment. Absolute diagnosis necessitates darkfield examination of umbilical vein blood or lesion drainage.

An infant with abnormal cerebrospinal fluid (CSF) may be treated with aqueous crystalline penicillin G, I.M. or I.V. (50,000 units/kg of body weight/day divided in two doses for at least 10 days), or aqueous penicillin G procaine I.M. (50,000 units/kg of body weight/day for at least 10 days). An infant with normal CSF may be treated with a single injection of penicillin G benzathine (50,000 units/kg of body weight).

When caring for a child with prenatal syphilis, record the extent of the rash, and watch for signs of systemic involvement, especially laryngeal swelling, jaundice, and decreasing urine output.

Primary syphilis

After an incubation period that generally lasts about 3 weeks, symptoms of primary syphilis develop.

Initially, one or more chancres (small, fluid-filled lesions) erupt on the genitalia; others may erupt on the anus, fingers, lips, tongue, nipples, tonsils, or eyelids. These chancres, which are usually painless, start as papules and then erode; they have indurated, raised edges and clear bases.

Chancres typically disappear after 3 to 6 weeks, even when untreated. They are usually associated with regional lymphadenopathy (unilateral or bilateral). In women, chancres are frequently overlooked because they often develop on internal structures — the cervix or the vaginal wall.

Secondary syphilis

The development of symmetrical mucocutaneous lesions and general lymphadenopathy signals the onset of secondary syphilis, which may develop within a few days or up to 8 weeks after the onset of initial chancres.

The rash of secondary syphilis can be macular, papular, pustular, or nodular. Lesions are of uniform size, well defined, and generalized. Macules often erupt between rolls of fat on the trunk and on the arms, palms, soles, face, and scalp. In warm, moist areas (perineum, scrotum, vulva, between rolls of fat), the lesions enlarge and erode, producing highly contagious, pink, or grayish-white lesions (condylomata lata).

Mild constitutional symptoms of syphilis appear in the second stage and may include headache, malaise, anorexia, weight loss, nausea, vomiting, sore throat and, possibly, slight fever. Alopecia may occur, with or without treatment, and is usually temporary. Nails become brittle and pitted.

Latent syphilis

Although no clinical symptoms occur in latent syphilis, it produces a reactive serologic test for syphilis. Because infectious mucocutaneous lesions may reappear when infection is of less than 4 years' duration, early latent syphilis is considered contagious.

Approximately two-thirds of patients remain asymptomatic in the late latent stage until death. The rest develop characteristic late-stage symptoms.

Late syphilis

The final, destructive, but noninfectious stage of the disease, late syphilis has three subtypes, any or all of which may affect the patient: late benign syphilis, cardiovascular syphilis, and neurosyphilis.

The lesions of *late benign syphilis* develop between 1 and 10 years after infection. They may appear on the skin, bones, mucous membranes, upper respiratory tract, liver, or stomach.

The typical lesion is a gumma — a chronic, superficial nodule or deep, granulomatous lesion that is solitary, asymmetric, painless, and indurated. Gummas can be found on any bone — particularly the long bones of the legs — and in any organ.

If late syphilis involves the liver, it can cause epigastric pain, tenderness, enlarged spleen, and anemia; if it involves the upper respiratory tract, it may cause perforation of the nasal septum or the palate. In severe cases, late benign syphilis results in destruction of bones or organs, which eventually causes death.

Cardiovascular syphilis develops about 10 years after the initial infection in approximately 10% of patients with late, untreated syphilis. It causes fibrosis of elastic tissue of the aorta and leads to aortitis, most often in the ascending and transverse sections of the aortic arch. Cardiovascular syphilis may be asymptomatic or may cause aortic regurgitation or aneurysm.

Symptoms of *neurosyphilis* develop in about 8% of patients with late, untreated syphilis and appear from 5 to 35 years after infection. These clinical effects consist of meningitis and widespread central nervous system damage that may include general paresis, personality changes, and arm and leg weakness.

Diagnosis

Identifying *T. pallidum* from a lesion on a dark-field examination provides immediate diagnosis of syphilis. This method is most effective when moist lesions are present, as in primary, secondary, and prenatal syphilis.

The fluorescent treponemal antibody-absorption test identifies antigens of *T. pallidum* in tissue, ocular fluid, cerebrospinal fluid (CSF), tracheobronchial secretions, and exudates from lesions. This is the most sensitive test available for detecting syphilis in all stages. Once reactive, it remains so permanently.

Other appropriate procedures include the following:

▶ Venereal Disease Research Laboratory (VDRL) slide test and rapid plasma reagin test detect nonspecific antibodies. Both tests, if positive, become reactive within 1 to 2 weeks after the primary lesion appears or 4 to 5 weeks after the infection begins.

▶ CSF examination identifies neurosyphilis when the total protein level is above 40 mg/100 ml, VDRL slide test is reactive, and CSF cell count exceeds 5 mononuclear cells/μl.

Treatment

Administration of penicillin I.M. is the treatment of choice. For early syphilis, treatment may consist of a single injection of penicillin G benzathine I.M. (2.4 million units). Syphilis of more than 1 year's duration should be treated with penicillin G benzathine I.M. (2.4 million units/week for 3 weeks).

Nonpregnant patients who are allergic to penicillin may be treated with oral tetracycline or doxycycline for 15 days for early syphilis; 30 days for late infections. Nonpenicillin therapy for latent or late syphilis should be used only after neurosyphilis has been excluded. Tetracycline is contraindicated in pregnant women.

Special considerations

▶ Stress the importance of completing the course of therapy even after symptoms subside.

▶ Check for a history of drug sensitivity before administering the first dose.

▶ Practice universal precautions.

▶ In secondary syphilis, keep lesions clean and dry. If they're draining, dispose of contaminated materials properly.

▶ In late syphilis, provide symptomatic care during prolonged treatment.

▶ In cardiovascular syphilis, check for signs of decreased cardiac output (decreased urine output, hypoxia, and decreased sensorium) and pulmonary congestion.

▶ In neurosyphilis, regularly check level of consciousness, mood, and coherence. Watch for signs of ataxia.

▶ Urge patients to seek VDRL testing after 3, 6, 12, and 24 months to detect possible relapse. Patients treated for latent or late syphilis should receive blood tests at 6-month intervals for 2 years.

▶ Be sure to report all cases of syphilis to local public health authorities. Urge the patient to inform sexual partners of his infection so that they can receive treatment also.

▶ Refer the patient and his sexual partners for HIV testing.

T

TAENIASIS

Also called tapeworm disease or cestodiasis, taeniasis is a parasitic infestation by *Taenia saginata* (beef tapeworm), *Taenia solium* (pork tapeworm), *Diphyllobothrium latum* (fish tapeworm), or *Hymenolepis nana* (dwarf tapeworm).

Taeniasis is usually a chronic, benign intestinal disease; however, infestation with *T. solium* may cause dangerous systemic and central nervous system (CNS) symptoms if larvae invade the brain and striated muscle of vital organs. (See *Common tapeworm infestations.*)

Causes

T. saginata, T. solium, and *D. latum* are transmitted to humans by ingestion of beef, pork, or fish that contains tapeworm cysts. Gastric acids break down these cysts in the stomach, liberating them to mature. Mature tapeworms fasten to the intestinal wall and produce ova that are passed in the stools.

Transmission of *H. nana* is direct from person to person and requires no intermediate host; it completes its life cycle in the intestine.

Signs and symptoms

Taeniasis may produce mild symptoms, such as nausea, flatulence, hunger sensations, weight loss, diarrhea, and increased appetite, or no symptoms at all. Occasionally, worm segments may exit through the anus and appear on bedclothes.

Diagnosis

Tapeworm infestations are diagnosed by laboratory observation of tapeworm ova or body segments in stools. Because ova aren't excreted continuously, confirmation may require multiple specimens. A supporting dietary or travel history aids confirmation.

Treatment

Niclosamide offers a cure in up to 95% of patients. In beef, pork, and fish tapeworm infestation, the drug is given once; in severe dwarf tapeworm infestation, twice (5 to 7 days each time, spaced 2 weeks apart). Another anthelmintic agent, praziquantel, may also be effective.

After drug treatment, all types of tapeworm infestation require a follow-up laboratory examination of stool specimens during the next 3 to 5 weeks to check for any remaining ova or worm segments. Of course, persistent infestation typically requires a second course of medication.

Special considerations

▶ Obtain a complete history, including recent travel to endemic areas, dietary habits, and physical symptoms.
▶ Dispose of the patient's excretions carefully. Wear gloves when giving personal care and handling fecal excretions, bedpans, and bed linens; wash your hands thoroughly and instruct the patient to do the same.
▶ Tell the patient not to consume anything after midnight on the day niclosamide therapy is to start because the drug must be given on an empty stomach. After ad-

COMMON TAPEWORM INFESTATIONS

TYPE AND SOURCE OF INFECTION	INCIDENCE	CLINICAL FEATURES
Diphyllobothrium latum (fish tapeworm) Uncooked or undercooked infected freshwater fish, such as pike, trout, salmon, and turbot	Finland, parts of the former Soviet Union, Japan, Alaska, Australia, the Great Lakes region (U.S.), Switzerland, Chile, and Argentina	Anemia (hemoglobin level as low as 6 to 8 g)
Hymenolepis nana (dwarf tapeworm) No intermediate host; parasite passes directly from person to person via ova passed in stool; inadequate hand washing facilitates its spread	Most common tapeworm in humans; particularly prevalent among institutionalized mentally retarded children and in underdeveloped countries	Dependent on patient's nutritional status and number of parasites; commonly no symptoms with mild infestation; with severe infestation, anorexia, diarrhea, restlessness, dizziness, and apathy
Taenia saginata (beef tapeworm) Uncooked or undercooked infected beef	Worldwide, but prevalent in Europe and East Africa	Crawling sensation in the perianal area caused by worm segments that have been passed rectally; intestinal obstruction and appendicitis due to long worm segments that have twisted in the intestinal lumen
Taenia solium (pork tapeworm) Uncooked or undercooked infected pork	Highest in Mexico and Latin America; lowest among Muslims and Jews	Seizures, headaches, personality changes; commonly overlooked in adults

ministering the drug, document passage of strobilae.

▶ In pork tapeworm infestation, use standard precautions. Avoid procedures and drugs that may cause vomiting or gagging. If the patient is a child or is incontinent, he requires a private room. Obtain a list of contacts.

▶ Document level of consciousness and be alert for changes. If CNS symptoms appear, keep an artificial airway or padded tongue blade close at hand, raise side rails, keep the bed low, and help with walking as needed.

 PREVENTION TIP To prevent reinfestation, teach proper handwashing technique and the need to cook meat and fish thoroughly. Stress the need for follow-up evaluations to monitor the success of therapy and to detect possible reinfestation.

TETANUS

Lockjaw or tetanus is an acute exotoxin-mediated infection caused by the anaerobic, spore-forming, gram-positive bacillus *Clostridium tetani.* Usually, such infection is systemic; less often, localized.

Tetanus is fatal in up to 60% of unimmunized persons, usually within 10 days of onset. When symptoms develop within 3 days after exposure, the prognosis is poor.

Causes

Normally, transmission is through a puncture wound that is contaminated by soil, dust, or animal excreta containing *C. tetani,* or by way of burns and minor wounds. After *C. tetani* enters the body, it causes local infection and tissue necrosis. It also produces toxins that then enter the bloodstream and lymphatics and eventually spread to central nervous system tissue.

Tetanus occurs worldwide, but it's more prevalent in agricultural regions and developing countries that lack mass immunization programs. It's one of the most common causes of neonatal deaths in developing countries, where infants of unimmunized mothers are delivered under unsterile conditions. In such infants, the unhealed umbilical cord is the portal of entry.

In America, about 75% of all cases occur between April and September.

Signs and symptoms

The incubation period varies from 3 to 4 weeks in mild tetanus to less than 2 days in severe tetanus. When symptoms occur within 3 days after injury, death is more likely. If tetanus remains localized, signs of onset are spasm and increased muscle tone near the wound.

If tetanus is generalized (systemic), indications include marked muscle hyper-

tonicity, hyperactive deep tendon reflexes, tachycardia, profuse sweating, low-grade fever, and painful, involuntary muscle contractions:

▶ neck and facial muscles, especially cheek muscles — locked jaw (trismus) and a grotesque, grinning expression called *risus sardonicus*

▶ somatic muscles — arched-back rigidity (opisthotonos), boardlike abdominal rigidity

▶ intermittent tonic convulsions lasting several minutes, which may result in cyanosis and sudden death by asphyxiation.

Despite such pronounced neuromuscular symptoms, cerebral and sensory functions remain normal. Complications include atelectasis, pneumonia, pulmonary emboli, acute gastric ulcers, flexion contractures, and cardiac arrhythmias.

Neonatal tetanus is always generalized. The first clinical sign is difficulty in sucking, which usually appears 3 to 10 days after birth. It progresses to total inability to suck, with excessive crying, irritability, and nuchal rigidity.

Diagnosis

Frequently, diagnosis must rest on clinical features and a history of trauma and no previous tetanus immunization. Blood cultures and tetanus antibody tests are often negative; only a third of patients have a positive wound culture. Cerebrospinal fluid pressure may rise above normal. Diagnosis also must rule out meningitis, rabies, phenothiazine or strychnine toxicity, and other conditions that mimic tetanus.

Treatment

Within 72 hours after a puncture wound, a patient with no previous history of tetanus immunization first requires tetanus immune globulin (TIG) or tetanus antitoxin to confer temporary protection. Next, he needs active immunization with tetanus toxoid. A patient who has not received tetanus immunization within 5 years needs a booster injection of tetanus toxoid.

If tetanus develops despite immediate postinjury treatment, the patient will require airway maintenance and a muscle relaxant, such as diazepam, to decrease muscle rigidity and spasm. If muscle contractions aren't relieved by muscle relaxants, a neuromuscular blocker may be needed. The patient with tetanus needs high-dose antibiotics (penicillin administered I.V., if he's not allergic to it).

Special considerations

When caring for the patient with a puncture wound:

▶ Thoroughly debride and cleanse the injury site with 3% hydrogen peroxide, and check the patient's immunization history. Record the cause of injury. If it's a dog bite, report the case to local public health authorities.

▶ Before giving penicillin and TIG, antitoxin, or toxoid, obtain an accurate history of allergies to immunizations or penicillin. If the patient has a history of any allergies, keep epinephrine 1:1,000 and resuscitative equipment available.

▶ Stress the importance of maintaining active immunization with a booster dose of tetanus toxoid every 10 years.

After tetanus develops:

▶ Maintain an adequate airway and ventilation to prevent pneumonia and atelectasis. Suction often and watch for signs of respiratory distress. Keep emergency airway equipment on hand because the patient may require artificial ventilation or oxygen administration.

▶ Maintain an I.V. line for medications and emergency care if necessary.

▶ Monitor electrocardiography frequently for arrhythmias. Accurately record intake and output, and check vital signs often.

▶ Turn the patient frequently to prevent pressure sores and pulmonary stasis.

▶ Because even minimal external stimulation provokes muscle spasms, keep the patient's room dark and quiet. Warn visitors not to upset or overly stimulate the patient.

▶ If urinary retention develops, insert an indwelling urinary catheter.

▶ Give muscle relaxants and sedatives as ordered, and schedule patient care to coincide with heaviest sedation.

▶ Insert an artificial airway, if necessary, to prevent tongue injury and maintain airway during spasms.

▶ Provide adequate nutrition to meet the patient's increased metabolic needs. The patient may need nasogastric feedings or hyperalimentation.

THROAT ABSCESS

Abscess of the throat may be peritonsillar (quinsy) or retropharyngeal. Peritonsillar abscess forms in the connective tissue space between the tonsil capsule and constrictor muscle of the pharynx.

Retropharyngeal abscess, or abscess of the potential space, forms between the posterior pharyngeal wall and prevertebral fascia. With treatment, the prognosis for both types of abscesses is good.

Causes

Peritonsillar abscess is a complication of acute tonsillitis, usually after streptococcal or staphylococcal infection. It occurs more often in adolescents and young adults than in children.

Acute retropharyngeal abscess results from infection in the retropharyngeal lymph glands, which may follow an upper respiratory tract bacterial infection. Because these lymph glands, present at birth, begin to atrophy after age 2, acute retropharyngeal abscess most commonly affects infants and children under age 2.

Chronic retropharyngeal abscess may result from tuberculosis of the cervical spine (Pott's disease) and may occur at any age.

Signs and symptoms

Peritonsillar abscess and retropharyngeal abscess have different signs and symptoms.

Peritonsillar abscess

Key symptoms of peritonsillar abscess include severe throat pain, occasional ear pain on the same side as the abscess, and tenderness of the submandibular gland. Dysphagia causes drooling. Trismus may occur as a result of edema and infection spreading from the peritonsillar space to the pterygoid muscles.

Other effects include fever, chills, malaise, rancid breath, nausea, muffled speech, dehydration, cervical adenopathy, and localized or systemic sepsis.

Retropharyngeal abscess

Clinical features of retropharyngeal abscess include pain, dysphagia, fever and, when the abscess is located in the upper pharynx, nasal obstruction; with a low-positioned abscess, dyspnea, progressive inspiratory stridor (from laryngeal obstruction), neck hyperextension and, in children, drooling and muffled crying.

A very large abscess may press on the larynx, causing edema, or may erode into major vessels, causing sudden death from asphyxia or aspiration.

Diagnosis

Diagnosing peritonsillar abscess is based on a patient history of bacterial pharyngitis. Examination of the throat shows swelling of the soft palate on the abscessed side, with displacement of the uvula to the opposite side; red, edematous mucous membranes; and tonsil displacement toward the midline. Culture may reveal streptococcal or staphylococcal infection.

Peritonsillar abscess can also be caused by an aerobic microorganism such as bacteroides.

Diagnosis of retropharyngeal abscess is based on patient history of nasopharyn-

gitis or pharyngitis, and on physical examination revealing a soft, red bulging of the posterior pharyngeal wall. X-rays show the larynx pushed forward and a widened space between the posterior pharyngeal wall and vertebrae.

If neck pain or stiffness occurs, look for extension to epidural space or cervical vertebrae. Culture and sensitivity tests isolate the causative organism and determine the appropriate antibiotic.

Treatment

For early-stage peritonsillar abscess, large doses of penicillin or another broad-spectrum antibiotic are necessary. If the patient is immunocompromised or has been repeatedly hospitalized, antibiotic therapy should include coverage for staphylococci and gram-negative organisms.

For late-stage peritonsillar abscess, with cellulitis of the tonsillar space, primary treatment is usually incision and drainage under a local anesthetic, followed by antibiotic therapy for 7 to 10 days. Tonsillectomy, scheduled no sooner than 1 month after healing, prevents recurrence but is recommended only after several episodes.

In acute retropharyngeal abscess, the primary treatment is incision and drainage through the pharyngeal wall. In chronic retropharyngeal abscess, drainage is performed through an external incision behind the sternomastoid muscle. During incision and drainage, strong, continuous mouth suction is necessary to prevent aspiration of pus. Postoperative drug therapy includes antibiotics (usually penicillin) and analgesics.

Special considerations

 ALERT Be alert for signs of respiratory obstruction (inspiratory stridor, dyspnea, increasing restlessness, or cyanosis). Keep emergency airway equipment nearby.

▶ Be aware that these infections can extend to the mediastinum, worsening sepsis and chest pain, and increasing breathing difficulty.

▶ Explain the drainage procedure to the patient or his parents. Because the procedure is generally done under a local anesthetic, the patient may be apprehensive.

▶ Perform incision and drainage. To allow easy expectoration and suction of pus and blood, place the patient in a semirecumbent or sitting position.

After incision and drainage:

▶ Give antibiotics, analgesics, and antipyretics. Stress the importance of completing the full course of prescribed antibiotic therapy.

▶ Monitor vital signs, and watch for any significant changes or bleeding. Assess pain and treat accordingly.

▶ If the patient is unable to swallow, ensure adequate hydration with I.V. therapy. Monitor fluid intake and output, and watch for dehydration.

▶ Provide meticulous mouth care. Apply petrolatum to the patient's lips. Promote healing with warm saline gargles or throat irrigations for 24 to 36 hours after incision and drainage. Encourage adequate rest.

TICK PARALYSIS

Tick paralysis is caused by over 40 species of ticks worldwide (5 in North America, including the deer tick) and can occur in almost any region where ticks are found. The disease has killed thousands of animals, mainly cows and sheep, in other parts of the world. Although tick paralysis is of concern in domestic animals and livestock in the United States as well, human cases are rare and usually occur in children under age 10 during April to June— when nymphs and mature wood ticks are most prevalent—especially in the Northwest.

Onset of symptoms usually occurs after a tick has fed for several days. Unlike Lyme disease, ehrlichiosis, and babesio-

sis, which are caused by systemic proliferation and expansion of parasites in the body long after the offending tick is gone, tick paralysis is chemically induced by the tick and can therefore continue only in its presence. Once the tick is removed, symptoms usually diminish rapidly. However, in some cases, profound paralysis can develop and even become fatal before anyone becomes aware of a tick's presence.

Causes

Tick paralysis occurs when an engorged and pregnant female tick produces a neurotoxin in its salivary glands, which blocks the release of acetylcholine at the synapse and inhibits motor-stimulus conduction, and transmits it to an animal or human during feeding. Experiments show that the greatest amount of toxin is produced between the fifth and seventh day of attachment (often initiating or increasing the severity of symptoms), although the timing may vary depending on the species of tick.

Signs and symptoms

Symptoms of tick paralysis generally begin from five to seven days after a tick becomes attached, beginning with fatigue, numbness of the legs, and muscle pains. The tick usually attaches itself on the scalp. Paralysis rapidly develops from the lower to the upper extremities and, if the tick is not removed, is followed by tongue and facial paralysis. There is little effect on sensory functions. The most severe complications may include convulsions, respiratory failure and, in up to 12% of untreated cases, death.

Diagnosis

Because of the inability of laboratory tests to indicate tick paralysis, diagnosis is based on symptoms and the rapid improvement of the patient once the engorged tick is removed.

Other conditions to consider include Guillain-Barré syndrome, botulism, poliomyelitis, polyneuritis, myelitis, and myasthenia gravis.

Treatment

 ALERT If unrecognized, tick paralysis can progress to respiratory failure. Prompt removal of the feeding tick(s) is essential. It is important to remove all the mouthparts, since they contain the salivary glands, which may continue to infect the patient even after the body of the tick has been removed.

Special considerations

❚ Provide frequent skin care, positioning, and toileting practices if the paralysis has advanced.
❚ Record accurate intake and output to prevent dehydration and skin breakdown.
❚ Perform careful observation of the affected tick bite area for potential infection, or any remaining toxin-producing glands.

 PREVENTION TIP To avoid tick bites, teach patients to:
❚ wear long pants, long-sleeved shirts, socks, and enclosed shoes
❚ use insect repellents
❚ inspect their body thoroughly after returning from any outing, even if they go no further than the front lawn. Prompt removal of ticks, preferably before they've had a chance to become engorged, will go a long way in preventing tick paralysis and other tick-borne diseases.

TINEA VERSICOLOR

A chronic, superficial, fungal infection, tinea versicolor (also known as pityriasis versicolor) may produce a multicolored rash, commonly on the upper trunk. This condition, primarily a cosmetic defect, usually affects young people, especially during warm weather, and is most prevalent in tropical countries. Recurrence is common.

Causes

The agent that causes tinea versicolor is *Malassezia furfur (Pityrosporum orbiculare)*. Whether this condition is infectious or merely a proliferation of normal skin fungi is uncertain.

Signs and symptoms

Tinea versicolor typically produces raised or macular, round or oval, slightly scaly lesions on the upper trunk, which may extend to the lower abdomen, neck, arms, and, rarely, the face. These lesions are usually tawny but may range from hypopigmented (white) patches in dark-skinned patients to hyperpigmented (brown) patches in fair-skinned patients. Some areas don't tan when exposed to sunlight, causing the cosmetic defect for which most persons seek medical help. Inflammation, burning, and itching are possible but usually absent.

Diagnosis

Visualization of lesions during Wood's light examination strongly suggests tinea versicolor.

Microscopic examination of skin scrapings prepared in potassium hydroxide solution confirms the disorder by showing hyphae, clusters of yeast, and large numbers of variously sized pores (a combination referred to as "spaghetti and meatballs").

Other conditions to consider include vitiligo, clear psoriasis, nummular eczema, and pityriasis rosea.

Treatment

The most economical and effective treatment is selenium sulfide lotion 2.5% applied once a day for 7 days. It's left on the skin for 10 minutes, then rinsed off thoroughly. In severe or persistent cases, therapy may require systemic ketoconazole. Topical treatment may cause temporary redness and irritation.

More expensive treatments for tinea versicolor include topical antifungals such as imidazole creams, which are applied twice daily for a month, and oral antifungals such as ketoconazole for extensive cases.

Special considerations

▶ Instruct the patient to apply selenium sulfide lotion, as ordered. Tell him that this medication may cause temporary adverse effects.

▶ Assure the patient that once his fungal infection is cured, discolored areas will gradually blend in after exposure to the sun or ultraviolet light.

▶ Because recurrence of tinea versicolor is common, advise the patient to watch for new areas of discoloration.

▶ Teach the patient proper hand-washing technique, and encourage good personal hygiene.

▶ Stress the importance of not scratching or picking lesions to avoid the risk of skin breaks and secondary bacterial infections.

▶ Provide written instructions for using prescribed medications. Tell the patient to contact the doctor if adverse reactions occur.

TONSILLITIS

Inflammation of the palatine tonsils, or tonsillitis, can be acute or chronic. The uncomplicated acute form usually lasts 4 to 6 days and commonly affects children between ages 5 and 10. The presence of proven chronic tonsillitis justifies tonsillectomy, the only effective treatment. Tonsils tend to hypertrophy during childhood and atrophy after puberty.

Causes

Tonsillitis generally results from infection with group A beta-hemolytic streptococci but can result from other bacteria or viruses, or from oral anaerobes.

Signs and symptoms

The acute form of tonsillitis commonly begins with a mild to severe sore throat

made worse by swallowing. A very young child, unable to complain about a sore throat, may stop eating. Tonsillitis may also produce dysphagia, fever, swelling and tenderness of the lymph glands in the submandibular area, muscle and joint pain, chills, malaise, headache, and pain (frequently referred to the ears).

Excess secretions may elicit the complaint of a constant urge to swallow; the back of the throat may feel constricted. Such discomfort usually subsides after 72 hours.

The chronic form of tonsillitis produces a recurrent sore throat and purulent drainage in the tonsillar crypts. Frequent attacks of acute tonsillitis may also occur. Complications include obstruction from tonsillar hypertrophy and peritonsillar abscess.

Diagnosis

Diagnostic confirmation requires a thorough throat examination that reveals:

▶ generalized inflammation of the pharyngeal wall

▶ swollen tonsils that project from between the pillars of the fauces and exude white or yellow exudate

▶ purulent drainage when pressure is applied to the tonsillar pillars

▶ possible edematous and inflamed uvula.

Culture may determine the infecting microbe and indicate appropriate antibiotic therapy. Leukocytosis is also usually present. Differential diagnosis rules out infectious mononucleosis, acute epiglottis, viral pharyngitis, Vincent's infection, and diphtheria.

Treatment

Effective treatment of acute tonsillitis requires rest, adequate fluid intake, administration of aspirin or acetaminophen and, for bacterial infection, antibiotics.

When the causative microbe is a group A beta-hemolytic streptococcus, penicillin is the drug of choice (another broad-spectrum antibiotic may be substituted). Most oral anaerobes will also respond to penicillin. To prevent complications, antibiotic therapy should continue for 10 to 14 days.

Chronic tonsillitis or the development of complications (obstructions from tonsillar hypertrophy, peritonsillar abscess) may require a tonsillectomy, but only after the patient has been free of tonsillar or respiratory tract infections for 3 to 4 weeks.

Special considerations

▶ Despite dysphagia, urge the patient to drink plenty of fluids, especially if he has a fever. Offer a child ice cream and flavored drinks and ices. Suggest gargling to soothe the throat, unless it exacerbates pain. Make sure the patient and parents understand the importance of completing the prescribed course of antibiotic therapy.

▶ Before tonsillectomy, explain to the adult patient that a local anesthetic prevents pain but allows a sensation of pressure during surgery. Warn the patient to expect considerable throat discomfort and some bleeding postoperatively.

▶ For the pediatric patient, keep your explanation simple and nonthreatening. Show the child the operating and recovery rooms, and briefly explain the hospital routine. Most facilities allow one parent to stay with the child.

▶ Advise the patient not to take aspirin or medications containing aspirin for 7 to 10 days before surgery to decrease the risk of bleeding.

▶ Postoperatively, maintain a patent airway. To prevent aspiration, place the patient on his side.

▶ Monitor vital signs frequently, and check for bleeding. Be alert for excessive bleeding, increased pulse rate, dropping blood pressure, or frequent swallowing.

▶ After the patient is fully alert and the gag reflex has returned, allow him to drink water.

▶ Urge the patient to drink plenty of nonirritating fluids.

▶ Before discharge, provide the patient or parents with written instructions on home care. Tell the patient to expect a white scab to form in the throat between 5 and 10 days postoperatively and to report bleeding, ear discomfort, or a fever that lasts longer than 3 days.

▶ Tell the patient that aspirin and medications containing aspirin are contraindicated postoperatively.

▶ Instruct the patient to avoid coughing or excessive clearing of the throat, which can irritate the throat and cause increased bleeding.

▶ Tell the patient that blood-tinged mucus is normal for 5 to 7 days after surgery.

TOXIC SHOCK SYNDROME

An acute bacterial infection, toxic shock syndrome (TSS) is caused by toxin-producing, penicillin-resistant strains of *Staphylococcus aureus,* such as TSS toxin-1 and staphylococcal enterotoxins B and C. The disease primarily affects menstruating women under age 30 and is associated with continuous use of tampons during the menstrual period.

TSS incidence peaked in the mid-1980s and has since declined, probably because of the withdrawal of high-absorbency tampons from the market.

Causes

Although tampons are clearly implicated in TSS, their exact role is uncertain. Theoretically, tampons may contribute to development of TSS by:

▶ introducing *S. aureus* into the vagina during insertion

▶ absorbing toxin from the vagina

▶ traumatizing the vaginal mucosa during insertion, thus leading to infection

▶ providing a favorable environment for the growth of *S. aureus.*

When TSS isn't related to menstruation, it seems to be linked to *S. aureus* infections, such as abscesses, osteomyelitis, and postsurgical infections.

Signs and symptoms

Typically, TSS produces intense myalgias, fever over 104° F (40° C), vomiting, diarrhea, headache, decreased level of consciousness, rigors, conjunctival hyperemia, and vaginal hyperemia and discharge. Severe hypotension occurs with hypovolemic shock. Within a few hours of onset, a deep red rash develops — especially on the palms and soles — and later desquamates.

Major complications include persistent neuropsychological abnormalities, mild renal failure, rash, and cyanotic arms and legs.

Diagnosis

A diagnosis of TSS is based on clinical findings and the presence of at least three of the following:

▶ GI effects, including vomiting and profuse diarrhea

▶ muscular effects, with severe myalgias or a fivefold or greater increase in creatine kinase

▶ mucous membrane effects, such as frank hyperemia

▶ renal involvement with elevated blood urea nitrogen or creatinine levels (at least twice the normal levels)

▶ liver involvement with elevated bilirubin, alanine aminotransferase, or aspartate aminotransferase levels (at least twice the normal levels)

▶ blood involvement with signs of thrombocytopenia and a platelet count of less than $100,000/\mu l$

▶ central nervous system effects, such as disorientation without focal signs.

In addition, isolation of *S. aureus* from vaginal discharge or lesions helps support the diagnosis. Negative results on blood tests for Rocky Mountain spotted fever, leptospirosis, and measles help rule out these disorders.

Treatment

TSS is treated with I.V. antistaphylococcal antibiotics that are beta-lactamase–resistant, such as oxacillin and nafcillin. To reverse shock, replace fluids with saline solution and colloids. Shock that doesn't respond to fluids may necessitate use of pressor agents such as dopamine.

Special considerations

▶ Monitor the patient's vital signs frequently.

▶ Administer antibiotics slowly and strictly on time. Be sure to watch for signs of penicillin allergy.

▶ Check the patient's fluid and electrolyte balance.

▶ Obtain specimens of vaginal and cervical secretions for culture of *S. aureus*.

▶ Tell the patient to avoid using tampons.

▶ Implement universal precautions.

TOXOPLASMOSIS

One of the most common infectious diseases, toxoplasmosis results from the protozoa *Toxoplasma gondii*. Distributed worldwide, it's less common in cold or hot arid climates and at high elevations. It usually causes localized infection but may produce significant generalized infection, especially in immunodeficient patients or neonates.

Congenital toxoplasmosis, characterized by lesions in the central nervous system, may result in stillbirth or serious birth defects.

Causes

T. gondii exists in trophozoite forms in the acute stages of infection and in cystic forms (tissue cysts and oocysts) in the latent stages. Ingestion of tissue cysts in raw or undercooked meat (heating, drying, or freezing destroys these cysts) or fecal-oral contamination from infected cats transmits toxoplasmosis. However, toxoplasmosis also occurs in vegetarians who aren't

OCULAR TOXOPLASMOSIS

Ocular toxoplasmosis (active retinochoroiditis), characterized by focal necrotizing retinitis, accounts for about 25% of all cases of granulomatous uveitis. It is usually the result of congenital infection, but may not appear until adolescence or young adulthood, when infection is reactivated. Symptoms include blurred vision, scotoma, pain, photophobia, and impairment or loss of central vision. Vision improves as inflammation subsides but usually without recovery of lost visual acuity. Ocular toxoplasmosis may subside after treatment with prednisone.

exposed to cats, so other means of transmission may exist.

Congenital toxoplasmosis follows transplacental transmission from a chronically infected mother or one who acquired toxoplasmosis shortly before or during pregnancy.

Signs and symptoms

The following signs and symptoms characterize congenital toxoplasmosis and acquired toxoplasmosis.

Toxoplasmosis acquired in the first trimester of pregnancy often results in stillbirth. About one-third of infants who survive have congenital toxoplasmosis. The later in pregnancy maternal infection occurs, the greater the risk of congenital infection in the infant.

Obvious signs of congenital toxoplasmosis include retinochoroiditis (see *Ocular toxoplasmosis*), hydrocephalus or microcephalus, cerebral calcification, seizures, lymphadenopathy, fever, hepatosplenomegaly, jaundice, and rash. Other defects, which may become apparent months or years later, include strabismus, blindness, epilepsy, and mental retardation.

Acquired toxoplasmosis may cause localized (mild lymphatic) or generalized (fulminating, disseminated) infection. Localized infection produces fever and a mononucleosis-like syndrome (malaise, myalgia, headache, fatigue, sore throat) and lymphadenopathy.

Generalized infection produces encephalitis, fever, headache, vomiting, delirium, seizures, and a diffuse maculopapular rash (except on the palms, soles, and scalp). Generalized infection may lead to myocarditis, pneumonitis, hepatitis, and polymyositis.

Diagnosis

Identification of *T. gondii* in an appropriate tissue specimen confirms toxoplasmosis. Serologic tests may be useful, and in patients with toxoplasmosis encephalitis, computed tomography and magnetic resonance imaging scans disclose lesions.

Treatment

Acute disease is treated with sulfonamides and pyrimethamine for about 4 weeks and, possibly, folinic acid to control side effects. In patients who also have acquired immunodeficiency syndrome, treatment continues indefinitely.

No safe, effective treatment exists for chronic toxoplasmosis or toxoplasmosis occurring in the first trimester of pregnancy.

Special considerations

▶ When caring for patients with toxoplasmosis, monitor drug therapy carefully and emphasize thorough patient teaching to prevent complications and control spread of the disease.

▶ Because sulfonamides cause blood dyscrasias and pyrimethamine depresses bone marrow, closely monitor the patient's hematologic values.

▶ Report all cases of toxoplasmosis to your local public health department.

PREVENTION TIP Instruct patients to wash hands after working with soil and to cover children's sandboxes (because soil and sand may be contaminated with cat oocysts). Change cat litter daily because cat oocytes don't become infective until 1 to 4 days after excretion. Cook meat thoroughly and freeze it promptly if it's not for immediate use.

TRACHEITIS

Tracheitis is an acute bacterial infection of the trachea that may lead to complete airway obstruction, sepsis, and death. Tracheitis occurs most commonly in children under age 3, but it can occur in children as old as age 8. Incidence of the disease is unknown, but it affects males and females equally.

Causes

Tracheitis is most often caused by *Staphylococcus aureus;* however, other bacterial organisms such as *Moraxella catarrhalis* and group A beta-hemolytic streptococci have also been implicated. The precipitating event is almost always a recent viral upper or lower respiratory tract infection. The decreased diameter of the child's trachea relative to the amount of swelling caused by the microbe may predispose the child to severe respiratory compromise. The microbes cause inflammation at the cricoid cartilage; mucosal edema; and copious, thick, purulent secretions.

Signs and symptoms

The child will exhibit an acute onset of high fever. A cough from a prior upper respiratory tract infection may still be present, but it rapidly worsens. The croup-like cough then progresses to the high-pitched, crowing sound of inspiratory stridor, signaling impending airway obstruction. Nasal flaring and intercostal retractions appear as respiratory compromise worsens. Odynophagia typically is not present. The child displays a toxic appearance. Signs and symptoms of toxic shock/sepsis may occur secondary to *S. aureus* infection.

Diagnosis

Endoscopy is the best diagnostic method, permitting direct visualization of the involved structures. Endoscopic symptoms include subglottic edema, ulceration, pseudomembrane formation, and intraluminal soft tissue irregularities.

Chest X-ray reveals the characteristic "steeple sign" (pencil-shaped configuration of subglottic edema) as well as patchy infiltrates with focal densities.

Tracheal or nasopharyngeal cultures will reveal the infecting pathogen. Arterial blood gases evaluate severity of oxygen deprivation, while a complete blood count reveals moderate leukocytosis with bands.

The differential diagnosis includes epiglottitis, foreign body, subglottic stenosis, tracheobronchitis, croup, and asthma. Failure to respond to croup treatments, such as humidity and racemic epinephrine, helps to differentiate tracheitis from croup.

Treatment

Treatment consists of maintaining a patent airway and antibiotic therapy. Most patients require endotracheal intubation or tracheostomy; for those who do not, supplemental oxygen should be provided. Intravenous cefuroxime is the drug of choice and should be administered empirically while awaiting culture results. In cases of toxic shock, hemodynamic monitoring and support may be required. Extubation can usually be accomplished after 3 to 7 days of antibiotic therapy.

Special considerations

▶ Monitor respiratory status closely in those patients who do not have an artificial airway via continuous pulse oximetry, ABGs, or both. Have a tracheostomy kit at the bedside.

▶ Suction intubated patients vigorously; obtain sputum cultures as ordered, preferably before antibiotic administration.

▶ Provide emotional support to the patient and family.

▶ Administer antipyretics as needed. Aspirin is not given to children under 18 years of age.

▶ Monitor complete blood counts.

▶ Monitor for signs of dehydration.

 PREVENTION TIP Parents should be carefully instructed regarding signs of respiratory distress in their young children, particularly after an upper respiratory infection. Stress that this is a true emergency requiring immediate medical treatment or death may quickly ensue. Parents who are unsure of the severity of their child's breathing difficulties should be encouraged to err on the side of caution and to seek immediate medical care.

TRACHOMA

The most common cause of preventable blindness in underdeveloped areas of the world, trachoma is a chronic form of keratoconjunctivitis. This infection is usually confined to the eye but may have a systemic component. Although trachoma itself is self-limiting, it causes permanent damage to the cornea and conjunctiva by scarring the lids; severe trachoma may lead to blindness, especially if a secondary bacterial infection develops. Early diagnosis and treatment (before trachoma results in scar formation) ensure recovery but without immunity to reinfection. Trachoma is prevalent in Africa, Latin America, and Asia, particularly in children; in the United States, it is prevalent among the Native Americans of the Southwest.

Causes

Trachoma results from infection by *Chlamydia trachomatis,* a gram-negative,

obligate intracellular bacteria. These microbes are transmitted from eye to eye by flies and gnats and by hand-eye contact in endemic areas.

Trachoma is spread by close contact between family members or among schoolchildren. Other predisposing factors include poverty and poor hygiene due to lack of water. Patients in hot, dusty climates are at greater risk.

Signs and symptoms

Trachoma begins with a mild infection resembling bacterial conjunctivitis (visible conjunctival follicles, red and edematous eyelids, pain, photophobia, tearing, and exudation).

After about 1 month, if the infection is untreated, conjunctival follicles enlarge into inflamed papillae that later become yellow or gray. At this stage, small blood vessels invade the cornea under the upper lid.

Eventually, severe scarring and contraction of the eyelids cause entropion; the eyelids turn inward and the lashes rub against the cornea, producing corneal scarring and visual distortion. In the later stages, severe conjunctival scarring may obstruct the lacrimal ducts and cause dry eyes. (See *What happens in trachoma.*)

Diagnosis

Follicular conjunctivitis with corneal infiltration and upper lid or conjunctival scarring suggest trachoma, especially in endemic areas, when these symptoms persist longer than 3 weeks.

Microscopic examination of a Giemsa-stained conjunctival scraping confirms the diagnosis by showing cytoplasmic inclusion bodies, some polymorphonuclear reaction, plasma cells, Leber's cells (large macrophages containing phagocytosed debris), and follicle cells.

Treatment

Primary treatment of trachoma consists of 3 to 4 weeks of topical or systemic antibiotic therapy with tetracycline, eryth-

WHAT HAPPENS IN TRACHOMA

Trachoma results from infection with *Chlamydia trachomatis* and its early stages resemble bacterial conjunctivitis. If untreated, this chronic infection can spread to the cornea and lead to scarring and, eventually, to blindness.

```
          Mild infection from close personal contact
                          │
                          ▼
                  Bilateral conjunctivitis
                          │
                          ▼
          Increasing edema, tearing, photophobia
                 │                        │
                 ▼                        ▼
  Development of conjunctival follicles   Inflammation of
                 │                        upper cornea
                 ▼                        │
  Scarring of conjunctival lining         ▼
  of the eyelid                     Superficial corneal
         │            │             vascularization
         ▼            ▼                    │
  Occlusion of    Entropion               ▼
  lacrimal ducts  (inversion of      Infiltration with
         │        the eyelid)        granulation tissue
         ▼            │
     Dry eyes         ▼
              Abrasion of the cornea
              by lashes
                      │
                      ▼
                  Ulcerations
                      │
                      ▼
              Scarring of cornea
                      │
                      ▼
                 Loss of vision
```

romycin, or sulfonamides. (Tetracycline is contraindicated in pregnant females because it may adversely affect the fetus, and in children under age 7, in whom it may discolor teeth permanently.) Severe entropion requires surgical correction.

Special considerations

▶ Because no definitive preventive measure exists (vaccines offer temporary and partial protection, at best), stress the need for strict compliance with the prescribed drug therapy.

If ordered, teach the patient or family members how to instill eyedrops correctly.

 PREVENTION TIP Emphasize the importance of hand washing and making the best use of available water supplies to maintain good personal hygiene. To prevent trachoma, warn patients not to allow flies or gnats to settle around the eyes.

TRICHINOSIS

An infection caused by larvae of the intestinal roundworm *Trichinella spiralis,* trichinosis (trichiniasis, trichinellosis) occurs worldwide, especially in populations that eat pork or bear meat. Trichinosis may produce multiple symptoms; respiratory, central nervous system (CNS), and cardiovascular complications; and, rarely, death.

Causes

Transmission is through ingestion of uncooked or undercooked meat that contains *T. spiralis* cysts. Such cysts are found primarily in swine, less often in dogs, cats, bears, foxes, wolves, and marine animals. These cysts result from the animals' ingestion of similarly contaminated flesh. In swine, such infection results from eating table scraps or raw garbage.

After gastric juices free the worm from the cyst capsule, it reaches sexual maturity in a few days. The female roundworm burrows into the intestinal mucosa and reproduces. Larvae are then transported through the lymphatic system and the bloodstream. They become embedded as cysts in striated muscle, especially in the diaphragm, chest, arms, and legs. Human-to-human transmission does not take place.

Signs and symptoms

In the United States, trichinosis is usually mild and seldom produces symptoms.

When symptoms do occur, they vary with the stage and degree of infection:

Stage 1 — Invasion: occurs 1 week after ingestion. Release of larvae and reproduction of adult *T. spiralis* cause anorexia, nausea, vomiting, diarrhea, abdominal pain, and cramps.

Stage 2 — Dissemination: occurs 7 to 10 days after ingestion. *T. spiralis* penetrates the intestinal mucosa and begins to migrate to striated muscle. Symptoms include edema, especially of the eyelids or face; muscle pain, particularly in extremities; and, occasionally, itching and burning skin, sweating, skin lesions, a temperature of 102° to 104° F (38.9° to 40° C), and delirium; and, in severe respiratory, cardiovascular, or CNS infections, palpitations and lethargy.

Stage 3 — Encystment: occurs during convalescence, generally 1 week later. *T. spiralis* larvae invade muscle fiber and become encysted.

Diagnosis

A history of ingestion of raw or improperly cooked pork or pork products, with typical clinical features, suggests trichinosis, but infection may be difficult to prove.

Stools may contain mature worms and larvae during the invasion stage.

Skeletal muscle biopsies can show encysted larvae 10 days after ingestion; and, if available, analyses of contaminated meat also show larvae.

Skin testing may show a positive histamine-like reactivity 15 minutes after intradermal injection of the antigen (within 17 to 20 days after ingestion). Positive histamine-like reactivity may remain positive for up to 5 years after exposure.

Elevated acute and convalescent antibody titers (determined by flocculation tests 3 to 4 weeks after infection) confirm this diagnosis.

Other abnormal results include elevated alanine aminotransferase, aspartate aminotransferase, creatine kinase, and lactate dehydrogenase levels during the acute stages and an elevated eosinophil count (up to 15,000/μl). A normal or increased cerebrospinal fluid lymphocyte level (to 300/μl) and increased protein levels indicate CNS involvement.

Treatment
Thiabendazole effectively combats this parasite during the intestinal stage; severe infection (especially CNS invasion) may warrant glucocorticoids to fight against possible inflammation.

Special considerations
▶ Question the patient about recent ingestion of pork products and the methods used to store and cook them.
▶ Reduce fever with alcohol rubs, tepid baths, cooling blankets, or antipyretics; relieve muscular pain with analgesics, enforced bed rest, and proper body alignment.
▶ Emphasize the importance of bed rest. Sudden death from cardiac involvement may occur in a patient with moderate to severe trichinosis infection who has resumed activity too soon. Warn the patient to continue bed rest into the convalescent stage to avoid a serious relapse and possible death.
▶ Tell the patient that possible adverse reactions to thiabendazole are nausea, vomiting, dizziness, dermatitis, and fever.
▶ Report all cases of trichinosis to local public health authorities.

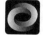 **PREVENTION TIP** Educate the public about proper cooking and storing methods, not only for pork and pork products but also for meat from carnivores. To kill trichinae, internal meat temperatures should reach 150° F (66° C) and its color should change from pink to gray unless the meat has been cured or frozen for at least 10 days at low temperatures. Warn travelers to foreign countries or to very poor areas in the United States to avoid eating pork; swine in these areas are often fed raw garbage.

TRICHOMONIASIS

A protozoal infection of the lower genitourinary tract, trichomoniasis affects about 15% of sexually active females and 10% of sexually active males. This infection, which occurs worldwide, may be acute or chronic in females. The risk of recurrence is minimized when sexual partners are treated concurrently.

Causes
Trichomonas vaginalis — a tetraflagellated, motile protozoan — causes trichomoniasis in females by infecting the vagina, the urethra and, possibly, the endocervix, bladder, Bartholin's glands, or Skene's glands; in males, it infects the lower urethra and, possibly, the prostate gland, seminal vesicles, or epididymis.

T. vaginalis grows best when the vaginal mucosa is more alkaline than normal (pH about 5.5 to 5.8). Therefore, factors that raise the vaginal pH — use of oral contraceptives, pregnancy, bacterial overgrowth, exudative cervical or vaginal lesions, or frequent douching, which disturbs lactobacilli that normally live in the vagina and maintain acidity — may predispose a woman to trichomoniasis.

Trichomoniasis is usually transmitted by intercourse; less often, by contaminated douche equipment or moist washcloths.

Signs and symptoms
Approximately 70% of females — including those with chronic infections — and most males with trichomoniasis are asymptomatic. In females, acute infection may produce variable signs, such as a gray or greenish yellow and possibly profuse and frothy, malodorous vaginal discharge. Its other effects include severe itching, redness, swelling, tenderness, dyspareunia, dysuria, urinary frequency and, occasionally, postcoital spotting, menorrhagia, or dysmenorrhea.

Such symptoms may persist for a week to several months and may be more pronounced just after menstruation or during pregnancy. If trichomoniasis is untreated, symptoms may subside, although *T. vaginalis* infection persists, possibly associated with an abnormal cytologic smear of the cervix.

In males, trichomoniasis may produce mild to severe transient urethritis, possibly with dysuria and frequency.

Diagnosis

Direct microscopic examination of vaginal or seminal discharge is decisive when it reveals *T. vaginalis,* a motile, pear-shaped organism. Examination of clear urine specimens may also reveal *T. vaginalis.*

Physical examination of symptomatic females shows vaginal erythema; edema; frank excoriation; a frothy, malodorous, greenish yellow vaginal discharge; and, rarely, a thin, gray pseudomembrane over the vagina. Cervical examination demonstrates punctate cervical hemorrhages, giving the cervix a strawberry appearance that is almost pathognomonic for this disorder.

Treatment

The treatment of choice for trichomoniasis is a single 2-g dose of oral metronidazole given to both sexual partners. Alternative treatment is 500 mg of oral metronidazole given twice daily for 7 days. Oral metronidazole has not been proven safe during the first trimester of pregnancy, but can be considered for use if symptoms are severe. Effective alternatives are not available for patients who are allergic to metronidazole. Sitz baths may be used to help relieve symptoms.

Special considerations

▶ Instruct the patient to refrain from douching before being examined for trichomoniasis.
▶ Urge abstinence from intercourse until the patient is cured. Refer partners for treatment. Tell the patient to avoid using tampons.

▶ Warn the patient to abstain from alcoholic beverages while taking metronidazole because alcohol consumption may provoke a disulfiram-type reaction (confusion, headache, cramps, vomiting, seizures). Also, tell the patient this drug may turn urine dark brown.
▶ Caution the patient to avoid over-the-counter douches and vaginal sprays because chronic use can alter vaginal pH.
▶ Advise the patient to scrub the bathtub with a disinfecting cleaner before and after sitz baths.

 PREVENTION TIP Tell the patient she can reduce the risk of genitourinary bacterial growth by wearing loose-fitting, cotton underwear, which allows ventilation; bacteria flourish in a warm, dark, moist environment.

TUBERCULOSIS

An acute or chronic infection caused by *Mycobacterium tuberculosis,* tuberculosis (TB) is characterized by pulmonary infiltrates, formation of granulomas with caseation, fibrosis, and cavitation. Globally, tuberculosis is the leading cause of morbidity and mortality. There are 8 to 10 million new cases each year. People living in crowded, poorly ventilated conditions are most likely to become infected.

In patients with strains that are sensitive to the usual antitubercular agents, the prognosis is excellent with correct treatment. However, in those with strains that are resistant to two or more of the major antitubercular agents, mortality is 50%.

Causes

After exposure to *M. tuberculosis,* roughly 5% of infected people develop active tuberculosis within 1 year; in the remainder, microbes cause a latent infection. The immune system usually controls the tubercle bacillus by killing it or walling it up in a tiny nodule (tubercle). However, the bacillus may lie dormant within the tubercle for years and later reactivate and spread.

Although the primary infection site is the lungs, mycobacteria commonly exist in other parts of the body. A number of factors increase the risk of infection reactivation: gastrectomy, uncontrolled diabetes mellitus, Hodgkin's disease, leukemia, silicosis, acquired immunodeficiency syndrome, and treatment with corticosteroids or immunosuppressives.

Tuberculosis is transmitted by droplet nuclei produced when infected persons cough or sneeze. Persons with a cavity lesion are particularly infectious because their sputum usually contains 1 million to 100 million bacilli per ml. After inhalation, if a tubercle bacillus settles in an alveolus, infection occurs. Cell-mediated immunity to the mycobacteria, which develops about 3 to 6 weeks later, usually contains the infection and arrests the disease.

If the infection reactivates, the body's response characteristically leads to caseation — the conversion of necrotic tissue to a cheeselike material. The caseum may localize, undergo fibrosis, or excavate and form cavities, the walls of which are studded with multiplying tubercle bacilli. If this happens, infected caseous debris may spread throughout the lungs by the tracheobronchial tree.

Sites of extrapulmonary TB include pleura, meninges, joints, lymph nodes, peritoneum, genitourinary tract, and bowel.

Signs and symptoms

In primary infection, after an incubation period of from 4 to 8 weeks, TB is usually asymptomatic but may produce nonspecific symptoms, such as fatigue, weakness, anorexia, weight loss, night sweats, and low-grade fever.

In reactivation, symptoms may include a cough that produces mucopurulent sputum, occasional hemoptysis, and chest pains.

Diagnosis

Diagnostic tests include chest X-rays, a tuberculin skin test, and sputum smears and cultures to identify *M. tuberculosis.* The following procedures aid diagnosis:

▶ Auscultation detects crepitant rales, bronchial breath sounds, wheezes, and whispered pectoriloquy.

▶ Chest percussion detects a dullness over the affected area, indicating consolidation or pleural fluid.

▶ Chest X-ray shows nodular lesions, patchy infiltrates (mainly in upper lobes), cavity formation, scar tissue, and calcium deposits; however, it may not be able to distinguish active from inactive TB.

▶ Tuberculin skin test detects TB infection. Intermediate-strength purified protein derivative (PPD) or 5 tuberculin units (0.1 ml) are injected intracutaneously on the forearm. The test results are read in 48 to 72 hours; a positive reaction (induration of 5 to 15 mm or more, depending on risk factors) develops 2 to 10 weeks after infection in both active and inactive TB. However, severely immunosuppressed patients may never develop a positive reaction.

▶ Stains and cultures (of sputum, cerebrospinal fluid, urine, drainage from abscess, or pleural fluid) show heat-sensitive, nonmotile, aerobic, acid-fast bacilli.

Treatment

Antitubercular therapy with daily oral doses of isoniazid, rifampin, and pyrazinamide (and sometimes ethambutol) for at least 6 months usually cures tuberculosis. After 2 to 4 weeks, the disease generally is no longer infectious. The patient can resume his lifestyle while taking medication.

Patients with atypical mycobacterial disease or drug-resistant TB may require treatment with second-line drugs, such as capreomycin, streptomycin, para-aminosalicylic acid, cycloserine, amikacin, and quinolone drugs. (See *Treating multiply drug-resistant TB,* page 320.) Because of

TREATING MULTIPLY DRUG-RESISTANT TB

The National Institute of Allergy and Infectious Disease (NIAID), a branch of the National Institutes of Health (NIH), is currently conducting a phase I/II, controlled, open label, dose escalation study to determine the tolerance, toxicity, and clinical effect of the administration of interferon-gamma on the clinical condition and immune function of patients with multiply drug-resistant M. tuberculosis infections (MDRTB). The study drug (interferon gamma) will be administered subcutaneously three times a week at three dose levels for one year, in addition to anti-tuberculosis medications.

▶ Be alert for adverse effects of medications. Because isoniazid sometimes leads to hepatitis or peripheral neuritis, monitor aspartate aminotransferase and alanine aminotransferase levels. To prevent or treat peripheral neuritis, give pyridoxine (vitamin B_6).

▶ If the patient receives ethambutol, watch for optic neuritis; if it develops, discontinue the drug. If he receives rifampin, watch for hepatitis and purpura. Also observe the patient for other complications such as hemoptysis.

▶ Emphasize the importance of regular follow-up examinations, and instruct the patient and his family concerning the signs and symptoms of recurring TB.

▶ Advise persons who have been exposed to infected patients to receive tuberculin tests and, if necessary, chest X-rays and prophylactic isoniazid.

the consequences of inadequate or incomplete treatment, direct observed therapy (DOT) to prevent noncompliance is increasingly being employed.

Special considerations

▶ Isolate the infectious patient in a quiet, well-ventilated room until he's no longer contagious.

▶ Teach the patient to cough and sneeze into tissues and to dispose of all secretions properly. Place a covered trash can nearby or tape a waxed bag to the side of the bed for used tissues.

▶ Instruct the patient to wear a mask when outside his room. Visitors and hospital personnel should wear masks when they are in the patient's room.

▶ Remind the patient to get plenty of rest and to eat balanced meals. If the patient is anorectic, urge him to eat small meals throughout the day. Record weight weekly.

U

URINARY TRACT INFECTION, LOWER

Cystitis and urethritis, the two forms of lower urinary tract infection (UTI), are nearly 10 times more common in women than in men; they affect approximately 10% to 20% of all women at least once. Lower UTI is also a prevalent bacterial disease in children, and girls are most commonly affected.

In men and children, lower UTIs are frequently related to anatomic or physiologic abnormalities and therefore require extremely close evaluation. UTIs often respond readily to treatment, but recurrence and resistant bacterial flare-up during therapy are possible.

Causes

Most lower UTIs result from ascending infection by a single gram-negative enteric bacteria, such as *Escherichia coli, Klebsiella, Proteus, Enterobacter, Pseudomonas,* or *Serratia.* However, in a patient with neurogenic bladder, an indwelling urinary catheter, or a fistula between the intestine and bladder, lower UTI may result from simultaneous infection with multiple pathogens.

Recent studies suggest that infection results from a breakdown in local defense mechanisms in the bladder that allow bacteria to invade the bladder mucosa and multiply. These bacteria cannot be readily eliminated by normal micturition.

During treatment, bacterial flare-up is generally caused by the microbe's resistance to the prescribed antimicrobial therapy. The presence of even a small number (less than 10,000/ ml) of bacteria in a midstream urine sample obtained during treatment casts doubt on the effectiveness of treatment.

In 99% of patients, recurrent lower UTI results from reinfection by the same microbe or from some new pathogen; in the remaining 1%, recurrence reflects persistent infection, usually from renal calculi, chronic bacterial prostatitis, or a structural anomaly that may become a source of infection.

The high incidence of lower UTI among women may result from the shortness of the female urethra (1¼" to 2" [3 to 5 cm]), which predisposes women to infection caused by bacteria from the vagina, perineum, rectum, or a sexual partner.

Men are less vulnerable because their urethras are longer (7¾" [19.68 cm]) and their prostatic fluid serves as an antibacterial shield. In both men and women, infection usually ascends from the urethra to the bladder.

Signs and symptoms

Lower UTI usually produces urgency, frequency, dysuria, cramps or spasms of the bladder, itching, a feeling of warmth during urination, nocturia, and possibly urethral discharge in males. Inflammation of the bladder wall also causes hematuria and fever.

Other common features include low back pain, malaise, nausea, vomiting, abdominal pain or tenderness over the bladder area, chills, and flank pain.

Diagnosis

Characteristic clinical features and a microscopic urinalysis showing red blood cells and white blood cells greater than 10/high-power field suggest lower UTI.

A clean, midstream urine specimen revealing a bacterial count of more than 100,000/ml confirms the diagnosis. Lower counts do not necessarily rule out infection, especially if the patient is voiding frequently, because bacteria require 30 to 45 minutes to reproduce in urine.

Careful midstream, clean-catch collection is preferred to catheterization, which can reinfect the bladder with urethral bacteria.

Sensitivity testing determines the appropriate therapeutic antimicrobial agent. Voiding cystoureterography or excretory urography may detect congenital anomalies that predispose the patient to recurrent UTIs.

If patient history and physical examination warrant, a blood test or a stained smear of the discharge rules out a sexually transmitted disease.

Treatment

Appropriate antimicrobials are the treatment of choice for most initial lower UTIs.

Females:

▶ For rare or infrequent uncomplicated UTIs or the first uncomplicated UTI without risk factors (diabetic, pregnant, immunocompromised), 3-day treatment with trimethoprim-sulfamethoxazole (TMP/SMX) or fluoroquinolone

▶ Postcoital UTI: single dose TMP/SMX or cephalexin

▶ Pregnant patients: 10 to 14 days of treatment with amoxicillin, augmentin, or nitrofurantoin

▶ All others: 10 to 14 days of treatment with TMP/SMX, fluoroquinolone, ofloxacin, or augmentin.

Males:

▶ First UTI, no risk factors: 7 to 10 days TMP/SMX or as indicated by culture and sensitivity

▶ Complicated or recurrent UTIs: 14 to 21 days of an antibiotic based on culture and sensitivity.

After 3 days of antibiotic therapy, urine culture should show no microbes.

If the urine is not sterile, bacterial resistance has probably occurred, making the use of a different antimicrobial necessary. Single-dose antibiotic therapy with amoxicillin or co-trimoxazole may be effective in women with acute, noncomplicated UTI. A urine culture taken 1 to 2 weeks later indicates whether the infection has been eradicated.

Recurrent infections due to infected renal calculi, chronic prostatitis, or structural abnormality may necessitate surgery; prostatitis also requires long-term antibiotic therapy. In patients without these predisposing conditions, long-term, low-dosage antibiotic therapy is the treatment of choice.

Special considerations

▶ Watch for GI disturbances from antimicrobial therapy.

▶ If sitz baths are not effective, apply heat sparingly to the perineum, but be careful not to burn the patient. Apply topical antiseptics, such as povidone-iodine ointment, on the urethral meatus as necessary.

▶ Collect all urine samples for culture and sensitivity testing carefully and promptly.

 PREVENTION TIP To prevent recurrent infections in women, teach the patient to carefully wipe the perineum from front to back and to clean thoroughly with soap and water after defecation; void immediately after sexual intercourse; drink plenty of fluids, especially water; drink cranberry juice, if suggested, for its acidic effects on urine, which inhibits the growth of some bacteria; and routinely avoid postponing urination. Recommend frequent comfort stops during long car trips and stress the need to empty the bladder completely.

COMPARING GRANULOMATOUS AND NONGRANULOMATOUS UVEITIS

FACTOR	GRANULOMATOUS	NONGRANULOMATOUS
Location	Usually, posterior part of the uveal tract	Anterior part of the iris and ciliary body
Onset	Insidious	Acute
Pain	None or slight	Marked
Photophobia	Slight	Marked
Course	Chronic	Acute
Prognosis	Fair to poor	Good
Recurrence	Occasional	Common
Blurred vision	Marked	Moderate

UVEITIS

Uveitis is inflammation of the uveal tract. It occurs as anterior uveitis, which affects the iris (iritis), or both the iris and the ciliary body (iridocyclitis); as posterior uveitis, which affects the choroid (choroiditis), or both the choroid and the retina (chorioretinitis); or as panuveitis, which affects the entire uveal tract. Although clinical distinction is not always possible, anterior uveitis occurs in two forms — granulomatous and nongranulomatous.

Granulomatous uveitis was once thought to be caused by tuberculosis bacilli; nongranulomatous uveitis, by streptococci. (See *Comparing granulomatous and nongranulomatous uveitis.*) Although this is not true, the terms are still used. Untreated anterior uveitis may result in elevated intraocular pressure resulting in visual loss. With immediate treatment, anterior uveitis usually subsides after a few days to several weeks; however, recurrence is likely.

Posterior uveitis may lead to visual loss if the macula is involved.

Causes

Typically, uveitis is idiopathic. But it can result from allergy, bacteria, viruses, fungi, chemicals, trauma, or surgery; or it may be associated with systemic diseases, such as rheumatoid arthritis, ankylosing spondylitis, and toxoplasmosis.

Signs and symptoms

Anterior uveitis produces moderate to severe unilateral eye pain; severe ciliary injection; photophobia; tearing; a small, nonreactive pupil; and blurred vision (due to the increased number of cells in the aqueous humor). It sometimes produces deposits called keratic precipitates on the back of the cornea that may be seen in the anterior chamber. The iris may adhere to the lens, causing posterior synechia and pupillary distortion; pain and photophobia may occur. Onset may be acute or insidious.

Posterior uveitis begins insidiously, with complaints of slightly decreased or blurred vision or floating spots. Posterior uveitis may be acute or chronic; and it may affect one or both eyes. Retinal damage, caused by lesions from toxoplasmosis, and retinal detachments may occur.

Diagnosis

In anterior uveitis, a slit-lamp examination shows a flare and cell pattern, which looks like particles dancing on a sunbeam. With a special lens, slit-lamp and ophthalmoscopic examination can also identify active inflammatory fundus lesions involving the retina and choroid.

In posterior uveitis, serologic tests may be used to rule out toxoplasmosis as the cause.

Treatment

Uveitis requires vigorous and prompt management, which includes treatment of any known underlying cause, application of a topical cycloplegic, such as 1% atropine sulfate, and of topical corticosteroids. For severe uveitis, therapy includes oral systemic corticosteroids. However, long-term steroid therapy can cause a rise in intraocular pressure (IOP) or cataracts. Carefully monitor IOP during acute inflammation. If IOP rises, therapy should include an antiglaucoma medication, such as an alpha agonist, or topical carbonic anhydrase inhibitor, such as dorozolamide.

 ALERT Refer to an ophthalmologist for a dilated fundus examination and treatment of local or systemic disease.

Special considerations

❯ Encourage rest during the acute phase.
❯ Teach the patient the proper method of instilling eyedrops.
❯ Suggest the use of dark glasses to ease the discomfort of photophobia.
❯ Instruct the patient to watch for and report adverse effects of systemic corticosteroid therapy (for example, edema, muscle weakness).
❯ Stress the importance of follow-up care. Tell the patient to seek treatment immediately at first signs of iritis.

V

VANCOMYCIN INTERMITTENTLY RESISTANT *STAPHYLOCOCCUS AUREUS* INFECTION

Vancomycin intermittently resistant *Staphylococcus aureus* (VIRSA) is a mutation of a bacterium that is spread easily by direct person-to-person contact. It was first discovered in mid-1996 when clinicians found the microbe in a Japanese infant's surgical wound. Similar isolates were reported in Michigan and New Jersey. Both patients had received multiple courses of vancomycin for methicillin-resistant *Staphylococcus aureus* (MRSA) infections.

Another mutation, vancomycin-resistant *Staphylococcus aureus* (VRSA) is fully resistant to vancomycin. Patients most at risk for infection by resistant microbes include:

▶ patients with a history of taking vancomycin, third-generation cephalosporins, or antibiotics targeted at anaerobic bacteria (such as *Clostridium difficile*)

▶ patients with indwelling urinary or central venous catheters

▶ elderly patients, especially those with prolonged or repeated hospital admissions

▶ patients with malignancies or chronic renal failure

▶ patients undergoing cardiothoracic or intra-abdominal surgery or organ transplants

▶ patients with wounds with an opening to the pelvic or intra-abdominal area, including surgical wounds, burns, and pressure ulcers

▶ patients with enterococcal bacteremia, often associated with endocarditis

▶ patients exposed to contaminated equipment or to a patient with the infecting microbe.

Causes

MRSA enters health care facilities through an infected or colonized patient or a colonized health care worker. It is thought that VIRSA/VRSA is colonized in a similar method. It is spread through direct contact between the patient and caregiver or between patients. It may also be spread through patient contact with contaminated surfaces such as an overbed table. It is capable of living for weeks on surfaces. It has been detected on patient gowns, bed linens, and handrails.

Signs and symptoms

There are no specific signs or symptoms related to infection by this microbe. The causative agent may be found incidentally when culture results show the microbe.

Diagnosis

Someone with no signs or symptoms of infection is considered colonized if VIRSA or VRSA can be isolated from stool or a rectal swab. A patient who is colonized is more than 10 times as likely to become infected with the organism (for example, through a breach in the immune system) than a patient who is not.

Treatment

There is virtually no antibiotic to combat VIRSA or VRSA. (See *Treating multidrug-resistant* Staphylococcus aureus, page 326.)

INVESTIGATIONAL THERAPY

TREATING MULTIDRUG-RESISTANT *STAPHYLOCOCCUS AUREUS*

Research is currently under way to develop an effective vaccine to prevent infection by *Staphylococcus aureus*. Studies have been completed on animals only, with promising results. The goal is to develop a vaccine to stimulate the production of antibodies against the *S. aureus* enterotoxin. The enterotoxin is one of the substances responsible for the severe virulence of this microbe.

Recently, the Centers for Disease Control and Prevention and the Hospital Infection Control Practices Advisory Committee proposed a two-level system of precautions to simplify isolation for resistant organisms. The first level calls for standard precautions, which incorporate features of universal blood and body fluid precautions, and body substance isolation precautions, to be used for all patient care. The second level calls for transmission-based precautions, implemented when a particular infection is suspected.

To prevent the spread of VIRSA and VRSA, some hospitals perform weekly surveillance cultures on at-risk patients in intensive care units or oncology units, and on patients who have been transferred from a long-term care facility. Any colonized patient is then placed in contact isolation until he's culture-negative or discharged. Colonization can last indefinitely, and no protocol has been established for the length of time a patient should remain in isolation.

Because no single antibiotic is currently available, the doctor may opt not to treat an infection at all. Instead, he may stop all antibiotics and simply wait for normal bacteria to repopulate and replace the strain. Combinations of various drugs may also be used, depending on the source of the infection.

Special considerations

▶ Personnel in contact with an infected patient should wash their hands before and after care of the patient.

▶ Good hand washing is the most effective way to prevent VIRSA and VRSA from spreading.

▶ Use an antiseptic soap such as chlorhexidine; bacteria have been cultured from workers' hands after they've washed with milder soap.

▶ Maintain contact isolation precautions when in contact with the patient. Provide a private room and dedicated equipment, and disinfect the environment.

▶ Change gloves when contaminated or when moving from a dirty area of the body to a clean one.

▶ Do not touch potentially contaminated surfaces, such as a bed or bed stand, after removing gown and gloves.

▶ Be particularly prudent in caring for a patient with an ileostomy, colostomy, or draining wound that is not contained by a dressing.

▶ Instruct family and friends to wear protective garb when they visit the patient, and teach them how to dispose of it.

▶ Provide teaching and emotional support to the patient and family members.

▶ Consider grouping infected patients together (known as cohorting) and having the same nursing staff care for them.

▶ Do not lay equipment used on the patient on the bed or bed stand; wipe it with appropriate disinfectant before leaving the room.

▶ Ensure judicious and careful use of antibiotics. Encourage doctors to limit the use of antibiotics.

▶ Instruct patients to take antibiotics for the full prescription period, even if they begin to feel better.

VANCOMYCIN-RESISTANT ENTEROCOCCUS INFECTION

Vancomycin-resistant enterococcus (VRE) is a mutation of a very common bacterium that spreads by direct person-to-person contact. Facilities in more than 40 states have reported VRE infections, with rates as high as 14% in oncology units of large teaching facilities. Patients most at risk for VRE infection include:

▶ immunosuppressed patients or those with severe underlying disease
▶ patients with a history of taking vancomycin, third-generation cephalosporins, or antibiotics targeted at anaerobic bacteria (such as *Clostridium difficile*)
▶ patients with indwelling urinary or central venous catheters
▶ elderly patients, especially those with prolonged or repeated hospital admissions
▶ patients with malignancies or chronic renal failure
▶ patients undergoing cardiothoracic or intra-abdominal surgery or organ transplants
▶ patients with wounds with an opening to the pelvic or intra-abdominal area, including surgical wounds, burns, and pressure ulcers
▶ patients with enterococcal bacteremia, often associated with endocarditis
▶ patients exposed to contaminated equipment or to a VRE-positive patient.

Causes

VRE enters health care facilities through an infected or colonized patient or a colonized health care worker. The microbe is spread through direct contact between the patient and caregiver or between patients. It can also be spread through patient contact with contaminated surfaces such as an overbed table. VRE is capable of living on surfaces for weeks, and has been detected on patient gowns, bed linens, and handrails.

Signs and symptoms

No specific signs and symptoms are related to VRE infection. The causative microbe may be found incidentally when culture results show the organism.

Diagnosis

Asymptomatic individuals are considered colonized if VRE can be isolated from stool or a rectal swab. Once colonized, a patient is more than 10 times as likely to become infected with VRE—for example, through a breach in the immune system.

Treatment

No specific treatment exists for eradicating VRE. The Centers for Disease Control and Prevention and the Hospital Infection Control Practices Advisory Committee have proposed a two-level system of precautions to simplify isolation. The first level calls for standard precautions, incorporating features of universal blood and body fluid precautions and body substance isolation precautions to be used for all patient care. The second level calls for transmission-based precautions, implemented when a particular infection is suspected.

To prevent the spread of VRE, some facilities perform weekly surveillance cultures on at-risk patients in intensive care units or oncology units and on patients who have been transferred from a long-term-care facility. Any colonized patient is then in contact isolation until culture-negative or until discharged. Colonization can last indefinitely, and no protocol has been established for the length of time a patient should remain in isolation.

Because no single antibiotic currently available can eradicate VRE, the doctor may, in some cases, opt not to treat an infection at all. Instead, he may stop all antibiotics and simply wait for normal bacteria to repopulate and replace the VRE strain. Combinations of various drugs may also be used, depending on the source of the infection.

Special considerations

▶ Hand washing before and after care of the patient is crucial.

▶ Use an antiseptic soap such as chlorhexidine; bacteria have been cultured from workers' hands after they've washed with milder soap.

▶ Use contact isolation precautions when in contact with the patient. Provide a private room and dedicated equipment for the patient. Disinfect the environment.

▶ Change gloves when contaminated or when moving from a dirty area of the body to a clean one.

▶ Do not touch potentially contaminated surfaces, such as a bed or bed stand, after removing gown and gloves.

▶ Be particularly prudent in caring for a patient with an ileostomy, colostomy, or draining wound that is not contained by a dressing.

▶ Instruct family and friends to wear protective garb when they visit the patient, and teach them how to dispose of it.

▶ Provide teaching and emotional support to the patient and family members.

▶ Consider grouping (cohorting) infected patients together and having the same nursing staff care for them.

▶ Do not lay equipment used on the patient on the bed or the bed stand. Wipe equipment with appropriate disinfectant before leaving the room.

▶ Ensure judicious and careful use of antibiotics. Encourage doctors to limit the use of antibiotics.

▶ Instruct patients to take antibiotics for the full prescription period, even if they begin to feel better.

VARICELLA

Also called chickenpox, varicella is a common, acute, and highly contagious infection caused by the herpesvirus varicella-zoster (V-Z), the same virus that, in its latent stage, causes herpes zoster (shingles). It can occur at any age, but it's most common in 2- to 8-year-olds.

Varicella vaccine prevents chickenpox in up to 90% of recipients. The American Academy of Pediatrics recommends the vaccine for all children and for adolescents and adults who haven't had chickenpox. It is unknown how the vaccine affects shingles.

Causes

Congenital varicella may affect infants whose mothers had acute infections in their first or early second trimester. Neonatal infection is rare, probably due to transient maternal immunity. Second attacks are also rare.

Chickenpox is transmitted by direct contact (primarily with respiratory secretions; less often with skin lesions) and indirect contact through the air. The incubation period lasts from 14 to 17 days. Chickenpox is probably communicable from 1 day before lesions erupt to 6 days after vesicles form (it's most contagious in the early stages of eruption of skin lesions).

Most children recover completely. Potentially fatal complications may affect children receiving corticosteroids, antimetabolites, or other immunosuppressant agents, and those with leukemia, other neoplasms, or immunodeficiency disorders. Congenital and adult varicella may also have severe effects.

This disease occurs worldwide and is endemic in large cities. Outbreaks occur sporadically, usually in areas with large groups of susceptible children. It affects all races and both sexes equally. Seasonal distribution varies; in temperate areas, incidence is higher during late autumn, winter, and spring.

Signs and symptoms

Chickenpox produces distinctive signs and symptoms, notably a pruritic rash. During the prodromal phase, the patient has slight fever, malaise, and anorexia. Within 24 hours, the rash typically begins as crops of small, erythematous macules on the trunk or scalp that progress to papules and then clear vesicles on an erythematous base (the so-called "dewdrop on a rose petal").

The vesicles become cloudy and break easily; then scabs form. The rash spreads to the face and, rarely, to the extremities. New vesicles continue to appear for 3 to 4 days, so the rash contains a combination of red papules, vesicles, and scabs in various stages. Occasionally, chickenpox also produces shallow ulcers on mucous membranes of the mouth, conjunctivae, and genitalia.

Congenital varicella causes hypoplastic deformity and scarring of a limb, retarded growth, and central nervous system and eye manifestations. In progressive varicella, an immunocompromised patient will have lesions and a high fever for more than 7 days.

Severe pruritus with this rash may provoke persistent scratching, which can lead to infection, scarring, impetigo, furuncles, and cellulitis. Rare complications include pneumonia, myocarditis, fulminating encephalitis (Reye's syndrome), bleeding disorders, arthritis, nephritis, hepatitis, and acute myositis.

Diagnosis

Chickenpox is diagnosed by characteristic clinical signs and usually doesn't require laboratory tests. However, the virus can be isolated from vesicular fluid within the first 3 to 4 days of the rash; Giemsa stain distinguishes V-Z from vaccinia-variola viruses. Serum contains antibodies 7 days after onset.

Treatment

Patients must remain in strict isolation until all the vesicles and most of the scabs disappear (usually for 1 week after the onset of the rash). Children can go back to school, however, if just a few scabs remain because, at this stage, chickenpox is no longer contagious. Congenital chickenpox requires no isolation.

Generally, treatment consists of the following:
▶ local or systemic antipruritics
▶ cool bicarbonate of soda baths
▶ calamine lotion
▶ diphenhydramine or another antihistamine
▶ antibiotics if bacterial infection develops.

Salicylates are contraindicated because of their link with Reye's syndrome.

Susceptible patients may need special treatment. When given up to 72 hours after exposure to varicella, varicella-zoster immune globulin may provide passive immunity. Acyclovir may slow vesicle formation, speed skin healing, and control the systemic spread of infection.

Special considerations

▶ A live attenuated varicella vaccine has been licensed for use in the United States.
▶ To help prevent chickenpox, don't admit a child exposed to chickenpox to a unit that contains children who receive immunosuppressant agents or who have leukemia or immunodeficiency disorders. A vulnerable child who's been exposed to chickenpox should receive varicella-zoster immune globulin to lessen its severity.

 PREVENTION TIP Teach the child and his family how to apply topical antipruritic medications correctly. Stress the importance of good hygiene. Tell the patient not to scratch the lesions. However, because the need to scratch may be overwhelming, parents should trim the child's fingernails or tie mittens on his hands. Warn parents to watch for and immediately report signs of complications. Severe skin pain and burning may indicate a serious secondary infection and require prompt medical attention.

VARIOLA

Variola, or smallpox, was an acute, highly contagious infectious disease caused by the poxvirus variola. After a global eradication program, the World Health Organization pronounced smallpox eradicated on October 26, 1979, two years after the last naturally occurring case was reported in Somalia. Vaccination is no longer recommended, except for certain laboratory workers. The last known case in the United States was reported in 1949. Although naturally occurring smallpox has been eradicated, variola virus preserved in laboratories remains an unlikely source of infection.

Smallpox developed in three major forms: variola major (classic smallpox), which carried a high mortality; variola minor, a mild form that occurred in nonvaccinated people and resulted from a less virulent strain; and varioloid, a mild variant of smallpox that occurred in previously vaccinated people who had only partial immunity.

Causes

Smallpox affected people of all ages. In temperate zones, incidence was highest during the winter; in the tropics, during the hot, dry months. Smallpox was transmitted directly by respiratory droplets or dried scales of virus-containing lesions, or indirectly through contact with contaminated linens or other objects. Variola major was contagious from onset until after the last scab was shed.

Signs and symptoms

Characteristically, after an incubation period of 10 to 14 days, smallpox caused an abrupt onset of chills (and possible seizures in children), high fever (above 104° F [40° C]), headache, backache, severe malaise, vomiting (especially in children), marked prostration and, occasionally, violent delirium, stupor, or coma. Two days after onset, symptoms became more severe, but by the 3rd day the patient began to feel better.

However, the patient soon developed a sore throat and cough as well as lesions on the mucous membranes of the mouth, throat, and respiratory tract. Within days, skin lesions also appeared, progressing from macular to papular, vesicular, and pustular (pustules were as large as ⅓″ [8 mm] in diameter). During the pustular stage, the patient's temperature again rose, and early symptoms returned. By day 10,

the pustules began to rupture, and eventually dried and formed scabs. Symptoms finally subsided about 14 days after onset. Desquamation of the scabs took another 1 to 2 weeks, caused intense pruritus, and commonly left permanently disfiguring scars.

In fatal cases, a diffuse dusky appearance came over the patient's face and upper chest. Death resulted from encephalitic manifestations, extensive bleeding from any or all orifices, or secondary bacterial infections.

Diagnosis

Smallpox was readily recognizable, especially during an epidemic or after known contact. The most conclusive laboratory test was a culture of variola virus isolated from an aspirate of vesicles and pustules. Other laboratory tests included microscopic examination of smears from lesion scrapings, and complement fixation to detect virus or antibodies to the virus in the patient's blood.

Treatment and special considerations

Treatment required hospitalization, with strict isolation, antimicrobial therapy to treat bacterial complications, vigorous supportive measures, and symptomatic treatment of lesions with antipruritics, starting during the pustular stage. Aspirin, codeine, or (as needed) morphine relieved pain; I.V. infusions and gastric tube feedings provided fluids, electrolytes, and calories because pharyngeal lesions made swallowing difficult.

VIBRIO PARAHAEMOLYTICUS INFECTION

A bacterium in the same family as those that cause cholera, *Vibrio parahaemolyticus* lives in brackish salt water and causes gastrointestinal illness in humans. It occurs naturally in coastal waters within the United States and Canada where oysters are cultivated. It is typically present in higher concentrations during summer, and is characterized as a halophilic or salt-requiring organism.

In Asia, *V. parahaemolyticus* is a common cause of foodborne disease. In the U.S., it is less commonly recognized as a cause of illness, partly because clinical laboratories rarely use the selective medium that is necessary to identify the organism. Not all states require this disease be reported to the state health department, but the Centers for Disease Control and Prevention collaborates with the Gulf Coast states of Alabama, Florida, Louisiana, and Texas to monitor the number of cases of *V. parahaemolyticus* infections in this region. From those states, about 30 to 40 cases are reported annually.

Causes

Most individuals become infected by eating contaminated shellfish, particularly oysters. Less commonly, this organism can cause an infection in the skin when an open wound is exposed to warm contaminated seawater.

Signs and symptoms

The principle symptoms that occur when *Vibrio parahaemolyticus* is ingested are watery diarrhea, abdominal cramping, nausea, vomiting, fever, and chills. Symptoms usually occur within 24 hours of ingestion. Illness is usually self-limited and lasts 3 days. Severe disease is rare and occurs more commonly in individuals with compromised immune systems. Open skin wounds can become infected when exposed to warm seawater.

Diagnosis

Vibrio parahaemolyticus can be isolated from cultures of stool, wound, or blood. For isolation from stool, the use of a selective medium containing thiosulfate, citrate, bile salts, and sucrose (TCBS agar) is recommended. If there is clinical suspicion for infection with this microbe, stool cultures should be performed.

Other diagnoses to consider are *Vibrio vulnificus,* cholera, viral gastroenteritis, or bacterial enteritis.

Treatment

Treatment is usually not required in most cases with this infection. There is presently no evidence that antibiotic therapy decreases the severity or length of illness. Fluid hydration is necessary to replace fluids lost through diarrhea. In severe or prolonged illness, antibiotics such as tetracycline, ampicillin, or ciprofloxacin can be used. The antibiotic of choice is based on the antimicrobial susceptibilities of the organism.

Special considerations

▶ Obtain a careful history of the patient's food intake, especially pertaining to seafood.
▶ Maintain adequate hydration.
▶ Carry out strict measurement of intake and output, including stools.
▶ Put on gloves and perform strict handwashing technique when handling body fluids and, especially, stool.
▶ Clean all open skin wounds and report any signs of inflammation or infection.
▶ Palpate abdomen and auscultate for bowel sounds. Report any abnormalities immediately.
▶ Administer antiemetics as required.
▶ Dispense antifever medications as directed to control fever.
▶ Notify local public health authorities of all confirmed cases of *Vibrio parahaemolyticus* infections.

VIBRIO VULNIFICUS INFECTION

Vibrio vulnificus is a bacterium found in the same family as those that cause cholera. It normally inhabits warm seawater and is part of a group of vibrios that are called halophilic because they require salt.

V. vulnificus is a rare cause of disease, but it is also underreported. Between 1988 and 1995, the Centers for Disease Control and Prevention (CDC) received reports of over 300 cases of this disease from the Gulf Coast states, where the majority of cases occur. There is no national surveillance system for *V. vulnificus,* but the CDC collaborates with the states of Alabama, Florida, Louisiana, Texas, and Mississippi to monitor the number of cases found in the Gulf Coast region.

This infection is an acute illness, and those who recover should not expect any long-term consequences. In immunocompromised patients this disease can be considered life-threatening.

Causes

Most individuals become infected by ingesting contaminated shellfish, particularly oysters, or by exposing an open wound to warm contaminated seawater. There is no evidence of person-to-person transmission of this microbe.

Signs and symptoms

In healthy individuals, ingestion of this microbe can cause vomiting, diarrhea, and abdominal pain. In immunosupressed patients, particularly those with chronic liver disease, *V. vulnificus* can infect the bloodstream, causing septic shock — characterized by fever and chills, hypotension, and blistering skin lesions. A recent study showed that individuals with these pre-existing medical conditions were 80 times more likely to develop *V. vulnificus* bloodstream infections than were healthy persons. *V. vulnificus* bloodstream infections are fatal about 50% of the time.

V. vulnificus can also cause an infection of the skin when open wounds are exposed to warm seawater; these infections may lead to skin breakdown and ulceration. Individuals who have compromised immune systems are at higher risk for invasion into the bloodstream as well as complications.

Diagnosis

Diagnosis is based on routine stool, wound, or blood cultures. The laboratory should be notified when this infection is suspected

by the doctor, since a special growth medium can be utilized to increase the diagnostic yield. Doctors should have a high suspicion for this microbe when patients present with gastrointestinal illness, fever, or shock following the ingestion of raw seafood, especially oysters, or with a wound infection after exposure to warm seawater.

Other diagnoses to consider would be *Vibrio parahaemolyticus,* cholera, gastroenteritis, and bacterial enteritis.

Treatment

The usual course of treatment is with antibiotics. Doxycycline or a third-generation cephalosporin (such as ceftazidime) is a suitable drug of choice.

Notify the laboratory if *V. vulnificus* is suspected so the appropriate growth medium can be used for testing.

Special considerations

▶ Obtain a careful history of the patient's food intake, especially of oysters and other seafood.

▶ Maintain adequate hydration.

▶ Carry out strict measurement of intake and output, including stools.

▶ Put on gloves and perform strict hand-washing technique when handling body fluids and, especially, stool.

▶ Perform a complete physical assessment.

▶ Palpate abdomen and auscultate for bowel sounds. Report any abnormalities immediately.

▶ Clean all open wounds and report signs of infection.

▶ Administer antiemetics as required.

▶ Dispense antipyretic medications as directed to control fever.

▶ Notify local public health authorities of confirmed cases of *V. vulnificus.*

 PREVENTION TIP To prevent *Vibrio vulnificus* infections, instruct patients to cook shellfish thoroughly and eat it promptly. Avoid cross contamination of cooked seafood and other foods with raw seafood or juices from raw seafood.

WXYZ

WEST NILE ENCEPHALITIS

West Nile encephalitis is an infectious disease that primarily causes an inflammation or encephalitis of the brain. The etiology stems from the West Nile virus (WNV), a flavivirus commonly found in humans, birds, and other vertebrates in Africa, West Asia, and the Middle East. This disease is part of a family of vector-borne diseases that also include malaria, yellow fever, and Lyme disease.

WNV had not been previously documented in the Western Hemisphere until August 1999, when a virus found in numerous dead birds in the New York, New Jersey, and Connecticut region was definitively identified by genetic sequencing as the West Nile virus. Scientists in the United States discovered the rare strain initially in birds at the Bronx Zoo and believe the birds may have carried the disease that has been spread as mosquitoes fed on the infected birds.

In the temperate areas of the world, West Nile encephalitis occurs mainly in the late summer or early fall. In the southern climates where temperatures are milder, West Nile encephalitis can occur all year round.

Health officials at the Centers for Disease Control and Prevention (CDC) reported that as of November 17, 1999, 56 cases (31 confirmed and 25 probable) of WNV infection have been identified, including seven deaths.

The risk of contracting West Nile encephalitis is greater for all residents of areas where active cases have been identified, but persons age 50 or older or those with compromised immune systems are at greatest risk.

Currently there is no documented evidence that a pregnant woman's fetus is at risk due to an infection with WNV. The mortality rate of West Nile encephalitis, as measured by case-fatality rates, ranges from 3% to 15% and is higher in the elderly.

Causes

The West Nile virus is transmitted to humans by the bite of a mosquito (primarily the *Culex* species) infected with the virus. The insects are considered the primary vector for WNV and the source of the August 1999 outbreak in New York, New Jersey, and Connecticut. Mosquitoes become infected by feeding on birds contaminated with WNV, and then transmit the virus to humans and animals when taking a blood meal or a "bite." (See *Routes of transmission of West Nile virus,* page 334.)

Ticks have been found infected with WNV in Africa and Asia only. The role of ticks in the transmission and maintenance of the virus remains uncertain, and so far they are not considered vectors in the United States.

The CDC has reported that there is no evidence that a person can contract the virus from handling live or dead infected birds. However, avoid barehanded contact when handling dead animals, including dead birds, and use gloves or double plastic bags to place the carcass in a garbage can, and report the finding to the nearest Emergency Management Office.

ROUTES OF TRANSMISSION OF WEST NILE VIRUS

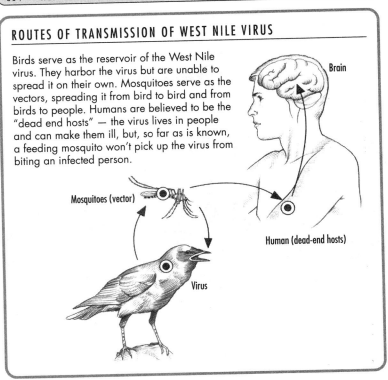

Birds serve as the reservoir of the West Nile virus. They harbor the virus but are unable to spread it on their own. Mosquitoes serve as the vectors, spreading it from bird to bird and from birds to people. Humans are believed to be the "dead end hosts" — the virus lives in people and can make them ill, but, so far as is known, a feeding mosquito won't pick up the virus from biting an infected person.

Brain

Mosquitoes (vector)

Human (dead-end hosts)

Virus

Signs and symptoms

Mild infections of the virus are more common and include fever, headache, and body aches, often accompanied by a skin rash, and swollen lymph glands. Severe infections can be manifested by headache, high fever, neck stiffness, stupor, disorientation, coma, tremors, occasional convulsions, paralysis, and, rarely, death.

The incubation period for West Nile encephalitis is anywhere from 5 to 15 days after exposure.

Most patients who are bitten by an infected mosquito will develop no symptoms at all. It is estimated that only one in 300 people who are bitten by an infected mosquito will actually get sick.

Diagnosis

The enzyme-linked immunosorbent assay (ELISA or MAC-ELISA) is the test of choice for rapid definitive diagnosis. The major advantage of MAC-ELISA lab analysis is the high probability of accurate diagnosis of WNV infection when performed only with acute serum or cerebrospinal fluid specimens obtained while the patient is still hospitalized.

Other conditions to consider include St. Louis encephalitis, which is symptomatically similar. Because the term "encephalitis" (brain inflammation) can be caused by numerous viral and bacterial infections, all data must be examined to confirm a diagnosis.

Treatment

There is no specific therapy for West Nile encephalitis, no vaccine, and no known cure. Treatment aims to control the specific symptoms. Supportive care, such as intravenous fluids, fever control, and respiratory support, is rendered when necessary. Steroids may be used to control brain swelling and pain killers for milder symptoms.

Special considerations

▶ Obtain an extensive history of the patient's recent whereabouts within the last 2 to 3 weeks (especially around bodies of water, such as lakes and ponds), presence of dead birds, and recent mosquito bites.

▶ Perform a comprehensive physical assessment and report signs of headache, fever, lymphadenopathy, and a maculopapular rash.

▶ Perform a complete neurological examination and report any signs of confusion, lethargy, weakness, or slurred speech.

▶ Maintain adequate hydration with I.V. fluids.

▶ Monitor strict intake and output.

▶ Utilize fever control methods.

▶ Utilize respiratory support measures when applicable.

▶ West Nile encephalitis is not transmitted from person to person, but use universal precautions.

▶ Report any suspected cases of West Nile encephalitis to the applicable state Department of Health.

 PREVENTION TIP To reduce the risk of becoming infected with West Nile encephalitis, teach patients the following points:

▶ Stay indoors at dawn, dusk, and in the early evening.

▶ Wear long-sleeved shirts and long pants whenever you are outdoors.

▶ Apply insect repellent sparingly to exposed skin. An effective repellent will contain 20% to 30% DEET (N, N-diethyl-meta-toluamide). DEET in high concentrations (greater than 30%) may cause side effects, particularly in children; avoid products containing more than 30% DEET.

▶ Repellents may irritate the eyes and mouth, so avoid applying repellant to the hands of children. Insect repellants should not be applied to children under age 3.

▶ Spray clothing with repellents containing DEET, as mosquitoes may bite through thin clothing.

▶ Whenever you use an insecticide or insect repellent, be sure to read and follow the manufacturer's directions for use, as printed on the product.

▶ Vitamin B and "ultrasonic" devices are not effective in preventing mosquito bites.

GUIDE TO
ANTI-INFECTIVE DRUGS

atovaquone
chloroquine hydrochloride
(See Antimalarials.)
chloroquine phosphate
(See Antimalarials.)
metronidazole
metronidazole hydrochloride
pentamidine isethionate

COMBINATION PRODUCTS

Helidac: metronidazole 250 mg (with povidone), tetracycline 500 mg, bismuth subsalicylate 262.4 mg (with povidone)

---

atovaquone

Mepron, Wellvone§

Pregnancy Risk Category C

HOW SUPPLIED

Suspension: 750 mg/5 ml

ACTION

Unknown. Appears to interfere with electron transport in protozoal mitochondria, inhibiting enzymes needed for the synthesis of nucleic acids and adenosine triphosphate.

Route	Onset	Peak	Duration
P.O.	Unknown	1 hr-days	Unknown

INDICATIONS & DOSAGE

Acute, mild to moderate Pneumocystis carinii *pneumonia in patients who can't tolerate co-trimoxazole —*
Adults: 750 mg P.O. b.i.d. with food for 21 days.
Prevention of P. carinii *pneumonia in patients who can't tolerant co-trimoxazole —*
Adults and adolescents ages 13 to 16: 1,500 mg (10 ml) P.O. daily with food.

ADVERSE REACTIONS

CNS: *headache, insomnia,* asthenia, anxiety, dizziness.
CV: hypotension.
EENT: *cough,* sinusitis, rhinitis, taste perversion, *oral candidiasis.*
GI: *nausea, diarrhea, vomiting,* constipation, *abdominal pain,* anorexia, dyspepsia.
Hematologic: anemia, *neutropenia.*
Hepatic: elevated liver function tests.
Metabolic: hypoglycemia, hyponatremia.
Skin: *rash,* pruritus, *diaphoresis,* sweating.
Other: *fever, pain.*

INTERACTIONS

Drug-drug. *Rifabutin, rifampin:* decreases atovaquone's steady-state concentration. Avoid concurrent use.

EFFECTS ON DIAGNOSTIC TESTS

None reported.

CONTRAINDICATIONS

Contraindicated in patients with hypersensitivity to drug.

SPECIAL CONSIDERATIONS

▶ Use cautiously in breast-feeding patients. Drug has appeared in breast milk.
▶ Because drug is highly bound to plasma protein (over 99.9%), use cautiously with other highly protein-bound drugs.
▶ *Alert:* Because of risk of other concurrent pulmonary infections, patient must be monitored closely during therapy.

Patient teaching

▶ Drug is taken with meals because food enhances absorption significantly.

Reactions may be *common,* uncommon, *life-threatening,* or COMMON AND LIFE-THREATENING.

metronidazole

Apo-Metronidazole , Flagyl,
Flagyl ER, Metrogyl‡, Novo-
Nidazol , Protostat, Trikacide

metronidazole hydrochloride

Flagyl IV RTU, Novo-Nidazol

Pregnancy Risk Category B

HOW SUPPLIED

Tablets: 200 mg‡, 250 mg, 375 mg,
400 mg‡, 500 mg
Tablets (extended-release): 750 mg
Oral suspension (benzoyl metronidazole):
200 mg/5 ml‡
Injection: 500 mg/100 ml ready to use
Powder for injection: 500-mg single-dose
vials

ACTION

A direct-acting trichomonacide and amebicide that works at both intestinal and extraintestinal sites. It is thought to enter the
cells of microorganisms that contain nitro-
reductase. Unstable compounds are then
formed that bind to DNA and inhibit synthesis, causing cell death.

Route	Onset	Peak	Duration
P.O.	Unknown	2 hr	Unknown
I.V.	Immediate	1 hr	Unknown

INDICATIONS & DOSAGE

Amoebic hepatic abscess —
Adults: 500 to 750 mg P.O. t.i.d. for 5 to
10 days.
Children: 30 to 50 mg/kg daily (in three
divided doses) for 10 days.
Intestinal amebiasis —
Adults: 750 mg P.O. t.i.d. for 5 to 10 days.
Children: 30 to 50 mg/kg daily (in three
divided doses) for 10 days.

Therapy for adults or children is fol-
lowed by oral iodoquinol.
Trichomoniasis —
Adults: 250 mg P.O. t.i.d. for 7 days or
2 g P.O. in single dose (may give the 2-g
dose in two 1-g doses, each on the same
day); 4 to 6 weeks should elapse between
courses of therapy.
Children: 5 mg/kg P.O. t.i.d. for 7 days.
Refractory trichomoniasis —
Adults: 250 mg P.O. b.i.d. for 10 days.
Or, 500 mg P.O. b.i.d. for 7 days.
*Bacterial infections due to anaerobic
microorganisms —*
Adults: loading dose is 15 mg/kg I.V. infused over 1 hour (about 1 g for a 70-kg
[154-lb] adult). Maintenance dose is
7.5 mg/kg I.V. or P.O. q 6 hours (about
500 mg for a 70-kg adult). First maintenance dose should be given 6 hours after
loading dose. Maximum dose not to exceed 4 g daily.
*Prevention of postoperative infection
in contaminated or potentially contaminated colorectal surgery —*
Adults: 15 mg/kg I.V. infused over 30 to
60 minutes and completed about 1 hour
before surgery. Then, 7.5 mg/kg I.V. infused over 30 to 60 minutes at 6 and 12
hours after initial dose.
Bacterial vaginosis —
Adults: 500 mg P.O. b.i.d. for 7 days.

ADVERSE REACTIONS

CNS: vertigo, *headache,* ataxia, dizziness,
syncope, incoordination, confusion, irritability, depression, weakness, insomnia,
seizures, peripheral neuropathy.
CV: flattened T wave, edema.
EENT: rhinitis, sinusitis, pharyngitis,
metallic taste.
GI: abdominal cramping or pain, stomatitis, epigastric distress, *nausea,* vomiting,
anorexia, diarrhea, constipation, proctitis,
dry mouth.
GU: darkened urine, polyuria, dysuria,
cystitis, decreased libido, dyspareunia,

dryness of vagina and vulva, vaginal candidiasis, *vaginitis,* genital pruritus.
Hematologic: transient leukopenia, ***neutropenia,*** thrombophlebitis after I.V. infusion.
Musculoskeletal: fleeting joint pains.
Respiratory: upper respiratory infection.
Skin: flushing, rash.
Other: fever, overgrowth of nonsusceptible organisms, especially *Candida.*

INTERACTIONS

Drug-drug. *Cimetidine:* increased risk of metronidazole toxicity because of inhibited hepatic metabolism. Monitor closely.
Disulfiram: acute psychoses and confusional states. Don't use within 2 weeks of last disulfiram dose.
Lithium: increased lithium levels resulting in possible toxicity. Monitor serum lithium levels closely.
Oral anticoagulants: increased anticoagulant effects. Monitor closely.
Phenobarbital, phenytoin: decreased metronidazole effectiveness. Total phenytoin clearance may be reduced. Monitor closely.
Drug-lifestyle. *Alcohol use:* disulfiram-like reaction (nausea, vomiting, headache, cramps, flushing). Don't use together or for 3 days after completion of drug therapy.

EFFECTS ON DIAGNOSTIC TESTS

Metronidazole may interfere with the chemical analyses of aminotransferases and triglycerides, leading to falsely decreased values.

CONTRAINDICATIONS

Contraindicated in patients with hypersensitivity to drug or other nitroimidazole derivatives and during first trimester of pregnancy.

SPECIAL CONSIDERATIONS

▸ Use cautiously in patients with history of blood dyscrasia or CNS disorder and in those with retinal or visual field changes. Also, use cautiously in patients with hepatic disease or alcoholism and in conjunction with hepatotoxic drugs.
▸ Monitor liver function tests carefully in elderly patients. If test results are altered, monitor metronidazole levels closely to prevent toxicity.
▸ Drug is contraindicated in first trimester of pregnancy. However, if indicated during pregnancy for trichomoniasis, be aware that the 7-day regimen is preferred over the 2-g, single-dose regimen.
▸ Oral form is taken with meals.
▸ Patient, especially one receiving corticosteroids, should be observed for edema; Flagyl I.V. RTU (ready to use) may cause sodium retention.
▸ Number and character of stools should be recorded when drug is used to treat amebiasis. Metronidazole should be used only after confirming *Trichomonas vaginalis* infection is confirmed by wet smear or culture or *Entamoeba histolytica* is identified. Asymptomatic sexual partners of patients being treated for *T. vaginalis* infection should be treated simultaneously to avoid reinfection.

I.V. administration

▸ No preparation is needed for Flagyl I.V. RTU.
▸ To prepare lyophilized vials of metronidazole, 4.4 ml of sterile water for injection, bacteriostatic water for injection, sterile normal saline for injection, or bacteriostatic normal saline for injection is added to the vial. Reconstituted drug contains 100 mg/ml. The contents of vial is added to 100 ml of D_5W, lactated Ringer's injection, or normal saline for a final concentration of 5 mg/ml. The resulting highly acidic solution must be neutralized before administration. For each 500 mg metronidazole, 5 mEq sodium bicarbonate is carefully added; carbon dioxide gas will form and may need to be vented.

Reactions may be *common,* uncommon, *life-threatening*, or COMMON AND LIFE-THREATENING.

▶ **Alert:** Drug is infused over at least 1 hour. Drug is not given via I.V. push.

▶ The neutralized diluted solution should not be refrigerated because precipitation may occur. If Flagyl I.V. RTU is refrigerated, crystals may form. These disappear after the solution warms to room temperature.

Patient teaching

▶ Take oral form with food to minimize GI upset, although extended-release tablets should be taken at least 1 hour before or 2 hours after meals.

▶ Sexual partners should be treated simultaneously to avoid reinfection.

▶ Proper hygiene is essential.

▶ Avoid alcohol and alcohol-containing medications during therapy and for at least 3 days after completing therapy.

▶ Metallic taste and dark or red-brown urine may occur.

pentamidine isethionate

NebuPent, Pentacarinat, Pentam 300

Pregnancy Risk Category C

HOW SUPPLIED

Injection, aerosol: 300-mg vial

ACTION

Unknown. Believed to interfere with biosynthesis of DNA, RNA, phospholipids, and proteins in susceptible organisms.

Route	Onset	Peak	Duration
I.V.	Unknown	1 hr	Unknown
I.M., inhalation	Unknown	0.5 hr	Unknown

INDICATIONS & DOSAGE

Pneumocystis carinii *pneumonia* —
Adults and children: 3 to 4 mg/kg I.V. or I.M. once daily for 14 to 21 days.

Prevention of P. carinii *pneumonia in high-risk patients* —
Adults: 300 mg by inhalation (using a Respirgard II nebulizer) once q 4 weeks.

ADVERSE REACTIONS

CNS: confusion, hallucinations, *fatigue, dizziness,* headache.
CV: *hypotension, ventricular tachycardia,* chest pain.
EENT: burning in throat (with inhaled form), *pharyngitis.*
GI: *nausea, metallic taste, decreased appetite, vomiting,* diarrhea, abdominal pain, anorexia, pancreatitis.
GU: *elevated BUN and serum creatinine levels,* **acute renal failure.**
Hematologic: *leukopenia, thrombocytopenia,* anemia.
Hepatic: elevated AST and ALT levels.
Metabolic: *hypoglycemia,* hyperglycemia, hypocalcemia.
Musculoskeletal: myalgia.
Respiratory: *cough, bronchospasm, shortness of breath,* pneumothorax, *congestion.*
Skin: rash, *Stevens-Johnson syndrome.*
Other: *night sweats, chills,* edema, *sterile abscess, pain, induration at injection site.*

INTERACTIONS

Drug-drug. *Aminoglycosides, amphotericin B, capreomycin, cisplatin, colistin, methoxyflurane, polymyxin B, vancomycin:* increased risk of nephrotoxicity. Monitor closely.
Antineoplastics: additive bone marrow suppression. Use together cautiously.

EFFECTS ON DIAGNOSTIC TESTS

None reported.

CONTRAINDICATIONS

Contraindicated in patients with a history of an anaphylactic reaction to drug.

SPECIAL CONSIDERATIONS

▶ Use cautiously in patients with hypertension, hypotension, hypoglycemia, hypocalcemia, leukopenia, thrombocytopenia, anemia, diabetes, pancreatitis, Stevens-Johnson syndrome, or hepatic or renal dysfunction.

▶ Aerosol form is only administered using the Respirgard II nebulizer. Dosage recommendations are based on particle size and delivery rate of this device. To administer aerosol, the contents of one vial is mixed in 6 ml sterile water for injection. Normal saline solution is not used. The drug should not be mixed with other drugs.

▶ Low-pressure (less than 20 pounds per square inch [psi]) compressors must not be used. The flow rate should be 5 to 7 L/minute from a 40- to 50-psi air or oxygen source.

▶ For I.M. injection, drug is reconstituted with 3 ml of sterile water for a solution containing 100 mg/ml; drug should be administered deeply. Expect patient to report pain and induration at injection site.

▶ Monitor blood glucose, serum calcium, serum creatinine, and BUN levels daily. After parenteral administration, blood glucose level may decrease initially; hypoglycemia may be severe in 5% to 10% of patients. This may be followed by hyperglycemia and type 1 diabetes mellitus, which may be permanent because of pancreatic cell damage.

▶ In patients with AIDS, pentamidine may produce less severe adverse reactions than co-trimoxazole.

I.V. administration

▶ Drug is reconstituted with 3 ml of sterile water for injection; then diluted in 50 to 250 ml of D_5W. Solution is infused over at least 60 minutes.

▶ *Alert:* To minimize risk of hypotension when drug is given I.V., the drug is infused slowly with patient lying down. Blood pressure must be closely monitored.

Patient teaching

▶ Use the aerosol device until the chamber is empty, which may take up to 45 minutes.

▶ I.M. injection is painful.

▶ Complete full course of pentamidine therapy, even if feeling better.

Reactions may be *common*, uncommon, *life-threatening*, or COMMON AND LIFE-THREATENING.

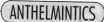

mebendazole
pyrantel pamoate
thiabendazole

COMBINATION PRODUCTS
None.

mebendazole

Vermox

Pregnancy Risk Category C

HOW SUPPLIED
Tablets (chewable): 100 mg

ACTION
Selectively and irreversibly inhibits uptake of glucose and other nutrients in susceptible helminths.

Route	Onset	Peak	Duration
P.O.	Unknown	2-4 hr	Variable

INDICATIONS & DOSAGE
Pinworm—
Adults and children over age 2: 100 mg P.O. as a single dose; repeated if infection persists 2 to 3 weeks later.
Roundworm, whipworm, hookworm —
Adults and children over age 2: 100 mg P.O. b.i.d. for 3 days; repeated if infection persists 3 weeks later.

ADVERSE REACTIONS
CNS: *seizures.*
GI: occasional, transient abdominal pain and diarrhea in massive infection and expulsion of worms.
Skin: urticaria.
Other: fever.

INTERACTIONS
Drug-drug. *Carbamazepine, hydantoins:*
reduced plasma mebendazole levels, potentially decreasing its effect. Monitor closely.
Cimetidine: increased plasma mebendazole levels. Monitor closely.

EFFECTS ON DIAGNOSTIC TESTS
None reported.

CONTRAINDICATIONS
Contraindicated in patients with hypersensitivity to drug.

SPECIAL CONSIDERATIONS
▶ Tablets may be chewed, swallowed whole, or crushed and mixed with food.
▶ Drug is administered to all family members to decrease the risk of spreading the infection.
▶ Dietary restrictions, laxatives, or enemas aren't necessary.
▶ Safe use in children under age 2 hasn't been established.

Patient teaching
▶ Personal hygiene, especially good handwashing technique is important. Refrain from preparing food for others.
▶ To avoid reinfection, wash perianal area daily, change undergarments and bedclothes daily, and wash hands and clean fingernails before meals and after bowel movements.

pyrantel pamoate
Antiminth, Combantrin , Pin-Rid, Pin-X, Reese's Pinworm Medicine

Pregnancy Risk Category C

HOW SUPPLIED
Tablets: 62.5 mg
Capsules (soft-gel): 180 mg

---

*Liquid contains alcohol.   **May contain tartrazine.   †Canada   ‡Australia   §U.K.   ◇OTC

Oral suspension: 50 mg/ml

ACTION
Blocks neuromuscular action, paralyzing the worm and causing its expulsion by normal peristalsis.

Route	Onset	Peak	Duration
P.O.	Variable	1-3 hr	Variable

INDICATIONS & DOSAGE
Roundworm, pinworm —
Adults and children ages 2 and older: 11 mg/kg P.O. as a single dose. Maximum dose is 1 g. For pinworm, dose should be repeated in 2 weeks.

ADVERSE REACTIONS
CNS: headache, dizziness, drowsiness, insomnia.
GI: anorexia, nausea, vomiting, gastralgia, abdominal cramps, diarrhea, tenesmus.
Hepatic: transient elevation of AST.
Skin: rash.
Other: fever, weakness.

INTERACTIONS
Drug-drug. *Piperazine salts:* possible antagonism. Don't give together.

EFFECTS ON DIAGNOSTIC TESTS
None reported.

CONTRAINDICATIONS
Contraindicated in patients with hypersensitivity to drug.

SPECIAL CONSIDERATIONS
▶ Drug is used cautiously in patients with severe malnutrition or anemia and in patients with hepatic dysfunction.
▶ Dietary restrictions, laxatives, or enemas aren't needed.
▶ Drug should be given to all family members.

Patient teaching
▶ Drug may be taken with food, milk, or fruit juices. Shake suspension well.
▶ Personal hygiene is important, especially good hand-washing technique. To avoid reinfection, wash perianal area daily, change undergarments and bedclothes daily, and wash hands and clean fingernails before meals and after bowel movements.
▶ Refrain from preparing food for others.
▶ Take entire dose as prescribed.

thiabendazole
Mintezol

Pregnancy Risk Category C

HOW SUPPLIED
Tablets (chewable): 500 mg
Oral suspension: 500 mg/5 ml

ACTION
Unknown. Appears to inhibit the helminth-specific enzyme fumarate reductase.

Route	Onset	Peak	Duration
P.O.	Unknown	1-2 hr	Unknown

INDICATIONS & DOSAGE
Cutaneous infestations with larva migrans (creeping eruption) —
Adults and children: 25 mg/kg P.O. b.i.d. for 2 to 5 days. Maximum dose is 3 g daily. If lesions persist 2 days after completion of a 2-day course of therapy, course is repeated.
Roundworm, threadworm, whipworm —
Adults and children: 25 mg/kg P.O. in two doses daily for 2 successive days.
Trichinosis —
Adults and children: 25 mg/kg P.O. in two doses daily for 2 to 4 successive days.

ADVERSE REACTIONS
CNS: impaired mental alertness, impaired

coordination, numbness, *seizures, drowsiness, fatigue,* giddiness, *headache,* dizziness.

CV: *hypotension,* flushing.

EENT: tinnitus, blurry vision, dry mouth and eyes, xanthopsia.

GI: *anorexia, nausea, vomiting,* diarrhea, epigastric distress, cholestasis.

GU: hematuria, enuresis, crystalluria, malodorous urine.

Hematologic: *leukopenia.*

Hepatic: jaundice, transient elevations of AST levels, *parenchymal liver damage.*

Skin: *rash, pruritus, erythema multiforme, Stevens-Johnson syndrome.*

Other: lymphadenopathy, fever, chills, *angioedema, anaphylaxis.*

INTERACTIONS

Drug-drug. *Theophylline:* may impair hepatic metabolism of theophylline, increasing risk of toxicity. Monitor patient closely.

EFFECTS ON DIAGNOSTIC TESTS

None reported.

CONTRAINDICATIONS

Contraindicated in patients with hypersensitivity to drug.

SPECIAL CONSIDERATIONS

▶ Use cautiously in patients with hepatic or renal dysfunction, severe malnutrition, and anemia, and in patients who are vomiting.

▶ Drug should be administered to all family members to prevent risk of spreading infection.

▶ Dietary restrictions, laxatives, or enemas aren't necessary. However, supportive therapy is indicated for anemic, dehydrated, or malnourished patients.

Patient teaching

▶ Take drug after meals. Shake oral suspension before measuring dose. Chew tablets before swallowing.

▶ Avoid hazardous activities such as driving because drug may cause drowsiness.

▶ Personal hygiene is important, especially good hand-washing technique. To avoid reinfection, wash perianal area daily, change undergarments and bedclothes daily, and wash hands and clean fingernails before meals and after bowel movements. Refrain from preparing food for others during infestation.

amphotericin B
amphotericin B cholesteryl
    sulfate complex
amphotericin B lipid complex
amphotericin B liposomal
fluconazole
flucytosine
griseofulvin microsize
griseofulvin ultramicrosize
itraconazole
ketoconazole
nystatin
terbinafine hydrochloride

COMBINATION PRODUCTS
None.

amphotericin B
Amphocin, Amphotericin B for
Injection, Fungilin†, Fungizone
Intravenous

Pregnancy Risk Category B

HOW SUPPLIED
Tablets: 100 mg‡
Oral suspension: 100 mg/ml‡
Lozenges: 10 mg‡
Powder for injection: 50 mg

ACTION
Binds to sterol in the fungal cell membrane, altering cell permeability and allowing leakage of intracellular components. Fungal cell death occurs in part as a result of membrane permeability changes.

Route	Onset	Peak	Duration
P.O.	Unknown	Unknown	Unknown
I.V.	Immediate	Unknown	Unknown

INDICATIONS & DOSAGE
Systemic fungal infections (histoplasmosis, coccidioidomycosis, blastomycosis, cryptococcosis, disseminated candidiasis, aspergillosis, phycomycosis, zygomycosis), meningitis —
Adults: initially, a test dose of 1 mg in 20 ml of D5W infused I.V. over 20 to 30 minutes may be recommended. If tolerated, daily dose is then initiated as 0.25 to 0.3 mg/kg daily by slow I.V. infusion (0.1 mg/ml) over 2 to 6 hours. Dose is gradually increased to maximum 1 mg/kg daily. If drug is discontinued for 1 week or more, drug is resumed with initial dose and increased gradually.
Infections of the GI tract due to Candida albicans —
Adults: 100 mg P.O. q.i.d. for 2 weeks.
Oral and perioral candidal infections—
Adults: 1 lozenge q.i.d. for 7 to 14 days. Lozenge should dissolve slowly.

ADVERSE REACTIONS
CNS: *headache,* peripheral neuropathy, *malaise,* **seizures.**
CV: hypotension, ***arrhythmias, asystole,*** hypertension, tachycardia, flushing, *phlebitis, thrombophlebitis.*
EENT: hearing loss, tinnitus, transient vertigo, blurred vision, diplopia.
GI: *anorexia, weight loss, nausea, vomiting, dyspepsia, diarrhea, epigastric pain, cramping,* melena, steatorrhea, **hemorrhagic gastroenteritis.**
GU: *abnormal renal function with hypokalemia, azotemia, hyposthenuria, renal tubular acidosis, nephrocalcinosis;* **permanent renal impairment;** anuria; oliguria; increased BUN and serum creatinine.
Hematologic: *normochromic anemia, normocytic anemia,* **thrombocytopenia, leukopenia, agranulocytosis,** eosinophilia, leukocytosis.
Hepatic: hepatitis, jaundice, ***acute liver***

Reactions may be *common*, uncommon, *life-threatening*, or COMMON AND LIFE-THREATENING.

346

failure, elevated alkaline phosphatase, ALT, AST, GGT, LD, and bilirubin levels.

Metabolic: hypokalemia, hypoglycemia, hyperglycemia, hyperuricemia, hypomagnesemia.

Musculoskeletal: arthralgia, myalgia.

Respiratory: dyspnea, tachypnea, bronchospasm, wheezing.

Skin: maculopapular rash, pruritus (without rash).

Other: tissue damage with extravasation, *fever, chills, generalized pain,* **anaphylactoid reaction,** *pain at injection site.*

INTERACTIONS

Drug-drug. *Antineoplastics (mechlorethamine):* may cause renal toxicity, bronchospasm, and hypotension. Use cautiously.

Cardiac glycosides: increased risk of digitalis toxicity in potassium-depleted patients. Monitor closely.

Corticosteroids: enhanced potassium depletion. Serum potassium levels must be monitored.

Flucytosine: synergistic effect; may cause increased toxicity of flucytosine. Monitor closely.

Other nephrotoxic drugs (such as antibiotics, pentamidine): may cause additive renal toxicity. These drugs must be administered cautiously.

Thiazides: may intensify electrolyte depletion, especially potassium. Patient must be monitored for hypokalemia.

Drug-herb. *Gossypol:* enhanced or increased risk of renal toxicity when administered together. Avoid concomitant use.

EFFECTS ON DIAGNOSTIC TESTS
None reported.

CONTRAINDICATIONS
Contraindicated in patients with hypersensitivity to drug.

SPECIAL CONSIDERATIONS
▸ Use drug cautiously in patients with impaired renal function.

▸ *Alert:* Note that different amphotericin B preparations are not interchangeable and that dosages will vary.

▸ *Alert:* To reduce severe adverse reactions, patient may receive premedication with antipyretics, antihistamines, antiemetics, or small doses of corticosteroids and be given an alternate-day schedule. For severe reactions, discontinue drug.

▸ Fluid intake and output must be monitored for change in urine appearance or volume. BUN and serum creatinine (or creatinine clearance) should be monitored at least weekly. Kidney damage is typically reversible if drug is stopped at first sign of dysfunction.

▸ Obtain liver and renal function studies weekly. Drug may be stopped if alkaline phosphatase or bilirubin levels increase. If BUN exceeds 40 mg/100 ml, or if serum creatinine level exceeds 3 mg/100 ml, health care provider may reduce or stop drug until renal function improves. Monitor CBC weekly.

▸ Potassium levels should be monitored closely; and patient assessed for signs of hypokalemia. Calcium and magnesium levels should be checked twice weekly.

I.V. administration
▸ An initial test dose should be given. Patient's pulse, respiratory rate, temperature, and blood pressure must be monitored for at least 4 hours.

▸ An infusion pump and in-line filter with mean pore diameter larger than 1 micron should be used. Rapid infusion may cause CV collapse.

▸ Sites in distal veins are best. If veins become thrombosed, administration sites must be alternated.

▸ Vital signs must be monitored every 30 minutes; fever, shaking chills, and hypotension may appear 1 to 2 hours after start of I.V. infusion and should subside within 4 hours of stopping drug.

❭ Antibiotics are given separately, not mixed or piggybacked with amphotericin B.

❭ Amphotericin B appears to be compatible with limited amounts of heparin sodium, hydrocortisone sodium succinate, and methylprednisolone sodium succinate.

❭ Dry form is stored at 35.6° to 46.4° F (2° to 8° C). Protect from light. Amphotericin B is reconstituted with 10 ml of sterile water only. To avoid precipitation, solutions containing sodium chloride, other electrolytes, or bacteriostatic agents (such as benzyl alcohol) are not mixed with the drug. If solution contains precipitate or foreign matter, it should not be used.

❭ Reconstituted solution is stable for 1 week under refrigeration or 24 hours at room temperature. It has 8-hour stability in room light.

Patient teaching

❭ Possible discomfort at I.V. site and other potential adverse reactions may occur. Report signs and symptoms of hypersensitivity immediately.

❭ Therapy may take several months. Stress importance of compliance and recommended follow-up.

amphotericin B cholesteryl sulfate complex

Amphotec

Pregnancy Risk Category B

HOW SUPPLIED

Injection: 50 mg/20 ml, 100 mg/50 ml

ACTION

Binds to sterols in cell membranes of sensitive fungi, resulting in leakage of intracellular contents and causing cell death due to changes in membrane permeability. The spectrum of activity includes *Aspergillus fumigatus, Candida albicans, Coccidioides immitis,* and *Cryptococcus neoformans.*

Route	Onset	Peak	Duration
I.V.	Unknown	3 hr	Unknown

INDICATIONS & DOSAGE

Invasive aspergillosis in patients in whom renal impairment or unacceptable toxicity precludes use of amphotericin B deoxycholate in effective doses and in those with invasive aspergillosis in whom prior amphotericin B deoxycholate therapy has failed —

Adults and children: 3 to 4 mg/kg/day I.V. Dilute in D_5W and administer by continuous infusion at 1 mg/kg/hour. Perform a test dose before commencing new courses of treatment; infuse a small amount of drug (10 ml of final preparation containing 1.6 to 8.3 mg of drug) over 15 to 30 minutes and monitor for next 30 minutes. Can shorten infusion time to 2 hours or lengthen infusion time based on patient tolerance.

ADVERSE REACTIONS

CNS: abnormal thinking, anxiety, agitation, confusion, depression, dizziness, hallucinations, headache, hypertonia, neuropathy, nervousness, paresthesia, psychosis, *seizures,* somnolence, speech disorder, stupor, asthenia.

CV*: arrhythmias, atrial fibrillation, bradycardia, cardiac arrest, heart failure, hemorrhage,* hypertension, *hypotension,* phlebitis, chest pain, orthostatic hypotension, *shock, supraventricular tachycardia,* syncope, *tachycardia,* vasodilation, *ventricular extrasystoles.*

EENT: amblyopia, deafness, epistaxis, eye hemorrhage, pharyngitis, tinnitus, rhinitis, sinusitis.

GI: anorexia, diarrhea, dry mouth, GI hemorrhage, gingivitis, glossitis, hematemesis, melena, mouth ulceration, *nausea,* oral candidiasis, stomatitis, *vomiting,* weight gain or loss, abdominal pain.

GU: albuminuria, dysuria, glycosuria, *increased creatinine,* increased BUN, hematuria, oliguria, urinary incontinence or urine retention, ***renal failure.***

Hematologic: anemia, coagulation disorders, ecchymosis, hypochromic anemia, leukocytosis, ***leukopenia,*** petechiae, decreased prothrombin, ***thrombocytopenia.***

Hepatic: jaundice, *abnormal liver function test results,* ***hepatic failure.***

Metabolic: acidosis, dehydration, *hypokalemia,* hypocalcemia, hypoglycemia, hypoproteinemia, hyperglycemia, hypervolemia, hypophosphatemia, hyponatremia, hyperkalemia, hyperlipemia, hypernatremia, *hyperbilirubinemia,* hypomagnesemia.

Musculoskeletal: arthralgia, myalgia, neck or back pain.

Respiratory: ***apnea,*** asthma, dyspnea, hemoptysis, hyperventilation, hypoxia, increased cough, lung or respiratory disorders, pleural effusion, ***pulmonary edema.***

Skin: acne, pruritus, rash, sweating, skin discoloration, nodule, ulcer, urticaria.

Other: ***allergic reaction,*** alopecia, ***anaphylaxis,*** *chills,* edema, *fever,* peripheral or facial edema, infection, mucous membrane disorder, pain or reaction at injection site, ***sepsis.***

INTERACTIONS

Drug-drug. *Antineoplastics:* may enhance renal toxicity, bronchospasm, and hypotension. Use cautiously.

Cardiac glycosides: can enhance potassium excretion and may potentiate digitalis toxicity. Serum potassium levels must be monitored closely.

Corticosteroids: enhanced potassium depletion, which could predispose patient to cardiac dysfunction. Electrolytes must be monitored closely.

Cyclosporine, tacrolimus: may possibly increase serum creatinine levels. Renal function must be monitored.

Flucytosine: toxicity may be increased by amphotericin. Use together cautiously.

Imidazoles (clotrimazole, fluconazole, ketoconazole, miconazole): may antagonize effects of amphotericin, although their significance has not been determined. Monitor closely.

Nephrotoxic drugs (such as aminoglycosides, pentamidine): may enhance renal toxicity. Renal function must be monitored closely.

Skeletal muscle relaxants: amphotericin B-induced hypokalemia may enhance the effects of skeletal muscle relaxants. Serum potassium must be monitored closely.

EFFECTS ON DIAGNOSTIC TESTS

None reported.

CONTRAINDICATIONS

Contraindicated in patients with hypersensitivity to drug or its components unless the benefits outweigh risks.

SPECIAL CONSIDERATIONS

▶ It's unknown if drug appears in breast milk. Because of the potential for serious adverse reactions in breast-fed infants, a decision should be made to discontinue breast-feeding or to stop treatment, taking into account the importance of drug to the mother.

▶ Intake and output must be monitored for changes in urine appearance or volume.

▶ Renal and hepatic function tests, serum electrolytes (especially potassium, magnesium, and calcium), CBC, and PT must be monitored.

▶ ***Alert:*** Note that different amphotericin B preparations aren't interchangeable and that dosages will vary.

I.V. administration

▶ Unopened vials are stored at room temperature. A 50-mg vial is reconstituted with rapid addition of 10 ml of sterile water for injection, and 100-mg vial with rapid addition of 20 ml sterile water. Vial is shaken gently. A diluent other than sterile water for injection should not be used. Reconstituted drug is clear or opalescent liquid and is stable for 24 hours refrigerated. Partially used vials are discarded. Undiluted drug is not administered.

⬧ For infusion, the reconstituted drug is added to bag of D₅W to final concentration of approximately 0.6 mg/ml. Drug is incompatible with saline, electrolyte solutions, and bacteriostatic agents. A filter or an in-line filter is not used, and the mixture should not be frozen.

⬧ Drug is infused over at least 2 hours. It should not be mixed with other drugs. If administered through an existing I.V. line, the line is flushed with D₅W before infusion or a separate line is used.

⬧ **Alert:** Vital signs must be monitored every 30 minutes during initial therapy. Acute infusion-related reactions (fever, chills, hypotension, nausea, tachycardia) usually occur 1 to 3 hours after starting I.V. infusion. These reactions are usually more severe after initial doses and usually diminish with subsequent doses. If severe respiratory distress occurs, stop infusion immediately and don't treat further with drug.

⬧ Pretreatment with antihistamines and corticosteroids or reducing the rate of infusion (or both) may reduce the acute infusion-related reactions.

Patient teaching

⬧ Immediately report symptoms of hypersensitivity.

⬧ Discomfort at I.V. site may occur.

⬧ Fever, chills, nausea, and vomiting may occur; these can be severe with initial treatment but usually subside with repeated doses.

amphotericin B lipid complex

Abelcet

Pregnancy Risk Category B

HOW SUPPLIED
Suspension for injection: 100 mg/20-ml vial

ACTION
Binds to sterols of fungal cell membranes. Fungal cell damage or death is due to increased membrane permeability and leakage of intracellular contents.

Route	Onset	Peak	Duration
I.V.	Unknown	Unknown	Unknown

INDICATIONS & DOSAGE
Invasive fungal infections, including Aspergillus sp. *and* Candida sp., *in patients who are refractory to or intolerant of conventional amphotericin B therapy —*
Adults and children: 5 mg/kg daily I.V. as a single infusion administered at rate of 2.5 mg/kg/hour.

ADVERSE REACTIONS
CNS: headache, pain.
CV: chest pain, ***cardiac arrest,*** hypertension, hypotension.
GI: abdominal pain, diarrhea, ***GI hemorrhage***, nausea, vomiting.
GU: *increased serum creatinine level,* ***kidney failure.***
Hematologic: anemia, ***leukopenia, thrombocytopenia.***
Hepatic: bilirubinemia.
Metabolic: hypokalemia.
Respiratory: dyspnea, respiratory disorder, ***respiratory failure.***
Skin: rash.
Other: *chills, fever,* infection, **MULTIPLE ORGAN FAILURE,** *sepsis.*

INTERACTIONS

Drug-drug. *Antineoplastics:* increased risk of renal toxicity, bronchospasm, and hypotension. Use cautiously.

Cardiac glycosides: increased risk of digitalis toxicity due to amphotericin B-induced hypokalemia. Serum potassium levels must be monitored closely.

Clotrimazole, fluconazole, itraconazole, ketoconazole, miconazole: may antagonize amphotericin B. Monitor closely.

Corticosteroids, corticotropin: enhanced hypokalemia, which may lead to cardiac toxicity. Serum electrolyte levels and cardiac function must be monitored.

Cyclosporine: increased renal toxicity. Monitor closely.

Flucytosine: increased risk of flucytosine toxicity due to increased cellular uptake or impaired renal excretion. Use cautiously.

Nephrotoxic drugs (such as aminoglycosides, pentamidine): increased risk of renal toxicity. Use cautiously. Renal function must be monitored closely.

Skeletal muscle relaxants: enhanced effects of skeletal muscle relaxants resulting from amphotericin B-induced hypokalemia. Serum potassium levels must be monitored closely.

Zidovudine: increased myelotoxicity and nephrotoxicity. Renal and hematologic function must be monitored.

EFFECTS ON DIAGNOSTIC TESTS

None reported.

CONTRAINDICATIONS

Contraindicated in patients with hypersensitivity to amphotericin B or its components.

SPECIAL CONSIDERATIONS

▶ Use cautiously in patients with renal impairment. Need for dosage adjustment should be based on overall clinical status of patient. Renal toxicity is more common at higher dosages.

▶ **Alert:** Note that different amphotericin B preparations aren't interchangeable and dosages will vary.

▶ Patient is premedicated with acetaminophen, antihistamines, and corticosteroids to prevent or lessen severity of infusion-related reactions, such as fever, chills, nausea, and vomiting, which occur 1 to 2 hours after start of infusion.

▶ Leukocyte transfusions are not given with drug because acute pulmonary toxicity has been reported with concurrent administration.

▶ Serum creatinine and electrolyte levels (especially magnesium and potassium), liver function, and CBC during therapy must be monitored.

▶ It's unknown if drug appears in breast milk; therefore, a decision to administer drug or discontinue breast-feeding should be made.

I. V. administration

▶ To prepare, vial is shaken gently until no yellow sediment remains. Using aseptic technique, the calculated dose is withdrawn into one or more 20-ml syringes, using an 18-gauge needle. More than one vial will be required. A 5-micron filter needle is attached to the syringe and the dose is injected into an I.V. bag of D_5W. One filter needle can be used for up to four vials of amphotericin B lipid complex. The volume of D_5W should be sufficient to yield a final concentration of 1 mg/ml.

▶ For pediatric patients and patients with cardiovascular disease, recommended final concentration is 2 mg/ml.

▶ Drug must not be mixed with saline or infused in same I.V. line as other drugs. An in-line filter is not used.

▶ Any unused drug is discarded; it does not contain a preservative.

▶ An infusion pump is used to administer the drug by continuous infusion at a rate of 2.5 mg/kg/hour. If infusion time exceeds 2 hours, contents are mixed by shaking infusion bag every 2 hours.

▶ For infusion through an existing I.V. line, the line must first be flushed with D_5W.

▶ If severe respiratory distress occurs, the infusion must be discontinued and supportive therapy for anaphylaxis provided. Drug shouldn't be reinstituted in this situation.

▶ Vital signs must be monitored closely. Fever, shaking chills, and hypotension may appear within 2 hours of initiating infusion. Slowing infusion rate may decrease incidence of infusion-related reactions.

▶ Infusions are stable for up to 48 hours if refrigerated (36° to 46° F [2° to 8° C]) and up to 6 hours at room temperature.

Patient teaching

▶ Fever, chills, nausea, and vomiting may occur during infusion; these reactions usually subside with subsequent doses.

▶ Report any redness or pain at infusion site.

▶ Report any symptoms of acute hypersensitivity, such as respiratory distress.

▶ Therapy may take several months.

▶ Frequent laboratory testing to monitor kidney and liver function is necessary.

amphotericin B liposomal

AmBisome

Pregnancy Risk Category B

HOW SUPPLIED

Injection: 50-mg vial

ACTION

Antifungal activity is derived from amphotericin B, which binds to the sterol component of a fungal cell membrane, leading to alterations in cell permeability and cell death.

Route	Onset	Peak	Duration
I.V.	Unknown	Unknown	Unknown

INDICATIONS & DOSAGE

Empirical therapy for presumed fungal infection in febrile, neutropenic patients —

Adults and children: 3 mg/kg I.V. infusion daily.

Systemic fungal infections due to Aspergillus sp., Candida sp., *or* Cryptococcus sp. *refractory to amphotericin B deoxycholate or in patients in whom renal impairment or unacceptable toxicity precludes use of amphotericin B deoxycholate—*

Adults and children: 3 to 5 mg/kg I.V. infusion daily.

Visceral leishmaniasis in immunocompetent patients —

Adults and children: 3 mg/kg I.V. infusion daily on days 1 to 5, 14, and 21. A repeat course of therapy may be beneficial if initial treatment fails to achieve parasitic clearance.

Visceral leishmaniasis in immunocompromised patients —

Adults and children: 4 mg/kg I.V. infusion daily on days 1 to 5, 10, 17, 24, 31, and 38. Expert advice regarding further treatment is recommended if initial therapy fails or patient experiences relapse.

ADVERSE REACTIONS

CNS: *anxiety, confusion, headache, insomnia, asthenia.*

CV: *chest pain, hypotension, tachycardia, hypertension, edema.*

EENT: *epistaxis, rhinitis.*

GI: *nausea, vomiting, abdominal pain, diarrhea,* **GI hemorrhage,**

GU: *hematuria, elevated creatinine and BUN levels.*

Hepatic: *elevated ALT and AST levels, increased alkaline phosphatase level, bilirubinemia.*

Metabolic: *hyperglycemia,* hypernatremia,

Reactions may be *common,* uncommon, *life-threatening*, or COMMON AND LIFE-THREATENING.

hypocalcemia, hypokalemia, hypomagnesemia.
Musculoskeletal: *back pain.*
Respiratory: *increased cough, dyspnea,* hypoxia, *pleural effusion, lung disorder,* hyperventilation.
Skin: *pruritus, rash, sweating.*
Other: *chills, infection, flushing,* **anaphylaxis,** *pain,* **sepsis,** *fever, blood product infusion reaction.*

INTERACTIONS

Drug-drug. *Antineoplastics:* may enhance potential for renal toxicity, bronchospasm, and hypotension. Use cautiously.
Cardiac glycosides: increased risk of digitalis toxicity due to amphotericin B-induced hypokalemia. Serum potassium level must be monitored closely.
Clotrimazole, fluconazole, ketoconazole, miconazole: may induce fungal resistance to amphotericin B. Use together cautiously.
Corticosteroids, corticotropin: may potentiate potassium depletion, which could result in cardiac dysfunction. Serum electrolyte levels and cardiac function must be monitored.
Flucytosine: may increase flucytosine toxicity by increasing cellular reuptake or impairing renal excretion of flucytosine. Use cautiously.
Other nephrotoxic drugs, such as antibiotics, antineoplastics: may cause additive nephrotoxicity. Administer cautiously. Renal function must be monitored closely.
Skeletal muscle relaxants: enhanced effects of skeletal muscle relaxants resulting from amphotericin B-induced hypokalemia. Serum potassium levels must be monitored.

EFFECTS ON DIAGNOSTIC TESTS
None reported.

CONTRAINDICATIONS
Contraindicated in patients with hypersensitivity to drug or its components.

SPECIAL CONSIDERATIONS
▸ Use drug cautiously in patients with impaired renal function, in elderly patients, and in pregnant women.
▸ Patients concomitantly receiving chemotherapy or bone marrow transplantation are at greater risk for additional adverse reactions, including seizures, arrhythmias, and thrombocytopenia.
▸ Leukocyte transfusions are not given with drug because acute pulmonary toxicity has been reported with concurrent administration.
▸ *Alert:* Note that different amphotericin B preparations aren't interchangeable and dosages will vary.
▸ To lessen risk or severity of adverse reactions, patient is premedicated with antipyretics, antihistamines, antiemetics, or corticosteroids.
▸ BUN and serum creatinine and electrolyte levels (particularly magnesium and potassium), liver function, and CBC must be monitored.
▸ Therapy may take several weeks to months.
▸ Patient should be monitored for signs of hypokalemia (ECG changes, muscle weakness, cramping, drowsiness).
▸ Patients treated with amphotericin B liposomal had a lower incidence of chills, elevated BUN, hypokalemia, hypertension, and vomiting than patients treated with conventional amphotericin B.
▸ It's unknown if drug appears in human milk. Because of potential for serious adverse reactions in breast-fed infants, a decision should be made whether to discontinue breast-feeding or discontinue drug, taking into account importance of drug to mother.

I.V. administration
▸ Each 50-mg vial of amphotericin B liposomal is reconstituted with 12 ml of sterile water for injection to yield a solution of 4 mg amphotericin B/ml.

---

*Liquid contains alcohol.   **May contain tartrazine.   †Canada   ‡Australia   §U.K.   ◇OTC

◗ **Alert:** Drug should not be reconstituted with bacteriostatic water for injection, and no bacteriostatic agents should be allowed in the solution. The drug should not be reconstituted with saline or saline added to reconstituted concentration or mixed with other drugs.

◗ After reconstitution, vial is shaken vigorously for 30 seconds or until particulate matter is dispersed.

◗ The calculated amount of reconstituted solution is then withdrawn into a sterile syringe and injected through a 5-micron filter into the appropriate amount of D_5W to further dilute to a final concentration of 1 to 2 mg/ml. Lower concentrations (0.2 to 0.5 mg/ml) may be appropriate for pediatric patients to provide sufficient volume of infusion.

◗ An existing I.V. line must be flushed with D_5W before infusion of drug. If this isn't feasible, drug should be administered through a separate line.

◗ A controlled infusion device and an inline filter with a mean pore diameter larger than 1 micron should be used. Initially, drug is infused over at least 2 hours. Infusion time may be reduced to 1 hour if treatment is well tolerated. If patient experiences discomfort during infusion, duration of infusion may be increased.

◗ Patient must be observed closely for adverse reactions during infusion. If anaphylaxis occurs, infusion is stopped immediately and supportive therapy provided.

◗ An unopened vial is stored at 36° to 46° F (2° to 8° C). Once reconstituted, concentrate is stored for up to 24 hours at 36° to 46° F. Don't freeze.

Patient teaching

◗ Immediately report signs and symptoms of hypersensitivity.

◗ Therapy may take several months; personal hygiene and other measures to prevent spread and recurrence of lesions are important.

◗ Report any adverse reactions that occur while receiving drug, especially signs of hypokalemia (muscle weakness, cramping, drowsiness).

◗ Frequent laboratory testing is necessary.

fluconazole

Diflucan

Pregnancy Risk Category C

HOW SUPPLIED

Tablets: 50 mg, 100 mg, 150 mg, 200 mg
Powder for oral suspension: 10 mg/ml, 40 mg/ml
Injection: 200 mg/100 ml, 400 mg/200 ml

ACTION

Inhibits fungal cytochrome P-450 (responsible for fungal sterol synthesis) and weakens fungal cell walls.

Route	Onset	Peak	Duration
P.O.	Unknown	1-2 hr	30 hr
I.V.	Immediate	Immediate	Unknown

INDICATIONS & DOSAGE

Oropharyngeal candidiasis —
Adults: 200 mg P.O. or I.V. on first day, followed by 100 mg once daily. Therapy should last at least 2 weeks.
Children: 6 mg/kg P.O. or I.V. on first day, followed by 3 mg/kg daily for 2 weeks.
Esophageal candidiasis —
Adults: 200 mg P.O. or I.V. on first day, followed by 100 mg once daily. Higher doses (up to 400 mg daily) have been used, depending on patient's condition and tolerance of treatment. Patients should receive drug for at least 3 weeks and for 2 weeks after symptoms resolve.
Children: 6 mg/kg P.O. or I.V. on first day followed by 3 mg/kg daily for at least 3 weeks, and for at least 2 weeks after symp-

---

toms resolve. Doses up to 12 mg/kg may be used based on clinical judgment.

Vulvovaginal candidiasis —
Adults: 150 mg P.O. for one dose only or 50 mg P.O. daily for 3 days.

Systemic candidiasis —
Adults: 400 mg P.O. or I.V. on first day, followed by 200 mg once daily. Treatment should continue for at least 4 weeks and for 2 weeks after symptoms resolve.
Children: 6 to 12 mg/kg/day P.O. or I.V.

Cryptococcal meningitis —
Adults: 400 mg P.O. or I.V. on first day, followed by 200 mg once daily. Higher doses (up to 400 mg daily) may be used. Treatment should continue for 10 to 12 weeks after CSF cultures are negative.
Children: 12 mg/kg/day P.O. or I.V. on first day, followed by 6 mg/kg daily for 10 to 12 weeks after CSF culture is negative.

Prevention of candidiasis in bone marrow transplant —
Adults: 400 mg P.O. or I.V. once daily. Start prophylaxis several days before anticipated agranulocytosis. Continue therapy for 7 days after neutrophil count rises above 1,000 cells/mm³.

Suppression of relapse of cryptococcal meningitis in patients with AIDS —
Adults: 200 mg P.O. or I.V. daily.
Children: 3 to 6 mg/kg/day P.O. or I.V.
Dosage adjustment: For renally impaired patients, if creatinine clearance is 11 to 50 ml/minute, dosage is reduced by 50%. Patients receiving regular hemodialysis treatment should receive the usual dose after each dialysis session.

ADVERSE REACTIONS

CNS: headache, dizziness.
EENT: taste perversion.
GI: *nausea,* vomiting, abdominal pain, diarrhea, dyspepsia.
Hematologic: *leukopenia, thrombocytopenia.*
Hepatic: *hepatotoxicity* (rare), elevated liver enzymes.

Skin: rash, ***Stevens-Johnson syndrome*** (rare).
Other: *anaphylaxis.*

INTERACTIONS

Drug-drug. *Cyclosporine, phenytoin, theophylline:* may increase plasma concentrations of these drugs. Serum cyclosporine or phenytoin levels must be monitored.
Isoniazid, oral sulfonylureas, phenytoin, rifampin, valproic acid: increased incidence of elevated hepatic transaminases. Monitor closely.
Oral antidiabetics (glipizide, glyburide, tolbutamide): may increase plasma concentrations of these drugs. Enhanced hypoglycemic effect may occur.
Rifampin: enhanced metabolism of fluconazole. Lack of response may occur.
Warfarin: increased risk of bleeding. PT and INR must be monitored.
Zidovudine: zidovudine activity may be increased. Monitor closely.
Drug-food. *Caffeine:* may increase caffeine plasma levels. Ofloxacin or lomefloxacin are alternative drugs.

EFFECTS ON DIAGNOSTIC TESTS

None reported.

CONTRAINDICATIONS

Contraindicated in patients with hypersensitivity to drug.

SPECIAL CONSIDERATIONS

▶ Use drug cautiously in patients with hypersensitivity to other antifungal azole compounds; no data exist regarding cross-sensitivity.
▶ Liver function tests are periodically monitored during prolonged therapy.
▶ If patient develops mild rash, it must be monitored closely. Drug is discontinued if lesions progress.
▶ Incidence of adverse reactions appears to be greater in HIV-infected patients.

I.V. administration

▶ Protective overwrap from I.V. bags must not be removed until just before use to ensure product sterility. The plastic container may show some opacity from moisture absorbed during sterilization. This does not affect the drug and diminishes over time. Other drugs should not be added to the I.V. bag.

▶ *Alert:* The drug is administered by continuous infusion at a rate not to exceed 200 mg/hour. An infusion pump is used. To prevent air embolism, connecting in a series with other infusions is not recommended. Other drugs are not added to the solution.

Patient teaching

▶ Take drug as directed, even after he feels better.

▶ Report adverse reactions promptly.

flucytosine (5-fluorocytosine, 5-FC)
Ancobon, Ancotil‡

Pregnancy Risk Category C

HOW SUPPLIED
Capsules: 250 mg, 500 mg

ACTION
Unknown. Appears to penetrate fungal cells and cause defective protein synthesis.

Route	Onset	Peak	Duration
P.O.	Unknown	1-2 hr	Unknown

INDICATIONS & DOSAGE
Severe fungal infections due to susceptible strains of Candida *(including septicemia, endocarditis, urinary tract and pulmonary infections) and* Cryptococcus *(meningitis, pulmonary infection, and possible urinary tract infection) —*

Adults: 50 to 150 mg/kg daily P.O. in four equally divided doses q 6 hours.

ADVERSE REACTIONS
CNS: headache, vertigo, sedation, fatigue, weakness, confusion, hallucinations, psychosis, ataxia, hearing loss, paresthesia, parkinsonism, peripheral neuropathy.
CV: *cardiac arrest,* chest pain.
GI: nausea, vomiting, diarrhea, abdominal pain, dry mouth, duodenal ulcer, *hemorrhage,* ulcerative colitis, anorexia.
GU: azotemia, elevated creatinine and BUN levels, crystalluria, *renal failure.*
Hematologic: anemia, *leukopenia, bone marrow suppression, thrombocytopenia,* eosinophilia, *agranulocytosis, aplastic anemia.*
Hepatic: elevated liver enzymes, elevated serum alkaline phosphatase, jaundice.
Metabolic: hypoglycemia, hypokalemia.
Respiratory: *respiratory arrest,* dyspnea.
Skin: occasional rash, pruritus, urticaria, photosensitivity.

INTERACTIONS
Drug-drug. *Amphotericin B:* synergistic effects and possibly enhanced toxicity when used together. Monitor closely.

EFFECTS ON DIAGNOSTIC TESTS
Flucytosine falsely elevates creatinine values on iminohydrolase enzymatic assay.

CONTRAINDICATIONS
Contraindicated in patients with hypersensitivity to drug.

SPECIAL CONSIDERATIONS
▶ Use with extreme caution in patients with impaired hepatic or renal function or bone marrow suppression.
▶ Capsules are administered over 15 minutes to reduce adverse GI reactions.
▶ Blood, liver, and renal function studies are monitored frequently during therapy; susceptibility tests are obtained weekly to monitor drug resistance.

▶ If possible, blood level assays of drug are regularly performed to maintain flucytosine at therapeutic level (25 to 120 mcg/ml). Higher blood levels may be toxic.

▶ Fluid intake and output should be monitored and marked changes reported.

Patient teaching
▶ Therapeutic response may take weeks or months.
▶ Report adverse reactions promptly.

---

griseofulvin microsize

Fulcin‡, Fulvicin-U/F, Grifulvin V, Grisactin 500, Grisovin‡, Grisovin, Grisovin FP

griseofulvin ultramicrosize

Fulvicin P/G, Grisactin Ultra, Griseostatin‡, Gris-PEG

Pregnancy Risk Category C

HOW SUPPLIED
griseofulvin microsize
Tablets: 250 mg, 500 mg
Capsules: 125 mg, 250 mg
Oral suspension: 125 mg/5 ml
griseofulvin ultramicrosize
Tablets: 125 mg, 165 mg, 250 mg, 330 mg

ACTION
Arrests fungal cell activity by disrupting mitotic spindle structure.

Route	Onset	Peak	Duration
P.O.	Unknown	4-8 hr	Unknown

INDICATIONS & DOSAGE
Ringworm infections of skin, hair, nails (tinea corporis, tinea capitis, tinea cruris)

when due to Trichophyton, Microsporum, *or* Epidermophyton —
Adults: 500 mg of microsize P.O. daily in single or divided doses. Severe infections may require up to 1 g daily. Or, 330 to 375 mg ultramicrosize P.O. daily in single or divided doses. Duration of therapy is 2 to 8 weeks depending on site of infection.
    Tinea pedis, tinea unguium —
Adults: 0.75 to 1 g of microsize P.O. daily. Or, 660 to 750 mg of ultramicrosize P.O. daily in divided doses. Duration of therapy is 4 weeks to 1 year.
Children: 11 mg/kg/day of microsize P.O. Or, 7.3 mg/kg/day of ultramicrosize P.O.

ADVERSE REACTIONS
CNS: headache (in early stages of treatment), fatigue (with large doses), occasional mental confusion, impaired performance of routine activities, psychotic symptoms, dizziness, insomnia, paresthesia of hands and feet (after extended therapy).
EENT: transient decrease in hearing, oral thrush.
GI: nausea, vomiting, flatulence, diarrhea, epigastric distress, *bleeding.*
GU: proteinuria, menstrual irregularities.
Hematologic: leukopenia, *agranulocytosis,* porphyria.
Hepatic: *hepatic toxicity.*
Skin: *rash, urticaria,* photosensitivity, angioedema.
Other: hypersensitivity reactions, lupus erythematosus.

INTERACTIONS
Drug-drug. *Coumarin anticoagulants:* decreased effectiveness. PT and INR must be monitored when used concurrently.
Cyclosporine: decreased serum cyclosporine levels. Monitor closely.
Oral contraceptives: decreased effectiveness. Alternative methods of contraception should be suggested.
Phenobarbital: decreased griseofulvin

---

blood levels due to decreased absorption or increased metabolism. Avoid using together or griseofulvin is administered t.i.d.

Drug-food. *High-fat meals:* increased absorption. Drug and meal are administered together.

Drug-lifestyle. *Alcohol use:* may cause tachycardia, diaphoresis, and flushing. Avoid alcohol consumption.

Sun exposure: may increase risk of photosensitivity reaction. Avoid unprotected sun exposure.

EFFECTS ON DIAGNOSTIC TESTS
None reported.

CONTRAINDICATIONS
Contraindicated in patients hypersensitive to drug and in those with porphyria or hepatocellular failure. Also contraindicated in pregnant patients or women who intend to become pregnant during therapy.

SPECIAL CONSIDERATIONS
▶ Use drug cautiously in penicillin-sensitive patients.
▶ *Alert:* Because of potential toxicity, drug is used only when topical treatment fails.
▶ Laboratory tests are obtained to confirm diagnosis. Drug is continued until clinical and laboratory examinations confirm eradication.
▶ *Alert:* Because griseofulvin ultramicrosize is dispersed in polyethylene glycol, it's absorbed more rapidly and completely than microsize preparations and is effective at one-half to two-thirds the usual griseofulvin dose. Preparations are not interchangable.
▶ Drug is administered after a high-fat meal to enhance absorption and minimize GI distress.
▶ Hematologic, renal, and hepatic function need to be assessed periodically during prolonged therapy.
▶ Discontinue drug in patients who experience agranulocytosis.
▶ Effective treatment of tinea pedis may require concomitant use of a topical drug.

▶ Safety in children under age 2 hasn't been established.

Patient teaching
▶ Take drug after a high-fat meal.
▶ Prolonged treatment may be needed to control infection and prevent relapse, even if symptoms abate in first few days of therapy.
▶ Keep skin clean and dry and to maintain good hygiene.
▶ Avoid intense sunlight. Unprotected sun exposure may cause photosensitivity reactions.

itraconazole
Sporanox

Pregnancy Risk Category C

HOW SUPPLIED
Capsules: 100 mg
Oral solution: 10 mg/ml

ACTION
Interferes with fungal cell-wall synthesis by inhibiting the formation of ergosterol and increasing cell-wall permeability that makes the fungus susceptible to osmotic instability.

Route	Onset	Peak	Duration
P.O.	Unknown	3-4 hr	Unknown

INDICATIONS & DOSAGE
Pulmonary and extrapulmonary blastomycosis, nonmeningeal histoplasmosis —
Adults: 200 mg P.O. daily. Dosage increased as needed and tolerated in 100-mg increments to a maximum of 400 mg daily. Doses that exceed 200 mg daily should be given in two divided doses. Treatment should continue for a minimum of 3 months. In life-threatening illness, a loading dose of 200 mg t.i.d. is given for 3 days.

Aspergillosis —
Adults: 200 to 400 mg P.O. daily.

Onychomycosis (fungal nail disease) from dermatophytes of the toenail —
Adults: 200 mg P.O. once daily for 12 consecutive weeks.

Onychomycosis of the fingernail —
Adults: initially, 200 mg P.O. b.i.d. for 1 week; after 3 weeks, dosage is repeated.

Oropharyngeal candidiasis —
Adults: 200 mg swished in mouth vigorously and swallowed daily, for 1 to 2 weeks.

Oropharyngeal candidiasis in patients unresponsive to fluconazole tablets —
Adults: 100 mg swished in mouth vigorously and swallowed b.i.d., for 2 to 4 weeks.

Esophageal candidiasis —
Adults: 100 to 200 mg swished in mouth vigorously and swallowed daily, for a minimum treatment of 3 weeks. Treatment should continue for 2 weeks after symptoms resolve.

ADVERSE REACTIONS
CNS: headache, dizziness, somnolence, fatigue, malaise.
CV: hypertension.
GI: *nausea,* vomiting, diarrhea, abdominal pain, anorexia.
GU: albuminuria, impotence.
Hepatic: impaired hepatic function.
Metabolic: hypokalemia.
Skin: rash, pruritus.
Other: edema, fever, decreased libido.

INTERACTIONS
Drug-drug. *Antacids, H_2-receptor antagonists, phenytoin, rifampin:* possible lowered itraconazole plasma levels. Avoid concomitant use.
Cisapride: inhibited metabolism of these drugs, resulting in elevated blood levels and risk of serious cardiac toxicity. Never administer together.
Cyclosporine, digoxin, tacrolimus: possible increased plasma levels of these drugs.

Plasma levels should be monitored closely.
Isoniazid: may decrease plasma levels of itraconazole. Monitor closely.
Oral anticoagulants: possible enhanced anticoagulant effects. PT and INR should be monitored closely.
Oral antidiabetics: similar antifungals have caused hypoglycemia. Blood glucose levels should be monitored closely.

EFFECTS ON DIAGNOSTIC TESTS
None reported.

CONTRAINDICATIONS
Contraindicated in patients with hypersensitivity to drug; in those receiving astemizole, cisapride, triazolam, or midazolam (orally); and in breast-feeding patients.

SPECIAL CONSIDERATIONS
▶ Use cautiously in patients with hypochlorhydria because they may not absorb drug readily. Because hypochlorhydria can accompany HIV infection, use cautiously in HIV-infected patients.
▶ Also use cautiously in patients receiving other highly bound medications because drug and its metabolites are more than 99% bound to plasma proteins.
▶ Baseline liver function tests are performed initially and monitored periodically.

Patient teaching
▶ Report all medications to avoid potential drug interactions.
▶ Report signs and symptoms of liver disease (anorexia, dark urine, pale stools, unusual fatigue, or jaundice).
▶ Oral solution must not be used interchangeably with itraconazole capsules.
▶ Take capsule with food to ensure maximal absorption.
▶ Solution is taken without food and should be used 10 ml at a time.

---

*Liquid contains alcohol.   **May contain tartrazine.   †Canada   ‡Australia   §U.K.   ◇OTC

ketoconazole

Nizoral

Pregnancy Risk Category C

HOW SUPPLIED

Tablets: 200 mg
Oral suspension: 100 mg/5 ml

ACTION

Inhibits purine transport and DNA, RNA, and protein synthesis; increases cell-wall permeability, making the fungus more susceptible to osmotic pressure.

Route	Onset	Peak	Duration
P.O.	Unknown	1-2 hr	Unknown

INDICATIONS & DOSAGE

Systemic candidiasis, chronic mucocandidiasis, oral thrush, candiduria, coccidioidomycosis, blastomycosis, histoplasmosis, chromomycosis, and paracoccidioidomycosis; severe cutaneous dermatophyte infections resistant to therapy with topical or oral griseofulvin —
Adults and children over 40 kg (88 lb): initially, 200 mg P.O. daily in a single dose. Dose may be increased to 400 mg once daily in patients who don't respond.
Children ages 2 and older: 3.3 to 6.6 mg/kg P.O. daily as a single dose.

ADVERSE REACTIONS

CNS: headache, nervousness, dizziness, somnolence, photophobia, ***suicidal tendencies,*** severe depression.
GI: *nausea, vomiting,* abdominal pain, diarrhea.
GU: impotence, gynecomastia with tenderness.
Hematologic: ***thrombocytopenia,*** hemolytic anemia, ***leukopenia.***
Hepatic: elevated liver enzymes, ***fatal hepatotoxicity.***
Metabolic: hyperlipidemia.
Skin: pruritus.

Other: fever, chills.

INTERACTIONS

Drug-drug. *Antacids, anticholinergics, H_2 blockers:* decreased absorption of ketoconazole. These drugs should not be administered until at least 2 hours after ketoconazole dose.
Anticoagulants: effects may be enhanced. INR, PT, and PTT must be monitored and the dose adjusted as needed.
Cisapride: may cause ventricular arrhythmias. Avoid concomitant use.
Cyclosporine: may increase cyclosporine plasma levels. Serum levels must be monitored.
Isoniazid, rifampin: increased ketoconazole metabolism. A decreased antifungal effect may occur.
Paclitaxel: metabolism inhibited. Use together cautiously.
Theophylline: may decrease theophylline plasma levels. Serum levels must be monitored.
Drug-herb. *Yew:* inhibits ketoconazole metabolism. Avoid concomitant use.

EFFECTS ON DIAGNOSTIC TESTS

None reported.

CONTRAINDICATIONS

Contraindicated in patients with hypersensitivity to drug.

SPECIAL CONSIDERATIONS

▶ Use cautiously in patients with hepatic disease and in those who are taking other hepatotoxic drugs.
▶ Because of the potential for serious hepatotoxicity, don't use ketoconazole for less serious conditions, such as fungus infections of the skin or nails.
▶ Elevated liver enzymes and nausea that does not subside as well as unusual fatigue, jaundice, dark urine, or pale stool should be monitored; all are signs or symptoms of possible hepatotoxicity.
▶ Note that much larger doses (up to

800 mg/day) can be used to treat fungal meningitis and intracerebral fungal lesions.

Patient teaching

▸ If you have achlorhydria, dissolve each tablet in 4 ml aqueous solution of 0.2 N hydrochloric acid, sip mixture through a glass or plastic straw (to avoid contact with teeth), and finish by drinking a glass of water because ketoconazole requires gastric acidity for dissolution and absorption.

▸ Treatment must continue until all tests indicate that active fungal infection has subsided. If drug is discontinued too soon, infection will recur. Minimum treatment for candidiasis is 7 to 14 days; for other systemic fungal infections, 6 months; for resistant dermatophyte infections, at least 4 weeks.

▸ Nausea, common early in therapy, will subside. To minimize, divide daily dose into two doses or take dose with meals.

nystatin

Mycostatin*, Nadostine , Nilstat, Nystat-Rx, Nystex*

Pregnancy Risk Category NR

HOW SUPPLIED

Tablets: 500,000 U
Oral suspension: 100,000 U/ml; 50, 150, or 500 million U; 1 or 2 billion U
Powder: 50, 150, or 500 million U; 1, 2, or 5 billion U
Troches: 200,000 U
Vaginal suppositories: 100,000 U

ACTION

Unknown. Probably binds to sterols in fungal cell membrane, altering cell permeability and allowing leakage of intracellular components.

Route	Onset	Peak	Duration
P.O., topical	Unknown	Unknown	Unknown

INDICATIONS & DOSAGE

GI infections —
Adults: 500,000 to 1 million U as oral tablets t.i.d.

Oral, vaginal, and intestinal infections due to Candida albicans (Monilia) *and other Candida species —*
Adults: 400,000 to 600,000 U oral suspension q.i.d. for oral candidiasis.
Children and infants ages 3 months and older: 250,000 to 500,000 U oral suspension q.i.d.
Neonates and premature infants: 100,000 U oral suspension q.i.d.
Vaginal infections —
Adults: 100,000 U, as vaginal tablets, inserted high into vagina, daily or b.i.d. for 14 days.

ADVERSE REACTIONS

GI: transient nausea, vomiting, diarrhea.

INTERACTIONS

None significant.

EFFECTS ON DIAGNOSTIC TESTS

None reported.

CONTRAINDICATIONS

Contraindicated in patients with hypersensitivity to drug.

SPECIAL CONSIDERATIONS

▸ Drug is not effective against systemic infections.

▸ Pregnant patients can use vaginal tablets up to 6 weeks before term to treat maternal infection that may cause thrush in neonates.

▸ For treatment of oral candidiasis (thrush): After the mouth is clean of food debris, the patient must hold suspension in mouth for several minutes before swallowing. When treating infants, medication is

---

*Liquid contains alcohol.   **May contain tartrazine.   †Canada   ‡Australia   §U.K.   ◇OTC

swabbed on oral mucosa. Immunosuppressed patients are sometimes instructed by the doctor to suck on vaginal tablets (100,000 U) because this provides prolonged contact with oral mucosa.

Patient teaching
▶ Continue medication for at least 2 days after symptoms disappear. Health care provider determines exact length of therapy.
▶ Continue therapy during menstruation.
▶ Predisposing factors of vaginal infection include use of antibiotics, oral contraceptives, and corticosteroids; diabetes; reinfection by sexual partner; and tight-fitting pantyhose. Wear cotton (not synthetic) underwear.
▶ Careful hygiene for affected areas, including cleaning perineal area from front to back after defecation, is necessary.
▶ Report redness, swelling, or irritation.
▶ Overusing mouthwash or wearing poorly fitting dentures, especially in older patients, may promote infection.

terbinafine hydrochloride
Lamisil

Pregnancy Risk Category B

HOW SUPPLIED
Tablets: 250 mg

ACTION
Inhibits squalene epoxidase, a key enzyme in sterol biosynthesis of fungi. This enzyme inhibition results in a deficiency of ergosterol and a corresponding accumulation of sterol within the fungal cell.

Route	Onset	Peak	Duration
P.O.	Unknown	2 hr	Unknown

INDICATIONS & DOSAGE
Fingernail onychomycosis due to dermatophytes (tinea unguium) —
Adults: 250 mg P.O. once daily for 6 weeks.
   Toenail onychomycosis due to dermatophytes (tinea unguium) —
Adults: 250 mg P.O. once daily for 12 weeks.

ADVERSE REACTIONS
CNS: *headache.*
EENT: taste disturbances, visual disturbances.
GI: diarrhea, dyspepsia, abdominal pain, nausea, flatulence.
Hepatic: hepatobiliary dysfunction (including cholestatic jaundice).
Hematologic: *neutropenia,* decrease in absolute lymphocyte counts.
Skin: rash, pruritus, urticaria, *Stevens-Johnson syndrome, toxic epidermal necrolysis.*
Other: *hypersensitivity reactions, anaphylaxis.*

INTERACTIONS
Drug-drug. *Cimetidine:* decreases drug clearance by one-third. Avoid concomitant use.
Cyclosporine: drug increases clearance of cyclosporine. Serum levels must be monitored.
Rifampin: increases terbinafine clearance by 100%. Monitor patient.
Drug-food. *Caffeine:* I.V. caffeine clearance is decreased. Use together cautiously.

EFFECTS ON DIAGNOSTIC TESTS
None reported.

CONTRAINDICATIONS
Contraindicated in patients with hypersensitivity to drug.

SPECIAL CONSIDERATIONS
▶ Drug is not recommended in patients

---

with preexisting liver disease or renal impairment (creatinine clearance below 50 ml/minute), or in pregnant or breast-feeding patients.

▶ CBC and hepatic enzymes must be monitored in patients receiving drug for over 6 weeks. Drug should be discontinued if hepatobiliary dysfunction or cholestatic hepatitis develops.

▶ Safety in children has not been established.

▶ *Alert:* Don't confuse terbinafine with terbutaline.

Patient teaching

▶ Successful treatment of nail infections may not be observed for 4 weeks for fingernail infections and 10 weeks for toenail infections.

**chloroquine hydrochloride
chloroquine phosphate
doxycycline**
(See Tetracyclines.)
**hydroxychloroquine sulfate
mefloquine hydrochloride
primaquine phosphate
pyrimethamine
pyrimethamine with
  sulfadoxine**

COMBINATION PRODUCTS
None.

chloroquine hydrochloride
Aralen HCl, Chlorquin†

chloroquine phosphate
Aralen Phosphate, Avloclor§,
Chlorquin†

Pregnancy Risk Category C

HOW SUPPLIED
chloroquine hydrochloride
Injection: 50 mg/ml (40-mg/ml base)
chloroquine phosphate
Tablets: 250 mg (150-mg base), 500 mg
(300-mg base)
Injection: 5 mg (200-mg base)

ACTION
Unknown. May bind to and alter the properties of DNA in susceptible parasites.

Route	Onset	Peak	Duration
P.O.	Unknown	1-3 hr	Unknown
I.M.	Unknown	0.5 hr	Unknown

INDICATIONS & DOSAGE
Acute malarial attacks due to Plasmodium vivax, P. malariae, P. ovale, *and susceptible strains of* P. falciparum —
Adults: initially, 600 mg (base) P.O.; then
300 mg at 6, 24, and 48 hours. Or 160 to
200 mg (base) I.M. initially, repeated in
6 hours p.r.n. Switch patient to oral therapy as soon as possible.
Children: initially, 10 mg (base)/kg
P.O.; then 5 mg (base)/kg at 6, 24, and 48
hours (don't exceed adult dose). Or 5 mg
(base)/kg I.M. initially, repeated in 6 hours
p.r.n. Don't exceed 10 mg (base)/kg/24
hours. Switch patient to oral therapy as
soon as possible.
  Malaria prophylaxis —
Adults and children: 5 mg (base)/kg P.O.
(not to exceed 300 mg) weekly on the same
day (begun 1 to 2 weeks before probable
exposure and continued for 4 to 6 weeks
after leaving endemic area). If treatment
begins after exposure, initial dose is doubled (10 mg/kg) in two divided doses P.O.
6 hours apart.
  Extraintestinal amebiasis —
Adults: 1 g (600-mg base) chloroquine
phosphate P.O. daily for 2 days; then
500 mg (300-mg base) daily for 2 to 3
weeks. Treatment is usually combined
with an intestinal amebicide. When oral
therapy is unfeasible, administer 4 to 5 ml
chloroquine hydrochloride (200 to
250 mg; 160- to 200-mg base) I.M. daily
for 10 to 12 days. Resume oral therapy as
soon as possible.
Children: 16.7 mg/kg chloroquine phosphate (10-mg/kg base) P.O. once daily for
2 to 3 weeks. Maximum dose is 500 mg
chloroquine phosphate (300-mg base) daily.

ADVERSE REACTIONS
CNS: mild and transient headache, psy-
chic stimulation, *seizures,* dizziness, neuropathy.
CV: hypotension, ECG changes.

Reactions may be *common,* uncommon, *life-threatening,* or COMMON AND LIFE-THREATENING.

EENT: blurred vision; difficulty in focusing; reversible corneal changes; typically irreversible, sometimes progressive or delayed retinal changes such as narrowing of arterioles; macular lesions; pallor of optic disk; optic atrophy; patchy retinal pigmentation, typically leading to blindness, ototoxicity (nerve deafness, vertigo, tinnitus).

GI: anorexia, abdominal cramps, diarrhea, nausea, vomiting, stomatitis.

Hematologic: *agranulocytosis, aplastic anemia,* hemolytic anemia, *thrombocytopenia.*

Skin: pruritus, lichen planus eruptions, skin and mucosal pigmentary changes, pleomorphic skin eruptions.

INTERACTIONS

Drug-drug. *Cimetidine:* decreased hepatic metabolism of chloroquine. Toxicity may occur; monitor for toxicity.
Kaolin, magnesium and aluminum salts: decreased GI absorption. Administration times must be separated.
Drug-lifestyle. *Sun exposure:* may exacerbate drug-induced dermatoses. Avoid excessive sun exposure.

EFFECTS ON DIAGNOSTIC TESTS
None reported.

CONTRAINDICATIONS
Contraindicated in patients with hypersensitivity to drug, retinal or visual field changes, or porphyria.

SPECIAL CONSIDERATIONS
▶ Use with extreme caution in patients with severe GI, neurologic, or blood disorders.
▶ Use cautiously in patients with hepatic disease or alcoholism because drug concentrates in the liver, and in those with G6PD deficiency or psoriasis because drug may exacerbate these conditions.
▶ *Alert:* Drug dosage may be discussed in mg or mg-base; be aware of the difference.

▶ Baseline and periodic ophthalmic examinations should be performed. Ocular muscle weakness should be checked periodically after long-term use.
▶ Patient should have audiometric examinations before, during, and after therapy, especially if therapy is long-term.
▶ CBC and liver function studies should be performed periodically during long-term therapy; if a severe blood disorder not attributable to the disease develops, drug may need to be discontinued.
▶ *Alert:* Patient should be monitored for possible overdose, which can quickly lead to toxic signs and symptoms: headache, drowsiness, visual disturbances, CV collapse, and seizures, followed by cardiopulmonary arrest. Children are extremely susceptible to toxicity; avoid long-term treatment.

Patient teaching
▶ For prophylaxis, take drug immediately before or after meals on same day each week.
▶ Avoid excessive sun exposure to prevent exacerbation of drug-induced dermatoses.
▶ Report adverse reactions promptly, especially blurred vision, increased sensitivity to light, or muscle weakness.

hydroxychloroquine sulfate
Plaquenil Sulfate

Pregnancy Risk Category C

HOW SUPPLIED
Tablets: 200 mg (155-mg base)

ACTION
Unknown. May bind to and alter the properties of DNA in susceptible organisms.

Route	Onset	Peak	Duration
P.O.	Unknown	2-4.5 hr	Unknown

INDICATIONS & DOSAGE

Suppressive prophylaxis of malaria attacks due to Plasmodium vivax, P. malariae, P. ovale, *and susceptible strains of* P. falciparum —

Adults: 400 mg (310-mg base) P.O. weekly on same day of week (begin 1 to 2 weeks before entering endemic area and continue for 4 weeks after leaving endemic area). If not started before exposure, initial dose is doubled to 800 mg (620-mg base) in two divided doses.

Children: 5 mg/kg (base) P.O. weekly on same day of week (begin 1 to 2 weeks before entering endemic area and continue for 4 weeks after leaving endemic area). Don't exceed adult dose. If not started before exposure, initial dose is doubled to 10 mg/kg (base) in two divided doses.

Acute malarial attacks —

Adults: initially, 800 mg (sulfate) P.O.; then 400 mg after 6 to 8 hours; then 400 mg daily for 2 days (total 2 g sulfate salt).

Children: 13 mg/kg (sulfate) P.O.; then 6.5 mg/kg 6 hours later; then 6.5 mg/kg daily for 2 days.

Lupus erythematosus (chronic discoid and systemic) —

Adults: 400 mg (sulfate) P.O. daily or b.i.d., continued for several weeks or months, depending on response. For prolonged maintenance dose, 200 to 400 mg (sulfate) daily.

Rheumatoid arthritis —

Adults: initially, 400 to 600 mg (sulfate) P.O. daily. When good response occurs (usually in 4 to 12 weeks), dosage is cut in half.

ADVERSE REACTIONS

CNS: irritability, nightmares, ataxia, *seizures,* psychosis, vertigo, nystagmus, dizziness, hypoactive deep tendon reflexes, lassitude, skeletal muscle weakness, headache.

CV: T wave inversion or depression, widening of the QRS complex.

EENT: blurred vision; difficulty in focusing; reversible corneal changes; typically irreversible, sometimes progressive or delayed retinal changes such as narrowing of arterioles; macular lesions; pallor of optic disk; optic atrophy; visual field defects; patchy retinal pigmentation, commonly leading to blindness, ototoxicity.

GI: anorexia, abdominal cramps, diarrhea, nausea, vomiting.

Hematologic: *agranulocytosis, leukopenia, thrombocytopenia, hemolysis in patients with G6PD deficiency, aplastic anemia.*

Skin: pruritus, lichen planus eruptions, skin and mucosal pigmentary changes, pleomorphic skin eruptions, worsened psoriasis.

Other: weight loss, alopecia, bleaching of hair.

INTERACTIONS

Drug-drug. *Cimetidine:* decreased hepatic metabolism of hydroxychloroquine. Toxicity may occur.

Kaolin, magnesium and aluminum salts: decreased GI absorption. Administration times must be separated.

EFFECTS ON DIAGNOSTIC TESTS

None reported.

CONTRAINDICATIONS

Contraindicated in patients with retinal or visual field changes, porphyria, or hypersensitivity to drug and in long-term therapy for children.

SPECIAL CONSIDERATIONS

▶ Use with extreme caution in patients with severe GI, neurologic, or blood disorders.

▶ Use cautiously in patients with hepatic disease or alcoholism because drug concentrates in liver, and in those with G6PD deficiency or psoriasis because drug may exacerbate these conditions.

▶ *Alert:* Drug dosage may be discussed in mg or mg-base; be aware of the difference.

▶ Baseline and periodic ophthalmic examinations should be performed. Tests for ocular muscle weakness should periodically be checked after long-term use.

▶ Patient should undergo audiometric examinations before, during, and after therapy, especially if therapy is long-term.

▶ CBC and liver function studies should be monitored periodically during long-term therapy; if severe blood disorder not attributable to disease develops, drug may need to be discontinued.

▶ *Alert:* Patient should be monitored for possible overdose, which can quickly lead to toxic signs or symptoms: headache, drowsiness, visual disturbances, CV collapse, and seizures, followed by cardiopulmonary arrest. Children are extremely susceptible to toxicity; long-term treatment should be avoided.

Patient teaching

▶ For prophylaxis, take hydroxychloroquine immediately before or after meals on same day each week.

▶ Report adverse reactions promptly.

mefloquine hydrochloride
Lariam

Pregnancy Risk Category C

HOW SUPPLIED
Tablets: 250 mg

ACTION
Unknown. Antimalarial action may be related to drug's ability to form complexes with hemin; may also act by raising intravesicular pH in parasite acid vesicles.

Route	Onset	Peak	Duration
P.O.	Unknown	7-24 hr	Unknown

INDICATIONS & DOSAGE
Acute malaria infections due to

mefloquine-sensitive strains of Plasmodium falciparum *or* P. vivax —
Adults: 1,250 mg P.O. as a single dose. Patients with *P. vivax* infections should receive subsequent therapy with primaquine or other 8-aminoquinolines to avoid relapse after treatment of the initial infection.

Malaria prophylaxis —
Adults: 250 mg P.O. once weekly. Prophylaxis should be initiated 1 week before entering endemic area and continued for 4 weeks after returning. If patient returns to an area without malaria after a prolonged stay in an endemic area, prophylaxis should end after three doses.

ADVERSE REACTIONS
CNS: dizziness, syncope, headache, psychotic manifestations, hallucinations, confusion, anxiety, fatigue, vertigo, depression, *seizures.*
EENT: tinnitus, visual disturbances.
GI: anorexia, vomiting, *nausea,* loose stools, diarrhea, abdominal discomfort or pain.
Hematologic: decreased hematocrit, *leukopenia,* and *thrombocytopenia.*
Hepatic: transient elevations of transaminases.
Musculoskeletal: myalgia.
Skin: rash.
Other: fever, chills.

INTERACTIONS
Drug-drug. *Beta blockers, quinidine, quinine:* ECG abnormalities and cardiac arrest may occur. Avoid concomitant use.
Chloroquine, quinine: increased risk of seizures. Avoid concomitant use.
Valproic acid: decreased valproic acid blood levels and loss of seizure control at start of mefloquine therapy. Anticonvulsant blood levels should be monitored.

EFFECTS ON DIAGNOSTIC TESTS
None reported.

CONTRAINDICATIONS
Contraindicated in patients with hypersensitivity to mefloquine or related compounds.

SPECIAL CONSIDERATIONS
▶ Use cautiously in patients with cardiac disease or seizure disorders.
▶ Because the health risks from concomitant administration of quinine and mefloquine are great, mefloquine therapy shouldn't begin sooner than 12 hours after the last dose of quinine or quinidine.
▶ Patients with *P. vivax* infections are at high risk for relapse because the drug does not eliminate the hepatic phase (exo-erythrocytic parasites). Follow-up therapy with primaquine is advisable.
▶ Liver function tests should be monitored periodically.
▶ If overdose is suspected, vomiting should be induced or gastric lavage performed as appropriate because of potential for cardiotoxicity. Mefloquine has produced cardiac actions similar to quinidine and quinine.

Patient teaching
▶ For prophylaxis, take drug on the same day of each week.
▶ Always take drug with a full glass (at least 8 oz [240 ml]) of water, never on an empty stomach.
▶ Use caution when performing activities that require alertness and coordination because dizziness, disturbed sense of balance, and neuropsychiatric reactions may occur.
▶ If taking mefloquine prophylactically, discontinue drug and notify health care provider if signs or symptoms of impending toxicity (such as unexplained anxiety, depression, confusion, or restlessness) occur.
▶ If undergoing long-term therapy, have periodic ophthalmic examinations because drug may cause ocular lesions.

primaquine phosphate
Pregnancy Risk Category C

HOW SUPPLIED
Tablets: 15 mg (base)

ACTION
Unknown. May bind to and alter the properties of DNA in susceptible parasites.

Route	Onset	Peak	Duration
P.O.	Unknown	1-3 hr	Unknown

INDICATIONS & DOSAGE
Radical cure of relapsing vivax malaria, eliminating symptoms and infection completely; prevention of relapse —
Adults: 15 mg (base) P.O. daily for 14 days. (A 26.3-mg tablet provides 15 mg of base.) Begin therapy during the last 2 weeks of, or following, a course of suppression with chloroquine or comparable agent.
Children: 0.5 mg/kg/day (0.3-mg base/kg/day; maximum 15-mg base/dose) P.O. for 14 days.

ADVERSE REACTIONS
GI: nausea, vomiting, epigastric distress, abdominal cramps.
Hematologic: decreases or increases in WBC counts, decreases in RBC counts, *hemolytic anemia* (in G6PD deficiency), methemoglobinemia (in NADH methemoglobin reductase deficiency).

INTERACTIONS
Drug-drug. *Magnesium and aluminum salts:* decreased GI absorption. Administration times should be separated.
Quinacrine: enhanced toxicity of primaquine. Don't use together.

EFFECTS ON DIAGNOSTIC TESTS
None reported.

CONTRAINDICATIONS

Contraindicated in patients with systemic diseases in which agranulocytosis may develop (such as lupus erythematosus or rheumatoid arthritis) and in those taking bone marrow suppressants and potentially hemolytic drugs. Concomitant administration of quinacrine and primaquine is contraindicated.

SPECIAL CONSIDERATIONS

▶ Use cautiously in patients with previous idiosyncratic reaction (manifested by hemolytic anemia, methemoglobinemia, or leukopenia), in those with a family or personal history of favism, and in those with erythrocytic G6PD deficiency or NADH methemoglobin reductase deficiency.

▶ *Alert:* Drug dosage may be discussed in mg or mg-base; be aware of the difference.

▶ Drug is administered with meals.

▶ Keep in mind that when administering drug, a fast-acting antimalarial (such as chloroquine) is used to reduce possibility of drug-resistant strains.

▶ Frequent blood studies and urine examinations should be obtained in light-skinned patients taking more than 30 mg (base) daily, dark-skinned patients taking more than 15 mg (base) daily, and patients with severe anemia or suspected sensitivity.

▶ Patient should be monitored for sudden fall in hemoglobin level or erythrocyte or leukocyte count, or marked darkening of the urine, which suggest impending hemolytic reactions. Drug must be discontinued immediately.

Patient teaching

▶ Take drug with meals to minimize stomach upset (nausea, vomiting, or stomach pain). If stomach upset persists, notify health care provider.

▶ Stop drug therapy and notify health care provider immediately if marked darkening of urine occurs.

▶ Complete full course of therapy.

pyrimethamine
Daraprim

pyrimethamine with sulfadoxine
Fansidar

Pregnancy Risk Category C

HOW SUPPLIED

pyrimethamine
Tablets: 25 mg
pyrimethamine with sulfadoxine
Tablets: pyrimethamine 25 mg, sulfadoxine 500 mg

ACTION

Inhibits the enzyme dihydrofolate reductase, thereby impeding reduction of dihydrofolic acid to tetrahydrofolic acid. Sulfadoxine competitively inhibits use of PABA.

Route	Onset	Peak	Duration
P.O.	Unknown	1.5-8 hr	2 wk

INDICATIONS & DOSAGE

Malaria prophylaxis and transmission control (pyrimethamine) —
Adults and children ages 10 and older: 25 mg P.O. weekly.
Children ages 4 to 10: 12.5 mg P.O. weekly.
Children under age 4: 6.25 mg P.O. weekly.

Needs to be continued in all age-groups for at least 6 to 10 weeks after leaving endemic areas.

Acute attacks of malaria (Fansidar) —
Adults and children ages 14 and older: 2 to 3 tablets as a single dose, either alone or in sequence with quinine or primaquine.
Children ages 9 to 13: 2 tablets.
Children ages 4 to 8: 1 tablet.
Children under age 4: ½ tablet.

Malaria prophylaxis (Fansidar) —
Adults and children ages 14 and older:
1 tablet weekly, or 2 tablets q 2 weeks.
Children ages 9 to 13: ¾ tablet weekly,
or 1½ tablets q 2 weeks.
Children ages 4 to 8: ½ tablet weekly, or
1 tablet q 2 weeks.
Children under age 4: ¼ tablet weekly,
or ½ tablet q 2 weeks.
Acute attacks of malaria (pyrimethamine) —
Adults and children ages 15 and older:
50 mg P.O. daily for 2 days; then once
weekly, with doses as described above.
Children under age 15: 25 mg P.O. daily for 2 days; then once weekly, with doses as described above.

Not recommended alone in nonimmune patients; drug should be used with faster-acting antimalarials such as chloroquine for 2 days to initiate transmission control and suppressive cure.
Toxoplasmosis (pyrimethamine) —
Adults: initially, 50 to 75 mg P.O. with 1 to 4 g sulfadiazine; continue for 1 to 3 weeks. Reduce after 3 weeks by half and continue for 4 to 5 weeks.
Children: initially, 1 mg/kg/day P.O. (not to exceed 100 mg) in two equally divided doses for 2 to 4 days; then 0.5 mg/kg daily for 4 weeks, along with 100 mg sulfadiazine/kg P.O. daily, divided q 6 hours.

ADVERSE REACTIONS
CNS: headache, peripheral neuritis, mental depression, *seizures,* ataxia, hallucinations, fatigue.
CV: *arrhythmias,* allergic myocarditis.
EENT: scleral irritation, periorbital edema.
GI: anorexia, vomiting, atrophic glossitis.
Hematologic: *agranulocytosis, aplastic anemia,* megaloblastic anemia, *leukopenia, thrombocytopenia, pancytopenia.*
Skin: *Stevens-Johnson syndrome,* generalized skin eruptions, urticaria, pruritus, photosensitivity.

Note: Adverse drug reactions related to sulfadiazine are similar to sulfonamides.

INTERACTIONS
Drug-drug. *Co-trimoxazole, methotrexate, sulfonamides:* increased risk of bone marrow suppression. Avoid concomitant use.
Lorazepam: increased risk of hepatotoxicity. Avoid concomitant use.
PABA: decreased antitoxoplasmic effects. May require dosage adjustment.

EFFECTS ON DIAGNOSTIC TESTS
None reported.

CONTRAINDICATIONS
Pyrimethamine is contraindicated in patients with hypersensitivity to drug and in those with megaloblastic anemia due to folic acid deficiency. Fansidar is contraindicated in patients with porphyria.

Repeated use of Fansidar is contraindicated in patients with severe renal insufficiency, marked parenchymal damage to the liver, blood dyscrasias, known hypersensitivity to pyrimethamine or sulfonamides, or documented megaloblastic anemia due to folate deficiency. Also contraindicated in infants under age 2 months and in pregnant (at term) and breast-feeding women.

SPECIAL CONSIDERATIONS
▶ Use cautiously in patients with impaired hepatic or renal function, severe allergy or bronchial asthma, G6PD deficiency, or seizure disorders (smaller doses may be needed), and after treatment with chloroquine.
▶ Twice-weekly blood counts, including platelets must be obtained for the patient with toxoplasmosis because dosages used approach toxic levels. If signs of folic acid or folinic acid deficiency develop, dosage should be reduced or discontinued while the patient receives parenteral folinic acid

(leucovorin) until blood counts become normal.

▶ When used to treat toxoplasmosis in patients with AIDS, therapy may be lifelong.

▶ Fansidar should be used only in areas where chloroquine-resistant malaria is prevalent and only if the traveler plans to stay longer than 3 weeks.

Patient teaching

▶ Take drug with meals.

▶ If you have toxoplasmosis, be aware of the importance of frequent laboratory studies and compliance with therapy. There is a potential need for long-term therapy.

▶ If taking Fansidar, stop drug and notify health care provider at first sign of rash.

▶ Take first prophylactic dose 1 to 2 days before traveling.

clofazimine
cycloserine
dapsone
ethambutol hydrochloride
isoniazid
pyrazinamide
rifabutin
rifampin
rifapentine
streptomycin sulfate
(See Aminoglycosides.)

COMBINATION PRODUCTS
Rifamate: isoniazid 150 mg and rifampin 300 mg.
Rifater: isoniazid 50 mg, rifampin 120 mg, and pyrazinamide 300 mg.
Rimactane/INH Dual Pack: 30 300-mg isoniazid tablets and 60 300-mg rifampin capsules.

clofazimine

Lamprene

Pregnancy Risk Category C

HOW SUPPLIED
Capsules: 50 mg

ACTION
Unknown. Thought to inhibit mycobacterial growth by binding preferentially to mycobacterial DNA. Also has anti-inflammatory effects that suppress skin reactions of erythema nodosum leprosum.

Route	Onset	Peak	Duration
P.O.	Unknown	1-6 hr	Unknown

INDICATIONS & DOSAGE
Dapsone-resistant leprosy (Hansen's disease) —
Adults: 100 mg P.O. daily with other antileprotics for 3 years. Then, clofazimine *alone,* 100 mg daily.
Erythema nodosum leprosum —
Adults: 100 to 200 mg P.O. daily for up to 3 months; when prolonged, concomitant corticosteroid therapy is necessary. Dose is tapered to 100 mg daily as soon as possible. Doses above 200 mg daily are not recommended.

ADVERSE REACTIONS
EENT: *conjunctival and corneal pigmentation, dryness, burning, itching, irritation.*
GI: *epigastric pain, diarrhea, nausea, vomiting, GI intolerance, **bowel obstruction, bleeding.***
Hematologic: eosinophilia.
Hepatic: elevated albumin, serum bilirubin, and AST.
Metabolic: hypokalemia, elevated blood glucose level.
Skin: *pink to brownish black pigmentation, ichthyosis and dryness,* rash, pruritus.
Other: ***splenic infarction,*** discolored body fluids and excrement.

INTERACTIONS
Drug-drug. *Dapsone:* impaired anti-inflammatory effects of clofazimine. No intervention appears necessary.
Isoniazid: may decrease level of drug in the skin and increase serum and urine levels of clofazimine. Patient should be monitored for decreased effectiveness.
Rifampin: decreased rifampin bioavailability. Patient should be monitored for decreased effectiveness.

EFFECTS ON DIAGNOSTIC TESTS
None reported.

CONTRAINDICATIONS
No known contraindications.

Reactions may be *common*, uncommon, *life-threatening*, or COMMON AND LIFE-THREATENING.

SPECIAL CONSIDERATIONS

▶ Use cautiously in patients with GI dysfunction, such as abdominal pain and diarrhea.

▶ Doses exceeding 100 mg should be given daily for as short a period as possible and only under close medical supervision.

▶ If patient complains of colic, burning abdominal pain, or other GI symptoms, a reduced dose or an increased interval between doses may be necessary.

Patient teaching

▶ Take drug with meals or milk.

▶ Clofazimine may discolor skin, body fluids, and excrement. The color ranges from pink to brownish black. The unsightly skin discoloration is reversible, but may not disappear until several months or years after drug treatment ends.

▶ Apply skin oil or cream to help reverse skin dryness or ichthyosis.

cycloserine

Seromycin

Pregnancy Risk Category C

HOW SUPPLIED

Capsules: 250 mg

ACTION

Inhibits cell-wall biosynthesis by interfering with the bacterial use of amino acids. Action may be bacteriostatic or bactericidal, depending on the concentration of drug attained at the site of infection and the susceptibility of the infecting organism.

Route	Onset	Peak	Duration
P.O.	Unknown	4-8 hr	Unknown

INDICATIONS & DOSAGE

Adjunctive treatment in pulmonary or extrapulmonary tuberculosis —

Adults: initially, 250 mg P.O. q 12 hours for 2 weeks; then, if blood levels are below 25 to 30 mcg/ml and no toxicity has developed, dose is increased to 250 mg q 8 hours for 2 weeks. If optimum blood levels are still not achieved and no toxicity has developed, then dose is increased to 250 mg q 6 hours. Maximum dose is 1 g/day. If CNS toxicity occurs, drug is discontinued for 1 week, then resumed at 250 mg daily for 2 weeks. If no serious toxic effects occur, dose is increased by 250-mg increments q 10 days until blood level of 25 to 30 mcg/ml is obtained.
Children: 10 to 20 mg/kg/day P.O. in two divided doses (maximum of 0.75 to 1 g).
Acute urinary tract infections —
Adults: 250 mg P.O. q 12 hours for 2 weeks.

ADVERSE REACTIONS

CNS: *seizures,* drowsiness, somnolence, headache, tremor, dysarthria, vertigo, confusion, loss of memory, *possible suicidal tendencies,* psychosis, hyperirritability, paresthesia, paresis, hyperreflexia, *coma.*
CV: *sudden heart failure.*
Hepatic: elevated transaminase level.
Other: hypersensitivity reactions (allergic dermatitis).

INTERACTIONS

Drug-drug. *Ethionamide:* increased risk of CNS toxicity (seizures). Monitor patient closely.
Isoniazid: CNS toxicity (dizziness or drowsiness). Monitor patient closely.
Drug-lifestyle. *Alcohol use:* increased risk of CNS toxicity (seizures). Monitor patient closely.

EFFECTS ON DIAGNOSTIC TESTS

None reported.

CONTRAINDICATIONS

Contraindicated in patients hypersensitive to drug and in those with seizure disorders, depression or severe anxiety, psychosis, and severe renal insufficiency. Also contraindicated in patients who use alcohol excessively.

SPECIAL CONSIDERATIONS

▶ Use cautiously in patients with impaired renal function; reduced dose is required.
▶ A specimen for culture and sensitivity tests should be obtained before therapy begins and periodically thereafter to detect possible resistance.
▶ Cycloserine is considered a "second-line" drug in the treatment of tuberculosis and should always be administered with other antituberculotics to prevent the development of resistant organisms.
▶ Serum cycloserine levels must be monitored periodically, especially in patients receiving high doses (over 500 mg daily) because toxic reactions may occur with blood levels above 30 mcg/ml.
▶ Hematologic tests and renal and liver function studies must be monitored.
▶ Patient should be watched for psychotic symptoms, hallucinations, and possible suicidal tendencies.
▶ Pyridoxine, an anticonvulsant, tranquilizer, or sedative may be given to relieve adverse reactions.

Patient teaching

▶ Avoid alcohol, which may cause serious neurologic reactions.
▶ Do not perform hazardous activities if drowsiness occurs.
▶ Report adverse reactions promptly because dosage adjustment may be necessary or other medications may be prescribed to relieve adverse reactions.

dapsone

Avlosulfon , Dapsone 100‡
Pregnancy Risk Category C

HOW SUPPLIED

Tablets: 25 mg, 100 mg

ACTION

Unknown. May inhibit folic acid biosynthesis in susceptible organisms.

Route	Onset	Peak	Duration
P.O.	Unknown	4-8 hr	Unknown

INDICATIONS & DOSAGE

All forms of leprosy (Hansen's disease) —
Adults: 100 mg P.O. daily, indefinitely; give with rifampin 600 mg P.O. monthly for 6 months.
Children: 1 to 2 mg/kg P.O. daily for minimum of 3 years.
 Dermatitis herpetiformis —
Adults: 50 mg P.O. daily; increased to 300 mg daily, p.r.n.

ADVERSE REACTIONS

CNS: insomnia, psychosis, headache, paresthesia, peripheral neuropathy, vertigo.
CV: tachycardia.
EENT: tinnitus, blurred vision.
GI: anorexia, abdominal pain, nausea, vomiting, pancreatitis.
GU: albuminuria, nephrotic syndrome, renal papillary necrosis, male infertility.
Hematologic: *hemolytic anemia, agranulocytosis, aplastic anemia.*
Respiratory: pulmonary eosinophilia.
Skin: lupus erythematosus, phototoxicity, *exfoliative dermatitis, toxic erythema, erythema multiforme, toxic epidermal necrolysis,* morbilliform and scarlatiniform reactions, urticaria, *erythema nodosum.*
Other: fever, infectious mononucleosis-like syndrome, *sulfone syndrome.*

Reactions may be *common,* uncommon, *life-threatening,* or COMMON AND LIFE-THREATENING.

INTERACTIONS

Drug-drug. *Activated charcoal:* may decrease dapsone's GI absorption and enterohepatic recycling. Monitor closely.
Didanosine: possible therapeutic failure of dapsone, leading to an increase in infection. Avoid concomitant use.
Folic acid antagonists (such as methotrexate): increased risk of adverse hematologic reactions. Avoid concomitant use.
PABA: may antagonize the effect of dapsone by interfering with the primary mechanism of action. Patient is monitored for lack of efficacy.
Probenecid: reduces urinary excretion of dapsone metabolites, increasing plasma concentrations. Monitor closely.
Rifampin: increased hepatic metabolism of dapsone. Patient is monitored for lack of efficacy.
Trimethoprim: increased serum levels of both drugs may occur, possibly increasing the pharmacologic and toxic effects of each drug. Monitor closely.
Drug-lifestyle. *Sun exposure:* may cause photosensitivity. Patient must avoid prolonged exposure to sunlight or sunlamps.

EFFECTS ON DIAGNOSTIC TESTS

None reported.

CONTRAINDICATIONS

Contraindicated in patients with hypersensitivity to drug. Also contraindicated in breast-feeding women because of risk of tumorigenicity.

SPECIAL CONSIDERATIONS

▶ Use cautiously in patients with chronic renal, hepatic, or CV disease; refractory types of anemia; and G6PD deficiency.
▶ A baseline CBC should be obtained. CBC is monitored weekly for the first month, monthly for 6 months, and semiannually thereafter.
▶ Reduce or temporarily discontinue dapsone if hemoglobin falls below 9 g/dl, WBC count falls below 5,000/mm³, or

RBC count falls below 2.5 million/mm³ or remains low.
▶ If generalized, diffuse dermatitis occurs, therapy may need to be interrupted.
▶ Antihistamines may be used to combat allergic dermatitis.
▶ Patient should be monitored for signs and symptoms of erythema nodosum reaction (malaise, fever, painful inflammatory induration in the skin and mucosa, iritis, and neuritis), which may occur during therapy as a result of *Mycobacterium leprae* bacilli. In severe cases, therapy should be stopped and glucocorticoids given cautiously.
▶ Patient should be observed for signs and symptoms of sulfone syndrome, including fever, malaise, jaundice (with hepatic necrosis), lymphadenopathy, methemoglobinemia, and hemolytic anemia.

Patient teaching

▶ *Alert:* Because of the risk of tumorigenicity, breast-feeding should be discontinued during therapy. If breast-feeding, immediately notify health care provider if cyanosis occurs in infant.
▶ Long-term therapy is needed. Complete the full course of drug therapy.
▶ Avoid unprotected exposure to sunlight or sunlamps.

ethambutol hydrochloride
Etibi, Myambutol

Pregnancy Risk Category C

HOW SUPPLIED

Tablets: 100 mg, 400 mg

ACTION

Unknown. Appears to interfere with the synthesis of one or more metabolites of susceptible bacteria, altering cellular metabolism during cell division (bacteriostatic).

Route	Onset	Peak	Duration
P.O.	Unknown	2-4 hr	Unknown

INDICATIONS & DOSAGE

Adjunctive treatment in pulmonary tuberculosis —

Adults and children over age 13: in patients who have not received previous antitubercular therapy, 15 mg/kg P.O. as a single daily dose.

Retreatment: 25 mg/kg P.O. daily as a single dose for 60 days (or until bacteriologic smears and cultures become negative) with at least one other antituberculotic; then decreased to 15 mg/kg/day as a single dose.

ADVERSE REACTIONS

CNS: headache, dizziness, mental confusion, possible hallucinations, malaise, peripheral neuritis.
CV: *thrombocytopenia.*
EENT: optic neuritis, bloody sputum.
GI: anorexia, nausea, vomiting, abdominal pain, GI upset.
Hepatic: abnormal liver function test results.
Musculoskeletal: joint pain.
Skin: dermatitis, pruritus, *toxic epidermal necrolysis.*
Other: *anaphylactoid reactions,* fever, elevated uric acid level, precipitation of acute gout.

INTERACTIONS

Drug-drug. *Aluminum salts:* may delay and reduce absorption of ethambutol. Separate administration times by several hours.

EFFECTS ON DIAGNOSTIC TESTS

None reported.

CONTRAINDICATIONS

Contraindicated in patients with optic neuritis or hypersensitivity to drug and in children under age 13.

SPECIAL CONSIDERATIONS

▶ Use cautiously in patients with impaired renal function, cataracts, recurrent eye inflammations, gout, and diabetic retinopathy.
▶ Visual acuity and color discrimination tests should be performed before and during therapy.
▶ AST and ALT levels must be obtained before therapy, and these levels are monitored every 3 to 4 weeks.
▶ Dosage reduction is necessary in patients with impaired renal function.
▶ Other antituberculotics must always be administered with ethambutol to prevent the development of resistant organisms.
▶ Serum uric acid level should be monitored and the patient is monitored for signs of gout.

Patient teaching

▶ Visual disturbances will generally disappear several weeks to months after drug is stopped. Optic neuritis is related to dose and duration of treatment.
▶ Drug is administered concurrently with other antituberculotics.
▶ Complete the full course of drug therapy.

isoniazid (isonicotinic acid hydrazide, INH)

Isotamine , Laniazid, Nydrazid**,
PMS-Isoniazid
Pregnancy Risk Category C

HOW SUPPLIED

Tablets: 100 mg, 300 mg
Oral solution: 50 mg/5 ml
Injection: 100 mg/ml

ACTION

Unknown. Appears to inhibit cell-wall biosynthesis by interfering with lipid and DNA synthesis (bactericidal).

Route	Onset	Peak	Duration
P.O., I.M.	Unknown	1-2 hr	Unknown

INDICATIONS & DOSAGE

Actively growing tubercle bacilli —
Adults: 5 mg/kg P.O. or I.M. daily in a single dose, up to 300 mg/day, continued for 6 months to 2 years.
Infants and children: 10 to 20 mg/kg P.O. or I.M. daily in a single dose, up to 300 mg/day, continued long enough to prevent relapse. Coadministration of at least one other antituberculotic is recommended.

Prevention of tubercle bacilli in those exposed to tuberculosis or those with positive skin test whose chest X-rays and bacteriologic studies are consistent with nonprogressive tuberculosis —
Adults: 300 mg P.O. daily in a single dose, continued for 6 months to 1 year.
Infants and children: 10 mg/kg P.O. daily in a single dose, up to 300 mg/day, continued for 1 year.

ADVERSE REACTIONS

CNS: *peripheral neuropathy, **seizures,*** toxic encephalopathy, memory impairment, toxic psychosis.
EENT: optic neuritis and atrophy.
GI: nausea, vomiting, epigastric distress.
GU: gynecomastia.
Hematologic: *agranulocytosis,* hemolytic anemia, ***aplastic anemia,*** eosinophilia, ***thrombocytopenia,*** sideroblastic anemia.
Hepatic: *hepatitis*, jaundice, *elevated serum transaminase levels,* bilirubinemia.
Metabolic: hyperglycemia, metabolic acidosis, hypocalcemia, hypophosphatemia.
Skin: irritation at I.M. injection site.
Other: rheumatic and lupus-like syndromes, ***hypersensitivity reactions,*** pyridoxine deficiency.

INTERACTIONS

Drug-drug. *Aluminum-containing antacids and laxatives:* may decrease the rate and amount of isoniazid absorbed. Isoni-

azid is given at least 1 hour before antacid or laxative.
Benzodiazepines: isoniazid may inhibit the metabolic clearance of benzodiazepines that undergo oxidative metabolism (diazepam, triazolam), possibly increasing the activity of the benzodiazepine. Monitor closely.
Carbamazepine, halothane: increased risk of isoniazid hepatotoxicity. Use together cautiously.
Carbamazepine, phenytoin: increased plasma levels of these anticonvulsants. Monitor closely.
Cycloserine, meperidine: may increase CNS adverse reactions and hypotension (meperidine only). Safety precautions should be instituted.
Disulfiram: may cause neurologic symptoms, including changes in behavior and coordination. Avoid concomitant use.
Enflurane: in rapid acetylators of isoniazid, high-output renal failure may occur because of nephrotoxic levels of inorganic fluoride. Renal function must be monitored.
Ketoconazole: serum concentrations of ketoconazole may be decreased. The patient should be monitored for lack of efficacy.
Oral anticoagulants: anticoagulant activity may be enhanced. Monitor patient closely.
Drug-food. *Foods containing tyramine:* may cause hypertensive crisis. Avoid such foods or eat in small quantities.
Drug-lifestyle. *Alcohol use:* may be associated with increased incidence of isoniazid-related hepatitis. Avoid concomitant use.

EFFECTS ON DIAGNOSTIC TESTS

Isoniazid alters results of urine glucose tests that use cupric sulfate method (Benedict's reagent or Diastix).

CONTRAINDICATIONS
Contraindicated in patients with acute hepatic disease or isoniazid-associated liver damage.

SPECIAL CONSIDERATIONS
▶ Use cautiously in patients with chronic non-isoniazid-associated liver disease, seizure disorders (especially in those taking phenytoin), severe renal impairment, and chronic alcoholism and in elderly patients.
▶ Isoniazid must be given with other antituberculotics to prevent the development of resistant organisms.
▶ Keep in mind that isoniazid pharmacokinetics may vary among patients because drug is metabolized in the liver by genetically controlled acetylation. Fast acetylators metabolize the drug up to five times as fast as slow acetylators. About 50% of blacks and whites are slow acetylators; over 80% of Chinese, Japanese, and Inuits are fast acetylators.
▶ Peripheral neuropathy is more common in patients who are slow acetylators or who are malnourished, alcoholic, or diabetic.
▶ Hepatic function must be monitored closely for changes. Elevated liver function study results occur in about 15% of patients; most abnormalities are mild and transient, but some may persist throughout treatment.
▶ Pyridoxine may be given to prevent peripheral neuropathy, especially in malnourished patients.

Patient teaching
▶ Take drug exactly as prescribed; don't discontinue it without health care provider's approval.
▶ Take drug with food if GI irritation occurs.
▶ Notify health care provider immediately if signs and symptoms of liver impairment (anorexia, fatigue, malaise, jaundice, dark urine) occur.

▶ Avoid alcoholic beverages while taking drug. Also, avoid certain foods (fish, such as skipjack and tuna, and tyramine-containing products, such as aged cheese, beer, and chocolate) because drug has some MAO inhibitor activity.
▶ Complete the full course of drug treatment, which may take months or years.

pyrazinamide
pms-Pyrazinamide, Tebrazid, Zinamide†

Pregnancy Risk Category C

HOW SUPPLIED
Tablets: 500 mg

ACTION
Unknown.

Route	Onset	Peak	Duration
P.O.	Unknown	1-2 hr	Unknown

INDICATIONS & DOSAGE
Adjunctive treatment of tuberculosis (when primary and secondary antituberculotics can't be used or have failed) —
Adults: 15 to 30 mg/kg P.O. once daily. Maximum dose is 3 g daily. Or, when compliance is a problem, 50 to 70 mg/kg (based on lean body mass) P.O. twice weekly.

ADVERSE REACTIONS
CNS: malaise.
GI: anorexia, nausea, vomiting.
GU: dysuria, interstitial nephritis.
Hematologic: sideroblastic anemia, *thrombocytopenia.*
Hepatic: *hepatotoxicity, hepatitis.*
Metabolic: hyperuricemia, gout.
Musculoskeletal: *arthralgia, myalgia.*
Skin: rash, urticaria, pruritus, photosensitivity.

Reactions may be *common*, uncommon, *life-threatening*, or COMMON AND LIFE-THREATENING.

Other: fever, porphyria.

INTERACTIONS
None significant.

EFFECTS ON DIAGNOSTIC TESTS
Pyrazinamide may interfere with urine ketone determinations. Drug's systemic effects may temporarily decrease 17-ketosteroid levels. Drug may increase protein-bound iodine and urate levels.

CONTRAINDICATIONS
Contraindicated in patients with severe hepatic disease, acute gout, or hypersensitivity to drug.

SPECIAL CONSIDERATIONS
▶ Use cautiously in patients with diabetes mellitus, renal failure, or gout.
▶ Pyrazinamide must always be administered with other antituberculotics to prevent the development of resistant organisms.
▶ Drug is administered for the initial 2 months of a 6-month or longer treatment regimen for drug-susceptible patients. Patients with HIV infection may require longer courses of therapy.
▶ A reduced dosage is needed in patients with renal impairment because nearly 100% of the drug is excreted in urine.
▶ Doses that exceed 35 mg/kg may cause liver damage.
▶ Hematopoietic studies and serum uric acid levels must be monitored.
▶ Liver function studies must be monitored; the patient must also be assessed for jaundice and liver tenderness or enlargement before and frequently during therapy.
▶ Signs and symptoms of gout and liver impairment (anorexia, fatigue, malaise, jaundice, dark urine, and liver tenderness) must be brought to the attention of the health care provider.
▶ When used with surgical management of tuberculosis, pyrazinamide is started 1 to 2 weeks before surgery and continued for 4 to 6 weeks postoperatively.

Patient teaching
▶ Other antituberculotics will be required concomitantly.
▶ Report adverse reactions promptly.
▶ Complete full course of drug therapy. If daily therapy poses a problem, ask about twice-weekly dosing.

rifabutin
Mycobutin

Pregnancy Risk Category B

HOW SUPPLIED
Capsules: 150 mg

ACTION
Inhibits DNA-dependent RNA polymerase in susceptible bacteria, blocking bacterial protein synthesis.

Route	Onset	Peak	Duration
P.O.	Unknown	2-4 hr	Unknown

INDICATIONS & DOSAGE
Prevention of disseminated Mycobacterium avium *complex in patients with advanced HIV infection —*
Adults: 300 mg P.O. daily as a single dose or divided b.i.d.

ADVERSE REACTIONS
CNS: headache.
GI: dyspepsia, eructation, flatulence, diarrhea, nausea, vomiting, abdominal pain, anorexia, taste perversion.
GU: discolored urine.
Hematologic: NEUTROPENIA, LEUKOPENIA, *thrombocytopenia,* eosinophilia.
Hepatic: increased aminotransferases.
Musculoskeletal: myalgia.
Skin: *rash.*
Other: fever.

INTERACTIONS

Drug-drug. *Drugs metabolized by the liver, zidovudine:* may alter serum levels of these drugs. Dosage adjustments may be necessary.

Oral contraceptives: decreased effectiveness. Nonhormonal forms of birth control should be used.

Drug-food. *High-fat foods:* reduced rate but not extent of absorption. Avoid concurrent administration.

EFFECTS ON DIAGNOSTIC TESTS

None reported.

CONTRAINDICATIONS

Contraindicated in patients with hypersensitivity to drug or other rifamycin derivatives (such as rifampin). Also contraindicated in patients with active tuberculosis because single-agent therapy with rifabutin increases the risk of inducing bacterial resistance to both rifabutin and rifampin.

SPECIAL CONSIDERATIONS

▶ Use cautiously in patients with pre-existing neutropenia and thrombocytopenia. Baseline hematologic studies should be done and repeated periodically.

▶ Drug may be mixed with soft foods such as applesauce for patients who have difficulty swallowing.

▶ Dose may be divided twice daily to decrease GI adverse effects.

▶ *Alert:* Don't confuse rifabutin, rifampin, and rifapentine.

Patient teaching

▶ Take drug for as long as prescribed, exactly as directed, even after feeling better.

▶ Drug or its metabolites may color urine, feces, sputum, saliva, tears, and skin brownish orange. Avoid wearing soft contact lenses because they may be permanently stained.

▶ Report photophobia, excessive lacrima-

tion, or eye pain immediately; drug may cause uveitis (rare).

rifampin (rifampicin)

Rifadin, Rifadin IV, Rimactane, Rimycin†, Rofact

Pregnancy Risk Category C

HOW SUPPLIED

Capsules: 150 mg, 300 mg
Injection: 600 mg

ACTION

Inhibits DNA-dependent RNA polymerase, thus impairing RNA synthesis (bactericidal).

Route	Onset	Peak	Duration
P.O.	Unknown	2-4 hr	Unknown
I.V.	Unknown	Unknown	Unknown

INDICATIONS & DOSAGE

Pulmonary tuberculosis —

Adults: 600 mg P.O. or I.V. daily in single dose 1 hour before or 2 hours after meals.

Children over age 5: 10 to 20 mg/kg P.O. or I.V. daily in single dose 1 hour before or 2 hours after meals. Maximum daily dose is 600 mg. Administration with other antituberculotics is recommended.

Meningococcal carriers —

Adults: 600 mg P.O. or I.V. q 12 hours for 2 days; or 600 mg P.O. or I.V. once daily for 4 days.

Children ages 1 month to 12 years: 10 mg/kg P.O. or I.V. q 12 hours for 2 days, not to exceed 600 mg/day; or 20 mg/kg once daily for 4 days.

Neonates: 5 mg/kg P.O. or I.V. q 12 hours for 2 days.

ADVERSE REACTIONS

CNS: headache, fatigue, drowsiness, be-

havioral changes, dizziness, mental confusion, generalized numbness, ataxia.
CV: *shock.*
EENT: visual disturbances, exudative conjunctivitis.
GI: epigastric distress, anorexia, nausea, vomiting, abdominal pain, diarrhea, flatulence, sore mouth and tongue, pseudomembranous colitis, pancreatitis.
GU: hemoglobinuria, hematuria, *acute renal failure,* menstrual disturbances.
Hematologic: eosinophilia, *thrombocytopenia,* transient leukopenia, hemolytic anemia.
Hepatic: *hepatotoxicity, transient abnormalities in liver function tests.*
Musculoskeletal: osteomalacia.
Respiratory: shortness of breath, wheezing.
Skin: pruritus, urticaria, rash.
Other: flulike syndrome, discoloration of body fluids, hyperuricemia, porphyria exacerbation.

INTERACTIONS

Drug-drug. *Acetaminophen, analgesics, anticoagulants, anticonvulsants, barbiturates, beta blockers, cardiac glycosides, clofibrate, chloramphenicol, corticosteroids, cyclosporine, dapsone, diazepam, disopyramide, methadone, mexiletine, narcotics, oral contraceptives, progestins, quinidine, sulfonylureas, theophylline, verapamil:* reduced effectiveness of these drugs. Monitor closely.
Halothane: may increase risk of hepatotoxicity of both drugs. Liver function must be monitored closely.
Ketoconazole, para-aminosalicylate sodium: may interfere with absorption of rifampin. These drugs are given 8 to 12 hours apart.
Probenecid: may increase rifampin levels. Use cautiously.
Drug-lifestyle. *Alcohol use:* may increase risk of hepatotoxicity. Avoid use of alcohol during therapy.

EFFECTS ON DIAGNOSTIC TESTS

Rifampin alters standard serum folate and vitamin B_{12} assays. Rifampin may cause temporary retention of sulfobromophthalein in the liver excretion test. It may also interfere with contrast material in gallbladder studies and urinalysis based on spectrophotometry.

CONTRAINDICATIONS

Contraindicated in patients with hypersensitivity to rifampin or related drugs.

SPECIAL CONSIDERATIONS

▶ Use cautiously in patients with liver disease.
▶ Treatment with at least one other antituberculotic is recommended.
▶ Drug is given 1 hour before or 2 hours after meals for optimal absorption; however, if GI irritation occurs, patient may take rifampin with meals.
▶ Hepatic function, hematopoietic studies, and serum uric acid levels must be monitored. Drug's systemic effects may cause asymptomatic elevation of liver function tests (14%) and serum uric acid.
▶ Signs of hepatic impairment must be watched for and reported to appropriate heath care personnel.
▶ Drug may cause hemorrhage in neonates of rifampin-treated mothers.
▶ *Alert:* Don't confuse rifabutin, rifampin, and rifapentine.

I.V. administration

▶ Drug is reconstituted with 10 ml of sterile water for injection to make a solution containing 60 mg/ml. 100 ml of D_5W is added and then the mixture is infused over 30 minutes, or 500 ml of D_5W is added and the mixture is infused over 3 hours. Once prepared, the solution must be used within a 4-hour period. When dextrose is contraindicated, drug may be diluted with normal saline for injection. Other I.V. solutions must not be used.

Patient teaching

▶ Take drug with meals if GI upset occurs.

▶ Drowsiness and possible red-orange discoloration of urine, feces, saliva, sweat, sputum, and tears may occur. Avoid wearing soft contact lenses because they may be permanently stained.

▶ Avoid alcoholic beverages during drug therapy.

rifapentine

Priftin

Pregnancy Risk Category C

HOW SUPPLIED

Tablets (film-coated): 150 mg

ACTION

Inhibits DNA-dependent RNA polymerase in susceptible strains of *Mycobacterium tuberculosis.* Drug demonstrates bactericidal activity against the organism both intra- and extracellularly.

Route	Onset	Peak	Duration
P.O.	Unknown	5-6 hr	Unknown

INDICATIONS & DOSAGE

Pulmonary tuberculosis, with at least one other antituberculotic to which the isolate is susceptible —

Adults: during the intensive phase of short-course therapy, 600 mg P.O. twice weekly for 2 months, with an interval between doses of not less than 3 days (72 hours).

During the continuation phase of short-course therapy, 600 mg P.O. once weekly for 4 months with isoniazid or another agent to which the isolate is susceptible.

ADVERSE REACTIONS

CNS: headache, dizziness, pain.
CV: hypertension.

GI: anorexia, nausea, vomiting, dyspepsia, diarrhea.
GU: pyuria, proteinuria, hematuria, urinary casts.
Hematologic: *neutropenia,* lymphopenia, anemia, *leukopenia,* thrombocytosis.
Hepatic: elevated AST and ALT.
Musculoskeletal: arthralgia.
Respiratory: hemoptysis.
Skin: rash, pruritus, acne, maculopapular rash.
Other: *hyperuricemia.*

INTERACTIONS

Drug-drug. *Antiarrhythmics (disopyramide, mexiletine, quinidine, tocainide), antibiotics (chloramphenicol, clarithromycin, dapsone, doxycycline, fluoroquinolones), anticonvulsants (phenytoin), antifungals (fluconazole, itraconazole, ketoconazole), barbiturates, benzodiazepines (diazepam), beta blockers, calcium channel blockers (diltiazem, nifedipine, verapamil), cardiac glycosides, clofibrate, corticosteroids, haloperidol, HIV protease inhibitors (indinavir, nelfinavir, ritonavir, saquinavir), immunosuppressants (cyclosporine, tacrolimus), levothyroxine, narcotic analgesics (methadone), oral anticoagulants (warfarin), oral hypoglycemics (sulfonylureas), oral or other systemic hormonal contraceptives progestins, quinine, reverse transcriptase inhibitors (delavirdine, zidovudine), sildenafil, theophylline, tricyclic antidepressants (amitriptyline, nortriptyline):* rifapentine induces metabolism of the hepatic cytochrome P-450 enzyme system, decreasing the activity of these drugs. Dosage adjustments may be needed

EFFECTS ON DIAGNOSTIC TESTS

May alter serum assays for folate and vitamin B_{12}.

CONTRAINDICATIONS

Contraindicated in patients with history of hypersensitivity to a rifamycin (rifapentine, rifampin, or rifabutin).

SPECIAL CONSIDERATIONS

▶ Use cautiously and with frequent monitoring in patients with liver disease.

▶ Rifamycin antibiotics have been associated with hepatotoxicity. Liver function test results must be monitored before beginning drug therapy.

▶ Drug therapy may affect liver function test results, CBC, and platelet counts; these must be monitored carefully.

▶ Coadministration of pyridoxine (vitamin B$_6$) is recommended in malnourished patients, in those predisposed to neuropathy (alcoholics, diabetics), and in adolescents.

▶ *Alert:* Drug must be given with appropriate daily companion drugs. Compliance with all medications, especially with daily companion drugs on the days when rifapentine isn't given, is crucial for early sputum conversion and protection from relapse of tuberculosis.

▶ Administration of drug during the last 2 weeks of pregnancy may lead to postnatal hemorrhage in the mother or infant. Clotting parameters must be monitored closely if drug is given.

▶ Rifapentine can turn body tissues and fluids red-orange and can permanently stain contact lenses.

▶ Appropriate health care personnel must be made aware of persistent or severe diarrhea.

▶ *Alert:* Don't confuse rifabutin, rifampin, and rifapentine.

Patient teaching

▶ Complete the full course of drug therapy and daily companion medications exactly as prescribed, as well as necessary follow-up visits and laboratory tests.

▶ Use nonhormonal methods of birth control.

▶ Take drug with food if nausea, vomiting, or GI upset occurs.

▶ Notify health care provider if any of the following occurs: fever, loss of appetite, malaise, nausea, vomiting, darkened urine, yellowish discoloration of the skin and eyes, pain or swelling of the joints, or excessive loose stools or diarrhea.

▶ Protect pills from excessive heat.

▶ Rifapentine can turn body fluids red-orange. Avoid wearing contact lenses because these can become permanently stained.

amikacin sulfate
gentamicin sulfate
neomycin sulfate
streptomycin sulfate
tobramycin sulfate

COMBINATION PRODUCTS

Neosporin G.U. Irrigant: 40 mg neomycin sulfate and 200,000 U polymyxin B sulfate/ml.

amikacin sulfate

Amikin

Pregnancy Risk Category D

HOW SUPPLIED

Injection: 50 mg/ml, 250 mg/ml

ACTION

Inhibits protein synthesis by binding directly to the 30S ribosomal subunit. Generally bactericidal.

Route	Onset	Peak	Duration
I.V.	Immediate	Immediate	8-12 hr
I.M.	Unknown	1 hr	8-12 hr

INDICATIONS & DOSAGE

Serious infections due to sensitive strains of Pseudomonas aeruginosa, Escherichia coli, Proteus, Klebsiella, Serratia, Enterobacter, Acinetobacter, Providencia, Citrobacter, *or* Staphylococcus —
Adults and children: 15 mg/kg/day divided q 8 to 12 hours I.M. or I.V. infusion.
Neonates: initially, 10 mg/ kg I.V. loading dose; then 7.5 mg/kg q 12 hours.
    Uncomplicated urinary tract infection —
Adults: 250 mg I.M. or I.V. b.i.d.
Dosage adjustment: For adult patients with impaired renal function, initially, 7.5 mg/kg.

Subsequent doses and frequency determined by blood amikacin levels and renal function studies.

ADVERSE REACTIONS
CNS: *neuromuscular blockade.*
EENT: *ototoxicity.*
GU: *azotemia, nephrotoxicity;* possible elevation in BUN, nonprotein nitrogen, or serum creatinine levels; possible increase in urinary excretion of casts.
Musculoskeletal: arthralgia.
Respiratory: *apnea.*

INTERACTIONS
Drug-drug. *Acyclovir, amphotericin B, cisplatin, methoxyflurane, vancomycin, other aminoglycosides:* increased nephrotoxicity. Use together cautiously.
Cephalosporins: increased nephrotoxicity. Use together cautiously.
Dimenhydrinate: may mask symptoms of ototoxicity. Use with caution.
General anesthetics, neuromuscular blockers: may potentiate neuromuscular blockade. Monitor closely.
Indomethacin: may increase serum trough and peak levels of amikacin. Serum amikacin level must be monitored closely.
I.V. loop diuretics (such as furosemide): increased ototoxicity. Use cautiously.
Parenteral penicillins (such as ticarcillin): amikacin inactivation in vitro. Drugs must not be mixed together.

EFFECTS ON DIAGNOSTIC TESTS
None reported.

CONTRAINDICATIONS
Contraindicated in patients with hypersensitivity to drug or other aminoglycosides.

SPECIAL CONSIDERATIONS
▶ Use cautiously in patients with impaired

Reactions may be *common*, uncommon, *life-threatening*, or COMMON AND LIFE-THREATENING.

384

renal function or neuromuscular disorders, in neonates and infants, and in elderly patients.

▶ A specimen for culture and sensitivity tests should be obtained before giving first dose. Therapy may begin pending results.

▶ Patient's hearing should be evaluated before and during therapy. Patient complaints of tinnitus, vertigo, or hearing loss are important.

▶ Patient's weight and renal function studies should be reviewed before therapy begins.

▶ Blood for peak amikacin level is obtained 1 hour after I.M. injection and 30 minutes to 1 hour after I.V. infusion ends; for trough levels, blood is drawn just before next dose. Blood must not be collected in a heparinized tube; heparin is incompatible with aminoglycosides.

▶ Peak blood levels over 35 mcg/ml and trough levels over 10 mcg/ml may be associated with higher incidence of toxicity.

▶ Renal function (output, specific gravity, urinalysis, BUN and creatinine levels, and creatinine clearance) must be monitored.

▶ Superinfection (continued fever and other signs and symptoms of new infection, especially of upper respiratory tract) may occur.

▶ Therapy is usually continued for 7 to 10 days. If no response occurs after 3 to 5 days, therapy may be stopped and new specimens obtained for culture and sensitivity testing.

▶ *Alert:* Don't confuse Amikin with Amicar.

I.V. administration

▶ I.V. drug is diluted in 100 to 200 ml of D_5W or normal saline solution and infused over 30 to 60 minutes.

▶ After I.V. infusion, line is flushed with normal saline solution or D_5W.

Patient teaching

▶ Report adverse reactions promptly.

▶ Maintain adequate fluid intake.

gentamicin sulfate

Cidomycin , Garamycin, Gentamicin Sulfate ADD-Vantage, Genticin§, Jenamicin

Pregnancy Risk Category D

HOW SUPPLIED

Injection: 40 mg/ml (adult), 10 mg/ml (pediatric)
I.V. infusion (premixed): 40 mg, 60 mg, 70 mg, 80 mg, 90 mg, 100 mg, 120 mg in normal saline solution

ACTION

Inhibits protein synthesis by binding directly to the 30S ribosomal subunit. Usually bactericidal.

Route	Onset	Peak	Duration
I.V.	Immediate	30-90 min	Unknown
I.M.	Unknown	30-90 min	Unknown

INDICATIONS & DOSAGE

Serious infections due to sensitive strains of Pseudomonas aeruginosa, Escherichia coli, Proteus, Klebsiella, Serratia, Enterobacter, Citrobacter, *or* Staphylococcus —
Adults: 3 mg/kg daily in divided doses I.M. or I.V. infusion q 8 hours. For life-threatening infections, patient may receive up to 5 mg/kg daily in three to four divided doses; dose should be reduced to 3 mg/kg daily as soon as clinically indicated.

Children: 2 to 2.5 mg/kg q 8 hours I.M. or by I.V. infusion.

Neonates over age 1 week or infants: 2.5 mg/kg q 8 hours I.M. or by I.V. infusion.

Neonates under age 1 week and preterm infants: 2.5 mg/kg q 12 hours I.M. or by I.V. infusion.

Meningitis —

Adults: systemic therapy as above.
Children: systemic therapy as above.
Endocarditis prophylaxis for GI or GU procedure or surgery —
Adults: 1.5 mg/kg I.M. or I.V. 30 minutes before procedure or surgery. Maximum dose is 80 mg. Given with ampicillin (vancomycin in penicillin-allergic patients).
Children: 2 mg/kg I.M. or I.V. 30 minutes before procedure or surgery. Maximum dose is 80 mg. Given with ampicillin (vancomycin in penicillin-allergic patients).
After hemodialysis to maintain therapeutic blood levels —
Adults: 1 to 1.7 mg/kg I.M. or by I.V. infusion after each dialysis.
Children: 2 to 2.5 mg/kg I.M. or by I.V. infusion after each dialysis.
Dosage adjustment: For adult patients with impaired renal function, doses and frequency are determined by serum gentamicin levels and renal function.

ADVERSE REACTIONS

CNS: headache, lethargy, encephalopathy, confusion, dizziness, *seizures,* numbness, peripheral neuropathy, vertigo, ataxia, tingling.
CV: hypotension.
EENT: *ototoxicity,* blurred vision, tinnitus.
GI: vomiting, nausea.
GU: *nephrotoxicity;* possible elevation in BUN, nonprotein nitrogen, or serum creatinine levels; possible increase in urinary excretion of casts.
Hematologic: anemia, eosinophilia, *leukopenia, thrombocytopenia, agranulocytosis.*
Hepatic: increased ALT, AST, bilirubin, LD.
Musculoskeletal: muscle twitching, myasthenia gravis-like syndrome.
Respiratory: *apnea.*
Skin: rash, urticaria, pruritus.
Other: fever, *anaphylaxis;* injection site pain.

INTERACTIONS

Drug-drug. *Acyclovir, amphotericin B, cisplatin, methoxyflurane, vancomycin, other aminoglycosides:* increased ototoxicity and nephrotoxicity. Use together cautiously.
Cephalosporins: increased nephrotoxicity. Use together cautiously.
Dimenhydrinate: may mask symptoms of ototoxicity. Use with caution.
General anesthetics, neuromuscular blockers: may potentiate neuromuscular blockade. Monitor closely.
Indomethacin: may increase serum peak and trough levels of gentamicin. Serum gentamicin levels must be monitored closely.
I.V. loop diuretics (such as furosemide): increased ototoxicity. Use cautiously.
Parenteral penicillins (such as ampicillin and ticarcillin): gentamicin inactivation in vitro. Don't mix together.

EFFECTS ON DIAGNOSTIC TESTS
None reported.

CONTRAINDICATIONS
Contraindicated in hypersensitivity to drug or other aminoglycosides.

SPECIAL CONSIDERATIONS
▶ Use cautiously in neonates, infants, elderly patients, and patients with impaired renal function or neuromuscular disorders.
▶ A specimen for culture and sensitivity tests is obtained before first dose is given.
▶ Patient's hearing must be evaluated before and during therapy. Patient complaints of tinnitus, vertigo, or hearing loss are important.
▶ Patient's weight and renal function studies must be reviewed before therapy begins.
▶ *Alert:* Preservative-free formulations of gentamicin are used when the intrathecal route is ordered.
▶ Blood for peak gentamicin level is ob-

tained 1 hour after I.M. injection or 30 minutes after I.V. infusion finishes; for trough levels, blood is drawn just before next dose. Blood must not be collected in a heparinized tube; heparin is incompatible with aminoglycosides.

▶ Peak blood levels over 10 mcg/ml and trough levels over 2 mcg/ml may be associated with higher incidence of toxicity.

▶ Urine output, specific gravity, urinalysis, BUN and creatinine levels, and creatinine clearance must be monitored.

▶ Hemodialysis for 8 hours removes up to 50% of drug from blood.

▶ Superinfection (continued fever and other signs and symptoms of new infection, especially of upper respiratory tract) may occur.

▶ Therapy usually continues for 7 to 10 days. If no response occurs in 3 to 5 days, therapy may be stopped and new specimens obtained for culture and sensitivity testing.

I.V. administration

▶ When giving by intermittent I.V. infusion, the drug is diluted with 50 to 200 ml of D_5W or normal saline injection and infused over 30 minutes to 2 hours. After completing I.V. infusion, the line is flushed with normal saline solution or D_5W.

Patient teaching

▶ Maintain adequate fluid intake and report adverse reactions promptly.

▶ Don't perform hazardous activities if adverse CNS reactions occur.

neomycin sulfate

Mycifradin , Neo-fradin, Neosulf†, Neo-Tabs, Nivemycin§
Pregnancy Risk Category D

HOW SUPPLIED

Tablets: 500 mg
Oral solution: 125 mg/5 ml

ACTION

Inhibits protein synthesis by binding directly to the 30S ribosomal subunit. Generally bactericidal.

Route	Onset	Peak	Duration
P.O.	Unknown	1-4 hr	8 hr

INDICATIONS & DOSAGE

Infectious diarrhea due to enteropathogenic Escherichia coli —
Adults: 50 mg/kg daily P.O. in four divided doses for 2 to 3 days; maximum of 3 g daily is usually adequate.
Children: 50 to 100 mg/kg daily P.O. divided q 4 to 6 hours for 2 to 3 days.

Suppression of intestinal bacteria preoperatively —
Adults: 1 g P.O. q hour for four doses; then 1 g q 4 hours for the balance of the 24 hours. A saline cathartic should precede therapy.
Children: 40 to 100 mg/kg daily P.O. divided q 4 to 6 hours. First dose should follow saline cathartic.

Adjunct treatment in hepatic coma —
Adults: 1 to 3 g P.O. q.i.d. for 5 to 6 days; or 200 ml of 1% solution or 100 ml of 2% solution as enema retained for 20 to 60 minutes q 6 hours. In patients with chronic hepatic insufficiency, 4 g/day indefinitely may be needed.
Children: 50 to 100 mg/kg/day P.O. in divided doses for 5 to 6 days.

ADVERSE REACTIONS

EENT: *ototoxicity.*

GI: nausea, vomiting, diarrhea, malabsorption syndrome, *Clostridium difficile*-associated colitis.

GU: *nephrotoxicity;* possible elevation in BUN, nonprotein nitrogen, or serum creatinine levels; possible increase in urinary excretion of casts.

INTERACTIONS

Drug-drug. *Acyclovir, amphotericin B, cisplatin, methoxyflurane, vancomycin, other aminoglycosides:* increased nephrotoxicity. Use together cautiously.

Cephalosporins: increased nephrotoxicity. Use together cautiously.

Digoxin: decreased digoxin absorption. Monitor closely.

Dimenhydrinate: may mask symptoms of ototoxicity. Use with caution.

I.V. loop diuretics (such as furosemide): increased ototoxicity. Use cautiously.

Oral anticoagulants: inhibited vitamin K–producing bacteria; may potentiate anticoagulant effect. PT and INR must be monitored.

EFFECTS ON DIAGNOSTIC TESTS

None reported.

CONTRAINDICATIONS

Contraindicated in patients hypersensitive to other aminoglycosides and in those with intestinal obstruction.

SPECIAL CONSIDERATIONS

▶ Use cautiously in patients with impaired renal function, neuromuscular disorders, or ulcerative bowel lesions and in elderly patients. Drug is never administered parenterally.

▶ Renal function (output, specific gravity, urinalysis, BUN and creatinine levels, and creatinine clearance) must be monitored.

▶ Ototoxic and nephrotoxic properties of neomycin limit its usefulness.

▶ Patient's hearing must be evaluated before and during prolonged therapy. Patient complaints of tinnitus, vertigo, or hearing loss are important. Onset of deafness may occur several weeks after drug is stopped.

▶ Superinfection (fever or other signs and symptoms of new infection) may occur.

▶ In adjunctive treatment of hepatic coma, patient's dietary protein is decreased, and neurologic status is assessed frequently during therapy.

▶ For preoperative disinfection, a low-residue diet and a cathartic may be given immediately before oral administration of neomycin.

▶ Neomycin is nonabsorbable at the recommended dosage. However, more than 4 g/day may be systemically absorbed and lead to nephrotoxicity.

▶ Drug is available with polymyxin B as a urinary bladder irrigant.

Patient teaching

▶ Report adverse reactions promptly.
▶ Maintain adequate fluid intake.

streptomycin sulfate
Pregnancy Risk Category D

HOW SUPPLIED

Injection: 1 g/2.5-ml ampules

ACTION

Inhibits protein synthesis by binding directly to the 30S ribosomal subunit. Generally bactericidal.

Route	Onset	Peak	Duration
I.M.	Unknown	1-2 hr	Unknown

INDICATIONS & DOSAGE

Streptococcal endocarditis —
Adults: 1 g q 12 hours I.M. for 1 week; then 500 mg I.M. q 12 hours for 1 week, given with penicillin.
Elderly: 500 mg I.M. q 12 hours for entire 2 weeks, given with penicillin.

Primary and adjunctive treatment in tuberculosis —

Adults: 15 mg/kg (maximum of 1 g) I.M. daily for 2 to 3 months; then 1 g I.M. two or three times weekly.

Children: 20 to 40 mg/kg (maximum of 1 g) I.M. daily in divided doses injected deeply into large muscle mass. Given with other antituberculotics, but not with capreomycin; continued until sputum specimen becomes negative.

Elderly: 10 mg/kg I.M. daily.

Enterococcal endocarditis —

Adults: 1 g I.M. q 12 hours for 2 weeks; then 500 mg I.M. q 12 hours for 4 weeks, given with penicillin.

Tularemia —

Adults: 1 to 2 g I.M. daily in divided doses injected deeply into upper outer quadrant of buttocks; continued for 7 to 14 days or until patient is afebrile for 5 to 7 days.

ADVERSE REACTIONS

CNS: *neuromuscular blockade,* vertigo, paresthesia of the face.

EENT: *ototoxicity.*

GI: vomiting, nausea.

GU: some nephrotoxicity (not as frequently as with other aminoglycosides); possible elevation in BUN, nonprotein nitrogen, or serum creatinine levels; possible increase in urinary excretion of casts.

Hematologic: eosinophilia, *leukopenia, thrombocytopenia, hemolytic anemia.*

Respiratory: *apnea.*

Skin: *exfoliative dermatitis.*

Other: hypersensitivity reactions, *anaphylaxis.*

INTERACTIONS

Drug-drug. *Acyclovir, amphotericin B, cisplatin, methoxyflurane, vancomycin, other aminoglycosides:* increased nephrotoxicity. Use together cautiously.

Cephalosporins: increased nephrotoxicity. Use together cautiously.

Dimenhydrinate: may mask symptoms of streptomycin-induced ototoxicity. Use together cautiously.

General anesthetics, neuromuscular blockers: may potentiate neuromuscular blockade. The patient should be monitored closely.

I.V. loop diuretics (such as furosemide): increased ototoxicity. Use together cautiously.

EFFECTS ON DIAGNOSTIC TESTS

Streptomycin may cause a false-positive reaction in copper sulfate tests for urine glucose (Benedict's reagent or Diastix).

CONTRAINDICATIONS

Contraindicated in patients with hypersensitivity to drug or other aminoglycosides.

SPECIAL CONSIDERATIONS

▶ Use cautiously in patients with impaired renal function or neuromuscular disorders and in elderly patients.

▶ A specimen for culture and sensitivity tests should be obtained before first dose is given except when treating tuberculosis. Therapy may begin pending results.

▶ Patient's hearing should be evaluated before therapy and for 6 months afterward. Patient complaints of hearing loss, roaring noises, or fullness in ears are important.

▶ *Alert:* Streptomycin is never administered I.V.

▶ Hands must be protected when preparing the medication because drug is irritating.

▶ For I.M. administration, drug is injected deeply into upper outer quadrant of buttocks. Injection sites are rotated.

▶ Blood for peak streptomycin level is obtained 1 to 2 hours after I.M. injection; for trough levels, blood is drawn just before next dose. A heparinized tube must not be used because heparin is incompatible with aminoglycosides.

▶ Signs and symptoms of superinfection

(continued fever and other signs of new infection) may occur.

▶ In primary treatment of tuberculosis, drug is discontinued when sputum becomes negative.

Patient teaching

▶ Report adverse reactions promptly.

▶ Maintain adequate fluid intake.

▶ Blood tests are necessary to monitor streptomycin levels and determine the effectiveness of therapy.

tobramycin sulfate

Nebcin, TOBI

Pregnancy Risk Category D

HOW SUPPLIED

Multidose vials: 80 mg/2 ml, 20 mg/2 ml (pediatric)
Powder for injection: 1.2 g
Premixed parenteral injection for I.V. infusion: 60 mg or 80 mg in normal saline solution
Nebulizer solution (for inhalation): 300 mg/5 ml

ACTION

Inhibits protein synthesis by binding directly to the 30S ribosomal subunit. Generally bactericidal.

Route	Onset	Peak	Duration
I.V.	Immediate	Immediate	8 hr
I.M.	Unknown	30-90 min	8 hr
Inhalation	Unknown	Unknown	Unknown

INDICATIONS & DOSAGE

Serious infections due to sensitive strains of Escherichia coli, Proteus, Klebsiella, Enterobacter, Serratia, Morganella morganii, Staphylococcus aureus, Pseudomonas, Citrobacter, *or* Providencia —
Adults: 3 mg/kg I.M. or I.V. daily in divided doses. Up to 5 mg/kg daily divided

q 6 to 8 hours for life-threatening infections; dose should be reduced to 3 mg/kg daily as soon as clinically indicated.
Children: 6 to 7.5 mg/kg I.M. or I.V. daily in three or four divided doses.
Neonates under age 1 week or premature infants: up to 4 mg/kg/day I.V. or I.M. in two equal doses q 12 hours.
Dosage adjustment: For patients with renal impairment, loading dose is 1 mg/kg; then decreased doses at 8-hour intervals or same dose at prolonged intervals.

Management of cystic fibrosis patients with Pseudomonas aeruginosa —
Adults and children ages 6 and older: 300 mg via nebulizer q 12 hours for 28 days (cycle of 28 days on drug and 28 days off).

ADVERSE REACTIONS

CNS: headache, lethargy, confusion, disorientation, ***seizures.***
EENT: *ototoxicity, hoarseness, pharyngitis.*
GI: vomiting, nausea, diarrhea.
GU: *nephrotoxicity;* possible elevation in BUN, nonprotein nitrogen, or serum creatinine levels; possible increase in urinary excretion of casts.
Hematologic: anemia, eosinophilia, ***leukopenia, thrombocytopenia, agranulocytosis.***
Musculoskeletal: muscle twitching.
Respiratory: bronchospasm.
Skin: rash, urticaria, pruritus.
Other: electrolyte imbalances, fever.

INTERACTIONS

Drug-drug. *Acyclovir, amphotericin B, cisplatin, methoxyflurane, vancomycin, other aminoglycosides:* increased nephrotoxicity. Use together cautiously.
Cephalosporins: increased nephrotoxicity. Use together cautiously.
Dimenhydrinate: may mask symptoms of ototoxicity. Use with caution.
General anesthetics, neuromuscular blockers: may potentiate neuromuscular block-

ade. Patient should be monitored closely.

I.V. loop diuretics (such as furosemide): increased ototoxicity. Use together cautiously.

Parenteral penicillins (such as ticarcillin): tobramycin inactivation in vitro. Medications should not be mixed together.

EFFECTS ON DIAGNOSTIC TESTS

None reported.

CONTRAINDICATIONS

Contraindicated in patients with hypersensitivity to drug or other aminoglycosides.

SPECIAL CONSIDERATIONS

▶ Use cautiously in patients with impaired renal function or neuromuscular disorders and in elderly patients.

▶ A specimen for culture and sensitivity tests is obtained before first dose is given. Therapy may begin pending results.

▶ Patient's weight and renal function studies are reviewed before therapy.

▶ Patient's hearing must be evaluated before and during therapy. Patient complaints of tinnitus, vertigo, or hearing loss are important.

▶ Nebulizer solution is administered over 10 to 15 minutes using hand-held Pari LC Plus reusable nebulizer with DeVilbiss Pulmo-Aide compressor.

▶ TOBI is should not be diluted or mixed with dornase alpha in the nebulizer.

▶ Blood for peak level is obtained 1 hour after I.M. injection or 30 minutes after the infusion stops; blood is drawn for trough level just before next dose. Blood must not be collected in a heparinized tube; heparin is incompatible with aminoglycosides.

▶ *Alert:* Peak blood levels over 12 mcg/ml and trough levels over 2 mcg/ml may be associated with increased toxicity.

▶ Renal function (output, specific gravity, urinalysis, creatinine clearance, and BUN and creatinine levels) must be monitored.

▶ Signs and symptoms of superinfection (continued fever and other signs of new infection) may occur.

▶ If no response occurs in 3 to 5 days, therapy may be stopped and new specimens obtained for culture and sensitivity testing.

▶ *Alert:* Don't confuse tobramycin with Trobicin.

I.V. administration

▶ For adults, drug is diluted in 50 to 100 ml of normal saline solution or D_5W; a smaller volume is used for children. Drug is infused over 20 to 60 minutes. After I.V. infusion, line is flushed with normal saline solution or D_5W.

Patient teaching

▶ Report adverse reactions promptly.

▶ Don't perform hazardous activities if adverse CNS reactions occur.

▶ Maintain adequate fluid intake.

▶ Learn proper use and maintenance of the nebulizer.

▶ If undergoing multiple inhaled therapies, use TOBI last.

▶ Don't use TOBI if it's cloudy, has particles in the solution, or has been stored at room temperature for more than 28 days.

amoxicillin/clavulanate
  potassium
amoxicillin trihydrate
ampicillin
ampicillin sodium
ampicillin trihydrate
ampicillin sodium/
  sulbactam sodium
cloxacillin sodium
dicloxacillin sodium
mezlocillin sodium
nafcillin sodium
oxacillin sodium
penicillin G benzathine
penicillin G potassium
penicillin G procaine
penicillin G sodium
penicillin V potassium
piperacillin sodium
piperacillin sodium/
  tazobactam sodium
ticarcillin disodium
ticarcillin disodium/
  clavulanate potassium

COMBINATION PRODUCTS
None.

amoxicillin/clavulanate potassium (amoxycillin/clavulanate potassium)
Augmentin, Clavulin

Pregnancy Risk Category B

HOW SUPPLIED
Tablets (chewable): 125 mg amoxicillin trihydrate, 31.25 mg clavulanic acid; 200 mg amoxicillin trihydrate, 28.5 mg clavulanic acid; 250 mg amoxicillin trihydrate, 62.5 mg clavulanic acid
Tablets (film-coated): 250 mg amoxicillin trihydrate, 125 mg clavulanic acid; 500 mg amoxicillin trihydrate, 125 mg clavulanic acid; 875 mg amoxicillin trihydrate, 125 mg clavulanic acid
Oral suspension: 125 mg amoxicillin trihydrate and 31.25 mg clavulanic acid/ 5 ml (after reconstitution); 200 mg amoxicillin trihydrate and 28.5 mg clavulanic acid/5 ml (after reconstitution); 250 mg amoxicillin trihydrate and 62.5 mg clavulanic acid/5 ml (after reconstitution); 400 mg amoxicillin trihydrate and 57 mg clavulanic acid/5 ml (after reconstitution)

ACTION
An aminopenicillin that prevents bacterial cell-wall synthesis during replication. Clavulanic acid increases amoxicillin effectiveness by inactivating beta-lactamases, which destroy amoxicillin.

Route	Onset	Peak	Duration
P.O.	Unknown	1-2.5 hr	6-8 hr

INDICATIONS & DOSAGE
Lower respiratory infections, otitis media, sinusitis, skin and skin-structure infections, and urinary tract infections due to susceptible strains of gram-positive and gram-negative organisms —
Adults and children weighing 40 kg (88 lb) or over: 250 mg (based on the amoxicillin component) P.O. q 8 hours; or 500 mg q 12 hours. For more severe infections, 500 mg q 8 hours or 875 mg P.O. q 12 hours.
Children ages 3 months and older and weighing under 40 kg: 20 to 45 mg/kg (based on the amoxicillin component and severity of infection) P.O. daily in divided doses q 8 to 12 hours.
Children under age 3 months: 30 mg/ kg/day P.O. divided q 12 hours based on the amoxicillin component. The 125 mg/ 5-ml oral suspension is recommended.

Reactions may be *common*, uncommon, *life-threatening*, or COMMON AND LIFE-THREATENING.

Dosage adjustment: Don't give the 875-mg tablet to patients with renal impairment and creatinine clearance under 30 ml/minute. If creatinine clearance is 10 to 30 ml/minute, dosage is 250 to 500 mg P.O. q 12 hours. If creatinine clearance is under 10 ml/minute, dosage is 250 to 500 mg P.O. q 24 hours. Give hemodialysis patients 250 to 500 mg P.O. q 24 hours with an additional dose both during and at the end of dialysis.

ADVERSE REACTIONS

CNS: agitation, anxiety, insomnia, confusion, behavioral changes, dizziness.
GI: *nausea,* vomiting, *diarrhea,* indigestion, gastritis, stomatitis, glossitis, black "hairy" tongue, enterocolitis, pseudomembranous colitis.
GU: vaginitis.
Hematologic: anemia, ***thrombocytopenia,*** thrombocytopenic purpura, eosinophilia, ***leukopenia, agranulocytosis.***
Other: ***hypersensitivity reactions, anaphylaxis,*** overgrowth of nonsusceptible organisms.

INTERACTIONS

Drug-drug. *Allopurinol:* increased incidence of rash. Monitor patient.
Oral contraceptives: efficacy of oral contraceptives may be decreased. Additional form of contraception should be recommended during penicillin therapy.
Probenecid: increased blood levels of amoxicillin and other penicillins. Probenecid may be used for this purpose.

EFFECTS ON DIAGNOSTIC TESTS

Amoxicillin/clavulanate potassium alters results of urine glucose tests that use cupric sulfate (Benedict's reagent or Clinitest). Make urine glucose determinations with glucose oxidase methods (Chemstrip uG). Positive Coombs' tests have occurred with other clavulanate combinations.

CONTRAINDICATIONS

Contraindicated in patients with hyper-sensitivity to drug or other penicillins and in those with a previous history of amoxicillin-associated cholestatic jaundice or hepatic dysfunction.

SPECIAL CONSIDERATIONS

▶ Use cautiously in patients with other drug allergies, especially to cephalosporins (possible cross-sensitivity), and in those with mononucleosis (high incidence of maculopapular rash).
▶ Before drug is given, patient must be asked about previous allergic reactions to penicillin. However, a negative history of penicillin allergy is no guarantee against a future allergic reaction.
▶ A specimen for culture and sensitivity tests is obtained before giving first dose. Therapy may begin pending results.
▶ Drug is given at least 1 hour before a bacteriostatic antibiotic.
▶ Patient should be observed closely. With large doses and prolonged therapy, bacterial or fungal superinfection may occur, especially in elderly, debilitated, or immunosuppressed patients.
▶ Avoid use of 250-mg tablet in children under 40 kg. Use chewable form instead.
▶ ***Alert:*** Both 250-mg and 500-mg film-coated tablets contain the same amount of clavulanic acid (125 mg). Therefore, two 250-mg tablets are not equivalent to one 500-mg tablet.
▶ This drug combination is particularly useful in clinical settings with a high prevalence of amoxicillin-resistant organisms.
▶ Oral suspension should be refrigerated after reconstitution, discarded after 10 days.
▶ ***Alert:*** Don't confuse amoxicillin with amoxapine.

Patient teaching

▶ Take entire quantity of drug exactly as prescribed, even after feeling better.
▶ Drug may be taken with food to prevent GI upset. If taking the oral suspension, keep it refrigerated, shake it well before

---

*Liquid contains alcohol.   **May contain tartrazine.   †Canada   ‡Australia   §U.K.   ◊OTC taking it, and discard remaining drug after 10 days.

▶ Inform health care provider if a rash occurs because rash is a sign of an allergic reaction.

amoxicillin trihydrate (amoxycillin trihydrate)

Alphamox‡, Amoxil, Apo-Amoxi , Cilamox‡, Moxacin‡, Novamoxin , Nu-Amoxi , Trimox, Wymox

Pregnancy Risk Category B

HOW SUPPLIED

Tablets (chewable): 125 mg, 250 mg
Capsules: 250 mg, 500 mg
Oral suspension: 50 mg/ml (pediatric drops), 125 mg/5 ml, 250 mg/5 ml (after reconstitution)

ACTION

An aminopenicillin that inhibits cell-wall synthesis during bacterial multiplication. Bacteria resist amoxicillin by producing penicillinases — enzymes that hydrolyze amoxicillin.

Route	Onset	Peak	Duration
P.O.	Unknown	1-2 hr	6-8 hr

INDICATIONS & DOSAGE

Systemic infections, acute and chronic urinary tract infections due to susceptible strains of gram-positive and gram-negative organisms —
Adults and children weighing 20 kg (44 lb) or over: 250 to 500 mg P.O. q 8 hours.
Children weighing under 20 kg: 20 mg/kg P.O. daily in divided doses q 8 hours; in severe infection, 40 mg/kg P.O. daily in divided doses q 8 hours or 500 mg to 1 g/m^2 P.O. in divided doses q 8 hours.

Uncomplicated gonorrhea —
Adults and children weighing over 45 kg (99 lb): 3 g P.O. with 1 g probenecid given as a single dose.
Children ages 2 and older weighing under 45 kg: 50 mg/kg (maximum of 3 g) P.O. with 25 mg/kg (up to 1 g) of probenecid as a single dose. Don't give probenecid to children under age 2.
Endocarditis prophylaxis for dental and GI/GU procedures —
Adults: 2 g P.O. 1 hour before procedure.
Children: 50 mg/kg P.O. 1 hour before procedure.

ADVERSE REACTIONS

CNS: lethargy, hallucinations, *seizures,* anxiety, confusion, agitation, depression, dizziness, fatigue.
GI: *nausea,* vomiting, *diarrhea,* glossitis, stomatitis, gastritis, abdominal pain, enterocolitis, pseudomembranous colitis, black "hairy" tongue.
GU: interstitial nephritis, nephropathy, vaginitis.
Hematologic: anemia, *thrombocytopenia,* thrombocytopenic purpura, eosinophilia, *leukopenia,* hemolytic anemia, *agranulocytosis.*
Other: *hypersensitivity reactions, anaphylaxis,* overgrowth of nonsusceptible organisms.

INTERACTIONS

Drug-drug. *Allopurinol:* increased incidence of rash. Monitor patient.
Oral contraceptives: efficacy of oral contraceptives may be decreased. Additional form of contraception should be recommended during penicillin therapy.
Probenecid: increased blood levels of amoxicillin and other penicillins. Probenecid may be used for this purpose.

EFFECTS ON DIAGNOSTIC TESTS

Amoxicillin may alter results of urine glucose tests that use cupric sulfate (Benedict's reagent or Clinitest). Make urine

---

glucose determinations with glucose oxidase methods (Diastix or Chemstrip uG). Amoxicillin may falsely cause a positive Coombs' test.

CONTRAINDICATIONS
Contraindicated in patients with hypersensitivity to drug or other penicillins.

SPECIAL CONSIDERATIONS
▶ Use cautiously in patients with other drug allergies, especially to cephalosporins (possible cross-sensitivity), and in those with mononucleosis (high incidence of maculopapular rash).
▶ Before drug is given, patient must be asked about previous allergic reactions to penicillin. However, a negative history of penicillin allergy is no guarantee against a future allergic reaction.
▶ A specimen for culture and sensitivity tests is obtained before giving first dose. Therapy may begin pending results.
▶ Amoxicillin is given at least 1 hour before a bacteriostatic antibiotic.
▶ Patient must be observed closely. With large doses and prolonged therapy, superinfection may occur, especially in elderly, debilitated, or immunosuppressed patients.
▶ Trimox oral suspension may be stored at room temperature for up to 2 weeks. Individual product labels should be checked for storage information.
▶ Amoxicillin generally causes fewer cases of diarrhea than does ampicillin.
▶ *Alert:* Don't confuse amoxicillin with amoxapine.

Patient teaching
▶ Take entire quantity exactly as prescribed, even after feeling better.
▶ Drug may be taken with food.
▶ Notify health care provider if rash, fever, or chills develops. Rash is the most common allergic reaction, especially if allopurinol is also being taken.
▶ If patient is a child, parent should place pediatric drops directly on child's tongue for swallowing or add to formula, milk, fruit juice, water, ginger ale, or a cold drink; patient should take immediately and consume entirely.

ampicillin
Apo-Ampi , Novo Ampicillin , Nu-Ampi , Omnipen-N

ampicillin sodium
Ampicin , Ampicyn‡, Omnipen-N, Penbritin , Totacillin-N

ampicillin trihydrate
Omnipen, Penbritin , Principen, Totacillin
Pregnancy Risk Category B

HOW SUPPLIED
Capsules: 250 mg, 500 mg
Oral suspension: 125 mg/5 ml, 250 mg/5 ml
Injection: 125 mg, 250 mg, 500 mg, 1 g, 2 g

ACTION
An aminopenicillin that inhibits cell-wall synthesis during microorganism multiplication. Bacteria resist ampicillin by producing penicillinases — enzymes that hydrolyze ampicillin.

Route	Onset	Peak	Duration
P.O.	Unknown	2 hr	6-8 hr
I.V.	Immediate	Immediate	Unknown
I.M.	Unknown	1 hr	Unknown

INDICATIONS & DOSAGE
Systemic infections and acute and chronic urinary tract infections due to susceptible strains of gram-positive and gram-negative organisms —
Adults and children weighing 40 kg (88

lb) or more: 250 to 500 mg P.O. q 6 hours; or 1 to 12 g I.M. or I.V. daily in divided doses q 4 to 6 hours.

Children weighing under 40 kg: 25 to 100 mg/kg/day P.O. in equally divided doses q 6 hours; or 25 to 50 mg/kg/day I.M. or I.V. in divided doses q 6 to 8 hours. Pediatric dosages shouldn't exceed recommended adult dosages.

Meningitis —
Adults: 150 to 200 mg/kg/day I.V. in divided doses q 3 to 4 hours. May be given I.M. after 3 days of I.V. therapy.
Children: 100 to 200 mg/kg I.V. daily in divided doses q 3 to 4 hours. Give I.V. for 3 days; then give I.M.

Uncomplicated gonorrhea —
Adults and children weighing over 45 kg (99 lb): 3.5 g P.O. with 1 g probenecid given as a single dose.

Endocarditis prophylaxis for dental and GI/GU procedures —
Adults: 2 g I.M. or I.V. within 30 minutes before procedure.
Children: 50 mg/kg I.M. or I.V. within 30 minutes before procedure.
Note: Give drug with gentamicin in high-risk procedures.

ADVERSE REACTIONS

CNS: lethargy, hallucinations, *seizures,* anxiety, confusion, agitation, depression, dizziness, fatigue.
CV: vein irritation, thrombophlebitis.
GI: *nausea,* vomiting, *diarrhea,* glossitis, stomatitis, gastritis, abdominal pain, enterocolitis, pseudomembranous colitis, black "hairy" tongue.
GU: interstitial nephritis, nephropathy, vaginitis.
Hematologic: anemia, *thrombocytopenia,* thrombocytopenic purpura, eosinophilia, *leukopenia,* hemolytic anemia, *agranulocytosis.*
Other: *hypersensitivity reactions (erythematous maculopapular rash, urticaria, anaphylaxis),* overgrowth of nonsusceptible organisms, pain at injection site.

INTERACTIONS

Drug-drug. *Allopurinol:* increased incidence of rash. Monitor patient.
Oral contraceptives: efficacy of oral contraceptives may be decreased. Additional forms of contraception should be recommended during penicillin therapy.
Probenecid: increased blood levels of ampicillin and other penicillins. Probenecid may be used for this purpose.

EFFECTS ON DIAGNOSTIC TESTS

Drug alters results of urine glucose tests that use cupric sulfate (Benedict's reagent or Clinitest). Make urine glucose determinations with glucose oxidase methods (Diastix or Chemstrip uG). Ampicillin may falsely decrease serum aminoglycoside levels.

CONTRAINDICATIONS

Contraindicated in patients with hypersensitivity to drug or other penicillins.

SPECIAL CONSIDERATIONS

▶ Use cautiously in patients with other drug allergies, especially to cephalosporins (possible cross-sensitivity), and in those with mononucleosis (high incidence of maculopapular rash).
▶ Before drug is given, patient must be asked about previous allergic reactions to penicillin. However, a negative history of penicillin allergy is no guarantee against a future allergic reaction.
▶ A specimen for culture and sensitivity tests should be obtained before giving first dose. Therapy may begin pending results.
▶ Drug is usually given only I.M. or I.V. if the infection is severe or if patient can't take oral dose.
▶ Drug is administered 1 to 2 hours before or 2 to 3 hours after meals. When given orally, drug may cause GI disturbances. Food may interfere with absorption.
▶ Ampicillin is given at least 1 hour before a bacteriostatic antibiotic.
▶ Patient must be observed closely. With

large doses or prolonged therapy, bacterial or fungal superinfection may occur, especially in elderly, debilitated, or immunosuppressed patients.

▶ Dosage should be decreased in patients with impaired renal function.

▶ In pediatric meningitis, ampicillin may be given with parenteral chloramphenicol for 24 hours pending cultures.

I.V. administration

▶ For I.V. injection, drug is reconstituted with bacteriostatic water for injection. 5 ml is used for the 125-mg, 250-mg, or 500-mg vials; 7.4 ml is used for the 1-g vials; or 14.8 ml is used for the 2-g vials. Direct I.V. injections are given over 3 to 5 minutes for doses of 500 mg or less; over 10 to 15 minutes for larger doses. A rate of 100 mg/minute should not be exceeded. Or, the drug is diluted in 50 to 100 ml of normal saline for injection and give by intermittent infusion over 15 to 30 minutes.

▶ **Alert:** Drug should not be mixed with solutions containing dextrose or fructose because these substances promote rapid breakdown of ampicillin.

▶ Initial dilution should be used within 1 hour. Manufacturer's directions should be followed for stability data when ampicillin is further diluted for I.V. infusion.

▶ I.V. infusion is given intermittently to prevent vein irritation, and site is changed every 48 hours.

Patient teaching

▶ Take entire quantity of medication exactly as prescribed, even after feeling better.

▶ Take oral form on an empty stomach 1 hour before or 2 hours after meals.

▶ Report discomfort at I.V. injection site.

▶ Notify health care provider if rash, fever, or chills develop. Rash is the most common allergic reaction, especially if allopurinol is also being taken.

ampicillin sodium/ sulbactam sodium

Unasyn

Pregnancy Risk Category B

HOW SUPPLIED

Injection: vials and piggyback vials containing 1.5 g (1 g ampicillin sodium with 0.5 g sulbactam sodium), 3 g (2 g ampicillin sodium with 1 g sulbactam sodium), and 10 g (10 g ampicillin sodium with 5 g sulbactam sodium)

ACTION

An aminopenicillin that inhibits cell-wall synthesis during microorganism multiplication. Sulbactam inactivates bacterial beta-lactamase, which inactivates ampicillin, causing bacterial resistance to it.

Route	Onset	Peak	Duration
I.V.	15 min	Immediate	Unknown
I.M.	Unknown	Unknown	Unknown

INDICATIONS & DOSAGE

Intra-abdominal, gynecologic, and skin-structure infections due to susceptible strains —

Adults and children weighing over 40 kg (88 lb): dosage expressed as total drug (each 1.5-g vial contains 1 g ampicillin sodium and 0.5 g sulbactam sodium) — 1.5 to 3 g I.M. or I.V. q 6 hours. Maximum daily dose is 4 g sulbactam and 8 g ampicillin (12 g of combined drugs).

Children ages 1 and older weighing below 40 kg: 300 mg/kg/day (200 mg ampicillin/100 mg sulbactam) I.V. in divided doses q 6 hours. Don't exceed 4 g daily.

Dosage adjustment: For renally impaired patients with creatinine clearance of 15 to 29 ml/minute, give 1.5 to 3 g q 12 hours; if creatinine clearance is 5 to 14 ml/minute, give 1.5 to 3 g q 24 hours.

---

*Liquid contains alcohol.   **May contain tartrazine.   †Canada   ‡Australia   §U.K.   ◇OTC

ADVERSE REACTIONS

CV: vein irritation, thrombophlebitis.

GI: *nausea,* vomiting, *diarrhea,* glossitis, stomatitis, gastritis, black "hairy" tongue, enterocolitis, pseudomembranous colitis.

GU: increased BUN, creatinine.

Hematologic: anemia, ***thrombocytopenia,*** thrombocytopenic purpura, eosinophilia, ***leukopenia, agranulocytosis.***

Hepatic: increased liver function tests.

Other: *hypersensitivity reactions, anaphylaxis, overgrowth of nonsusceptible organisms, pain* at injection site.

INTERACTIONS

Drug-drug. *Allopurinol:* increased incidence of rash. Monitor patient.

Oral contraceptives: efficacy of oral contraceptives may be decreased. An additional form of contraception should be recommended during penicillin therapy.

Probenecid: increased levels of ampicillin. Probenecid may be used for this purpose.

EFFECTS ON DIAGNOSTIC TESTS

Ampicillin alters results of urine glucose tests that use cupric sulfate (Benedict's reagent or Clinitest). Make urine glucose determinations with glucose oxidase methods (Diastix). In pregnant women, transient decreases in serum estradiol, conjugated estrone, conjugated estriol, and estriol glucuronide levels may occur.

CONTRAINDICATIONS

Contraindicated in patients with hypersensitivity to drug or other penicillins.

SPECIAL CONSIDERATIONS

▶ Use cautiously in patients with other drug allergies, especially to cephalosporins (possible cross-sensitivity), and in those with mononucleosis (high incidence of maculopapular rash).

▶ Before drug is given, patient must be asked about previous allergic reactions to penicillin. However, a negative history of penicillin allergy is no guarantee against a future allergic reaction.

▶ A specimen for culture and sensitivity tests is obtained before giving first dose. Therapy may begin pending results.

▶ Liver function tests must be monitored during therapy, especially in patients with impaired liver function.

▶ I.M. route is not used in children.

▶ For I.M. injection, the drug is reconstituted with sterile water for injection or 0.5% or 2% lidocaine hydrochloride injection. 3.2 ml is added to a 1.5-g vial (or 6.4 ml to a 3-g vial) to yield a concentration of 375 mg/ml. Drug is administered deeply.

▶ Patient must be observed closely. With large doses and prolonged therapy, bacterial or fungal superinfection may occur, especially in elderly, debilitated, or immunosuppressed patients.

▶ Dosage should be decreased in patients with impaired renal function.

I.V. administration

▶ To prepare I.V. injection, powder is reconstituted with one of the following diluents: normal saline solution, sterile water for injection, D_5W, lactated Ringer's injection, 1/6 M sodium lactate, dextrose 5% or half-normal saline for injection, and 10% invert sugar. Stability varies with diluent, temperature, and concentration of solution.

▶ After reconstitution, vials should stand for a few minutes to allow foam to dissipate. This will permit visual inspection of contents for particles.

▶ When given I.V., drug should not be added to or mixed with other drugs because they might prove incompatible.

▶ Drug is given at least 1 hour before a bacteriostatic antibiotic.

▶ *Alert:* I.V. dose is given by slow injection (over 10 to 15 minutes) or diluted in 50 to 100 ml of a compatible diluent, and infused over 15 to 30 minutes. If permitted, drug is given intermittently to prevent vein irritation. Site is changed every 48 hours.

Patient teaching
▶ Report any rash, fever, or chills. Rash is the most common allergic reaction.
▶ I.M. injection may cause pain at injection site.
▶ Report discomfort at I.V. insertion site.

cloxacillin sodium
Apo-Cloxi, Cloxapen,
Novo-Cloxin, Nu-Cloxi,
Orbenin

Pregnancy Risk Category B

HOW SUPPLIED
Capsules: 250 mg, 500 mg
Oral solution: 125 mg/5 ml (after reconstitution)

ACTION
A penicillinase-resistant penicillin that inhibits cell-wall synthesis during microorganism multiplication. Bacteria resist penicillins by producing penicillinases — enzymes that convert penicillins to inactive penicillic acid. Cloxacillin resists these enzymes.

Route	Onset	Peak	Duration
P.O.	Unknown	2 hr	6 hr

INDICATIONS & DOSAGE
Systemic infections due to penicillinase-producing staphylococci —
Adults and children weighing over 20 kg (44 lb): 250 to 500 mg P.O. q 6 hours.
Children weighing 20 kg or less: 50 to 100 mg/kg P.O. daily, in divided doses q 6 hours (maximum of 4 g daily).

ADVERSE REACTIONS
CNS: lethargy, hallucinations, *seizures,* anxiety, confusion, agitation, depression, dizziness, fatigue.
GI: *nausea,* vomiting, *epigastric distress, diarrhea,* enterocolitis, pseudomembranous colitis, black "hairy" tongue, abdominal pain.
GU: interstitial nephritis, nephropathy.
Hematologic: eosinophilia, anemia, *thrombocytopenia, leukopenia,* hemolytic anemia, *agranulocytosis,* transient reductions in RBC, WBC, and platelet counts.
Hepatic: transient elevations in liver function tests.
Other: *hypersensitivity reactions, anaphylaxis,* overgrowth of nonsusceptible organisms.

INTERACTIONS
Drug-drug. *Oral contraceptives:* efficacy of oral contraceptives may be decreased. Additional form of contraception is recommended during penicillin therapy.
Probenecid: increased blood levels of cloxacillin and other penicillins. Probenecid may be used for this purpose.
Drug-food. *Any food:* may interfere with absorption. Drug should be given 1 to 2 hours before or 2 to 3 hours after meals. *Carbonated beverages, fruit juice:* inactivates drug. Don't give together.

EFFECTS ON DIAGNOSTIC TESTS
Drug alters test results for urine and serum proteins; it produces false-positive or elevated results in turbidimetric urine and serum protein tests using sulfosalicylic acid or trichloroacetic acid; it also reportedly produces false results on the Bradshaw screening test for Bence Jones protein.

CONTRAINDICATIONS
Contraindicated in patients with hypersensitivity to drug or other penicillins.

SPECIAL CONSIDERATIONS
▶ Use cautiously in patients with other

---

drug allergies, especially to cephalosporins (possible cross-sensitivity), and in those with mononucleosis (high incidence of maculopapular rash).

▶ Before the drug is given, the patient must be asked about previous allergic reactions to penicillin. However, a negative history of penicillin allergy is no guarantee against a future allergic reaction.

▶ A specimen for culture and sensitivity tests should be obtained before giving first dose. Therapy may begin pending results.

▶ Drug is given 1 to 2 hours before or 2 to 3 hours after meals. Drug may cause GI disturbances. Food may interfere with its absorption.

▶ Cloxacillin is given at least 1 hour before a bacteriostatic antibiotic.

▶ Renal, hepatic, and hematopoietic function must periodically be assessed in patients receiving long-term therapy.

▶ Elevated liver function test results may indicate drug-induced cholestasis or hepatitis.

▶ Patient must be observed closely. With large doses and prolonged therapy, bacterial or fungal superinfection may occur, especially in elderly, debilitated, or immunosuppressed patients.

Patient teaching

▶ Take entire quantity of drug exactly as prescribed, even after feeling better.

▶ Take drug on an empty stomach.

▶ *Alert:* Take each dose with a full glass of water, not with fruit juice or carbonated beverage because their acid will inactivate the drug.

▶ Notify health care provider if rash, fever, or chills develop. Rash is the most common allergic reaction.

dicloxacillin sodium

Diclocil‡, Dycill, Dynapen, Pathocil
Pregnancy Risk Category B

HOW SUPPLIED
Capsules: 125 mg, 250 mg, 500 mg
Oral suspension: 62.5 mg/5 ml (after reconstitution)

ACTION
A penicillinase-resistant penicillin that inhibits cell-wall synthesis during microorganism multiplication. Bacteria resist penicillins by producing penicillinases — enzymes that convert penicillins to inactive penicillic acid. Dicloxacillin resists these enzymes.

Route	Onset	Peak	Duration
P.O.	Unknown	2 hr	6 hr

INDICATIONS & DOSAGE
Systemic infections due to penicillinase-producing staphylococci —
Adults and children weighing over 40 kg (88 lb): 125 to 250 mg P.O. q 6 hours.
Children weighing 40 kg or less: 12.5 to 25 mg/kg P.O. daily, in divided doses q 6 hours depending on severity.

ADVERSE REACTIONS
CNS: neuromuscular irritability, *seizures,* lethargy, hallucinations, anxiety, confusion, agitation, depression, dizziness, fatigue.
GI: *nausea,* vomiting, *epigastric distress,* flatulence, *diarrhea,* enterocolitis, pseudomembranous colitis, black "hairy" tongue, abdominal pain.
GU: interstitial nephritis, nephropathy.
Hematologic: anemia, *thrombocytopenia,* eosinophilia, *leukopenia,* hemolytic anemia, *agranulocytosis.*
Hepatic: transient elevations in liver function test results.

Other: *hypersensitivity reactions (pruritus, urticaria, rash, anaphylaxis),* overgrowth of nonsusceptible organisms.

INTERACTIONS

Drug-drug. *Oral contraceptives:* efficacy of oral contraceptives may be decreased. An additional form of contraception should be recommended during penicillin therapy.

Probenecid: increased blood levels of dicloxacillin and other penicillins. Probenecid may be used for this purpose.

EFFECTS ON DIAGNOSTIC TESTS

Drug produces false-positive or elevated results in turbidimetric urine and serum protein tests using sulfosalicylic acid or trichloroacetic acid; it also reportedly produces false results on the Bradshaw screening test for Bence Jones protein.

CONTRAINDICATIONS

Contraindicated in patients with hypersensitivity to drug or other penicillins. It is not recommended for use in newborns.

SPECIAL CONSIDERATIONS

▶ Use cautiously in patients with other drug allergies, especially to cephalosporins (possible cross-sensitivity), and in those with mononucleosis (high incidence of maculopapular rash).

▶ Before the drug is given, the patient must be asked about previous allergic reactions to penicillin. However, a negative history of penicillin allergy is no guarantee against a future allergic reaction.

▶ A specimen for culture and sensitivity tests should be obtained before giving first dose. Therapy may begin pending results.

▶ The drug is given 1 to 2 hours before or 2 to 3 hours after meals. Drug may cause GI disturbances. Food may interfere with absorption.

▶ Dicloxacillin is given at least 1 hour before a bacteriostatic antibiotic.

▶ Renal, hepatic, and hematopoietic function must periodically be assessed in patients receiving long-term therapy.

▶ Elevated liver function test results may indicate drug-induced cholestasis or hepatitis.

▶ Patient must be observed closely. With large doses and prolonged therapy, bacterial or fungal superinfection may occur, especially in elderly, debilitated, or immunosuppressed patients.

Patient teaching

▶ Take entire quantity of drug exactly as prescribed, even after feeling better.

▶ Take drug on an empty stomach.

▶ Notify health care provider if rash, fever, or chills develop. Rash is the most common allergic reaction.

mezlocillin sodium

Mezlin

Pregnancy Risk Category B

HOW SUPPLIED

Injection: 1 g, 2 g, 3 g, 4 g, 20 g

ACTION

An extended-spectrum penicillin that inhibits cell-wall synthesis during microorganism multiplication. Bacteria resist mezlocillin by producing penicillinases — enzymes that hydrolyze mezlocillin.

Route	Onset	Peak	Duration
I.V.	Immediate	Immediate	Unknown
I.M.	Unknown	45-90 min	Unknown

INDICATIONS & DOSAGE

Systemic infections due to susceptible strains of gram-positive and especially gram-negative organisms (including Proteus *and* Pseudomonas aeruginosa*)* —

Adults: 100 to 300 mg/kg daily I.V. or I.M. in four to six divided doses. Usual dose is 3 g q 4 hours or 4 g q 6 hours. For serious infections, up to 24 g daily may be administered.

Children ages 1 month to 12 years: 50 mg/kg q 4 hours I.V. or I.M.

Dosage adjustment: For renally impaired patients with creatinine clearance of 10 to 30 ml/minute, 1.5 g q 6 hours for urinary tract infection or 3 g q 8 hours for serious infection; for creatinine clearance below 10 ml/minute, 1.5 g q 8 hours for urinary tract infection or 2 g q 8 hours for serious infection.

ADVERSE REACTIONS

CNS: neuromuscular irritability, *seizures.*
CV: vein irritation, phlebitis.
GI: nausea, diarrhea, vomiting, abnormal taste sensation, pseudomembranous colitis.
GU: interstitial nephritis.
Hematologic: *bleeding, neutropenia, thrombocytopenia,* eosinophilia, *leukopenia, hemolytic anemia.* **Hepatic:** transient elevations in liver function test results.
Metabolic: *hypokalemia.*
Other: *hypersensitivity reactions, anaphylaxis,* overgrowth of nonsusceptible organisms, pain at injection site.

INTERACTIONS

Drug-drug. *Aminoglycoside antibiotics (such as amikacin, gentamicin, tobramycin):* chemically incompatible. Drugs should not be mixed together in I.V. solution. Drugs should be given 1 hour apart, especially in patients with renal impairment.
Oral contraceptives: efficacy of oral contraceptives may be decreased. An additional form of contraception should be recommended during penicillin therapy.
Probenecid: increased blood levels of mezlocillin. Probenecid may be used for this purpose.
Vecuronium: prolonged neuromuscular blockade. Use with caution.

EFFECTS ON DIAGNOSTIC TESTS

Drug alters tests for urine or serum proteins; it interferes with turbidimetric methods that use sulfosalicylic acid, trichloroacetic acid, acetic acid, or nitric acid. Drug does not interfere with tests using bromphenol blue (Albustix, Albutest, Multistix). Positive Coombs' tests have been reported in patients taking mezlocillin.

CONTRAINDICATIONS

Contraindicated in patients with hypersensitivity to drug or other penicillins.

SPECIAL CONSIDERATIONS

▶ Use cautiously in patients with other drug allergies, especially to cephalosporins (possible cross-sensitivity), and in those with bleeding tendencies, uremia, or hypokalemia.

▶ Before drug is given, patient must be asked about previous allergic reactions to penicillin. However, a negative history of penicillin allergy is no guarantee against a future allergic reaction.

▶ A specimen for culture and sensitivity tests should be obtained before giving first dose. Therapy may begin pending results.

▶ When administering I.M., no more than 2 g should be given per injection. Drug must be injected deeply and slowly (12 to 15 seconds) into a large muscle.

▶ CBC and platelet counts are checked frequently. Drug may cause thrombocytopenia.

▶ Serum potassium level must be monitored.

▶ *Alert:* Seizure precautions must be instituted. Patients with high serum levels of drug may have seizures.

▶ Patient must be observed closely. With large doses and prolonged therapy, bacterial or fungal superinfection may occur, especially in elderly, debilitated, or immunosuppressed patients.

▶ Dosage should be altered in patients with impaired renal function.

Reactions may be *common,* uncommon, *life-threatening*, or COMMON AND LIFE-THREATENING.

▶ Drug is almost always used with another antibiotic such as gentamicin.
▶ **Alert:** Don't confuse methicillin with mezlocillin.

I.V. administration
▶ The drug is reconstituted with at least 10 ml/g of drug using sterile water for injection, D_5W, or normal saline for injection. Solutions with a concentration not exceeding 10% may be given by direct injection over 3 to 5 minutes. Or, the solution diluted in about 50 to 100 ml of suitable I.V. solution, and given by intermittent infusion over 30 minutes.
▶ I.V. infusion is given intermittently to prevent vein irritation. Site is changed every 48 hours.
▶ Drug is given at least 1 hour before bacteriostatic antibiotics.

Patient teaching
▶ Report adverse reactions promptly.
▶ Alert health care provider if discomfort occurs at I.V. site.
▶ Limit salt intake during mezlocillin therapy because of drug's high sodium content.

nafcillin sodium
Nallpen, Unipen

Pregnancy Risk Category B

HOW SUPPLIED
Capsules: 250 mg
Injection: 500 mg, 1 g, 2 g, 10 g
I.V. infusion piggyback: 1 g, 2 g

ACTION
A penicillinase-resistant penicillin that inhibits cell-wall synthesis during microorganism multiplication. Bacteria resist penicillins by producing penicillinases — enzymes that hydrolyze penicillins. Nafcillin resists these enzymes.

Route	Onset	Peak	Duration
P.O.	Unknown	0.5-2 hr	Unknown
I.V.	Immediate	Immediate	Unknown
I.M.	Unknown	0.5-1 hr	Unknown

INDICATIONS & DOSAGE
Systemic infections due to penicillinase-producing staphylococci —
Adults: 250 to 500 mg P.O. q 4 to 6 hours (more severe infections may be treated with 1 g P.O. q 4 to 6 hours); or 500 mg I.M. q 4 to 6 hours or I.V. q 4 hours, or (for more severe infections) 1 g I.M. or I.V. q 4 hours.
Children over age 1 month and weighing under 40 kg (88 lb): 25 to 50 mg/kg P.O. daily, in divided doses q 6 hours; or 25 mg/kg I.M. b.i.d. or 100 to 200 mg/kg I.M. or I.V. daily in divided doses q 4 to 6 hours.
Neonates: 10 mg/kg I.M. b.i.d. or 10 mg/kg P.O. t.i.d. or q.i.d.

ADVERSE REACTIONS
CV: vein irritation, thrombophlebitis.
GI: *nausea,* vomiting, diarrhea.
Hematologic: *neutropenia, agranulocytosis, thrombocytopenia.*
Other: *hypersensitivity reactions, anaphylaxis.*

INTERACTIONS
Drug-drug. *Aminoglycosides:* synergistic effect; monitor closely. Chemical and physical incompatibility. These drugs should not be mixed together in same I.V. solution.
Oral contraceptives: efficacy of oral contraceptives may be decreased. An additional form of contraception should be recommended during penicillin therapy.
Probenecid: increased blood levels of nafcillin. Probenecid may be used for this purpose.
Rifampin: dose-dependent antagonism. Monitor closely.
Warfarin: increased risk of bleeding when

used with I.V. nafcillin. PT and INR must be monitored closely.

EFFECTS ON DIAGNOSTIC TESTS

Turbidimetric urine and serum proteins are falsely positive or elevated in tests using sulfosalicylic acid or trichloroacetic acid.

CONTRAINDICATIONS

Contraindicated in patients with hypersensitivity to drug or other penicillins.

SPECIAL CONSIDERATIONS

▶ Use cautiously in patients with other drug allergies, especially to cephalosporins (possible cross-sensitivity), and in those with GI distress.

▶ Before drug is given, the patient must be asked about previous allergic reactions to penicillin. However, a negative history of penicillin allergy is no guarantee against a future allergic reaction.

▶ A specimen for culture and sensitivity tests should be obtained before giving first dose. Therapy may begin pending results.

▶ Dug is given 1 to 2 hours before or 2 to 3 hours after meals. When given orally, drug may cause GI disturbances. Food may interfere with absorption.

▶ Drug is given at least 1 hour before a bacteriostatic antibiotic.

▶ Patient must be observed closely. With large doses and prolonged therapy, bacterial or fungal superinfection may occur, especially in elderly, debilitated, or immunosuppressed patients.

▶ Serum sodium should be observed because each gram of nafcillin contains 2.9 mEq of sodium.

▶ An abnormal urinalysis result may indicate drug-induced interstitial nephritis.

I.V. administration

▶ Piggyback containers are reconstituted according to manufacturer's instructions. 500-mg, 1-g, or 2-g vials are reconstituted with sterile water for injection, D_5W, or normal saline for injection. 1.7 ml is added for each 500 mg of drug. Reconstituted drug may be given I.M. Or, drug may be diluted with 15 to 30 ml of sterile water for injection or half-normal or normal saline for injection, and given by direct injection into a vein or into the tubing of a free-flowing I.V. solution over 5 to 10 minutes. Or the drug may be diluted to a concentration of 2 to 40 mg/ml, and given by intermittent I.V. infusion over 30 to 60 minutes.

▶ Continuous I.V. infusions should be avoided to prevent vein irritation. Site is changed every 48 hours.

Patient teaching

▶ Take entire quantity of medication exactly as prescribed, even after feeling better.

▶ Take oral form of drug on an empty stomach.

▶ Notify health care provider if rash, fever, or chills develop. Rash is the most common allergic reaction.

---

oxacillin sodium

Bactocill

Pregnancy Risk Category B

HOW SUPPLIED

Capsules: 250 mg, 500 mg
Oral solution: 250 mg/5 ml (after reconstitution)
Injection: 250 mg, 500 mg, 1 g, 2 g, 4 g
I.V. infusion: 1 g, 2 g

ACTION

A penicillinase-resistant penicillin that inhibits cell-wall synthesis during microorganism multiplication. Bacteria resist penicillins by producing penicillinases—enzymes that convert penicillins to inactive penicillic acid. Oxacillin resists these enzymes.

Route	Onset	Peak	Duration
P.O.	Unknown	0.5-2 hr	Unknown
I.V.	Immediate	Immediate	Unknown
I.M.	Unknown	0.5 hr	Unknown

INDICATIONS & DOSAGE

Systemic infections due to penicillinase-producing staphylococci—

Adults and children weighing over 40 kg (88 lb): 500 mg to 1 g P.O. q 4 to 6 hours; or 250 mg to 1 g I.M. or I.V. q 4 to 6 hours.

Children over age 1 month weighing 40 kg or less: 50 to 100 mg/kg P.O. daily, in divided doses q 6 hours; or 50 to 200 mg/kg I.M. or I.V. daily in divided doses q 4 to 6 hours, depending on severity.

Premature infants and neonates: 25 mg/kg/day I.M. or I.V. in equally divided doses q 6 to 12 hours.

ADVERSE REACTIONS

CNS: neuropathy, neuromuscular irritability, *seizures,* lethargy, hallucinations, anxiety, confusion, agitation, depression, dizziness, fatigue.

CV: *thrombophlebitis.*

GI: oral lesions, nausea, vomiting, diarrhea, enterocolitis, pseudomembranous colitis.

GU: interstitial nephritis, nephropathy.

Hematologic: *thrombocytopenia,* eosinophilia, *hemolytic anemia, neutropenia,* anemia, *agranulocytosis.*

Hepatic: elevated liver enzymes.

Other: *hypersensitivity reactions, anaphylaxis,* overgrowth of nonsusceptible organisms.

INTERACTIONS

Drug-drug. *Aminoglycosides:* possible synergistic effect. Monitor closely. Chemical and physical incompatibility. These drugs should not be mixed together in same I.V. solution.

Oral contraceptives: efficacy of oral contraceptives may be decreased. Recommend additional form of contraception during penicillin therapy.

Probenecid: increased blood levels of oxacillin and other penicillins. Probenecid may be used for this purpose.

Rifampin: possible antagonism. Monitor closely.

EFFECTS ON DIAGNOSTIC TESTS

Turbidimetric urine and serum proteins are falsely positive or elevated in tests using sulfosalicylic acid or trichloroacetic acid.

CONTRAINDICATIONS

Contraindicated in patients with hypersensitivity to drug or other penicillins.

SPECIAL CONSIDERATIONS

‣ Use cautiously in patients with other drug allergies, especially to cephalosporins (possible cross-sensitivity), and in neonates and infants.

‣ Before drug is given, the patient must be asked about previous allergic reactions to penicillin. However, a negative history of penicillin allergy is no guarantee against a future allergic reaction.

‣ A specimen for culture and sensitivity tests must be obtained before giving first dose. Therapy may begin pending results.

‣ Drug is given I.M. or I.V. only if the infection is severe or if the patient can't take oral dose.

‣ Drug is given 1 to 2 hours before or 2 to 3 hours after meals. When given orally, drug may cause GI disturbances. Food may interfere with absorption.

‣ Drug is administered at least 1 hour before a bacteriostatic antibiotic.

‣ Periodic liver function studies should be completed to monitor for elevated AST and ALT levels. Elevations in liver function test results may indicate drug-induced hepatitis or cholestasis.

‣ Abnormal urinalysis results may indicate drug-induced interstitial nephritis.

‣ Patient must be observed closely. With

large doses and prolonged therapy, bacterial or fungal superinfection may occur, especially in elderly, debilitated, or immunosuppressed patients.

I.V. administration

▶ For direct I.V. injection, the drug is reconstituted with sterile water for injection or normal saline for injection. 5 ml of diluent is used for a 250- or 500-mg vial, 10 ml of diluent for a 1-g vial, 20 ml of diluent for a 2-g vial, or 40 ml of diluent for a 4-g vial. When the solution is clear, the ordered dose is withdrawn and injected over 10 minutes. When giving by piggyback injection, a 1-g piggyback vial is reconstituted with 20 to 100 ml of diluent; a 2-g vial is reconstituted with 19 to 99 ml of diluent. For intermittent infusion, drug is further diluted to a concentration of 5 to 40 mg/ml.

▶ To prevent vein irritation, continuous infusions should be avoided. Site should be changed every 48 hours.

Patient teaching

▶ Take entire quantity of drug exactly as prescribed, even after feeling better.
▶ Take drug on an empty stomach.
▶ Notify health care provider if rash, fever, or chills develop. Rash is the most common allergic reaction.

penicillin G benzathine (benzylpenicillin benzathine)

Bicillin L-A, Permapen

Pregnancy Risk Category B

HOW SUPPLIED

Injection: 300,000 U/ml, 600,000 U/ml, 1,200,000 U/2 ml, 2,400,000 U/4 ml

ACTION

A natural penicillin that inhibits cell-wall synthesis during microorganism multiplication. Bacteria resist penicillins by producing penicillinases—enzymes that convert penicillins to inactive penicillic acid.

Route	Onset	Peak	Duration
I.M.	Unknown	13-24 hr	1-4 wk

INDICATIONS & DOSAGE

Congenital syphilis —
Children under age 2: 50,000 U/kg I.M. as a single dose.
   Group A streptococcal upper respiratory infections —
Adults: 1.2 million U I.M. as a single injection.
Children weighing 27 kg (60 lb) or more: 900,000 U I.M. as a single injection.
Children weighing less than 27 kg: 300,000 to 600,000 U I.M. as a single injection.
   Prophylaxis of poststreptococcal rheumatic fever —
Adults and children: 1.2 million U I.M. once monthly.
   Syphilis of less than 1 year's duration —
Adults: 2.4 million U I.M. as a single dose.
Children: 50,000 U/kg (up to the adult dosage) I.M as a single dose.
   Syphilis of more than 1 year's duration —
Adults: 2.4 million U I.M. weekly for 3 successive weeks.
Children: 50,000 U/kg I.M. weekly for 3 successive weeks.

ADVERSE REACTIONS

CNS: neuropathy, *seizures,* lethargy, hallucinations, anxiety, confusion, agitation, depression, dizziness, fatigue.
GI: nausea, vomiting, enterocolitis, pseudomembranous colitis.
GU: interstitial nephritis, nephropathy.

Hematologic: eosinophilia, hemolytic anemia, *thrombocytopenia, leukopenia,* anemia, *agranulocytosis.*

Other: *hypersensitivity reactions, maculopapular and exfoliative dermatitis, anaphylaxis,* pain, sterile abscess at injection site.

INTERACTIONS

Drug-drug. *Aminoglycosides:* physical and chemical incompatibility. These drugs are administered separately.

Colestipol: decreased serum concentrations of penicillin G benzathine. Penicillin G benzathine is administered 1 hour before or 4 hours after colestipol.

Oral contraceptives: efficacy of oral contraceptives may be decreased. An additional form of contraception should be recommended during penicillin therapy.

Probenecid: increased blood levels of penicillin. Probenecid may be used for this purpose.

Tetracycline: may antagonize the effects. Avoid concurrent use.

EFFECTS ON DIAGNOSTIC TESTS

Penicillin G interferes with turbidimetric methods using sulfosalicylic acid, trichloracetic acid, acetic acid, and nitric acid. Drug does not interfere with tests using bromphenol blue (Albustix, Albutest, Multistix). It alters urine glucose testing using cupric sulfate (Benedict's reagent); use Diastix or Chemstrip uG instead. Penicillin G may cause falsely elevated results of urine specific gravity tests in patients with low urine output and dehydration and falsely elevated Norymberski and Zimmerman tests results for 17-ketogenic steroids. It causes false-positive CSF protein test results (Folin-Ciocalteau method) and may cause positive Coombs' test results. Drug may falsely decrease serum aminoglycoside levels. Adding betalactamase to the sample inactivates the penicillin, rendering the assay more accurate. Or, the sample can be spun down and frozen immediately after collection.

CONTRAINDICATIONS

Contraindicated in patients with hypersensitivity to drug or other penicillins.

SPECIAL CONSIDERATIONS

▶ Use cautiously in patients with other drug allergies, especially to cephalosporins (possible cross-sensitivity).

▶ Before the drug is given, the patient must be asked about previous allergic reactions to penicillin. However, a negative history of penicillin allergy is no guarantee against a future allergic reaction.

▶ A specimen for culture and sensitivity tests should be obtained before giving first dose. Therapy may begin pending results.

▶ Medication should be shaken well before injection.

▶ *Alert:* Drug is never given I.V. Inadvertent I.V. administration has caused cardiac arrest and death.

▶ Drug is injected deeply into upper outer quadrant of buttocks in adults; in midlateral thigh in infants and small children. Avoid injection into or near major nerves or blood vessels to prevent permanent neurovascular damage.

▶ Drug is given at least 1 hour before a bacteriostatic antibiotic.

▶ Drug's extremely slow absorption time makes allergic reactions difficult to treat.

▶ Patient must be observed closely. With large doses and prolonged therapy, bacterial or fungal superinfection may occur, especially in elderly, debilitated, or immunosuppressed patients.

▶ *Alert:* Don't confuse drug with polycillin, penicillamine, or the various types of penicillin.

Patient teaching

▶ Report adverse reactions promptly. Fever and eosinophilia are the most common reactions.

▶ I.M. injection may be painful, but ice applied to the site may ease discomfort.

penicillin G potassium (benzylpenicillin potassium)

Megacillin , Pfizerpen

Pregnancy Risk Category B

HOW SUPPLIED

Tablets: 500,000 U
Oral suspension: 250,000 U , 500,000 U
Injection: 1 million U, 5 million U, 10 million U, 20 million U
Premixed injection: 1 million U/50 ml, 2 million U/50 ml, 3 million U/50 ml

ACTION

A natural penicillin that inhibits cell-wall synthesis during microorganism multiplication. Bacteria resist penicillins by producing penicillinases—enzymes that convert penicillins to inactive penicillic acid.

Route	Onset	Peak	Duration
P.O.	Unknown	30-60 min	Unknown
I.V.	Immediate	Immediate	Unknown
I.M.	Unknown	15-30 min	Unknown

INDICATIONS & DOSAGE

Moderate to severe systemic infection —
Adults and children ages 12 and older: highly individualized; 1.6 to 3.2 million U P.O. daily in divided doses q 6 hours; 1.2 to 24 million U I.M. or I.V. daily in divided doses q 4 to 6 hours.
Children under age 12: 25,000 to 100,000 U/kg P.O. daily in divided doses q 6 hours; or 25,000 to 400,000 U/kg I.M. or I.V. daily in divided doses q 4 to 6 hours.

ADVERSE REACTIONS

CNS: neuropathy, *seizures,* lethargy, hallucinations, anxiety, confusion, agitation, depression, dizziness, fatigue.
CV: thrombophlebitis.

GI: nausea, vomiting, enterocolitis, pseudomembranous colitis.
GU: interstitial nephritis, nephropathy.
Hematologic: hemolytic anemia, *leukopenia, thrombocytopenia,* anemia, eosinophilia, *agranulocytosis.*
Metabolic: *possible severe potassium poisoning.*
Other: *hypersensitivity reactions, maculopapular eruptions, exfoliative dermatitis, anaphylaxis,* overgrowth of nonsusceptible organisms, pain at injection site.

INTERACTIONS

Drug-drug. *Aminoglycosides:* physical and chemical incompatibility. Drugs should be administered separately.
Colestipol: decreased serum levels of penicillin G potassium. Penicillin G potassium is administered 1 hour before or 4 hours after colestipol.
Oral contraceptives: efficacy of oral contraceptives may be decreased. An additional form of contraception should be recommended during penicillin therapy.
Potassium-sparing diuretics: possible increased risk of hyperkalemia. Don't use together.
Probenecid: increased blood levels of penicillin. Probenecid may be used for this purpose.

EFFECTS ON DIAGNOSTIC TESTS

Penicillin G interferes with turbidimetric methods using sulfosalicylic acid, trichloroacetic acid, acetic acid, and nitric acid. It does not interfere with tests using bromphenol blue (Albustix, Albutest, Multistix). Drug alters urine glucose testing using cupric sulfate (Benedict's reagent); use Diastix or Chemstrip uG instead. Penicillin G may cause falsely elevated results of urine specific gravity tests in patients with low urine output and dehydration and falsely elevated Norymberski and Zimmerman tests results for 17-ketogenic steroids. It causes false-positive CSF protein test results (Folin-Ciocalteau method) and may cause positive Coombs' test results. Drug may falsely decrease serum aminoglycoside levels. Adding beta-lactamase to the sample inactivates the penicillin, rendering the assay more accurate. Or, the sample can be spun down and frozen immediately after collection.

CONTRAINDICATIONS

Contraindicated in patients with hypersensitivity to drug or other penicillins.

SPECIAL CONSIDERATIONS

▶ Use cautiously in patients with other drug allergies, especially to cephalosporins (possible cross-sensitivity).
▶ Before drug is given, the patient must be asked about previous allergic reactions to penicillin. However, a negative history of penicillin allergy is no guarantee against a future allergic reaction.
▶ A specimen for culture and sensitivity tests should be obtained before giving first dose. Therapy may begin pending results.
▶ For I.M. injection, drug is administered deeply into large muscle; may be extremely painful.
▶ Drug is administered 1 to 2 hours before or 2 to 3 hours after meals. When given orally, drug may cause GI disturbances. Food may interfere with absorption.
▶ Penicillin G potassium is given at least 1 hour before a bacteriostatic antibiotic.
▶ Renal function should be monitored closely. Patients with poor renal function are predisposed to high blood levels of drug.
▶ Serum potassium and sodium levels must be monitored closely in patients receiving more than 10 million U I.V. daily.
▶ Patient must be monitored closely. With large doses and prolonged therapy, bacterial or fungal superinfection may occur, especially in elderly, debilitated, or immunosuppressed patients.
▶ *Alert:* Seizure precautions must be insti-

tuted. Patients with high blood levels of drug may develop seizures.
▶ *Alert:* Don't confuse drug with polycillin, penicillamine, or the various types of penicillin.

I.V. administration

▶ Drug is reconstituted with sterile water for injection, D_5W, or normal saline for injection. Volume of diluent varies with manufacturer.
▶ Drug is given via intermittent I.V. infusion over 30 minutes to 2 hours.

Patient teaching

▶ If taking oral form, take entire amount exactly as prescribed, even after feeling better.
▶ Take oral drug on empty stomach.
▶ Notify health care provider if rash, fever, or chills develop. Rash is the most common allergic reaction.
▶ I.M. injection may be painful, but ice applied to the site may help alleviate discomfort.

penicillin G procaine (benzylpenicillin procaine)
Ayercillin , Wycillin
Pregnancy Risk Category B

HOW SUPPLIED
Injection: 600,000U/ml, 1,200,000 U/ml, 2,400,000 U/ml

ACTION
A natural penicillin that inhibits cell-wall synthesis during microorganism multiplication. Bacteria resist penicillins by producing penicillinases—enzymes that convert penicillins to inactive penicillic acid.

Route	Onset	Peak	Duration
I.M.	Unknown	1-4 hr	1-5 days

INDICATIONS & DOSAGE

Moderate to severe systemic infection —
Adults: 600,000 to 1.2 million U I.M. daily in a single dose.
Children over age 1 month: 25,000 to 50,000 U/kg I.M. daily in a single dose.
Uncomplicated gonorrhea —
Adults and children weighing 45 kg (99 lb): 1 g probenecid P.O.; after 30 minutes, 4.8 million U of penicillin G procaine I.M., divided between two injection sites as a single dose.
Pneumococcal pneumonia —
Adults and children over age 12: 600,000 to 1 million U I.M. daily for 7 to 10 days.

ADVERSE REACTIONS

CNS: *seizures,* lethargy, hallucinations, anxiety, confusion, agitation, depression, dizziness, fatigue.
GI: nausea, vomiting, enterocolitis, pseudomembranous colitis.
GU: interstitial nephritis, nephropathy.
Hematologic: *thrombocytopenia, hemolytic anemia, leukopenia,* anemia, eosinophilia, *agranulocytosis.*
Musculoskeletal: arthralgia.
Other: *hypersensitivity reactions, anaphylaxis,* overgrowth of nonsusceptible organisms.

INTERACTIONS

Drug-drug. *Aminoglycosides:* physical and chemical incompatibility. Separate administration times.
Colestipol: decreased serum concentrations of penicillin G procaine. Penicillin G procaine should be administered 1 hour before or 4 hours after colestipol.
Oral contraceptives: efficacy of oral contraceptives may be decreased. Additional form of contraception is recommended during penicillin therapy.
Probenecid: increased blood levels of penicillin. Probenecid may be used for this purpose.

EFFECTS ON DIAGNOSTIC TESTS

Penicillin G interferes with turbidimetric methods using sulfosalicylic acid, trichloroacetic acid, acetic acid, and nitric acid. Drug does not interfere with tests using bromphenol blue (Albustix, Albutest, Multistix). Penicillin G alters urine glucose testing using cupric sulfate (Benedict's reagent); use Diastix instead. Penicillin G may cause falsely elevated results of urine specific gravity tests in patients with low urine output and dehydration and falsely elevated Norymberski and Zimmerman tests results for 17-ketogenic steroids. It causes false-positive CSF protein test results (Folin-Ciocalteau method) and may cause positive Coombs' test results. Drug may falsely decrease serum aminoglycoside levels. Adding beta-lactamase to the sample inactivates the penicillin, rendering the assay more accurate. Or, the sample can be spun down and frozen immediately after collection.

CONTRAINDICATIONS

Contraindicated in patients with hypersensitivity to drug or other penicillins.

SPECIAL CONSIDERATIONS

▶ Use cautiously in patients with other drug allergies, especially to cephalosporins (possible cross-sensitivity). Some formulations contain sulfites, which may cause allergic reactions in sensitive persons.
▶ Before drug is given, patient must be asked about previous allergic reactions to penicillin. However, a negative history of penicillin allergy is no guarantee against a future allergic reaction.
▶ A specimen for culture and sensitivity tests should be obtained before giving first dose. Therapy may begin pending results.
▶ Deep I.M. injections are given in upper outer quadrant of buttocks in adults; in midlateral thigh in small children. S.C. injections are not given. Injection site should not be massaged. Injection near major nerves or blood vessels should be avoid-

ed to prevent permanent neurovascular damage.

▶ **Alert:** Do not give drug I.V. Inadvertent I.V. administration has resulted in death due to CNS toxicity due to penicillin G procaine.

▶ Drug is given at least 1 hour before a bacteriostatic antibiotic.

▶ Allergic reactions are hard to treat because of drug's slow absorption rate.

▶ Renal and hematopoietic function must be monitored periodically.

▶ Patient must be observed closely. With large doses and prolonged therapy, bacterial or fungal superinfection may occur, especially in elderly, debilitated, or immunosuppressed patients.

▶ **Alert:** Don't confuse drug with polycillin, penicillamine, or the various types of penicillin.

Patient teaching
▶ Report adverse reactions promptly. Rash is the most common allergic reaction.

▶ I.M. injection may be painful, but ice applied to the site may help alleviate discomfort.

penicillin G sodium (benzylpenicillin sodium)
Crystapen
Pregnancy Risk Category B

HOW SUPPLIED
Injection: 5 million-U vial

ACTION
A natural penicillin that inhibits cell-wall synthesis during active multiplication. Bacteria resist penicillins by producing penicillinases — enzymes that convert penicillins to inactive penicillic acid.

Route	Onset	Peak	Duration
I.V.	Immediate	Immediate	Unknown
I.M.	Unknown	15-30 min	Unknown

INDICATIONS & DOSAGE
Moderate to severe systemic infection —
Adults and children ages 12 and older: 1.2 to 24 million U daily I.M. or I.V. in divided doses q 4 to 6 hours.
Children under age 12: 25,000 to 400,000 U/kg daily I.M. or I.V. in divided doses q 4 to 6 hours.

ADVERSE REACTIONS
CNS: neuropathy, *seizures,* lethargy, hallucinations, anxiety, confusion, agitation, depression, dizziness, fatigue.
CV: *heart failure,* thrombophlebitis, vein irritation.
GI: nausea, vomiting, enterocolitis, pseudomembranous colitis.
GU: interstitial colitis, nephropathy.
Hematologic: hemolytic anemia, *leukopenia, thrombocytopenia, agranulocytosis,* anemia, eosinophilia.
Musculoskeletal: arthralgia.
Other: *hypersensitivity reactions, anaphylaxis,* overgrowth of nonsusceptible organisms, pain at injection site.

INTERACTIONS
Drug-drug. *Aminoglycosides:* physical and chemical incompatibility. Separate administration times.
Colestipol: decreased serum levels of penicillin G sodium. Penicillin G sodium should be administered 1 hour before or 4 hours after colestipol.
Oral contraceptives: efficacy of oral contraceptives may be decreased. An additional form of contraception should be recommended during penicillin therapy.
Probenecid: increased blood levels of penicillin. Probenecid may be used for this purpose.

EFFECTS ON DIAGNOSTIC TESTS
Drug interferes with turbidimetric methods using sulfosalicylic acid, trichloroacetic acid, acetic acid, and nitric acid. Penicillin G does not interfere with tests using bromphenol blue (Albustix, Albutest,

Multistix). Penicillin G alters urine glucose testing using cupric sulfate (Benedict's reagent); use Diastix instead. It may cause falsely elevated results of urine specific gravity tests in patients with low urine output and dehydration and falsely elevated Norymberski and Zimmerman tests results for 17-ketogenic steroids. It causes false-positive CSF protein test results (Folin-Ciocalteau method) and may cause positive Coombs' test results. Drug may falsely decrease serum aminoglycoside levels. Adding beta-lactamase to the sample inactivates the penicillin, rendering the assay more accurate. Or, the sample can be spun down and frozen immediately after collection.

CONTRAINDICATIONS

Contraindicated in patients with hypersensitivity to drug or other penicillins and in those on sodium-restricted diets.

SPECIAL CONSIDERATIONS

▶ Use cautiously in patients with other drug allergies, especially to cephalosporins (possible cross-allergenicity).
▶ Before drug is given, the patient must be asked about previous allergic reactions to penicillin. However, a negative history of penicillin allergy is no guarantee against a future allergic reaction.
▶ A specimen for culture and sensitivity tests should be obtained before giving first dose. Therapy may begin pending results.
▶ Penicillin G sodium should be given at least 1 hour before a bacteriostatic antibiotic.
▶ Patient must be observed closely. With large doses and prolonged therapy, bacterial or fungal superinfection may occur, especially in elderly, debilitated, or immunosuppressed patients.
▶ *Alert:* Seizure precautions should be instituted. Patients with high blood levels of drug may develop seizures.
▶ *Alert:* Don't confuse drug with polycillin,

penicillamine, or the various types of penicillin.

I.V. administration

▶ Drug is reconstituted with sterile water for injection, normal saline for injection, or D_5W. Manufacturer's instructions for volume of diluent necessary to produce desired drug level should be followed.
▶ For intermittent I.V. infusion: Drug is diluted in 50 to 100 ml, and given over 30 minutes to 2 hours q 4 to 6 hours.
▶ In neonates and children, divided doses are given over 15 to 30 minutes.

Patient teaching

▶ Report adverse reactions promptly.
▶ Alert health care provider if discomfort occurs at I.V. site.
▶ I.M. injection may be painful, but ice applied to site may help alleviate discomfort.

penicillin V potassium (phenoxymethylpenicillin potassium)

Abbocillin VK‡, Apo-Pen VK, Beepen-VK, Cilicaine VK‡, Nadopen-V-200, Nadopen-V-400, Novo-Pen-VK, Nu-Pen-VK, Pen Vee, Pen Vee K, PVF K, PVK‡, V-Cillin K, Veetids**

Pregnancy Risk Category B

HOW SUPPLIED

Tablets: 250 mg, 500 mg
Tablets (film-coated): 250 mg, 500 mg
Capsules: 250 mg‡
Oral suspension: 125 mg/5 ml, 250 mg/5 ml (after reconstitution)

ACTION

A natural penicillin that inhibits cell-wall synthesis during microorganism multiplication. Bacteria resist penicillins by producing penicillinases—enzymes that convert penicillins to inactive penicillic acid.

Route	Onset	Peak	Duration
P.O.	Unknown	0.5-1 hr	Unknown

INDICATIONS & DOSAGE

Mild to moderate systemic infections —
Adults and children ages 12 and older: 125 to 500 mg (400,000 to 800,000 U) P.O. q 6 hours.
Children under age 12: 15 to 62.5 mg/kg (25,000 to 100,000 U/kg) P.O. daily in divided doses q 6 to 8 hours.

ADVERSE REACTIONS

CNS: neuropathy.
GI: *epigastric distress,* vomiting, diarrhea, *nausea,* black "hairy" tongue.
GU: nephropathy.
Hematologic: eosinophilia, hemolytic anemia, *leukopenia, thrombocytopenia.*
Other: *hypersensitivity reactions, anaphylaxis,* overgrowth of nonsusceptible organisms.

INTERACTIONS

Drug-drug. *Oral contraceptives:* efficacy of oral contraceptives may be decreased. An additional form of contraception is recommended during penicillin therapy.
Probenecid: increased blood levels of penicillin. Probenecid may be used for this purpose.

EFFECTS ON DIAGNOSTIC TESTS

Drug interferes with turbidimetric methods using sulfosalicylic acid, trichloroacetic acid, acetic acid, and nitric acid. It does not interfere with tests using bromphenol blue (Albustix, Albutest, Multistix).

CONTRAINDICATIONS

Contraindicated in patients with hypersensitivity to drug or other penicillins.

SPECIAL CONSIDERATIONS

▶ Use cautiously in patients with other drug allergies, especially to cephalosporins (possible cross-sensitivity), and in those with GI disturbances.
▶ Before drug is given, patient must be asked about previous allergic reactions to penicillins. However, a negative history of penicillin allergy is no guarantee against a future allergic reaction.
▶ A specimen for culture and sensitivity tests should be obtained before giving first dose. Therapy may begin pending results.
▶ Drug should be given at least 1 hour before a bacteriostatic antibiotic.
▶ Renal and hematopoietic function must periodically be assessed in patients receiving long-term therapy.
▶ Patient must be observed closely. With large doses and prolonged therapy, bacterial or fungal superinfection may occur, especially in elderly, debilitated, or immunosuppressed patients.
▶ The American Heart Association considers amoxicillin the preferred agent for endocarditis prophylaxis because GI absorption is better and serum levels are sustained longer. Penicillin V is considered an alternative agent.
▶ *Alert:* Don't confuse drug with polycillin, penicillamine, or the various types of penicillin.

Patient teaching

▶ Take entire quantity of drug exactly as prescribed, even after feeling better.
▶ Take drug with food if stomach upset occurs.
▶ Notify health care provider if rash, fever, or chills develop. Rash is the most common allergic reaction.

piperacillin sodium

Pipracil, Pipril‡

Pregnancy Risk Category B

HOW SUPPLIED
Injection: 2 g, 3 g, 4 g, 40 g

ACTION
Extended-spectrum penicillin that inhibits cell-wall synthesis during microorganism multiplication. Bacteria resist penicillins by producing penicillinases—enzymes that convert penicillins to inactive penicillic acid.

Route	Onset	Peak	Duration
I.V.	Immediate	Immediate	Unknown
I.M.	Unknown	30-50 min	Unknown

INDICATIONS & DOSAGE
Systemic infections due to susceptible strains of gram-positive and especially gram-negative organisms (including Proteus and Pseudomonas aeruginosa) —
Adults and children over age 12: 100 to 300 mg/kg (may go up to 600 mg/kg/day in cystic fibrosis patients) I.V. or I.M. daily in divided doses q 4 to 6 hours, not to exceed 24 g daily.
Prophylaxis of surgical infections —
Adults: 2 g I.V., given 30 to 60 minutes before surgery. Dose may be repeated during surgery and once or twice more after surgery.
Dosage adjustment: For patients with creatinine clearance of 20 to 40 ml/minute, 3 to 4 g I.V. q 8 hours; if creatinine clearance is below 20 ml/minute, 3 to 4 g I.V. q 12 hours depending on severity of infection.

ADVERSE REACTIONS
CNS: *seizures,* headache, dizziness, fatigue.
CV: vein irritation, phlebitis.
GI: nausea, diarrhea, vomiting, pseudomembranous colitis.

GU: interstitial nephritis.
Hematologic: *bleeding, neutropenia,* eosinophilia, *leukopenia, thrombocytopenia.*
Hepatic: transient elevations in liver function tests.
Metabolic: *hypokalemia,* hypernatremia.
Musculoskeletal: prolonged muscle relaxation.
Other: *hypersensitivity reactions, anaphylaxis,* overgrowth of nonsusceptible organisms, pain at injection site.

INTERACTIONS
Drug-drug. *Oral contraceptives:* efficacy of oral contraceptives may be decreased. An additional form of contraception should be recommended during penicillin therapy.
Probenecid: increased blood levels of piperacillin. Probenecid may be used for this purpose.
Vecuronium: prolonged neuromuscular blockade: Don't use together.

EFFECTS ON DIAGNOSTIC TESTS
Drug may falsely decrease serum aminoglycoside levels and may cause positive Coombs' tests.

CONTRAINDICATIONS
Contraindicated in patients with hypersensitivity to drug or other penicillins.

SPECIAL CONSIDERATIONS
▶ Use cautiously in patients with other drug allergies, especially to cephalosporins (possible cross-sensitivity), and in those with bleeding tendencies, uremia, and hypokalemia.
▶ Before drug is given, patient must be asked about previous allergic reactions to penicillin. However, a negative history of penicillin allergy is no guarantee against a future allergic reaction.
▶ A specimen for culture and sensitivity tests should be obtained before giving first dose. Therapy may begin pending results.

Reactions may be *common,* uncommon, *life-threatening,* or COMMON AND LIFE-THREATENING.

▶ Piperacillin should be given at least 1 hour before a bacteriostatic antibiotic.

▶ For I.M. injection, drug is reconstituted with sterile or bacteriostatic water for injection, normal saline for injection (with or without preservative), or 0.5% to 1% lidocaine hydrochloride. 2 ml of diluent is added for each gram of drug. Final solution will contain 1 g/2.5 ml.

▶ CBC and platelet counts are checked frequently. Drug may cause thrombocytopenia.

▶ Serum potassium and sodium levels should be monitored.

▶ INR must be monitored in patients receiving warfarin therapy because drug may prolong PT.

▶ *Alert:* Seizure precautions should be instituted. Patients with high serum levels of drug may have seizures.

▶ Patient must be observed closely. With large doses and prolonged therapy, bacterial or fungal superinfection may occur, especially in elderly, debilitated, or immunosuppressed patients.

▶ Patients with cystic fibrosis tend to be most susceptible to fever or rash.

▶ Drug may be better suited for patients on sodium-free diets than ticarcillin (piperacillin contains 1.85 mEq of sodium/g).

▶ Keep in mind that piperacillin is typically used with another antibiotic such as gentamicin.

I.V. administration

▶ Each gram of drug is reconstituted with 5 ml of diluent, such as sterile or bacteriostatic water for injection, normal saline for injection (with or without preservative), D_5W, or dextrose 5% in normal saline for injection. Mixture is shaken until dissolved. Reconstituted solution is then injected directly into a vein or into the tubing of a free-flowing I.V. solution over 3 to 5 minutes. Or, the solution may be diluted with at least 50 ml of a compatible I.V. solution, and given by intermittent infusion over 30 minutes.

▶ Continuous infusions should be avoided to prevent vein irritation. Site is changed every 48 hours.

▶ Aminoglycoside antibiotics, such as gentamicin and tobramycin, are chemically incompatible with piperacillin. These agents should not be mixed in the same I.V. container.

Patient teaching

▶ Report adverse reactions promptly.

▶ Report discomfort at I.V. site.

▶ Limit salt intake during therapy because drug contains 1.85 mEq of sodium/g.

piperacillin sodium/ tazobactam sodium

Zosyn

Pregnancy Risk Category B

HOW SUPPLIED

Powder for injection: 2 g piperacillin and 0.25 g tazobactam per vial, 3 g piperacillin and 0.375 g tazobactam per vial, 4 g piperacillin and 0.5 g tazobactam per vial

ACTION

Piperacillin is an extended-spectrum penicillin that inhibits cell-wall synthesis during microorganism multiplication. Tazobactam increases piperacillin's effectiveness by inactivating beta-lactamases, which destroy penicillins.

Route	Onset	Peak	Duration
I.V.	Immediate	Immediate	Unknown

INDICATIONS & DOSAGE

Appendicitis (complicated by rupture or abscess) and peritonitis due to Escherichia coli, Bacteroides fragilis, B. ovatus, B. thetaiotaomicron, *or* B. vulgatus; *skin and skin-structure infections due to* Staphylococcus aureus; *postpartum endometritis or pelvic inflammatory disease*

due to E. coli; *moderately severe community-acquired pneumonia due to* Haemophilus influenzae —
Adults: 3 g piperacillin and 0.375 g tazobactam I.V. q 6 hours.
Dosage adjustment: For renally impaired adults with creatinine clearance of 20 to 40 ml/minute, dosage is 2 g piperacillin and 0.25 g tazobactam I.V. q 6 hours; if it is below 20 ml/minute, 2 g piperacillin and 0.25 g tazobactam I.V. q 8 hours.

Nosocomial pneumonia (moderate to severe) due to piperacillin-resistant, beta-lactamase-producing strains of S. aureus —
Adults: initially, 3.375g I.V. over 30 minutes q 4 hours. Administer with an aminoglycoside.

ADVERSE REACTIONS

CNS: *headache, insomnia,* agitation, dizziness, anxiety.
CV: hypertension, tachycardia, chest pain, edema; inflammation, phlebitis at I.V. site.
EENT: rhinitis.
GI: *diarrhea, nausea, constipation,* vomiting, dyspepsia, stool changes, abdominal pain.
GU: interstitial nephritis, candidiasis.
Hematologic: *leukopenia,* anemia, eosinophilia, ***thrombocytopenia.***
Respiratory: dyspnea.
Skin: rash, pruritus.
Other: fever; pain, ***anaphylaxis.***

INTERACTIONS

Drug-drug. *Oral anticoagulants:* prolonged effectiveness. PT and INR must be monitored closely.
Oral contraceptives: efficacy of oral contraceptives may be decreased. An additional form of contraception should be recommended during penicillin therapy.
Probenecid: increased blood levels of piperacillin. Probenecid may be used for this purpose.
Vecuronium: prolonged neuromuscular blockade. Monitor closely.

EFFECTS ON DIAGNOSTIC TESTS

As with other penicillins, piperacillin/tazobactam may result in a false-positive reaction for urine glucose using a copper reduction method (such as Clinitest). Glucose tests based on enzymatic glucose oxidase reactions (such as Diastix) are recommended.

CONTRAINDICATIONS

Contraindicated in patients with hypersensitivity to drug or other penicillins.

SPECIAL CONSIDERATIONS

▶ Use cautiously in patients with other drug allergies, especially to cephalosporins (possible cross-sensitivity), and in those with bleeding tendencies, uremia, and hypokalemia.
▶ A specimen for culture and sensitivity tests should be obtained before giving first dose. Therapy may begin pending results.
▶ Because hemodialysis removes 6% of the piperacillin dose and 21% of the tazobactam dose, supplemental doses may be needed after hemodialysis.
▶ Patient must be observed closely. With large doses and prolonged therapy, bacterial and fungal superinfection may occur, especially in elderly, debilitated, or immunosuppressed patients.
▶ Drug contains 2.35 mEq sodium/g; patient's sodium intake needs to be monitored.
▶ There appears to be an increase of fever and rash in patients with cystic fibrosis.

I.V. administration

▶ Each gram of piperacillin is reconstituted with 5 ml of diluent, such as sterile or bacteriostatic water for injection, normal saline for injection, bacteriostatic normal saline for injection, D_5W, dextrose 5% in normal saline for injection, or dextran 6% in normal saline for injection. Lactated Ringer's injection is not used. Mixture is shaken until dissolved. The solution is further diluted to a final volume of 50 ml before infusion.

▶ Drug is infused over at least 30 minutes. Any primary infusion is discontinued during administration if possible. Piperacillin should not be mixed with other drugs. Aminoglycoside antibiotics (such as amikacin, gentamicin, and tobramycin) are chemically incompatible with this drug. These agents should not be mixed in the same I.V. container.

▶ The drug should be used immediately after reconstitution. Unused drug is discarded after 24 hours if stored at room temperature or 48 hours if refrigerated. Once diluted, drug is stable in I.V. bags for 24 hours at room temperature or 1 week if refrigerated.

▶ I.V. site is changed every 48 hours.

Patient teaching

▶ Report adverse reactions promptly.
▶ Alert health care provider if discomfort occurs at I.V. site.

ticarcillin disodium

Ticar

Pregnancy Risk Category B

HOW SUPPLIED

Injection: 1 g, 3 g, 6 g
I.V. infusion: 3 g

ACTION

An extended-spectrum penicillin that inhibits cell-wall synthesis during microorganism multiplication. Bacteria resist penicillins by producing penicillinases—enzymes that convert penicillins to inactive penicillic acid.

Route	Onset	Peak	Duration
I.V.	Immediate	Immediate	Unknown
I.M.	Unknown	30-75 min	Unknown

INDICATIONS & DOSAGE

Severe systemic infections due to susceptible strains of gram-positive and especially gram-negative organisms (including Pseudomonas *and* Proteus*) —*
Adults: 200 to 300 mg/kg I.V. daily in divided doses q 4 to 6 hours.
Children: 50 to 300 mg/kg I.V. daily in divided doses q 4 to 6 hours.
Dosage adjustment: For patients with renal failure, if creatinine clearance is 30 to 60 ml/minute, dosage is 2 g I.V. q 4 hours; if clearance is 10 to 29 ml/minute, 2 g I.V. q 8 hours; and if it is below 10 ml/minute, 2 g I.V. q 12 hours or 1 g I.M. q 6 hours.

ADVERSE REACTIONS

CNS: *seizures,* neuromuscular excitability.
CV: vein irritation, phlebitis.
GI: nausea, diarrhea, vomiting, pseudomembranous colitis.
Hematologic: *leukopenia, neutropenia,* eosinophilia, *thrombocytopenia,* hemolytic anemia.
Hepatic: transient elevations in liver function studies.
Metabolic: hypokalemia, hypernatremia.
Other: *hypersensitivity reactions, anaphylaxis,* overgrowth of nonsusceptible organisms, pain at injection site.

INTERACTIONS

Drug-drug. *Lithium:* altered renal elimination of lithium. Serum lithium levels should be monitored closely.
Oral contraceptives: efficacy of oral contraceptives may be decreased. An additional form of contraception should be recommended during penicillin therapy.
Probenecid: increased blood levels of ticarcillin and other penicillins. Probenecid may be used for this purpose.

EFFECTS ON DIAGNOSTIC TESTS

Ticarcillin interferes with turbidimetric methods that use sulfosalicylic acid, trichloroacetic acid, acetic acid, or nitric acid. Ticarcillin does not interfere with tests using bromphenol blue (Albustix, Albutest, Multistix). Ticarcillin may falsely decrease serum aminoglycoside concentrations. Systemic effects of ticarcillin may cause positive Coombs' test.

CONTRAINDICATIONS
Contraindicated in patients with hypersensitivity to drug or other penicillins.

SPECIAL CONSIDERATIONS
▶ Use cautiously in patients with other drug allergies, especially to cephalosporins (possible cross-sensitivity), and in those with impaired renal function, hemorrhagic conditions, hypokalemia, or sodium restrictions (drug contains 5.2 to 6.5 mEq sodium/g).
▶ Before drug is given, the patient must be asked about previous allergic reactions to penicillin. However, a negative history of penicillin allergy is no guarantee against a future allergic reaction.
▶ A specimen for culture and sensitivity tests should be obtained before giving first dose. Therapy may begin pending results.
▶ Ticarcillin should be given at least 1 hour before a bacteriostatic antibiotic.
▶ For I.M. injection, drug is reconstituted using sterile water for injection, normal saline for injection, or lidocaine 1% (without epinephrine). 2 ml diluent is used for each gram of drug. Drug is administered deep I.M. into large muscle. Don't exceed 2 g per injection.
▶ Serum potassium and sodium levels must be monitored.
▶ CBC and platelet counts are monitored frequently. Drug may cause thrombocytopenia.
▶ *Alert:* Seizure precautions should be instituted. Patients with high blood levels of ticarcillin may develop seizures.
▶ Ticarcillin is typically used with another antibiotic such as gentamicin.
▶ Patient must be observed closely. With large doses and prolonged therapy, bacte-

rial or fungal superinfection may occur, especially in elderly, debilitated, or immunosuppressed patients.
▶ INR is monitored in patients receiving warfarin therapy because drug may prolong PT.

I.V. administration
▶ Drug is reconstituted using D_5W, normal saline injection, sterile water for injection, or other compatible solution. 4 ml of diluent is added for each gram of drug. Mixture is further diluted to a maximum concentration of 50 mg/ml, and then injected slowly directly into a vein or into the tubing of a free-flowing I.V. solution. Or, solution may be diluted to a concentration of 10 to 100 mg/ml, and given by intermittent infusion over 30 to 120 minutes in adults or 10 to 20 minutes in neonates.
▶ Aminoglycoside antibiotics (such as amikacin, gentamicin, and tobramycin) are chemically incompatible with this drug. These agents should not be mixed in the same I.V. container.
▶ Continuous infusion should be avoided to prevent vein irritation. Site is changed every 48 hours.

Patient teaching
▶ Report adverse reactions promptly.
▶ Alert health care provider if discomfort occurs at I.V. insertion site.

ticarcillin disodium/ clavulanate potassium
Timentin
Pregnancy Risk Category B

HOW SUPPLIED
Injection: 3 g ticarcillin and 100 mg clavulanic acid in 3.1-g and 31-g vials
Premixed: 3.1 g/100 ml

ACTION

Ticarcillin is an extended-spectrum penicillin that inhibits cell-wall synthesis during microorganism replication. Clavulanic acid increases ticarcillin's effectiveness by inactivating beta-lactamases, which destroy ticarcillin.

Route	Onset	Peak	Duration
I.V.	Immediate	Immediate	Unknown

INDICATIONS & DOSAGE

Lower respiratory tract, urinary tract, bone and joint, and skin and skin-structure infections and septicemia when due to beta-lactamase-producing strains of bacteria or by ticarcillin-susceptible organisms —
Adults: 3.1 g (3 g ticarcillin and 100 mg clavulanic acid) administered by I.V. infusion q 4 to 6 hours.
Dosage adjustment: For patients with renal failure, if creatinine clearance is 30 to 60 ml/minute, dosage is 2 g I.V. q 4 hours; if it is 10 to 29 ml/minute, 2 g I.V. q 8 hours; and if it is below 10 ml/minute, 2 g I.V. q 12 hours (with hepatic dysfunction, q 24 hours).

ADVERSE REACTIONS

CNS: *seizures,* neuromuscular excitability, headache, giddiness.
CV: vein irritation, phlebitis.
GI: nausea, diarrhea, stomatitis, vomiting, epigastric pain, flatulence, pseudomembranous colitis, taste and smell disturbances.
Hematologic: *leukopenia, neutropenia,* eosinophilia, *thrombocytopenia,* hemolytic anemia, anemia.
Hepatic: transient elevations in liver function studies.
Metabolic: hypokalemia, hypernatremia.
Other: *hypersensitivity reactions, anaphylaxis,* overgrowth of nonsusceptible organisms, pain at injection site.

INTERACTIONS

Drug-drug. *Oral contraceptives:* efficacy of oral contraceptives may be decreased. An additional form of contraception should be recommended during penicillin therapy.
Probenecid: increased blood levels of ticarcillin. Probenecid may be used for this purpose.

EFFECTS ON DIAGNOSTIC TESTS

Drug interferes with turbidimetric methods that use sulfosalicylic acid, trichloroacetic acid, acetic acid, or nitric acid. Drug does not interfere with tests using bromphenol blue (Albustix, Albutest, Multistix). Systemic effects of drug may cause positive Coombs' test.

CONTRAINDICATIONS

Contraindicated in patients with hypersensitivity to drug or other penicillins.

SPECIAL CONSIDERATIONS

▶ Use cautiously in patients with other drug allergies, especially to cephalosporins (possible cross-sensitivity), and in those with impaired renal function, hemorrhagic conditions, hypokalemia, or sodium restrictions (drug contains 4.5 mEq sodium/g).
▶ Before drug is given, the patient must be asked about previous allergic reactions to penicillin. However, a negative history of penicillin allergy is no guarantee against a future allergic reaction.
▶ A specimen for culture and sensitivity tests should be obtained before giving first dose. Therapy may begin pending results.
▶ Drug should be given at least 1 hour before a bacteriostatic antibiotic.
▶ CBC and platelet counts are checked frequently. Drug may cause thrombocytopenia.
▶ Serum potassium must be monitored.
▶ The patient must be observed closely. With large doses and prolonged therapy, bacterial or fungal superinfection may occur, especially in elderly, debilitated, or immunosuppressed patients.

---

*Liquid contains alcohol.   **May contain tartrazine.   †Canada   ‡Australia   §U.K.   ◇OTC

I.V. administration

▶ Drug is reconstituted with 13 ml of sterile water for injection or normal saline for injection. The mixture is further diluted to a maximum of 10 to 100 mg/ml (based on ticarcillin component), and administered by I.V. infusion over 30 minutes. In fluid restricted patients, maximum dilution is of 48 mg/ml if using D_5W, 43 mg/ml if using normal saline for injection, or 86 mg/ml if using sterile water for injection.

▶ Drug is chemically incompatible with aminoglycoside antibiotics (amikacin, gentamicin, tobramycin). These agents should not be mixed in the same I.V. container.

Patient teaching

▶ Report adverse reactions promptly.
▶ Alert health care provider if discomfort occurs at I.V. site.
▶ Limit salt intake during drug therapy because of high sodium content.

cefaclor
cefadroxil
cefazolin sodium
cefdinir
cefepime hydrochloride
cefixime
cefmetazole sodium
cefonicid sodium
cefoperazone sodium
cefotaxime sodium
cefotetan disodium
cefoxitin sodium
cefpodoxime proxetil
cefprozil
ceftazidime
ceftibuten
ceftizoxime sodium
ceftriaxone sodium
cefuroxime axetil
cefuroxime sodium
cephalexin hydrochloride
cephalexin monohydrate
cephradine
loracarbef

COMBINATION PRODUCTS
None.

---

cefaclor

Ceclor, Distaclor§, Distaclor MR§

Pregnancy Risk Category B

HOW SUPPLIED
Capsules: 250 mg, 500 mg
Tablets (extended-release): 375 mg,
500 mg
Oral suspension: 125 mg/5 ml, 187 mg/
5 ml, 250 mg/5 ml, 375 mg/5 ml

ACTION
A second-generation cephalosporin that
inhibits cell-wall synthesis, promoting osmotic instability; usually bactericidal.

Route	Onset	Peak	Duration
P.O.	Unknown	0.5-1 hr	Unknown
P.O. (extended)	Unknown	1.5-2.5 hr	Unknown

INDICATIONS & DOSAGE
*Respiratory or urinary tract, skin, and
soft-tissue infections and otitis media due
to* Haemophilus influenzae, Streptococcus pneumoniae, S. pyogenes, Escherichia
coli, Proteus mirabilis, Klebsiella species,
and staphylococci —
Adults: 250 to 500 mg P.O. q 8 hours. For
pharyngitis or otitis media, daily dose may
be given in two equally divided doses
q 12 hours. For extended-release forms,
500 mg P.O. q 12 hours for 7 days for bronchitis; for pharyngitis or skin and skin-
structure infections, 375 mg P.O. q 12
hours for 10 days and 7 to 10 days, respectively.
Children: 20 mg/kg daily P.O. in divided doses q 8 hours. For pharyngitis or otitis media, daily dose may be given in two
equally divided doses q 12 hours. In more
serious infections, 40 mg/kg daily are
recommended, not to exceed 1 g daily.

ADVERSE REACTIONS
CNS: dizziness, headache, somnolence,
malaise.
GI: *nausea,* vomiting, *diarrhea,* anorexia, dyspepsia, abdominal cramps, pseudomembranous colitis, oral candidiasis.
GU: vaginal candidiasis, vaginitis.
Hematologic: *transient leukopenia,* anemia, eosinophilia, *thrombocytopenia,* lymphocytosis.
Hepatic: transient increases in liver enzymes.
Skin: *maculopapular rash,* dermatitis,
pruritus.

---

*Liquid contains alcohol.   **May contain tartrazine.   †Canada   ‡Australia   §U.K.   ◊OTC

Other: *hypersensitivity reactions (serum sickness, **anaphylaxis**), fever.*

INTERACTIONS

Drug-drug. *Antacids:* absorption of extended-release cefaclor is decreased if taken within 1 hour. Administration times are separated by 1 hour.
Chloramphenicol: antagonistic effect. Don't use together.
Probenecid: may inhibit excretion and increase blood levels of cefaclor. Monitor patient.

EFFECTS ON DIAGNOSTIC TESTS

Cefaclor may cause false-positive Coombs' test results and false-positive results in urine glucose tests using cupric sulfate (Benedict's reagent or Clinitest); use glucose oxidase tests (Diastix or Chemstrip uG) instead. Drug also causes false elevations in serum or urine creatinine levels in tests using Jaffé's reaction.

CONTRAINDICATIONS

Contraindicated in patients with hypersensitivity to drug or other cephalosporins.

SPECIAL CONSIDERATIONS

▶ Use cautiously in patients with impaired renal function or a history of sensitivity to penicillin and in breast-feeding women.
▶ A specimen for culture and sensitivity tests should be obtained before giving first dose. Therapy may begin pending results.
▶ With large doses or prolonged therapy, superinfection may occur, especially in high-risk patients.
▶ Reconstituted suspension is stored in the refrigerator. Suspension is stable for 14 days if refrigerated. Suspension is shaken well before use.
▶ **Alert:** Don't confuse drug with other cephalosporins that sound alike.

Patient teaching

▶ Take entire amount of drug exactly as prescribed, even after feeling better.

▶ Drug may be taken with meals. If taking the suspension, shake the container well before measuring dose, and keep the drug refrigerated.
▶ Notify health care provider if rash develops or signs and symptoms of superinfection appear.
▶ Don't crush, cut, or chew extended-release tablets.

---

cefadroxil

Duricef

Pregnancy Risk Category B

HOW SUPPLIED

Tablets: 1 g
Capsules: 500 mg
Oral suspension: 125 mg/5 ml, 250 mg/5 ml, 500 mg/5 ml

ACTION

A first-generation cephalosporin that inhibits cell-wall synthesis, promoting osmotic instability; usually bactericidal.

Route	Onset	Peak	Duration
P.O.	Unknown	1-2 hr	Unknown

INDICATIONS & DOSAGE

Urinary tract infections due to Escherichia coli, Proteus mirabilis, *and* Klebsiella *species; skin and soft-tissue infections due to staphylococci and streptococci; pharyngitis or tonsillitis due to group A beta-hemolytic streptococci —*
Adults: 1 to 2 g P.O. daily, depending on infection being treated. Usually given once daily or b.i.d.
Children: 30 mg/kg P.O. daily in two divided doses q 12 hours.
Dosage adjustment: For renally impaired patients with creatinine clearance of 25 to 50 ml/minute, 1 g P.O. followed by 500 mg q 12 hours; if clearance is between 10 and

---

24 ml/minute, 500 mg q 24 hours; and if it is below 10 ml/minute, 500 mg q 36 hours.

ADVERSE REACTIONS

CNS: *seizures.*
GI: pseudomembranous colitis, *nausea,* vomiting, *diarrhea,* glossitis, abdominal cramps, oral candidiasis.
GU: genital pruritus, candidiasis, vaginitis, renal dysfunction.
Hematologic: *transient neutropenia,* eosinophilia, *leukopenia,* anemia, *agranulocytosis, thrombocytopenia.*
Hepatic: transient increases in liver enzymes.
Respiratory: dyspnea.
Skin: *maculopapular and erythematous rashes,* urticaria.
Other: *hypersensitivity reactions, anaphylaxis, angioedema,* fever.

INTERACTIONS

Drug-drug. *Probenecid:* may inhibit excretion and increase blood levels of cefadroxil. Use together cautiously.

EFFECTS ON DIAGNOSTIC TESTS

Cefadroxil causes false-positive results in urine glucose tests using cupric sulfate (Benedict's reagent or Clinitest); use glucose oxidase test (Diastix or Chemstrip uG) instead. Drug causes false elevations in serum or urine creatinine levels in tests using Jaffé's reaction. Positive Coombs' test results occur in about 3% of patients taking cephalosporins.

CONTRAINDICATIONS

Contraindicated in patients with hypersensitivity to drug or other cephalosporins.

SPECIAL CONSIDERATIONS

▸ Use cautiously in patients with a history of sensitivity to penicillin and in breast-feeding women. Also, use cautiously in patients with impaired renal function; dosage adjustments may be necessary.
▸ A specimen for culture and sensitivity

tests should be obtained before giving first dose. Therapy may begin pending results.
▸ If creatinine clearance is below 50 ml/minute, dosage interval should be lengthened so drug doesn't accumulate. Renal function is monitored in patients with renal dysfunction.
▸ With large doses or prolonged therapy, superinfection may occur, especially in high-risk patients.
▸ *Alert:* Don't confuse drug with other cephalosporins that sound alike.

Patient teaching

▸ Take drug with food or milk to lessen GI discomfort.
▸ Take entire amount of drug exactly as prescribed, even after feeling better.
▸ Notify health care provider if rash develops or if signs and symptoms of superinfection, such as recurring fever, chills, and malaise appear.

cefazolin sodium

Ancef, Kefzol, Zolicef

Pregnancy Risk Category B

HOW SUPPLIED

Injection (parenteral): 250 mg, 500 mg, 1 g, 5 g, 10 g, 20 g
Infusion: 500 mg/50-ml vial, 1 g/50-ml vial

ACTION

A first-generation cephalosporin that inhibits cell-wall synthesis, promoting osmotic instability; usually bactericidal.

Route	Onset	Peak	Duration
I.V.	Immediate	Immediate	Unknown
I.M.	Unknown	1-2 hr	Unknown

INDICATIONS & DOSAGE

Perioperative prophylaxis in contaminated surgery —

Adults: 1 g I.M. or I.V. 30 to 60 minutes before surgery; then 0.5 to 1 g I.M. or I.V. q 6 to 8 hours for 24 hours. In long operations (over 2 hours), another 0.5- to 1-g I.M. or I.V. dose may be administered intraoperatively.

Note: In cases in which infection would be devastating, prophylaxis may be continued for 3 to 5 days.

Serious infections of respiratory, biliary, and GU tracts; skin, soft-tissue, bone, and joint infections; septicemia; endocarditis due to Escherichia coli, Enterobacteriaceae, gonococci, Haemophilus influenzae, Klebsiella, Proteus mirabilis, Staphylococcus aureus, Streptococcus pneumoniae, *and* group A beta-hemolytic streptococci —

Adults: 250 mg I.M. or I.V. q 8 hours to 1.5 g I.M. or I.V. q 6 hours. Maximum 12 g/day in life-threatening situations.

Children over age 1 month: 25 to 50 mg/kg/day I.M. or I.V. in three or four divided doses. In severe infections, dose may be increased to 100 mg/kg/day.

Dosage adjustment: For patients with renal failure with creatinine clearance of 35 to 54 ml/minute, give full dose q 8 hours; if clearance is 11 to 34 ml/minute, give 50% usual dose q 12 hours; if clearance is below 10 ml/minute, give 50% of usual dose q 18 to 24 hours.

ADVERSE REACTIONS

CV: *phlebitis, thrombophlebitis with I.V. injection.*

GI: pseudomembranous colitis, nausea, anorexia, vomiting, *diarrhea,* glossitis, dyspepsia, abdominal cramps, anal pruritus, oral candidiasis.

GU: genital pruritus, candidiasis, vaginitis.

Hematologic: neutropenia, leukopenia, eosinophilia, thrombocytopenia.

Hepatic: transient increases in liver enzymes.

Skin: *maculopapular and erythematous rashes, urticaria, pruritus, pain, indura-tion, sterile abscesses, tissue sloughing at injection site,* **Stevens-Johnson syndrome.**
Other: *hypersensitivity reactions, serum sickness, anaphylaxis.*

INTERACTIONS

Drug-drug. *Probenecid:* may inhibit excretion and increase blood levels of cefazolin. Use cautiously.

EFFECTS ON DIAGNOSTIC TESTS

Cephalosporins cause false-positive results in urine glucose tests using cupric sulfate (Benedict's reagent or Clinitest); use glucose oxidase tests (Diastix or Chemstrip uG) instead. Drug causes false elevations in serum or urine creatinine levels in tests using Jaffé's reaction. Drug also causes positive Coombs' test results.

CONTRAINDICATIONS

Contraindicated in patients with hypersensitivity to drug or other cephalosporins.

SPECIAL CONSIDERATIONS

▶ Use cautiously in patients with a history of sensitivity to penicillin and in breast-feeding women. Also, use cautiously and with dosage adjustments in patients with renal failure.
▶ A specimen for culture and sensitivity tests should be obtained before giving first dose. Therapy may begin pending results.
▶ Dose and dosing interval will be adjusted if creatinine clearance is below 55 ml/minute.
▶ After reconstitution, drug is injected I.M. without further dilution (this drug is not as painful as other cephalosporins). Injection is administered deeply into a large muscle mass, such as the gluteus maximus or lateral aspect of the thigh.
▶ With large doses or prolonged therapy, superinfection may occur, especially in high-risk patients.
▶ ***Alert:*** Don't confuse drug with other cephalosporins that sound alike.

I.V. administration

▶ Drug is reconstituted with sterile water, bacteriostatic water, or normal saline solution as follows: 2 ml to 500-mg vial; 2.5 ml to 1-g vial. Vial is shaken well until dissolved. Resultant concentration: 225 mg/ml or 330 mg/ml, respectively.

▶ Reconstituted cefazolin is stable for 24 hours at room temperature or 96 hours under refrigeration.

▶ For direct injection, Ancef is further diluted with 5 ml, or Kefzol with 10 ml, of sterile water for injection. Drug is injected into a large vein or into the tubing of a free-flowing I.V. solution over 3 to 5 minutes. For intermittent infusion, reconstituted drug is added to 50 to 100 ml of compatible solution or premixed solution is used. Commercially available frozen solutions of cefazolin in D_5W should be given only by intermittent or continuous I.V. infusion.

▶ Injection sites should be alternated if I.V. therapy lasts longer than 3 days. Use of small I.V. needles in larger available veins may be preferable.

Patient teaching

▶ Report adverse reactions promptly.
▶ Alert health care provider if discomfort occurs at I.V. injection site.

cefdinir

Omnicef

Pregnancy Risk Category B

HOW SUPPLIED

Capsules: 300 mg
Suspension: 125 mg/5 ml

ACTION

A third-generation cephalosporin whose bactericidal activity results from inhibition of cell-wall synthesis. Drug is stable in the presence of some beta-lactamase enzymes, causing some microorganisms resistant to penicillins and cephalosporins to be susceptible to cefdinir. Excluding *Pseudomonas, Enterobacter, Enterococcus,* and methicillin-resistant *Staphylococcus* species, cefdinir's spectrum of activity includes a broad range of gram-positive and gram-negative aerobic microorganisms.

Route	Onset	Peak	Duration
P.O.	Unknown	2-4 hr	Unknown

INDICATIONS & DOSAGE

Mild to moderate infections due to susceptible strains of microorganisms for conditions of community-acquired pneumonia, acute exacerbations of chronic bronchitis, acute maxillary sinusitis, acute bacterial otitis media, and uncomplicated skin and skin-structure infections —
Adults and children ages 13 and older: 300 mg P.O. q 12 hours; or 600 mg P.O. q 24 hours for 10 days. (Use q 12-hour dosages for pneumonia and skin infections.)

Children ages 6 months to 12 years: 7 mg/kg P.O. q 12 hours or 14 mg/kg P.O. q 24 hours for 10 days, up to maximum dose of 600 mg daily. (Use q 12-hour dosages for skin infections.)

Pharyngitis, tonsillitis —
Adults and children ages 13 and older: 300 mg P.O. q 12 hours for 5 to 10 days; or 600 mg P.O. q 24 hours for 10 days.

Children ages 6 months to 12 years: 7 mg/kg P.O. q 12 hours for 5 to 10 days; or 14 mg/kg P.O. q 24 hours for 10 days.

Dosage adjustment: If creatinine clearance is below 30 ml/minute, dosage is reduced to 300 mg P.O. once daily for adults and 7 mg/kg (up to 300 mg) P.O. once daily for children. In patients receiving chronic hemodialysis, dosage is 300 mg or 7 mg/kg P.O. at end of each dialysis session and subsequently every other day.

ADVERSE REACTIONS

CNS: headache.

GI: abdominal pain, *diarrhea,* nausea, vomiting.

GU: vaginal candidiasis, vaginitis, increased urine proteins and RBCs.

Hepatic: elevated GGT and alkaline phosphatase.

Skin: rash, cutaneous candidiasis.

INTERACTIONS

Drug-drug. *Antacids (magnesium- and aluminum-containing), iron supplements, multivitamins containing iron:* decrease cefdinir's rate of absorption and bioavailability; such preparations are administered 2 hours before or after cefdinir dose. *Probenecid:* inhibits the renal excretion of cefdinir. Monitor patient.

EFFECTS ON DIAGNOSTIC TESTS

False positive reaction for ketones (tests using nitroprusside only) and glucose (Clinitest, Benedict's or Fehling's solution) in urine may occur. Cephalosporins may occasionally induce a positive direct Coombs' test.

CONTRAINDICATIONS

Contraindicated in patients with known allergy to cephalosporins.

SPECIAL CONSIDERATIONS

▶ Use cautiously in patients with known hypersensitivity to penicillin because of the possibility of cross-sensitivity with other beta-lactam antibiotics. Also, use with caution in patients with history of colitis and renal insufficiency.

▶ Prolonged drug treatment may result in possible emergence and overgrowth of resistant organisms. Signs and symptoms of superinfection may occur.

▶ Pseudomembranous colitis has been reported with cefdinir and should be considered in patients with diarrhea subsequent to antibiotic therapy or in those with history of colitis.

▶ *Alert:* Don't confuse drug with other cephalosporins that sound alike.

Patient teaching

▶ Take antacids and iron supplements 2 hours before or after a dose of cefdinir.

▶ If diabetic, be aware that each teaspoon of suspension contains 2.86 g of sucrose.

▶ Drug may be taken without regard to meals.

▶ Report severe diarrhea or diarrhea accompanied by abdominal pain.

▶ Report adverse reactions or signs and symptoms of superinfection promptly.

cefepime hydrochloride

Maxipime

Pregnancy Risk Category B

HOW SUPPLIED

Injection: 500 mg/vial, 1 g/100-ml piggyback bottle, 1 g/ADD-Vantage vial, 1 g/15-ml vial, 2 g/100-ml piggyback bottle, 2 g/vial

ACTION

A fourth-generation cephalosporin that inhibits bacterial cell-wall synthesis, promotes osmotic instability, and destroys bacteria.

Route	Onset	Peak	Duration
I.V., I.M.	0.5 hr	1-2 hr	Unknown

INDICATIONS & DOSAGE

Mild to moderate urinary tract infections due to Escherichia coli, Klebsiella pneumoniae, *or* Proteus mirabilis, *including cases associated with concurrent bacteremia with these microorganisms —*

Adults and children ages 12 and older: 0.5 to 1 g I.M. (I.M. route used only for infections due to *E. coli*); or I.V. infused over 30 minutes q 12 hours for 7 to 10 days.

Severe urinary tract infections, including pyelonephritis, due to E. coli *or* K. pneumoniae —

Adults and children ages 12 and older: 2 g I.V. infused over 30 minutes q 12 hours for 10 days.

Moderate to severe pneumonia due to Streptococcus pneumoniae, Pseudomonas aeruginosa, K. pneumoniae, *or* Enterobacter species —

Adults and children ages 12 and older: 1 to 2g I.V. infused over 30 minutes q 12 hours for 10 days.

Moderate to severe skin infections, uncomplicated skin infections, and skin-structure infections due to Staphylococcus aureus *(methicillin-susceptible strains only) or* S. pyogenes —

Adults and children ages 12 and older: 2 g I.V. infused over 30 minutes q 12 hours for 10 days.

Complicated intra-abdominal infections (used with metronidazole) due to E. coli, *viridans group streptococci,* P. aeruginosa, K. pneumoniae, Enterobacter species, *or* B. fragilis —

Adults: 2 g I.V. infused over 30 minutes q 12 hours for 7 to 10 days.

Uncomplicated and complicated urinary tract infections (including pyelonephritis), uncomplicated skin and skin-structure infections, and pneumonia; as empiric therapy for febrile neutropenic children —

Children ages 2 months to 16 years weighing up to 40 kg (88 lb): 50 mg/kg/dose I.V. infused over 30 minutes q 12 hours (q 8 hours for febrile neutropenia) for 7 to 10 days; dosage shouldn't exceed the recommended adult dosage (2 g/dose).

Dosage adjustment: For renally impaired patients with creatinine clearance of 30 to 60 ml/minute, give full dose q 24 hours; if clearance is 11 to 29 ml/minute, give 50% usual dose q 24 hours; and if clearance is below 11 ml/minute, give 25% of usual dose q 24 hours.

ADVERSE REACTIONS
CNS: headache.
CV: phlebitis.
GI: colitis, diarrhea, nausea, vomiting, oral candidiasis.
GU: vaginitis.
Skin: rash, pruritus, urticaria.
Other: pain, inflammation, fever.

INTERACTIONS
Drug-drug. *Aminoglycosides:* may increase risk of nephrotoxicity. Renal function must be monitored closely.
Potent diuretics (such as furosemide): may increase risk of nephrotoxicity. Renal function must be monitored closely.

EFFECTS ON DIAGNOSTIC TESTS
Cefepime may cause a false-positive reaction for glucose in the urine when using Clinitest tablets. Glucose tests based on enzymatic glucose oxidase reactions (such as Diastix or Chemstrip uG) should be used instead. A positive direct Coombs' test may occur during treatment with drug.

CONTRAINDICATIONS
Contraindicated in patients with hypersensitivity to drug, other cephalosporins or beta-lactam antibiotics, or penicillins.

SPECIAL CONSIDERATIONS
▶ Use cautiously in patients with renal impairment, poor nutrition, or history of GI disease (particularly colitis); in those receiving a protracted course of antimicrobial therapy; and in breast-feeding women.
▶ Safety of drug in children under age 12 has not been established.
▶ Culture and sensitivity tests should be obtained before giving first dose, if appropriate. Therapy may begin pending results.
▶ Dosage adjustment is necessary in patients with impaired renal function. Renal function should be monitored.
▶ For I.M. administration, drug is consti-

tuted using sterile water for injection, normal saline for injection, 5% dextrose injection, 0.5% or 1% lidocaine hydrochloride, or bacteriostatic water for injection with parabens or benzyl alcohol. Manufacturer's guidelines should be followed for quantity of diluent to use.

 ▶ Solution is inspected for particulate matter before use. The powder and its solutions tend to darken, depending on storage conditions. Product potency is not adversely affected when stored as recommended.

 ▶ Superinfection may occur. Drug may cause overgrowth of nonsusceptible bacteria or fungi.

 ▶ Many cephalosporins can reduce PT activity. Patients at risk include those with renal or hepatic impairment or poor nutrition and those receiving prolonged cefepime therapy. PT and INR must be monitored in these patients. Exogenous vitamin K is administered as indicated.

 ▶ **Alert:** Don't confuse drug with other cephalosporins that sound alike.

I.V. administration

 ▶ The manufacturer's guidelines should be followed closely when reconstituting drug. Variations occur in constituting drug for administration, depending on concentration of drug ordered and how drug is packaged (piggyback vial, ADD-Vantage vial, or regular vial). Also be aware that the type of diluent used for constitution varies, depending on the product used. Only solutions recommended by the manufacturer should be used. The resulting solution should be administered over about 30 minutes.

 ▶ Intermittent I.V. infusion with a Y-type administration set can be accomplished with compatible solutions. However, during infusion of a solution containing cefepime, discontinuing the other solution is recommended.

Patient teaching
 ▶ Report pain at injection site.

 ▶ Report signs and symptoms of superinfection or GI disturbance.

cefixime
Suprax

Pregnancy Risk Category B

HOW SUPPLIED
Tablets: 200 mg, 400 mg
Oral suspension: 100 mg/5 ml (after reconstitution)

ACTION
A third-generation cephalosporin that inhibits cell-wall synthesis, promoting osmotic instability; usually bactericidal.

Route	Onset	Peak	Duration
P.O.	Unknown	3.1-4.4 hr	Unknown

INDICATIONS & DOSAGE
Uncomplicated urinary tract infections due to Escherichia coli *and* Proteus mirabilis; *otitis media due to* Haemophilus influenzae *(beta-lactamase positive and negative strains),* Moraxella (Branhamella) catarrhalis, *and* Streptococcus pyogenes; *pharyngitis and tonsillitis due to* S. pyogenes; *acute bronchitis and acute exacerbations of chronic bronchitis due to* S. pneumoniae *and* H. influenzae *(beta-lactamase positive and negative strains) —*
Adults and children over age 12 or weighing over 50 kg (110 lb): 400 mg/day P.O. as a single 400-mg tablet or 200mg q 12 hours.
Children ages 12 and less or weighing 50 kg or less: 8 mg/kg/day suspension P.O. as a single daily dose or 4 mg/kg q 12 hours.
 Uncomplicated gonorrhea due to Neisseria gonorrhoeae —
Adults: 400 mg P.O. as a single dose.
Dosage adjustment: For patients with re-

nal failure, if creatinine clearance is 21 to 60 ml/minute or patient undergoes hemodialysis, give 75% of dose at usual intervals; if less than 20 ml/minute, give 50% of usual dose at usual intervals.

ADVERSE REACTIONS
CNS: headache, dizziness.
GI: *diarrhea,* loose stools, abdominal pain, nausea, vomiting, dyspepsia, flatulence, pseudomembranous colitis.
GU: genital pruritus, vaginitis, genital candidiasis, transient increases in BUN and serum creatinine levels.
Hematologic: *thrombocytopenia, leukopenia,* eosinophilia.
Hepatic: transient increases in liver enzyme levels.
Skin: pruritus, rash, urticaria, *erythema multiforme, Stevens-Johnson syndrome.*
Other: drug fever, *hypersensitivity reactions, serum sickness, anaphylaxis.*

INTERACTIONS
Drug-drug. *Carbamazepine:* elevated carbamazepine levels reported when administered together. Avoid concomitant use.
Probenecid: may inhibit excretion and increase blood levels of cefixime. Use together cautiously.
Salicylates: may displace cefixime from plasma protein-binding sites. Clinical significance is unknown.

EFFECTS ON DIAGNOSTIC TESTS
Cefixime may cause false-positive results in urine glucose tests using cupric sulfate (Benedict's reagent or Clinitest); use glucose oxidase tests (Diastix or Chemstrip uG) instead. Drug may cause false-positive results in tests for urine ketones that utilize nitroprusside (but not nitroferricyanide). Positive direct Coombs' test results have been seen with other cephalosporins.

CONTRAINDICATIONS
Contraindicated in patients with hypersensitivity to drug or other cephalosporins.

SPECIAL CONSIDERATIONS
▶ *Alert:* Use cautiously and with reduced dosage in patients with renal dysfunction. Renal function must be monitored.
▶ Use cautiously in patients with a history of sensitivity to penicillin and in breast-feeding women.
▶ A specimen for culture and sensitivity tests should be obtained before giving first dose. Therapy may begin pending results.
▶ To prepare oral suspension, required amount of water is added to powder in two portions. The solution is shaken well after each addition. After mixing, suspension is stable for 14 days if kept tightly closed; no need to refrigerate. The solution should be shaken well before use.
▶ With large doses or prolonged therapy, superinfection may occur, especially in high-risk patients.
▶ *Alert:* Don't confuse drug with other cephalosporins that sound alike.

Patient teaching
▶ Take all of the drug prescribed, even after feeling better.
▶ If using oral suspension, shake container before measuring dose. Suspension does not need to be refrigerated.
▶ Notify health care provider if rash or signs and symptoms of superinfection develop.

cefmetazole sodium
Zefazone

Pregnancy Risk Category B

HOW SUPPLIED
Injection: 1-g vial, 2-g vial, 1 g/50 ml, 2 g/50 ml premixed solution

ACTION

A semisynthetic cephamycin antibiotic pharmacologically similar to second-generation cephalosporins that inhibit cell-wall synthesis, promoting osmotic instability; usually bactericidal.

Route	Onset	Peak	Duration
I.V.	Unknown	Immediate	Unknown

INDICATIONS & DOSAGE

Lower respiratory tract infections due to Streptococcus pneumoniae, Staphylococcus aureus *(penicillinase- and non-penicillinase-producing strains),* Escherichia coli, *and* Haemophilus influenzae *(non-penicillinase-producing strains); intra-abdominal infections due to* E. coli *or* Bacteroides fragilis; *skin and skin-structure infections due to* S. aureus *(penicillinase- and non-penicillinase-producing strains),* S. epidermidis, Streptococcus pyogenes, S. agalactiae, E. coli, Proteus mirabilis, Klebsiella pneumoniae, *and* B. fragilis —
Adults: 2 g I.V. q 6 to 12 hours for 5 to 14 days.
Urinary tract infections due to E. coli —
Adults: 2 g I.V. q 12 hours.
Prophylaxis in patients undergoing vaginal hysterectomy —
Adults: 2 g I.V. 30 to 90 minutes before surgery as a single dose; or 1 g I.V. 30 to 90 minutes before surgery, repeated in 8 and 16 hours.
Prophylaxis in patients undergoing abdominal hysterectomy —
Adults: 1 g I.V. 30 to 90 minutes before surgery, repeated in 8 and 16 hours.
Prophylaxis in patients undergoing cesarean section —
Adults: 2 g I.V. as a single dose after clamping cord; or 1 g I.V. after clamping cord, repeated in 8 and 16 hours.
Prophylaxis in patients undergoing colorectal surgery —
Adults: 2 g I.V. as a single dose 30 to 90 minutes before surgery. May follow with additional 2-g doses in 8 and 16 hours.
Prophylaxis in high-risk patients undergoing cholecystectomy —
Adults: 1 g I.V. 30 to 90 minutes before surgery, repeated in 8 and 16 hours.
Dosage adjustment: For patients with renal failure, if creatinine clearance is 50 to 90 ml/minute, give 1 to 2 g q 12 hours; if clearance is 30 to 49 ml/minute, give 1 to 2 g q 16 hours; if clearance is 10 to 29 ml/minute, give 1 to 2 g q 24 hours; if clearance is less than 10 ml/minute, give 1 to 2 g q 48 hours (administered after hemodialysis).

ADVERSE REACTIONS

CNS: headache.
CV: *shock,* hypotension, phlebitis, thrombophlebitis.
EENT: epistaxis, altered color perception.
GI: nausea, vomiting, *diarrhea,* epigastric pain, pseudomembranous colitis, candidiasis, bleeding.
GU: vaginitis, hot flashes.
Hepatic: elevated liver function test results.
Musculoskeletal: joint pain and inflammation.
Respiratory: pleural effusion, dyspnea, respiratory distress.
Skin: rash, pruritus, generalized erythema.
Other: fever, bacterial or fungal superinfection, *hypersensitivity reactions, serum sickness, anaphylaxis,* pain at injection site.

INTERACTIONS

Drug-drug. *Aminoglycosides:* potential increased risk of nephrotoxicity. Monitor closely.
Probenecid: may inhibit excretion and increase blood levels of cefmetazole. May be used for this effect.
Drug-lifestyle. *Alcohol use:* possible disulfiram-like reaction. Alcohol should be avoided for 24 hours before and after administration of cefmetazole.

Reactions may be *common,* uncommon, *life-threatening,* or COMMON AND LIFE-THREATENING.

EFFECTS ON DIAGNOSTIC TESTS
Drug causes false-positive results of urine glucose tests that use cupric sulfate (Benedict's reagent or Clinitest); use glucose oxidase tests (Diastix or Chemstrip uG) instead. Cefmetazole may cause positive Coombs' test results.

CONTRAINDICATIONS
Contraindicated in patients with hypersensitivity to drug or other cephalosporins.

SPECIAL CONSIDERATIONS
▶ Use cautiously in patients with a history of sensitivity to penicillin and in breastfeeding women.
▶ A specimen for culture and sensitivity tests should be obtained before giving first dose. Therapy may begin pending results.
▶ Patient is monitored for bacterial and fungal superinfections. Prolonged use may result in overgrowth of nonsusceptible organisms.
▶ INR is monitored in patients at risk (from renal or hepatic impairment, malnutrition, or prolonged therapy. Drug's chemical structure includes the methylthiotetrazole side chain that has been associated with bleeding disorders. However, such bleeding has not been reported with drug.
▶ In patients undergoing hemodialysis, dose is given at end of hemodialysis session.
▶ Renal function must be monitored.
▶ *Alert:* Don't confuse drug with other cephalosporins that sound alike.

I.V. administration
▶ Drug is reconstituted with bacteriostatic water for injection, sterile water for injection, or normal saline for injection. After reconstitution, drug may be further diluted to concentrations ranging from 1 to 20 mg/ml by adding it to normal saline injection, D_5W, or lactated Ringer's injection. Reconstituted or dilute solutions are stable for 24 hours at room temperature

(77° F [25° C]) or 1 week if refrigerated at 46° F (8° C).

Patient teaching
▶ Report adverse reactions promptly.
▶ Alert health care provider if discomfort occurs at I.V. insertion site.

cefonicid sodium
Monocid

Pregnancy Risk Category B

HOW SUPPLIED
Injection: 1 g
Infusion: 1 g/100 ml

ACTION
A second-generation cephalosporin that inhibits cell-wall synthesis, promoting osmotic instability; usually bactericidal.

Route	Onset	Peak	Duration
I.V.	Immediate	Immediate	Unknown
I.M.	Unknown	1-2 hr	Unknown

INDICATIONS & DOSAGE
Perioperative prophylaxis in contaminated surgery—
Adults: 1 g I.M. or I.V. 30 to 60 minutes before surgery; then 1 g I.M. or I.V. daily for 2 days after surgery. If used for prophylaxis in cesarean section, 1 g I.M. or I.V. after umbilical cord is clamped.

Serious infections of the lower respiratory and urinary tracts; skin and skin-structure infections; septicemia; bone and joint infections; preoperative prophylaxis. Susceptible microorganisms include Streptococcus pneumoniae, Klebsiella pneumoniae, Escherichia coli, Haemophilus influenzae, Proteus mirabilis, Staphylococcus aureus, S. epidermidis, *and* Streptococcus pyogenes —
Adults: usual dosage is 1 g I.V. or I.M. q 24 hours; in life-threatening infections,

2 g q 24 hours. For patients with renal failure, if creatinine clearance is 60 to 79 ml/minute, give 10 to 25 mg/kg q 24 hours; if clearance is 40 to 59 ml/minute, give 8 to 20 mg/kg q 24 hours; if clearance is 20 to 39 ml/minute, give 4 to 15 mg/kg q 24 hours; if clearance is 10 to 19 ml/minute, give 4 to 15 mg/kg q 48 hours; if clearance is 5 to 9 ml/minute, give 4 to 15 mg/kg q 3 to 5 days; if clearance is below 5 ml/minute, give 3 to 4 mg/kg q 3 to 5 days.

ADVERSE REACTIONS

CNS: dizziness, headache, malaise, paresthesia.
CV: *phlebitis, thrombophlebitis.*
GI: pseudomembranous colitis, diarrhea.
GU: *acute renal failure,* interstitial nephritis.
Hematologic: *neutropenia, leukopenia,* eosinophilia, anemia, thrombocytosis, *thrombocytopenia,* prolonged PT and INR.
Hepatic: elevated liver function test results.
Musculoskeletal: myalgia.
Skin: *maculopapular and erythematous rashes, urticaria, pain, induration, sterile abscesses, tissue sloughing at injection site.*
Other: *hypersensitivity reactions, serum sickness, anaphylaxis,* fever.

INTERACTIONS

Drug-drug. *Probenecid:* may inhibit excretion and increase blood levels of cefonicid. Use together cautiously.

EFFECTS ON DIAGNOSTIC TESTS

Cefonicid causes positive Coombs' test results and false-positive results in urine glucose tests using cupric sulfate (Benedict's reagent or Clinitest); use glucose oxidase tests (Diastix or Chemstrip uG) instead. Drug causes false elevations in serum or urine creatinine levels in tests using Jaffé's reaction.

CONTRAINDICATIONS

Contraindicated in patients with hypersensitivity to drug or other cephalosporins.

SPECIAL CONSIDERATIONS

▶ Use cautiously in patients with a history of sensitivity to penicillin and in breastfeeding women. Also, use cautiously and with dosage adjustments in patients with renal failure. Renal function must be monitored.
▶ A specimen for culture and sensitivity tests should be obtained before giving first dose. Therapy may begin pending results.
▶ Dosing interval will be adjusted for patients with renal impairment.
▶ For I.M. use, the 2-g I.M. doses are administered once daily; the dose is divided equally and injected deeply into large muscle masses, such as the gluteus maximus or the lateral aspect of the thigh.
▶ With large doses or prolonged therapy, superinfection may occur, especially in high-risk patients.
▶ The chemical structure of drug includes the methylthiotetrazole side chain that has been associated with bleeding disorders. However, such bleeding has not been reported with drug.
▶ *Alert:* Don't confuse drug with other cephalosporins that sound alike.

I.V. administration

▶ A 1-g vial is reconstituted with 2.5 ml of sterile water for injection (yields a concentration of 325 mg/ml). The vial is shaken well. Piggyback vials are reconstituted with 50 to 100 ml of sterile water for injection, bacteriostatic water for injection, or normal saline solution.
▶ The drug is infused over 20 to 30 minutes.

Patient teaching

▶ Report adverse reactions or signs and symptoms of superinfection promptly.
▶ Alert health care provider if discomfort occurs at I.V. insertion site.

Reactions may be *common*, uncommon, *life-threatening*, or COMMON AND LIFE-THREATENING.

cefoperazone sodium

Cefobid

Pregnancy Risk Category B

HOW SUPPLIED

Infusion: 1 g, 2 g piggyback
Parenteral: 1-g, 2-g vials; 1 g, 2 g pre-mixed

ACTION

A third-generation cephalosporin that inhibits cell-wall synthesis, promoting osmotic instability; usually bactericidal.

Route	Onset	Peak	Duration
I.V.	Immediate	Immediate	Unknown
I.M.	Unknown	1-2 hr	Unknown

INDICATIONS & DOSAGE

Serious infections of the respiratory tract; intra-abdominal, gynecologic, and skin infections; bacteremia; septicemia due to susceptible microorganisms (Streptococcus pneumoniae *and* S. pyogenes; Staphylococcus aureus *[penicillinase- and non-penicillinase-producing] and* S. epidermidis; enterococci; Escherichia coli; Klebsiella; Haemophilus influenzae; Enterobacter; Citrobacter; Proteus; *some* Pseudomonas, *including* P. aeruginosa; *and* Bacteroides fragilis) —

Adults: usual dosage is 1 to 2 g q 12 hours I.M. or I.V. In severe infections or in infections due to less sensitive organisms, total daily dose (or frequency) may be increased to 16 g/day.

Dosage adjustment: For patients with hepatic or biliary obstruction, total daily dose shouldn't exceed 4 g/day. In patients with hepatic and substantial renal impairment, total daily dose shouldn't exceed 2 g/day.

ADVERSE REACTIONS

CV: *phlebitis, thrombophlebitis.*
GI: pseudomembranous colitis, nausea, vomiting, *diarrhea.*

Hematologic: *transient neutropenia, eosinophilia,* anemia, hypoprothrombinemia, bleeding, elevated INR.
Hepatic: mildly elevated liver enzymes.
Skin: *maculopapular and erythematous rashes, urticaria, pain, induration, sterile abscesses, temperature elevation, tissue sloughing at I.M. injection site.*
Other: *hypersensitivity reactions, serum sickness, anaphylaxis,* fever.
Interactions
Drug-drug. *Probenecid:* may inhibit excretion and increase blood levels of cefoperazone. Use together cautiously.
Drug-lifestyle. *Alcohol use:* possible disulfiram-like reaction. Patient should not drink alcohol for several days after discontinuing cefoperazone.

EFFECTS ON DIAGNOSTIC TESTS

Cephalosporins cause false-positive results in urine glucose tests using cupric sulfate (Benedict's reagent or Clinitest); use glucose oxidase (Diastix or Chemstrip uG) instead. Cefoperazone may cause positive Coombs' test results.

CONTRAINDICATIONS

Contraindicated in patients with hypersensitivity to drug or other cephalosporins.

SPECIAL CONSIDERATIONS

▶ Use cautiously in patients with impaired renal function or with a history of sensitivity to penicillin. Also, use cautiously in breast-feeding women.
▶ Doses of 4 g/day should be given cautiously to patients with hepatic disease or biliary obstruction. Higher dosages require monitoring of serum levels.
▶ Liver and renal function are periodically monitored and compared to baseline.
▶ A specimen for culture and sensitivity tests should be obtained before giving first dose. Therapy may begin pending results.
▶ To prepare drug for I.M. injection: using the 1-g vial, drug is dissolved with 2 ml of sterile water for injection; then,

0.6 ml of 2% lidocaine hydrochloride is added for a final concentration of 333 mg/ml. Or, drug is dissolved with 2.8 ml of sterile water for injection; then 1 ml of 2% lidocaine hydrochloride is added for a final concentration of 250 mg/ml. When using the 2-g vial, drug is dissolved with 3.8 ml of sterile water for injection; then 1.2 ml of 2% lidocaine hydrochloride is added for final concentration of 333 mg/ml. Or, drug is dissolved with 5.4 ml of sterile water for injection; then 1.8 ml of 2% lidocaine hydrochloride is added for final concentration of 250 mg/ml.

▶ For I.M. administration, drug is injected deeply into a large muscle mass, such as the gluteus maximus or the lateral aspect of the thigh.

▶ With large doses or prolonged therapy, superinfection may occur, especially in high-risk patients.

▶ INR is monitored regularly. The drug's chemical structure includes the methylthiotetrazole side chain that has been associated with bleeding disorders. Vitamin K promptly reverses bleeding if it occurs.

▶ *Alert:* Don't confuse drug with other cephalosporins that sound alike.

I.V. administration

▶ The drug is reconstituted in a 1- or 2-g vial with a minimum of 2.8 ml of compatible I.V. solution; the manufacturer recommends using 5 ml/g. Drug is given by direct injection into a large vein or into the tubing of a free-flowing I.V. solution over 3 to 5 minutes. When giving by intermittent infusion, reconstituted drug is added to 20 to 40 ml of a compatible I.V. solution and infused over 15 to 30 minutes.

Patient teaching

▶ Report adverse reactions and signs and symptoms of superinfection promptly.

▶ Alert health care provider if discomfort occurs at I.V. insertion site.

cefotaxime sodium

Claforan
Pregnancy Risk Category B

HOW SUPPLIED

Injection: 500 mg, 1 g, 2-g vials, 10-g bottle
Infusion: 1-g, 2-g premixed package

ACTION

A third-generation cephalosporin that inhibits cell-wall synthesis, promoting osmotic instability; usually bactericidal.

Route	Onset	Peak	Duration
I.V.	Immediate	Immediate	Unknown
I.M.	Unknown	30 min	Unknown

INDICATIONS & DOSAGE

Perioperative prophylaxis in contaminated surgery —
Adults: 1 g I.M. or I.V. 30 to 60 minutes before surgery. Patients undergoing bowel surgery should receive preoperative mechanical bowel cleansing and a nonabsorbable anti-infective agent such as neomycin. Patients undergoing cesarean section should receive 1 g I.M. or I.V. as soon as the umbilical cord is clamped; then 1 g I.M. or I.V. 6 and 12 hours later.

Uncomplicated gonorrhea due to penicillinase-producing strains of Neisseria gonorrhoeae *or non-penicillinase-producing strains of the organism—*
Adults and adolescents: 500 mg I.M. as a single dose.

Serious infections of the lower respiratory and urinary tracts, CNS, skin, bone, and joints; gynecologic and intra-abdominal infections; bacteremia; septicemia due to susceptible microorganisms, such as streptococci (including Streptococcus pneumoniae *and* S. pyogenes*),* Staphylococcus aureus *(penicillinase- and non-penicillinase-producing) and* S. epidermidis, Escherichia coli, Klebsiella,

---

Haemophilus influenzae, Serratia marcescens, Pseudomonas species *(including P. aeruginosa)*, Enterobacter, Proteus, *and* Peptostreptococcus —

Adults: usual dose is 1 g I.V. or I.M. q 6 to 8 hours. Up to 12 g daily can be given in life-threatening infections.

Children weighing 50 kg (110 lb) or more: the usual adult dose, but dosage shouldn't exceed 12 g daily.

Children ages 1 month to 12 years weighing less than 50 kg: 50 to 180 mg/kg/day I.M. or I.V. in four to six divided doses.

Neonates ages 1 to 4 weeks: 50 mg/kg I.V. q 8 hours.

Neonates to age 1 week: 50 mg/kg I.V. q 12 hours.

Dosage adjustment: For patients with renal failure, if creatinine clearance is below 20 ml/minute, give half usual dose at usual interval.

ADVERSE REACTIONS

CNS: headache.

CV: *phlebitis, thrombophlebitis.*

GI: pseudomembranous colitis, nausea, vomiting, *diarrhea.*

GU: vaginitis, candidiasis, interstitial nephritis.

Hematologic: *transient neutropenia,* eosinophilia, hemolytic anemia, *thrombocytopenia, agranulocytosis.*

Hepatic: elevated liver function test results.

Skin: *maculopapular and erythematous rashes, urticaria, pain, induration, sterile abscesses, temperature elevation, tissue sloughing at I.M. injection site.*

Other: *hypersensitivity reactions, serum sickness, anaphylaxis,* elevated temperature.

INTERACTIONS

Drug-drug. *Aminoglycosides:* may increase risk of nephrotoxicity. Monitor closely.

Probenecid: may inhibit excretion and increase blood levels of cefotaxime. Use together cautiously.

EFFECTS ON DIAGNOSTIC TESTS

Cefotaxime may cause positive Coombs' test results.

CONTRAINDICATIONS

Contraindicated in patients with hypersensitivity to drug or other cephalosporins.

SPECIAL CONSIDERATIONS

▶ Use cautiously in patients with a history of sensitivity to penicillin and in breast-feeding women. Also, use cautiously and with dosage adjustments in patients with renal failure. Renal function must be monitored.

▶ A specimen for culture and sensitivity tests should be obtained before giving first dose. Therapy may begin pending results.

▶ For I.M. administration, drug is injected deeply into a large muscle mass, such as the gluteus maximus or the lateral aspect of the thigh.

▶ With large doses or prolonged therapy, superinfection may occur, especially in high-risk patients.

▶ *Alert:* Don't confuse drug with other cephalosporins that sound alike.

I.V. administration

▶ For direct injection, drug is reconstituted in 500-mg, 1-g, or 2-g vials with 10 ml of sterile water for injection. Solutions containing 1 g/14 ml are isotonic. Drug is injected into a large vein or into the tubing of a free-flowing I.V. solution over 3 to 5 minutes.

▶ For I.V. infusion, drug in infusion vials is reconstituted with 50 to 100 ml of D_5W or normal saline solution. Drug is infused over 20 to 30 minutes. Primary I.V. solution flow should be stopped during infusion.

Patient teaching

▶ Report adverse reactions and signs and symptoms of superinfection promptly.
▶ Alert health care provider if discomfort occurs at I.V. insertion site.

cefotetan disodium

Cefotan

Pregnancy Risk Category B

HOW SUPPLIED

Injection: 1 g, 2 g, 10 g
Infusion: 1 g, 2 g piggyback and premixed

ACTION

A second-generation cephalosporin that inhibits cell-wall synthesis, promoting osmotic instability; usually bactericidal.

Route	Onset	Peak	Duration
I.V.	Immediate	Immediate	Unknown
I.M.	Unknown	1.5-3 hr	Unknown

INDICATIONS & DOSAGE

Serious urinary tract and lower respiratory tract infections and gynecologic, skin and skin-structure, intra-abdominal, and bone and joint infections due to susceptible streptococci, Staphylococcus aureus *(penicillinase- and non-penicillinase-producing) and* S. epidermidis, Escherichia coli, Klebsiella, Enterobacter, Proteus, Haemophilus influenzae, Neisseria gonorrhoeae, *and* Bacteroides, *including* B. fragilis —
Adults: 1 to 2 g I.V. or I.M. q 12 hours for 5 to 10 days. Up to 6 g daily in life-threatening infections.
Perioperative prophylaxis —
Adults: 1 to 2 g I.V. given once 30 to 60 minutes before surgery. In cesarean section, dose should be administered as soon as umbilical cord is clamped.
Dosage adjustment: For patients with renal failure, if creatinine clearance is 10 to 30 ml/minute, give usual dose q 24 hours; if clearance is below 10 ml/minute, give usual dose q 48 hours.

ADVERSE REACTIONS

CV: *phlebitis, thrombophlebitis.*
GI: pseudomembranous colitis, nausea, *diarrhea.*
GU: *nephrotoxicity.*
Hematologic: *transient neutropenia,* eosinophilia, hemolytic anemia, hypoprothrombinemia, bleeding, thrombocytosis, *agranulocytosis, thrombocytopenia,* prolonged PT and INR.
Hepatic: elevated liver function test results.
Skin: *maculopapular and erythematous rashes, urticaria, pain, induration, sterile abscesses, tissue sloughing at injection site.*
Other: *hypersensitivity reactions, serum sickness, anaphylaxis,* elevated temperature.

INTERACTIONS

Drug-drug. *Aminoglycosides:* possible synergistic effect and possible increased risk of nephrotoxicity. Use with caution.
Probenecid: may inhibit excretion and increase blood levels of cefotetan. Sometimes used for this effect.
Drug-lifestyle. *Alcohol use:* possible disulfiram-like reaction. The patient should not drink alcohol for several days after discontinuing cefotetan.

EFFECTS ON DIAGNOSTIC TESTS

Cefotetan causes false-positive results in urine glucose tests using cupric sulfate (Benedict's reagent or Clinitest); use glucose oxidase tests (Diastix or Chemstrip uG) instead. Drug causes false elevations in serum or urine creatinine levels in tests using Jaffé's reaction and may cause positive Coombs' test results.

CONTRAINDICATIONS

Contraindicated in patients with hypersensitivity to drug or other cephalosporins.

SPECIAL CONSIDERATIONS

▶ Use cautiously in patients with history of sensitivity to penicillin and in breast-feeding women. Also, use cautiously and with dosage adjustments in patients with renal failure. Renal function must be monitored.

▶ A specimen for culture and sensitivity tests should be obtained before giving first dose. Therapy may begin pending results.

▶ For I.M. injection, the drug is reconstituted with sterile water or bacteriostatic water for injection, normal saline for injection, or 0.5% or 1% lidocaine hydrochloride. The solution is shaken to dissolve and let standing until clear.

▶ Reconstituted solution is stable for 24 hours at room temperature or 96 hours if refrigerated.

▶ With large doses or prolonged therapy, superinfection may occur, especially in high-risk patients.

▶ Drug's chemical structure includes the methylthiotetrazole side chain that has been associated with bleeding disorders. However, such bleeding has not been reported with this drug. PT and INR must be monitored.

▶ **Alert:** Don't confuse drug with other cephalosporins that sound alike.

I.V. administration

▶ The drug is reconstituted with sterile water for injection. Drug may then be mixed with 50 to 100 ml of D_5W or normal saline solution. Primary I.V. solution flow is stopped during cefotetan infusion.

▶ Infuse over 20 to 60 minutes.

Patient teaching

▶ Report adverse reactions and signs and symptoms of superinfection promptly.

▶ Alert health care provider if discomfort occurs at I.V. site.

▶ Notify health care provider if loose stool or diarrhea occurs.

cefoxitin sodium

Mefoxin

Pregnancy Risk Category B

HOW SUPPLIED

Injection: 1 g, 2 g, 10 g
Infusion: 1 g, 2 g in 50-ml or 100-ml container

ACTION

A second-generation cephalosporin that inhibits cell-wall synthesis, promoting osmotic instability; usually bactericidal.

Route	Onset	Peak	Duration
I.V.	Immediate	Immediate	Unknown
I.M.	Unknown	20-30 min	Unknown

INDICATIONS & DOSAGE

Serious infections of respiratory and GU tracts; skin; soft-tissue, bone, and joint infections; bloodstream and intra-abdominal infections due to susceptible organisms (such as Escherichia coli *and other coliform bacteria,* Staphylococcus aureus *[penicillinase- and non-penicillinase-producing] and* S. epidermidis, *strep-tococci,* Klebsiella, Haemophilus in-fluenzae, *and* Bacteroides, *including* B. fragilis); *perioperative prophylaxis —*
Adults: 1 to 2 g I.V. or I.M. q 6 to 8 hours for uncomplicated infections. Up to 12 g daily in life-threatening infections.
Children over age 3 months: 80 to 160 mg/kg daily I.V. or I.M., given in four to six equally divided doses. Maximum daily dose is 12 g.
Prophylaxis in surgery —
Adults: 2 g I.M. or I.V. 30 to 60 minutes before surgery, then 2 g I.M. or I.V. q 6 hours for 24 hours (72 hours after prosthetic arthroplasty).

Children ages 3 months and older: 30 to 40 mg/kg I.M. or I.V. 30 to 60 minutes before surgery, then 30 to 40 mg/kg q 6 hours for 24 hours (72 hours after prosthetic arthroplasty).

Dosage adjustment: For patients with renal failure, if creatinine clearance is 30 to 50 ml/minute, give 1 to 2 g q 8 to 12 hours; if clearance is 10 to 29 ml/minute, give 1 to 2 g q 12 to 24 hours; and if clearance is below 10 ml/minute, give 500 mg q 24 to 48 hours.

ADVERSE REACTIONS
CV: hypotension; *phlebitis, thrombophlebitis.*
GI: pseudomembranous colitis, nausea, vomiting, *diarrhea.*
GU: *acute renal failure.*
Hematologic: *transient neutropenia,* eosinophilia, hemolytic anemia, anemia, *thrombocytopenia.*
Hepatic: transient increases in liver enzyme levels.
Respiratory: dyspnea.
Skin: *maculopapular and erythematous rashes, urticaria, **exfoliative dermatitis,** pain, induration, sterile abscesses, tissue sloughing at injection site.*
Other: *hypersensitivity reactions, serum sickness, anaphylaxis,* elevated temperature.

INTERACTIONS
Drug-drug. *Nephrotoxic drugs:* possible increased risk of nephrotoxicity. Monitor closely.
Probenecid: may inhibit excretion and increase blood levels of cefoxitin. Sometimes used for this effect.

EFFECTS ON DIAGNOSTIC TESTS
Cefoxitin causes false-positive results in urine glucose tests using cupric sulfate (Benedict's reagent or Clinitest); use glucose oxidase tests (Diastix or Chemstrip uG) instead. Drug causes false elevations in serum or urine creatinine levels in tests using Jaffé's reaction and may cause positive Coombs' test results.

CONTRAINDICATIONS
Contraindicated in patients with hypersensitivity to drug or other cephalosporins.

SPECIAL CONSIDERATIONS
▶ Use cautiously in patients with a history of sensitivity to penicillin and in breast-feeding women. Also, use cautiously and with dosage adjustments in patients with renal failure. Renal function must be monitored.
▶ A specimen for culture and sensitivity tests should be obtained before giving first dose. Therapy may begin pending results.
▶ For I.M. use, each 1 g of drug is reconstituted with 2 ml of sterile water for injection or 0.5% or 1% lidocaine hydrochloride (without epinephrine) to minimize pain. Drug is injected deeply into a large muscle mass, such as the gluteus maximus or the lateral aspect of the thigh.
▶ After reconstitution, drug may be stored for 24 hours at room temperature or 1 week under refrigeration.
▶ With large doses or prolonged therapy, superinfection may occur, especially in high-risk patients.
▶ ***Alert:*** Don't confuse drug with other cephalosporins that sound alike.

I.V. administration
▶ 1 g is reconstituted with at least 10 ml of sterile water for injection and 2 g with 10 to 20 ml of sterile water for injection. Solutions of D_5W and normal saline for injection can also be used. For direct injection, drug is injected into a large vein or into the tubing of a free-flowing I.V. solution over 3 to 5 minutes. For intermittent infusion, reconstituted drug is added to 50 or 100 ml of D_5W or $D_{10}W$ or normal saline for injection. Primary I.V. solution is stopped during infusion.
▶ I.V. site is assessed frequently. Such use

has been linked to development of thrombophlebitis.

Patient teaching

▶ Report adverse reactions and signs and symptoms of superinfection promptly.
▶ Alert health care provider if discomfort is felt at I.V. site.
▶ Notify health care provider if loose stool or diarrhea occurs.

cefpodoxime proxetil
Vantin

Pregnancy Risk Category B

HOW SUPPLIED

Tablets (film-coated): 100 mg, 200 mg
Oral suspension: 50 mg/5 ml, 100 mg/5 ml in 100-ml bottles

ACTION

A third-generation cephalosporin that inhibits cell-wall synthesis, promoting osmotic instability; usually bactericidal.

Route	Onset	Peak	Duration
P.O.	Unknown	2-3 hr	Unknown

INDICATIONS & DOSAGE

Acute, community-acquired pneumonia due to non-beta-lactamase-producing strains of Haemophilus influenzae *or* Streptococcus pneumoniae —
Adults and children ages 13 and older: 200 mg P.O. q 12 hours for 14 days.

Acute bacterial exacerbation of chronic bronchitis due to S. pneumoniae, H. influenzae *(non-beta-lactamase-producing strains only), or* Moraxella (Branhamella) catarrhalis —
Adults and children ages 13 and older: 200 mg P.O. q 12 hours for 10 days.

Uncomplicated gonorrhea in men and women; rectal gonococcal infections in women —

Adults and children ages 13 and older: 200 mg P.O. as a single dose. Follow with doxycycline 100 mg P.O. b.i.d. for 7 days.

Uncomplicated skin and skin-structure infections due to Staphylococcus aureus *or* S. pyogenes —
Adults and children ages 13 and older: 400 mg P.O. q 12 hours for 7 to 14 days.

Acute otitis media due to S. pneumoniae, H. influenzae, *or* M. catarrhalis —
Children ages 6 months and older: 5 mg/kg (not to exceed 200 mg) P.O. q 12 hours or 10 mg/kg P.O. daily for 10 days.

Pharyngitis or tonsillitis due to S. pyogenes —
Adults: 100 mg P.O. q 12 hours for 10 days.
Children ages 6 months and older: 5 mg/kg (not to exceed 100 mg) P.O. q 12 hours for 10 days.

Uncomplicated urinary tract infections due to Escherichia coli, Klebsiella pneumoniae, Proteus mirabilis, *or* S. saprophyticus —
Adults: 100 mg P.O. q 12 hours for 7 days.

Mild to moderate acute maxillary sinusitis due to H. influenzae, S. pneumoniae, *or* M. catarrhalis —
Adults and adolescents ages 12 and older: 200 mg P.O. q 12 hours for 10 days.
Children ages 2 months to 11 years: 5 mg/kg P.O. q 12 hours for 10 days; maximum is 200 mg/dose.

Dosage adjustment: For patients with renal failure, if creatinine clearance is below 30 ml/minute, dosage interval should be increased to q 24 hours. Dialysis patients should receive drug three times weekly after dialysis.

ADVERSE REACTIONS

CNS: headache.
GI: *diarrhea,* nausea, vomiting, abdominal pain.
GU: vaginal fungal infections.
Skin: rash.
Other: *hypersensitivity reactions, anaphylaxis.*

INTERACTIONS

Drug-drug. *Antacids, H2 antagonists:* decreased absorption of cefpodoxime. Avoid concomitant use.

Probenecid: decreased excretion of cefpodoxime. Patient is monitored for toxicity.

Drug-food. *Any food:* increased absorption. Drug is given with food.

EFFECTS ON DIAGNOSTIC TESTS

Drug may induce a positive direct Coombs' test. Urine glucose determinations may be false-positive with copper sulfate tests (Clinitest); glucose enzymatic tests (Diastix or Chemstrip uG) are not affected.

CONTRAINDICATIONS

Contraindicated in patients with hypersensitivity to drug or other cephalosporins.

SPECIAL CONSIDERATIONS

▶ Use cautiously in patients with a history of penicillin hypersensitivity because of risk of cross-sensitivity and in patients receiving nephrotoxic drugs because other cephalosporins have been shown to have nephrotoxic potential. Because drug appears in breast milk, drug is used cautiously in breast-feeding women.

▶ Renal function is monitored and compared to baseline.

▶ A specimen for culture and sensitivity tests should be obtained before giving first dose. Therapy may begin pending results.

▶ Drug is administered with food to enhance absorption. Suspension is shaken well before using.

▶ Suspension is stored in the refrigerator (36° to 46° F [2° to 8° C]). Unused portion is discarded after 14 days.

▶ Superinfection may occur. Drug may cause overgrowth of nonsusceptible bacteria or fungi.

▶ *Alert:* Don't confuse drug with other cephalosporins that sound alike.

Patient teaching

▶ Take all of the drug as prescribed, even after feeling better.

▶ Take drug with food. If using suspension, shake container before measuring dose, and keep container refrigerated.

▶ Call health care provider if rash or signs and symptoms of superinfection develop.

▶ Notify health care provider if loose stool or diarrhea occurs.

cefprozil
Cefzil

Pregnancy Risk Category B

HOW SUPPLIED

Tablets: 250 mg, 500 mg
Oral suspension: 125 mg/5 ml, 250 mg/5 ml

ACTION

A second-generation cephalosporin that interferes with cell-wall synthesis during microorganism replication, leading to osmotic instability and cell lysis (bactericidal).

Route	Onset	Peak	Duration
P.O.	Unknown	1.5 hr	Unknown

INDICATIONS & DOSAGE

Pharyngitis or tonsillitis due to Streptococcus pyogenes —

Adults and children ages 13 and older: 500 mg P.O. daily for at least 10 days.

Otitis media due to S. pneumoniae, Haemophilus influenzae, *and* Moraxella (Branhamella) catarrhalis —

Infants and children ages 6 months to 12 years: 15 mg/kg P.O. q 12 hours for 10 days.

Secondary bacterial infections of acute bronchitis and acute bacterial exacerbation of chronic bronchitis due to S. pneumoniae, H. influenzae, *and* M. catarrhalis —

Adults and children ages 13 and older: 500 mg P.O. q 12 hours for 10 days.

Uncomplicated skin and skin-structure infections due to Staphylococcus aureus *and* S. pyogenes —

Adults and children ages 13 and older: 250 or 500 mg P.O. q 12 hours or 500 mg daily.

Acute sinusitis due to S. pneumoniae, H. influenzae *(beta-lactamase positive and negative strains), and* M. catarrhalis *(including beta-lactamase–producing strains)* —

Adults and children ages 13 and older: 250 mg P.O. q 12 hours for 10 days; for moderate to severe infection, 500 mg P.O. q 12 hours for 10 days.

Children ages 6 months to 12 years: 7.5 mg/kg P.O. q 12 hours for 10 days; for moderate to severe infections, 15 mg/kg P.O. q 12 hours for 10 days.

Dosage adjustment: For patients with renal failure, if creatinine clearance is below 30 ml/minute, give 50% of usual dose.

ADVERSE REACTIONS

CNS: dizziness, hyperactivity, headache, nervousness, insomnia, confusion, somnolence.

GI: *diarrhea, nausea,* vomiting, abdominal pain.

GU: elevated BUN level, elevated serum creatinine level, genital pruritus, vaginitis.

Hematologic: decreased leukocyte count, eosinophilia.

Hepatic: elevated liver enzymes, cholestatic jaundice (rare).

Skin: rash, urticaria, diaper rash.

Other: superinfection, *hypersensitivity reactions, serum sickness, anaphylaxis.*

INTERACTIONS

Drug-drug. *Aminoglycosides:* potential increased risk of nephrotoxicity. Monitor closely.

Probenecid: may inhibit excretion and increase blood levels of cefprozil. Use together cautiously.

EFFECTS ON DIAGNOSTIC TESTS

Cephalosporins may produce a false-positive result for urine glucose tests that use copper reduction method (Benedict's reagent, Fehling's solution, or Clinitest tablets); use enzymatic glucose oxidase methods instead. A false-negative reaction may occur in the ferricyanide test for blood glucose.

CONTRAINDICATIONS

Contraindicated in patients with hypersensitivity to drug or other cephalosporins.

SPECIAL CONSIDERATIONS

▶ Use cautiously in patients with history of sensitivity to penicillin and in breast-feeding women. Also, use cautiously in patients with impaired hepatic or renal function.

▶ Renal function and liver function test results are monitored.

▶ A specimen for culture and sensitivity tests should be obtained before giving first dose. Therapy may begin pending results.

▶ The drug is administered after hemodialysis treatment is completed; drug is removed by hemodialysis.

▶ Superinfection may occur. May cause overgrowth of nonsusceptible bacteria or fungi.

▶ ***Alert:*** Don't confuse drug with other cephalosporins that sound alike.

Patient teaching

▶ Take drug as prescribed, even after feeling better.

▶ Shake suspension well before measuring dose.

▶ Oral suspensions contain the drug in a bubble-gum-flavored form to improve palatability and promote compliance in children. Refrigerate reconstituted sus-

---

pension and discard unused drug after 14 days.

▶ Notify health care provider if rash or signs and symptoms of superinfection occur.

ceftazidime

Ceptaz, Fortaz, Fortum§, Kefadim§, Tazicef, Tazidime

Pregnancy Risk Category B

HOW SUPPLIED

Injection (with sodium carbonate): 500 mg, 1 g, 2 g, 6 g (pharmacy bulk package)
Injection (with arginine): 1 g, 2 g, 6 g, 10 g (pharmacy bulk package)
Infusion: 1 g, 2 g in 50-ml and 100-ml vials (premixed)

ACTION

A third-generation cephalosporin that inhibits cell-wall synthesis, promoting osmotic instability; usually bactericidal.

Route	Onset	Peak	Duration
I.V.	Immediate	Immediate	Unknown
I.M.	Unknown	1 hr	Unknown

INDICATIONS & DOSAGE

Serious infections of the lower respiratory and urinary tracts; gynecologic, intraabdominal, CNS, and skin infections; bacteremia; and septicemia due to susceptible microorganisms, such as streptococci (including Streptococcus pneumoniae *and* S. pyogenes), Staphylococcus aureus *(penicillinase- and non-penicillinase-producing),* Escherichia coli, Klebsiella, Proteus, Enterobacter, Haemophilus influenzae, Pseudomonas, *and some strains of* Bacteroides —
Adults and children ages 12 and older: 1 g I.V. or I.M. q 8 to 12 hours; up to 6 g daily in life-threatening infections.

Children ages 1 month to 11 years: 25 to 50 mg/kg I.V. q 8 hours (sodium carbonate formulation).
Neonates up to age 4 weeks: 30 mg/kg I.V. q 12 hours (sodium carbonate formulation).
Uncomplicated urinary tract infections —
Adults: 250 mg I.V. or I.M. q 12 hours.
Complicated urinary tract infections —
Adults and children ages 12 and older: 500 mg to 1 g I.V. or I.M. q 8 to 12 hours.
Dosage adjustment: For patients with renal failure, if creatinine clearance is 31 to 50 ml/minute, give 1 g q 12 hours; if clearance is 16 to 30 ml/minute, give 1 g q 24 hours; if clearance is 6 to 15 ml/minute, give 500 mg q 24 hours; if clearance is below 5 ml/minute, give 500 mg q 48 hours.

ADVERSE REACTIONS

CNS: headache, dizziness, paresthesia, *seizures.*
CV: *phlebitis, thrombophlebitis.*
GI: pseudomembranous colitis, nausea, vomiting, diarrhea, abdominal cramps.
GU: vaginitis, candidiasis.
Hematologic: eosinophilia; thrombocytosis, *leukopenia,* hemolytic anemia, *agranulocytosis, thrombocytopenia.*
Hepatic: transient elevation in liver enzyme levels.
Skin: *maculopapular and erythematous rashes, urticaria, pain, induration, sterile abscesses, tissue sloughing at injection site.*
Other: *hypersensitivity reactions, serum sickness, anaphylaxis.*

INTERACTIONS

Drug-drug. *Aminoglycosides:* additive or synergistic effect against some strains of *Pseudomonas aeruginosa* and Enterobacteriaceae. Patient is monitored for effects.
Chloramphenicol: antagonistic effect. Avoid concomitant use.
Probenecid: may inhibit excretion and in-

crease drug levels. May be used as a therapeutic effect.

EFFECTS ON DIAGNOSTIC TESTS
Drug causes false-positive results in urine glucose tests using cupric sulfate (Benedict's reagent or Clinitest); use glucose oxidase (Diastix or Chemstrip uG) instead. Ceftazidime may cause positive Coombs' test results.

CONTRAINDICATIONS
Contraindicated in patients with hypersensitivity to drug or other cephalosporins.

SPECIAL CONSIDERATIONS
▶ Use cautiously in patients with a history of sensitivity to penicillin and in breast-feeding women. Also, use cautiously and with dosage adjustments in patients with renal failure. Renal function is monitored.
▶ A specimen for culture and sensitivity tests should be obtained before giving first dose. Therapy may begin pending results.
▶ For I.M. administration, drug is injected deeply into a large muscle mass, such as the gluteus maximus or the lateral aspect of the thigh.
▶ With large doses or prolonged therapy, superinfection may occur, especially in high-risk patients.
▶ *Alert:* Commercially available preparations contain either sodium carbonate (Fortaz, Magnacef, Tazicef, Tazidime) or arginine (Ceptaz, Pentacef) to facilitate dissolution of drug. Safety and efficacy of arginine-containing solutions in children younger than age 12 have not been established.
▶ Ceftazidime is removed by hemodialysis; a supplemental dose of drug is indicated after each dialysis period.
▶ *Alert:* Don't confuse drug with other cephalosporins that sound alike.

I.V. administration
▶ Solutions containing sodium carbonate are reconstituted with sterile water for injection. 5 ml is added to a 500-mg vial; 10 ml to a 1-g or 2-g vial. The vial is shaken well to dissolve drug. Carbon dioxide is released during dissolution, and positive pressure will develop in the vial. A arginine-containing solutions are reconstituted with 10 ml of sterile water for injection. This formulation won't release gas bubbles. Each brand of ceftazidime includes specific instructions for reconstitution. They should be read carefully.
▶ Drug is infused over 15 to 30 minutes.

Patient teaching
▶ Report adverse reactions or signs and symptoms of superinfection promptly.
▶ Alert health care provider if discomfort occurs at I.V. insertion site.
▶ Notify health care provider if loose stool or diarrhea occurs.

---

ceftibuten
Cedax

Pregnancy Risk Category B

HOW SUPPLIED
Capsules: 400 mg
Oral suspension: 90 mg/5 ml, 180 mg/5 ml

ACTION
A third-generation cephalosporin that exerts its bacterial action by binding to essential target proteins of the bacterial cell wall, which leads to inhibition of cell-wall synthesis.

Route	Onset	Peak	Duration
P.O.	Unknown	2-4 hr	Unknown

INDICATIONS & DOSAGE
Acute bacterial exacerbation of chronic bronchitis due to Haemophilus influenzae, Moraxella catarrhalis, *or penicillin-*

susceptible strains of Streptococcus pneumoniae —

Adults and children weighing over 45 kg (99 lb): 400 mg P.O. daily for 10 days.

Pharyngitis and tonsillitis due to S. pyogenes; *acute bacterial otitis media due to* H. influenzae, M. catarrhalis, *or* S. pyogenes —
Adults and children weighing over 45 kg: 400 mg P.O. daily for 10 days.
Children under 45 kg: 9 mg/kg P.O. daily for 10 days.

Dosage adjustment: For adult patients with renal impairment, if creatinine clearance is 30 to 49 ml/minute, give 4.5 mg/kg or 200 mg P.O. q 24 hours; if clearance is 5 to 29 ml/minute, give 2.25 mg/kg or 100 mg P.O. q 24 hours. In patients undergoing hemodialysis two or three times weekly, give single dose of 400 mg (capsule) or 9 mg/kg (suspension) P.O. after each hemodialysis session. Maximum dose is 400 mg.

ADVERSE REACTIONS

CNS: headache, dizziness, aphasia, psychosis.
GI: nausea, vomiting, diarrhea, dyspepsia, abdominal pain, loose stools, pseudomembranous colitis.
GU: elevated BUN levels, toxic nephropathy, renal dysfunction.
Hematologic: elevated eosinophil levels, decreased hemoglobin levels, altered platelet count, *aplastic anemia,* hemolytic anemia, *hemorrhage, neutropenia, agranulocytosis, pancytopenia.*
Hepatic: hepatic cholestasis, elevated liver enzymes and bilirubin.
Skin: *Stevens-Johnson syndrome.*
Other: allergic reaction, *anaphylaxis,* drug fever.

INTERACTIONS

Drug-food. *Any food:* decreased bioavailability of drug, which slows its absorption. Drug is administered 2 hours before or 1 hour after a meal.

EFFECTS ON DIAGNOSTIC TESTS

Although drug isn't known to affect the direct Coombs' test, other cephalosporins have caused a false-positive direct Coombs' test. Some cephalosporins may cause a false-positive test for urinary glucose.

CONTRAINDICATIONS

Contraindicated in patients with hypersensitivity to cephalosporins.

SPECIAL CONSIDERATIONS

▶ Use cautiously in elderly patients and in patients with history of hypersensitivity to penicillin.
▶ Also, use cautiously in patients with impaired renal failure or GI disease, especially colitis. Renal function is monitored.
▶ Safety and effectiveness in infants under age 6 months have not been established.
▶ Drug should be used in pregnancy only if clearly needed. Not known if drug appears in breast milk; drug is used cautiously in breast-feeding women.
▶ A specimen for culture and sensitivity tests should be obtained before giving first dose. Therapy may begin pending test results.
▶ When preparing oral suspension, the bottle is first tapped to loosen powder. A chart supplied by manufacturer is followed for amount of water to add to powder when mixing oral suspension form. Water is added in two portions; the mixture is shaken well after each step. After mixing, suspension is stable for 14 days if refrigerated.
▶ Oral suspension must be shaken well before administering.
▶ *Alert:* If allergic reaction is suspected, drug should be discontinued. Emergency treatment may be required.
▶ Drug may cause overgrowth of nonsusceptible bacteria or fungi. Superinfection may occur.
▶ Pseudomembranous colitis has been re-

ported with nearly all antibacterial agents. Consider this diagnosis in patients who develop diarrhea secondary to therapy. Specimens for *Clostridium difficile* may be obtained.

▶ *Alert:* Don't confuse drug with other cephalosporins that sound alike.

Patient teaching

▶ Take all of the drug prescribed, even if feeling better.

▶ Take oral suspension at least 2 hours before or 1 hour after a meal, and shake the bottle well before measuring dose.

▶ Store oral suspension in the refrigerator, with lid tightly closed, and discard unused drug after 14 days.

▶ Consult health care provider if breastfeeding; it's unknown if drug appears in breast milk.

▶ If diabetic, be aware that suspension contains 1 g sucrose/teaspoon.

▶ Report adverse reactions or signs and symptoms of superinfection.

▶ Notify health care provider if loose stool or diarrhea occurs.

ceftizoxime sodium

Cefizox

Pregnancy Risk Category B

HOW SUPPLIED

Injection: 500 mg, 1 g, 2 g, 10g
Infusion: 1 g, 2 g in 100-ml vials or in 50 ml of D_5W

ACTION

A third-generation cephalosporin that inhibits cell-wall synthesis, promoting osmotic instability; usually bactericidal.

Route	Onset	Peak	Duration
I.V.	Immediate	Immediate	Unknown
I.M.	Unknown	0.5-1.5 hr	Unknown

INDICATIONS & DOSAGE

Serious infections of the lower respiratory and urinary tracts, gynecologic infections, bacteremia, septicemia, meningitis, intra-abdominal infections, bone and joint infections, and skin infections due to susceptible microorganisms, such as strep-tococci (including Streptococcus pneumoniae *and* S. pyogenes), Staphylococcus aureus *and* S. epidermidis, Escherichia coli, Klebsiella, Haemophilus influenzae, Enterobacter, Proteus, *some* Pseudomonas, *and* Peptostreptococcus —

Adults: usual dosage is 1 to 2 g I.V. or I.M. q 8 to 12 hours. In life-threatening infections, up to 2 g q 4 hours.

Children over age 6 months: 50 mg/kg I.V. q 6 to 8 hours. For serious infections, up to 200 mg/kg/day in divided doses may be used. Don't exceed 12 g/day.

Dosage adjustment: For patients with renal failure, if creatinine clearance is 50 to 79 ml/minute, give 500 mg to 1.5 g q 8 hours; if clearance is 5 to 49 ml/minute, give 250 mg to 1 g q 12 hours; if clearance is below 5 ml/minute or patient undergoes hemodialysis, give 500 mg to 1 g q 48 hours, or 250 to 500 mg q 24 hours.

ADVERSE REACTIONS

CV: *phlebitis, thrombophlebitis.*
GI: pseudomembranous colitis, nausea, anorexia, vomiting, *diarrhea.*
GU: vaginitis.
Hematologic: *transient neutropenia,* eosinophilia, hemolytic anemia, thrombocytosis, anemia, ***thrombocytopenia.***
Hepatic: transient elevation in liver enzymes.
Respiratory: dyspnea.
Skin: *maculopapular and erythematous rashes, urticaria,. pain, induration, sterile abscesses, tissue sloughing at injection site.*
Other: *hypersensitivity reactions, serum sickness, anaphylaxis,* elevated temperature.

INTERACTIONS

Drug-drug. *Aminoglycosides:* potential increase in nephrotoxicity. Avoid use. *Probenecid:* may inhibit excretion and increase blood levels of ceftizoxime. May be used for this effect.

EFFECTS ON DIAGNOSTIC TESTS

Ceftizoxime causes false-positive results in urine glucose tests using cupric sulfate (Benedict's reagent or Clinitest); use glucose oxidase (Diastix or Chemstrip uG) instead. Drug also causes false elevations in urine creatinine levels using Jaffé's reaction and may cause positive Coombs' test results.

CONTRAINDICATIONS

Contraindicated in patients with hypersensitivity to drug or other cephalosporins.

SPECIAL CONSIDERATIONS

▶ Use cautiously in patients with history of sensitivity to penicillin and in breast-feeding women. Also, use cautiously and with dosage adjustments in patients with renal failure. Renal function is monitored.
▶ A specimen for culture and sensitivity tests should be obtained before giving first dose. Therapy may begin pending results.
▶ To prepare I.M. injection, 1.5 ml of diluent is mixed per 500 mg of drug. For I.M. administration, drug is injected deeply into a large muscle mass, such as the gluteus maximus or the lateral aspect of the thigh. Larger doses (2 g) should be divided and administered at two separate sites.
▶ With large doses or prolonged therapy, superinfection may occur, especially in high-risk patients.
▶ *Alert:* Don't confuse drug with other cephalosporins that sound alike.

I.V. administration

▶ To reconstitute powder, 5 ml of sterile water is added to a 500-mg vial, 10 ml to a 1-g vial, or 20 ml to a 2-g vial.
▶ Drug is injected directly into vein over 3 to 5 minutes or slowly into I.V. tubing with free-flowing compatible solution.
▶ Drug in piggyback vials is reconstituted with 50 to 100 ml of normal saline solution or D_5W. Solution is shaken well.
▶ Drug is infused over 15 to 30 minutes.

Patient teaching

▶ Report adverse reactions and signs and symptoms of superinfection promptly.
▶ Alert health care provider if discomfort occurs at I.V. site.
▶ Notify health care provider if loose stool or diarrhea occurs.

ceftriaxone sodium
Rocephin

Pregnancy Risk Category B

HOW SUPPLIED

Injection: 250 mg, 500 mg, 1 g, 2 g, 10 g
Infusion: 1 g, 2 g piggyback; 1 g, 2 g/ 50 ml premixed

ACTION

A third-generation cephalosporin that inhibits cell-wall synthesis, promoting osmotic instability; usually bactericidal.

Route	Onset	Peak	Duration
I.V.	Immediate	Immediate	Unknown
I.M.	Unknown	1.5-4 hr	Unknown

INDICATIONS & DOSAGE

Uncomplicated gonococcal vulvovaginitis —
Adults: 125 mg I.M. as a single dose, plus azithromycin 1 g P.O. as a single dose or doxycycline 100 mg P.O. b.i.d. for 7 days. Alternatively, give ceftriaxone 250 mg I.M. as a single dose.
Most infections due to susceptible organisms; serious infections of the lower respiratory and urinary tracts; gyneco-

---

logic, bone and joint, intra-abdominal, and skin infections; bacteremia; septicemia; and Lyme disease due to such susceptible microorganisms as streptococci (including Streptococcus pneumoniae and S. pyogenes); Staphylococcus aureus (penicillinase- and non-penicillinase-producing) and S. epidermidis, Escherichia coli, Klebsiella, Haemophilus influenzae, Neisseria meningitidis, N. gonorrhoeae, Enterobacter, Proteus, Peptostreptococcus, Pseudomonas, and Serratia marcescens —

Adults and children over age 12: 1 to 2 g I.M. or I.V. daily or in equally divided doses q 12 hours. Total daily dosage shouldn't exceed 4 g.

Children ages 12 and younger: 50 to 75 mg/kg I.M. or I.V., not to exceed 2 g/day, given in divided doses q 12 hours.

Meningitis —

Adults and children: initially, 100 mg/kg I.M. or I.V. (not to exceed 4 g); thereafter, 100 mg/kg I.M. or I.V., given once daily or in divided doses q 12 hours, not to exceed 4 g, for 7 to 14 days.

Perioperative prophylaxis —

Adults: 1 g I.V. as a single dose 30 minutes to 2 hours before surgery.

Acute bacterial otitis media —

Children: 50 mg/kg (not to exceed 1 g) I.M. as a single dose.

ADVERSE REACTIONS

CNS: headache, dizziness.

CV: phlebitis.

GI: pseudomembranous colitis, nausea, vomiting, diarrhea.

GU: genital pruritus, candidiasis, elevated BUN levels.

Hematologic: eosinophilia, thrombocytosis, *leukopenia.*

Hepatic: elevated liver function test results.

Skin: pain, induration, tenderness at injection site, *rash;* pruritus.

Other: hypersensitivity reactions, serum sickness, anaphylaxis, elevated temperature, chills.

INTERACTIONS

Drug-drug. *Aminoglycosides:* additive or synergistic effect against some strains of *P. aeruginosa* and Enterobacteriaceae. Monitor patient.

Probenecid: high doses (1 or 2 g/day) may enhance hepatic clearance of ceftriaxone and shorten its half-life. Avoid concomitant use.

EFFECTS ON DIAGNOSTIC TESTS

Ceftriaxone causes false-positive results in urine glucose tests using cupric sulfate (Benedict's reagent or Clinitest); instead use glucose oxidase (Diastix or Chemstrip uG). Drug also causes false elevations in urine creatinine levels in tests using Jaffé's reaction, and may cause positive Coombs' test results.

CONTRAINDICATIONS

Contraindicated in patients with hypersensitivity to drug or other cephalosporins.

SPECIAL CONSIDERATIONS

▶ Use cautiously in patients with a history of sensitivity to penicillin and in breast-feeding women.

▶ A specimen for culture and sensitivity tests should be obtained before giving first dose. Therapy may begin pending results.

▶ A commercially available intramuscular kit containing 1% lidocaine as a diluent is available from the manufacturer.

▶ For I.M. administration, drug is injected deeply into a large muscle mass, such as the gluteus maximus or the lateral aspect of the thigh.

▶ With large doses or prolonged therapy, superinfection may occur, especially in high-risk patients.

▶ Drug is commonly used in home antibiotic programs for outpatient treatment of serious infections such as osteomyelitis.

▶ *Alert:* Don't confuse drug with other cephalosporins that sound alike.

I.V. administration
▶ Drug is reconstituted with sterile water for injection, normal saline injection, D$_5$W or D$_{10}$W injection, or a combination of NaCl and dextrose injection and other compatible solutions. Drug is reconstituted by adding 2.4 ml of diluent to the 250-mg vial, 4.8 ml to the 500-mg vial, 9.6 ml to the 1-g vial, and 19.2 ml to the 2-g vial. All reconstituted solutions yield a concentration that averages 100 mg/ml. After reconstitution, the drug is further diluted for intermittent infusion to desired concentration. I.V. dilutions are stable for 24 hours at room temperature.

Patient teaching
▶ Report adverse reactions promptly.
▶ Alert health care provider if discomfort occurs at I.V. insertion site.
▶ Home care patient and family will need to be taught how to prepare and administer drug.
▶ If home care patient is a diabetic who is testing his urine for glucose, the drug may affect results of cupric sulfate tests; an enzymatic test should be used instead.
▶ Notify health care provider if loose stool or diarrhea occurs.

---

cefuroxime axetil
Ceftin, Zinnat§

cefuroxime sodium
Kefurox, Zinacef

Pregnancy Risk Category B

HOW SUPPLIED
cefuroxime axetil
Tablets: 125 mg, 250 mg, 500 mg
Suspension: 125 mg/5 ml, 250 mg/5 ml

cefuroxime sodium
Injection: 750 mg, 1.5 g, 7.5 g
Infusion: 750 mg, 1.5-g premixed, frozen solution

ACTION
A second-generation cephalosporin that inhibits cell-wall synthesis, promoting osmotic instability; usually bactericidal.

Route	Onset	Peak	Duration
P.O.	Unknown	15-60 min	Unknown
I.V.	Immediate	Immediate	Unknown
I.M.	Unknown	2 hr	Unknown

INDICATIONS & DOSAGE
Injectable form: *Serious infections of the lower respiratory and urinary tracts; skin and skin-structure infections; bone and joint infections; septicemia; meningitis; and gonorrhea; and for perioperative prophylaxis.* Oral form: *Otitis media, pharyngitis, tonsillitis, infections of the urinary and lower respiratory tracts, and skin and skin-structure infections. Among susceptible organisms are* Streptococcus pneumoniae *and* S. pyogenes, Haemophilus influenzae, Klebsiella, Staphylococcus aureus, Escherichia coli, Moraxella (Branhamella) catarrhalis *(including beta-lactamase-producing strains),* Enterobacter, *and* Neisseria gonorrhoeae —
Adults and children ages 12 and older: usual dosage of cefuroxime sodium is 750 mg to 1.5 g I.M. or I.V. q 8 hours for 5 to 10 days. For life-threatening infections and infections due to less susceptible organisms, 1.5 g I.M. or I.V. q 6 hours; for bacterial meningitis, up to 3 g I.V. q 8 hours.

Or, administer 250 mg of cefuroxime axetil P.O. q 12 hours. For severe infections, dosage may be increased to 500 mg q 12 hours.
Children and infants over age 3 months: 50 to 100 mg/kg/day of cefuroxime sodium I.M. or I.V. in equally divided doses q 6 to 8 hours. Higher dosage of

---

100 mg/kg/day (not to exceed maximum adult dosage) should be used for more severe or serious infections. For bacterial meningitis, 200 to 240 mg/kg I.V. in divided doses q 6 to 8 hours. For other infections, 125 to 250 mg of cefuroxime axetil P.O. q 12 hours for a child who can swallow pills.

Uncomplicated urinary tract infections —
Adults: 125 to 250 mg P.O. q 12 hours.
Otitis media —
Children ages 2 and older: 250 mg P.O. q 12 hours.
Children under age 2: 125 mg P.O. q 12 hours.

Perioperative prophylaxis —
Adults: 1.5 g I.V. 30 to 60 minutes before surgery; in lengthy operations, 750 mg I.V. or I.M. q 8 hours. For open-heart surgery, 1.5 g I.V. at induction of anesthesia and then q 12 hours for a total dosage of 6 g.

Early Lyme disease (erythema migrans) due to Borrelia burgdorferi —
Adults and children ages 13 and older: 500 mg P.O. b.i.d. for 20 days.

Secondary bacterial infection of acute bronchitis —
Adults: 250 to 500 mg P.O. (tablets) b.i.d. for 5 to 10 days.

Dosage adjustment: For parenteral administration in patients with renal failure, if creatinine clearance is 10 to 20 ml/minute, give 750 mg I.M. or I.V. q 12 hours; if clearance is below 10 ml/minute, give 750 mg I.M. or I.V. q 24 hours.

ADVERSE REACTIONS

CV: *phlebitis, thrombophlebitis.*
GI: pseudomembranous colitis, nausea, anorexia, vomiting, *diarrhea.*
Hematologic: *transient neutropenia,* eosinophilia, *hemolytic anemia,* ***thrombocytopenia,*** decreased hematocrit and hemoglobin levels.
Hepatic: transient increases in liver enzymes.

Skin: *maculopapular and erythematous rashes, urticaria, pain, induration, sterile abscesses, temperature elevation, tissue sloughing at I.M. injection site.*
Other*: hypersensitivity reactions, serum sickness, anaphylaxis.*

INTERACTIONS

Drug-drug. *Aminoglycosides:* synergistic activity against some organisms; potential for increased nephrotoxicity. Monitor closely.
Diuretics: increased risk of adverse renal reactions. Monitor closely.
Probenecid: may inhibit excretion and increase blood levels of cefuroxime. Sometimes used for this effect.
Drug-food. *Any food:* increased absorption. Drug is given with food.

EFFECTS ON DIAGNOSTIC TESTS

Cefuroxime causes false-positive results in urine glucose tests using cupric sulfate (Benedict's reagent or Clinitest); use glucose oxidase tests (Diastix or Chemstrip uG) instead. Drug also causes false elevations in serum or urine creatinine levels in tests using Jaffé's reaction, and may cause positive Coombs' test results.

CONTRAINDICATIONS

Contraindicated in patients with hypersensitivity to drug or other cephalosporins.

SPECIAL CONSIDERATIONS

▶ Use cautiously in patients with history of sensitivity to penicillin and in breast-feeding women. Also, use cautiously and with reduced dosage in patients with impaired renal function. Renal function must be monitored.
▶ A specimen for culture and sensitivity tests should be obtained before giving first dose. Therapy may begin pending results.
▶ For I.M. administration, the drug is injected deeply into a large muscle mass, such as the gluteus maximus or the lateral aspect of the thigh.

▶ Absorption of cefuroxime axetil is enhanced by food.

▶ Keep in mind that cefuroxime axetil tablets may be crushed for patients who cannot swallow tablets. Tablets may be dissolved in small amounts of apple, orange, or grape juice or chocolate milk. However, the drug has a bitter taste that is difficult to mask, even with food.

▶ *Alert:* Cefuroxime axetil film-coated tablet and oral suspension aren't bioequivalent. Don't substitute on a mg/mg basis.

▶ With large doses or prolonged therapy, superinfection may occur, especially in high-risk patients.

▶ *Alert:* Don't confuse drug with other cephalosporins that sound alike.

I.V. administration

▶ For each 750-mg vial of Kefurox, 9 ml of sterile water for injection is used for reconstitution. Withdraw 8 ml from the vial for the proper dose. For each 1.5-g vial of Kefurox, 16 ml of sterile water for injection is used for reconstitution; entire contents of vial is withdrawn for a dose. For each 750-mg vial of Zinacef, 8 ml of sterile water for injection is used for reconstitution; for each 1.5-g vial, 16 ml is used for reconstitution. In each case, entire contents of vial is withdrawn for a dose.

▶ To give by direct injection, the drug is injected into a large vein or into the tubing of a free-flowing I.V. solution over 3 to 5 minutes.

▶ For intermittent infusion, reconstituted drug is added to 100 ml D_5W, normal saline for injection, or other compatible I.V. solution. Drug is infused over 15 to 60 minutes.

Patient teaching

▶ Take all of the drug as prescribed, even after feeling better.

▶ Take oral form with food. To aid swallowing, tablets may be dissolved or crushed, but bitter taste that results is hard to mask, even with food. If using suspen-sion, shake container well before measuring dose.

▶ Notify health care provider if rash or signs and symptoms of superinfection occur.

▶ If receiving drug I.V., alert health care provider if discomfort occurs at I.V. insertion site.

▶ Notify health care provider if loose stool or diarrhea occurs.

---

cephalexin hydrochloride
Keftab

cephalexin monohydrate
Apo-Cephalex , Biocef, Keflex,
Novo-Lexin , Nu-Cephalex

Pregnancy Risk Category B

HOW SUPPLIED
cephalexin hydrochloride
Tablets: 500 mg
cephalexin monohydrate
Tablets: 250 mg, 500 mg, 1 g
Capsules: 250 mg, 500 mg
Oral suspension: 125 mg/5 ml, 250 mg/5 ml

ACTION
A first-generation cephalosporin that inhibits cell-wall synthesis, promoting osmotic instability; usually bactericidal.

Route	Onset	Peak	Duration
P.O.	Unknown	1 hr	Unknown

INDICATIONS & DOSAGE
Respiratory tract, GI tract, skin, soft-tissue, bone, and joint infections and otitis media due to Escherichia coli *and other coliform bacteria, group A beta-hemolytic streptococci,* Klebsiella, Proteus mirabilis, Streptococcus pneumoniae, *and staphylococci —*

Adults: 250 mg to 1 g P.O. q 6 hours or 500 mg q 12 hours. Maximum 4 g daily.
Children: 6 to 12 mg/kg P.O. q 6 hours (monohydrate only). Maximum 25 mg/kg q 6 hours.
Dosage adjustment: For adults with impaired renal function, initial dose is the same. Recommended subsequent dosing for creatinine clearance below 5 ml/minute, 250 mg P.O. q 12 to 24 hours; for creatinine clearance of 5 to 10 ml/minute, 250 mg P.O. q 12 hours; and for creatinine clearance of 11 to 40 ml/minute, 500 mg P.O. q 8 to 12 hours.

ADVERSE REACTIONS
CNS: dizziness, headache, fatigue, agitation, confusion, hallucinations.
GI: pseudomembranous colitis, *nausea, anorexia,* vomiting, *diarrhea,* gastritis, glossitis, dyspepsia, abdominal pain, anal pruritus, tenesmus, oral candidiasis.
GU: genital pruritus, candidiasis, vaginitis, interstitial nephritis.
Hematologic: *neutropenia,* eosinophilia, anemia, *thrombocytopenia.*
Hepatic: transient increases in liver enzymes.
Musculoskeletal: arthritis, arthralgia, joint pain.
Skin: *maculopapular and erythematous rashes, urticaria.*
Other: *hypersensitivity reactions, serum sickness, anaphylaxis.*

INTERACTIONS
Drug-drug. *Probenecid:* may increase blood levels of cephalosporins. May be used for this effect.

EFFECTS ON DIAGNOSTIC TESTS
Cephalexin causes false-positive results in urine glucose tests using cupric sulfate (Benedict's reagent or Clinitest); use glucose oxidase tests (Diastix or Chemstrip uG) instead. Drug also causes false elevations in serum or urine creatinine levels in tests using Jaffé's reaction. Positive Coombs' test results occur in about 3% of patients taking cephalexin.

CONTRAINDICATIONS
Contraindicated in patients with hypersensitivity to cephalosporins.

SPECIAL CONSIDERATIONS
▶ Use cautiously in breast-feeding women and in patients with impaired renal function or history of sensitivity to penicillin. Renal function must be monitored.
▶ The patient must be asked about past reaction to cephalosporin or penicillin therapy before giving first dose.
▶ A specimen for culture and sensitivity tests should be obtained before giving first dose. Therapy may begin pending results.
▶ To prepare oral suspension: Required amount of water is added to powder in two portions. Solution is shaken well after each addition. After mixing, store in refrigerator. The mixture will remain stable for 14 days without significant loss of potency. The container should be kept tightly closed and shaken well before using.
▶ With large doses or prolonged therapy, superinfection may occur, especially in high-risk patients.
▶ Group A beta-hemolytic streptococcal infections should be treated for a minimum of 10 days.
▶ *Alert:* Don't confuse drug with other cephalosporins that sound alike.

Patient teaching
▶ Take all of the drug exactly as prescribed, even after feeling better.
▶ Take with food or milk to lessen GI discomfort. If taking suspension form, shake the container well before measuring dose, and store container in refrigerator.
▶ Notify health care provider if rash or signs and symptoms of superinfection develop.

cephradine
Velosef**
Pregnancy Risk Category B

HOW SUPPLIED
Capsules: 250 mg, 500 mg
Oral suspension: 125 mg/5 ml, 250 mg/ 5 ml

ACTION
First-generation cephalosporin that inhibits cell-wall synthesis, promoting osmotic instability; usually bactericidal.

Route	Onset	Peak	Duration
P.O.	Unknown	1 hr	Unknown

INDICATIONS & DOSAGE
Serious infections of respiratory, GU, or GI tract; skin and soft-tissue infections; bone and joint infections; septicemia; endocarditis; and otitis media due to such susceptible organisms as Escherichia coli *and other coliform bacteria, group A beta-hemolytic streptococci,* Klebsiella, Proteus mirabilis, Staphylococcus aureus, Streptococcus pneumoniae, S. viridans, *and staphylococci; perioperative prophylaxis —*
Adults: 250 to 500 mg P.O. q 6 hours or 500 mg to 1 g P.O. q 12 hours.
Children over age 9 months: 25 to 50 mg/kg P.O. daily in divided doses q 6 to 12 hours.
  Otitis media —
Children: 75 to 100 mg/kg P.O. daily in equally divided doses q 6 to 12 hours. Don't exceed 4 g daily.
  All patients, regardless of age and weight, may be given larger doses (up to 1 g q.i.d.) for severe or chronic infections.

ADVERSE REACTIONS
CNS: dizziness, headache, malaise, paresthesia.
GI: pseudomembranous colitis, *nausea, anorexia,* vomiting, heartburn, abdominal cramps, *diarrhea,* oral candidiasis.
GU: genital pruritus, candidiasis, vaginitis.
Hematologic: *transient neutropenia,* eosinophilia, *thrombocytopenia.*
Hepatic: transient increases in liver enzymes.
Skin: *maculopapular and erythematous rashes, urticaria.*
Other: *hypersensitivity reactions, serum sickness, anaphylaxis.*

INTERACTIONS
Drug-drug. *Probenecid:* may increase blood levels of cephalosporins. Sometimes used for this effect.

EFFECTS ON DIAGNOSTIC TESTS
Cephradine causes false-positive results in urine glucose tests using cupric sulfate (Benedict's reagent or Clinitest); instead use glucose oxidase tests (Diastix or Chemstrip uG). Drug also causes false elevations in serum or urine creatinine levels in tests using Jaffé's reaction, and may cause positive Coombs' test results.

CONTRAINDICATIONS
Contraindicated in patients with hypersensitivity to drug and to other cephalosporins.

SPECIAL CONSIDERATIONS
▶ Use cautiously in patients with impaired renal function or with a history of sensitivity to penicillin. Also, use cautiously in breast-feeding women.
▶ Renal function must be monitored.
▶ A specimen for culture and sensitivity tests should be obtained before giving first dose. Therapy may begin pending results.
▶ Group A beta-hemolytic streptococcal infections should be treated for a minimum of 10 days.
▶ With large doses or prolonged therapy, superinfection may occur, especially in high-risk patients.

▶ **Alert:** Don't confuse drug with other cephalosporins that sound alike.

Patient teaching

▶ Take all of the drug as prescribed, even after feeling better.

▶ Take drug with food or milk to lessen GI discomfort. If patient is taking suspension form, shake it well before measuring dose.

▶ Notify health care provider if rash or signs and symptoms of superinfection occur.

▶ Notify health care provider if loose stools or diarrhea occurs.

loracarbef

Lorabid

Pregnancy Risk Category B

HOW SUPPLIED

Pulvules: 200 mg, 400 mg
Powder for oral suspension: 100 mg/5 ml, 200 mg/5 ml in 50-ml, 75-ml and 100-ml bottles

ACTION

A synthetic beta-lactam antibiotic of the carbacephem class with actions similar to second-generation cephalosporins. Inhibits cell-wall synthesis, promoting osmotic instability; usually bactericidal.

Route	Onset	Peak	Duration
P.O.	Unknown	0.5-1 hr	Unknown

INDICATIONS & DOSAGE

Secondary bacterial infections of acute bronchitis —
Adults: 200 to 400 mg P.O. q 12 hours for 7 days.
Acute bacterial exacerbations of chronic bronchitis —
Adults: 400 mg P.O. q 12 hours for 7 days.

Pneumonia —
Adults: 400 mg P.O. q 12 hours for 14 days.
Pharyngitis, sinusitis, tonsillitis —
Adults: 200 to 400 mg P.O. q 12 hours for 10 days.
Children ages 6 months to 12 years: 15 mg/kg P.O. daily in divided doses q 12 hours for 10 days.
Acute otitis media —
Children ages 6 months to 12 years: 30 mg/kg (oral suspension) P.O. daily in divided doses q 12 hours for 10 days.
Uncomplicated skin and skin-structure infections —
Adults: 200 mg P.O. q 12 hours for 7 days.
Impetigo —
Children ages 6 months to 12 years: 15 mg/kg P.O. daily in divided doses q 12 hours for 7 days.
Uncomplicated cystitis —
Adults: 200 mg P.O. daily for 7 days.
Uncomplicated pyelonephritis —
Adults: 400 mg P.O. q 12 hours for 14 days.
Dosage adjustment: Patients with creatinine clearance of 50 ml/minute or more don't require dose and interval changes. If creatinine clearance is 10 to 49 ml/minute, give half of usual dose at same interval; if it is below 10 ml/minute, give usual dose q 3 to 5 days. Hemodialysis patients require an additional dose after dialysis.

ADVERSE REACTIONS

CNS: headache, somnolence, nervousness, insomnia, dizziness.
CV: vasodilation.
GI: diarrhea, nausea, vomiting, abdominal pain, anorexia, pseudomembranous colitis.
GU: vaginal candidiasis, transient increases in BUN and creatinine levels.
Hematologic: *transient thrombocytopenia, leukopenia,* eosinophilia, increased PT and INR, pancytopenia, *neutropenia.*
Hepatic: transient elevations in AST, ALT, and alkaline phosphatase levels.

Skin: rash, urticaria, pruritus, *erythema multiforme.*
Other: *hypersensitivity reactions, anaphylaxis.*

INTERACTIONS

Drug-drug. *Probenecid:* decreased excretion of loracarbef, causing increased plasma levels. Patient is monitored for toxicity.
Drug-food. *Any food:* decreased absorption. Drug is taken on an empty stomach at least 1 hour before or 2 hours after a meal.

EFFECTS ON DIAGNOSTIC TESTS

Drug can cause positive direct Coombs' test results.

CONTRAINDICATIONS

Contraindicated in patients with hypersensitivity to drug or other cephalosporins and in patients with diarrhea due to pseudomembranous colitis.

SPECIAL CONSIDERATIONS

▶ Use cautiously in pregnant or breast-feeding women. Safety and efficacy of drug have not been established in infants under age 6 months.
▶ A specimen for culture and sensitivity tests should be obtained before giving first dose. Therapy may begin pending results.
▶ To reconstitute powder for oral suspension, 30 ml of water is added in two portions to the 50-ml bottle or 60 ml of water in two portions to the 100-ml bottle; the bottle is shaken after each addition.
▶ After reconstitution, oral suspension may be stored for 14 days at room temperature (59° to 86° F [15° to 30° C]).
▶ Patient should be monitored for superinfection. May cause overgrowth of nonsusceptible bacteria or fungi.
▶ Renal function must be monitored.
▶ *Alert:* Patient must be monitored for seizures. Beta-lactam antibiotics may trigger seizures in susceptible patients, especially when given without dosage modification to those with renal impairment. If seizures occur, discontinue drug. Anticonvulsants may be administered.
▶ For otitis media, remember that the more rapidly absorbed oral suspension produces higher peak plasma levels than do the capsules.
▶ *Alert:* Don't confuse Lorabid with Lortab.

Patient teaching

▶ Take all of the drug prescribed, even after feeling better.
▶ Take drug on an empty stomach, at least 1 hour before or 2 hours after meals. Shake container well before measuring dose.
▶ Discard unused portion after 14 days.
▶ Notify health care provider if rash or signs and symptoms of superinfection appear.
▶ Notify health care provider if loose stool or diarrhea occurs.

Reactions may be *common*, uncommon, *life-threatening*, or COMMON AND LIFE-THREATENING.

demeclocycline hydrochloride
doxycycline calcium
doxycycline hyclate
doxycycline hydrochloride
doxycycline monohydrate
minocycline hydrochloride
tetracycline hydrochloride

COMBINATION PRODUCTS

Urobiotic-250: oxytetracycline hydrochloride 250 mg, sulfamethizole 250 mg, and phenazopyridine hydrochloride 50 mg.

Helidac: tetracycline 500 mg, bismuth salicylate 262.4 mg, and metronidazole 250 mg.

demeclocycline hydrochloride

Declomycin, Ledermycin‡
Pregnancy Risk Category D

HOW SUPPLIED

Tablets (film-coated): 150mg, 300 mg
Capsules: 150 mg

ACTION

Unknown. Thought to exert bacteriostatic effect by binding to the 30S and possibly 50S ribosomal subunits of microorganisms, thus inhibiting protein synthesis. May also alter the cytoplasmic membrane of susceptible microorganisms.

Route	Onset	Peak	Duration
P.O.	Unknown	3-4 hr	Unknown

INDICATIONS & DOSAGE

Infections due to susceptible gram-positive and gram-negative organisms (including Haemophilus ducreyi, Yersinia pestis, *and* Campylobacter fetus), Rick-ettsiae, Mycoplasma pneumoniae, Chlamydia trachomatis; *psittacosis; granuloma inguinale* —
Adults: 150 mg P.O. q 6 hours or 300 mg P.O. q 12 hours.
Children over age 8: 6.6 to 13.2 mg/kg P.O. daily, in divided doses q 6 to 12 hours.
    Gonorrhea —
Adults: initially, 600 mg P.O.; then 300 mg P.O. q 12 hours for 4 days (for total of 3 g).

ADVERSE REACTIONS

CNS: *intracranial hypertension,* dizziness.
CV: pericarditis.
EENT: dysphagia, tinnitus, visual disturbances.
GI: anorexia, *nausea, vomiting, diarrhea,* enterocolitis, glossitis, anogenital inflammation, pancreatitis.
GU: elevated serum BUN levels.
Hematologic: *neutropenia,* eosinophilia, *thrombocytopenia, hemolytic anemia.*
Hepatic: elevated liver enzymes.
Metabolic: diabetes insipidus syndrome.
Skin: *maculopapular and erythematous rashes, photosensitivity, increased pigmentation, urticaria.*
Other: *hypersensitivity reactions, anaphylaxis,* permanent tooth discoloration, bone growth retardation if used in children under age 9.

INTERACTIONS

Drug-drug. *Antacids (including sodium bicarbonate) and laxatives containing aluminum, magnesium, or calcium; antidiarrheals:* decreased antibiotic absorption. Antibiotic is given 1 hour before or 2 hours after any of these drugs.
Ferrous sulfate and other iron products, zinc: decreased antibiotic absorption. Antibiotic is given 2 hours before or 3 hours after iron administration.

---

*Liquid contains alcohol.   **May contain tartrazine.   †Canada   ‡Australia   §U.K.   ◇OTC

Methoxyflurane: may cause nephrotoxicity with tetracyclines. Avoid concurrent use.

Oral anticoagulants: increased anticoagulant effect. PT and INR must be monitored, and dosage adjusted as needed.

Oral contraceptives: decreased contraceptive effectiveness and increased risk of breakthrough bleeding. A nonhormonal birth control method should be recommended.

Penicillins: may interfere with bactericidal action of penicillins. Avoid use together.

Drug-food. *Milk, dairy products, other foods:* decreased antibiotic absorption. Antibiotic is given 1 hour before or 2 hours after any of the above.

Drug-lifestyle. *Sun exposure:* photosensitivity reactions may occur. Take precautions.

EFFECTS ON DIAGNOSTIC TESTS

Demeclocycline causes false-negative results in urine glucose tests using glucose oxidase reagent (Diastix or Chemstrip uG). Drug also causes false elevations in fluorometric tests for urine catecholamines.

CONTRAINDICATIONS

Contraindicated in patients with hypersensitivity to drug or other tetracyclines.

SPECIAL CONSIDERATIONS

‣ Use cautiously in patients with impaired renal or hepatic function.

‣ Use of these drugs during last half of pregnancy and in children under age 9 may cause permanent discoloration of teeth, enamel defects, and bone growth retardation.

‣ Signs and symptoms of diabetes insipidus syndrome include polyuria, polydipsia, and weakness.

‣ Renal and liver function test results must be monitored.

‣ Fluid balance and daily weights are monitored in patients with impaired kidney and liver function.

‣ A specimen for culture and sensitivity tests should be obtained before giving first dose. Therapy may begin pending test results.

‣ **Alert:** Expiration date needs to be checked. Outdated or deteriorated tetracyclines have been associated with reversible nephrotoxicity (Fanconi's syndrome).

‣ Drug should not be exposed to light or heat; store in tightly capped container.

‣ With large doses or prolonged therapy, superinfection is possible, especially in high-risk patients.

‣ Patient's tongue should be checked for signs of candidal infection. Stress good oral hygiene.

Patient teaching

‣ Take entire amount of drug, exactly as prescribed, even after feeling better.

‣ The drug's effectiveness is reduced when taken with milk or other dairy products, food, antacids, or iron products. Take each dose with a full glass of water on an empty stomach, at least 1 hour before or 2 hours after meals. Also, take drug at least 1 hour before bedtime to prevent esophageal irritation or ulceration.

‣ Avoid direct sunlight and ultraviolet light, wear protective clothing, and use sunscreen. Photosensitivity reactions may occur within a few minutes to several hours after sun exposure. Photosensitivity persists for some time after discontinuation of drug.

‣ Report signs and symptoms of superinfection.

---

doxycycline calcium
Vibramycin

doxycycline hyclate
Apo-Doxy , Doryx, Doxy Caps,
Doxy 100, Doxy 200, Doxycin ,
Novo-Doxylin , Vibramycin,
Vibra-Tabs

doxycycline hydrochloride
Doryx‡, Doxylin‡, Vibramycin‡

doxycycline monohydrate
Monodox, Vibramycin

Pregnancy Risk Category D

HOW SUPPLIED
doxycycline calcium
Oral suspension: 50 mg/5 ml
doxycycline hyclate
Tablets (film-coated): 100 mg
Capsules: 50 mg, 100 mg
Capsules (enteric-coated pellets): 100 mg
Injection: 100 mg, 200 mg
doxycycline hydrochloride
Tablets: 50 mg‡, 100 mg‡
Capsules: 50 mg‡, 100 mg‡
doxycycline monohydrate
Capsules: 50 mg, 100 mg
Oral suspension: 25 mg/5 ml

ACTION
Unknown. Thought to exert bacteriostatic effect by binding to the 30S and possibly 50S ribosomal subunits of microorganisms, thus inhibiting protein synthesis. May also alter the cytoplasmic membrane of susceptible microorganisms.

Route	Onset	Peak	Duration
P.O.	Unknown	1.5-4 hr	Unknown
I.V.	Immediate	Unknown	Unknown

INDICATIONS & DOSAGE
Infections due to susceptible gram-positive and gram-negative organisms (including Haemophilus ducreyi, Yersinia pestis, *and* Campylobacter fetus), Rickettsiae, Mycoplasma pneumoniae, Chlamydia trachomatis, *and* Borrelia burgdorferi *(Lyme disease); psittacosis; granuloma inguinale —*
Adults and children over age 8 weighing at least 45 kg (99 lb): 100 mg P.O. q 12 hours on first day; then 100 mg P.O. daily. Or, 200 mg I.V. on first day in one or two infusions; then 100 to 200 mg I.V. daily.
Children over age 8 and under 45 kg: 4.4 mg/kg P.O. or I.V. daily, in divided doses q 12 hours on first day; then 2.2 to 4.4 mg/kg daily in one or two divided doses.
    Give I.V. infusion slowly (minimum 1 hour). Infusion must be completed within 12 hours (within 6 hours in lactated Ringer's solution or dextrose 5% in lactated Ringer's solution).
Gonorrhea in patients allergic to penicillin —
Adults: 100 mg P.O. b.i.d. for 7 days (10 days for epididymitis).
Primary or secondary syphilis in patients allergic to penicillin —
Adults: 300 mg P.O. daily in divided doses for at least 10 days.
Uncomplicated urethral, endocervical, or rectal infections due to C. trachomatis *or* Ureaplasma urealyticum —
Adults: 100 mg P.O. b.i.d. for at least 7 days (10 days for epididymitis).
Prophylaxis of malaria —
Adults: 100 mg P.O. daily.
Children over age 8: 2 mg/kg P.O. once daily. Dose shouldn't exceed that of adults.
Note: Prophylaxis should begin 1 to 2 days before travel to endemic area and continued until 4 weeks after travel.
Pelvic inflammatory disease —
Adults: 100 mg I.V. q 12 hours with cefoxitin or cefotetan and continued for at

least 2 days after symptomatic improvement; thereafter, 100 mg P.O. q 12 hours for a total course of 14 days.

ADVERSE REACTIONS
CNS: *intracranial hypertension.*
CV: pericarditis, thrombophlebitis.
EENT: glossitis, dysphagia.
GI: anorexia, *epigastric distress, nausea,* vomiting, *diarrhea,* oral candidiasis, enterocolitis, anogenital inflammation.
Hematologic: *neutropenia,* eosinophilia, *thrombocytopenia,* hemolytic anemia.
Hepatic: elevated liver enzymes.
Musculoskeletal: bone growth retardation in children under age 9.
Skin: *maculopapular and erythematous rashes, photosensitivity, increased pigmentation, urticaria.*
Other: *hypersensitivity reactions, anaphylaxis,* superinfection; permanent discoloration of teeth, enamel defects.

INTERACTIONS
Drug-drug. *Antacids (including sodium bicarbonate) and laxatives containing aluminum, magnesium, or calcium; antidiarrheals:* decreased antibiotic absorption. Antibiotic is given 1 hour before or 2 hours after any of these drugs.
Carbamazepine, phenobarbital: decreased antibiotic effect. Avoid if possible.
Ferrous sulfate and other iron products, zinc: decreased antibiotic absorption. Drug is given 2 hours before or 3 hours after iron administration.
Methoxyflurane: may cause nephrotoxicity with tetracyclines. Monitor carefully.
Oral anticoagulants: increased anticoagulant effect. PT and INR must be monitored, and dosage adjusted as needed.
Oral contraceptives: decreased contraceptive effectiveness and increased risk of breakthrough bleeding. A nonhormonal form of birth control should be recommended.
Penicillins: may interfere with bactericidal action of penicillins. Avoid use together.
Drug-lifestyle. *Alcohol use:* decreased antibiotic effect. Avoid use together.
Sun exposure: photosensitivity reactions may occur. Take precautions.

EFFECTS ON DIAGNOSTIC TESTS
Drug causes false-negative results in urine glucose tests using glucose oxidase reagent (Diastix or Chemstrip uG). Parenteral dosage form may cause false-positive Clinitest results. Drug also causes false elevations in fluorometric tests for urine catecholamines.

CONTRAINDICATIONS
Contraindicated in patients with hypersensitivity to drug or other tetracyclines.

SPECIAL CONSIDERATIONS
▶ Use cautiously in patients with impaired renal or hepatic function.
▶ Use of these drugs during last half of pregnancy and in children under age 9 may cause permanent discoloration of teeth, enamel defects, and bone growth retardation.
▶ A specimen for culture and sensitivity tests should be obtained before giving first dose. Therapy may begin pending test results.
▶ *Alert:* Expiration date should be checked. Outdated or deteriorated tetracyclines have been associated with reversible nephrotoxicity (Fanconi's syndrome).
▶ Drug is administered with milk or food if adverse GI reactions develop.
▶ Reconstituted injectable solution is stable for 72 hours if refrigerated and protected from light.
▶ With large doses or prolonged therapy, there is a potential for superinfection, especially in high-risk patients.
▶ Patient's tongue should be checked for signs of fungal infection. Stress good oral hygiene.

▶ Drug is not indicated for the treatment of neurosyphilis.

▶ **Alert:** Don't confuse doxycycline, doxylamine, and dicyclomine.

I.V. administration

▶ Powder for injection is reconstituted with sterile water for injection. 10 ml is used in 100-mg vial and 20 ml in 200-mg vial. Solution is diluted to 100 to 1,000 ml for I.V. infusion. Extravasation must be avoided. Solutions that are more concentrated than 1 mg/ml should not be infused. Infusion time varies with dose, but usually ranges from 1 to 4 hours. I.V. infusion site is monitored for signs of thrombophlebitis, which may occur with I.V. administration.

▶ Drug should not be exposed to light or heat. Protect it from sunlight during infusion.

Patient teaching

▶ Take entire amount of drug exactly as prescribed, even after feeling better.

▶ Report adverse reactions promptly. If drug is being administered I.V., alert health care provider if discomfort occurs at I.V. site.

▶ Take oral form of drug with food or milk if stomach upset occurs. Don't take oral tablets or capsules within 1 hour of bedtime because of possible esophageal irritation or ulceration.

▶ Avoid direct sunlight and ultraviolet light, wear protective clothing, and use sunscreen. Photosensitivity reactions may occur within a few minutes to several hours after exposure. Photosensitivity persists for some time after therapy ends.

▶ Report signs and symptoms of superinfection to the health care provider.

minocycline hydrochloride
Apo-Minocycline , Dynacin, Minocin*, Minomycin†, Vectrin
Pregnancy Risk Category D

HOW SUPPLIED
Tablets (film-coated): 50 mg, 100 mg
Capsules (pellet-filled): 50 mg, 100 mg
Oral suspension: 50 mg/5 ml
Injection: 100 mg

ACTION
Unknown. Thought to exert bacteriostatic effect by binding to the 30S and possibly 50S ribosomal subunits of microorganisms, thus inhibiting protein synthesis. May also alter the cytoplasmic membrane of susceptible microorganisms.

Route	Onset	Peak	Duration
P.O.	Unknown	1-4 hr	Unknown
I.V.	Immediate	Immediate	Unknown

INDICATIONS & DOSAGE
Infections due to susceptible gram-negative and gram-positive organisms (including Haemophilus ducreyi, Yersinia pestis, *and* Campylobacter fetus*),* Rickettsiae, Mycoplasma pneumoniae, *and* Chlamydia trachomatis; psittacosis; granuloma inguinale —
Adults: initially — 200 mg I.V.; then 100 mg I.V. q 12 hours. Don't exceed 400 mg/day. Or, 200 mg P.O. initially; then 100 mg P.O. q 12 hours. May use 100 or 200 mg P.O. initially; then 50 mg q.i.d.
Children over age 8: initially, 4 mg/kg P.O. or I.V.; then 2 mg/kg q 12 hours.

Give I.V. in 500- to 1,000-ml solution without calcium and administer over 6 hours.

Gonorrhea in patients allergic to penicillin —
Adults: initially, 200 mg P.O.; then 100 mg q 12 hours for at least 4 days.

Syphilis in patients allergic to penicillin —
Adults: initially, 200 mg P.O.; then 100 mg q 12 hours for 10 to 15 days.

Meningococcal carrier state —
Adults: 100 mg P.O. q 12 hours for 5 days.

Uncomplicated urethral, endocervical, or rectal infection due to C. trachomatis *or* Ureaplasma urealyticum —
Adults: 100 mg P.O. b.i.d. for at least 7 days.

Uncomplicated gonococcal urethritis in men —
Adults: 100 mg P.O. b.i.d. for 5 days.

ADVERSE REACTIONS

CNS: headache, *intracranial hypertension,* light-headedness, dizziness, vertigo.
CV: pericarditis, *thrombophlebitis.*
EENT: dysphagia, glossitis.
GI: *anorexia,* epigastric distress, oral candidiasis, *nausea,* vomiting, *diarrhea,* enterocolitis, inflammatory lesions in anogenital region.
GU: elevated BUN.
Hematologic: *neutropenia,* eosinophilia, *thrombocytopenia,* hemolytic anemia.
Hepatic: elevated liver enzymes.
Musculoskeletal: bone growth retardation in children under age 9.
Skin: *maculopapular and erythematous rashes, photosensitivity, increased pigmentation, urticaria.*
Other: *hypersensitivity reactions, anaphylaxis,* superinfection; permanent discoloration of teeth, enamel defects.

INTERACTIONS

Drug-drug. *Antacids (including sodium bicarbonate) and laxatives containing aluminum, magnesium, or calcium; antidiarrheals:* decreased antibiotic absorption. Give antibiotic 1 hour before or 2 hours after any of these drugs.
Ferrous sulfate and other iron products, zinc: decreased antibiotic absorption. Give drug 2 hours before or 3 hours after iron administration.

Methoxyflurane: may cause nephrotoxicity when given with tetracyclines. Monitor carefully.
Oral anticoagulants: increased anticoagulant effect. PT and INR must be monitored, and dosage adjusted as needed.
Oral contraceptives: decreased contraceptive effectiveness and increased risk of breakthrough bleeding. A nonhormonal form of birth control should be recommended.
Penicillins: may interfere with bactericidal action of penicillins. Avoid use together.
Drug-lifestyle. *Sun exposure:* photosensitivity reactions may occur. Take precautions.

EFFECTS ON DIAGNOSTIC TESTS

Minocycline causes false-negative results in urine glucose tests using glucose oxidase reagent (Diastix or Chemstrip uG). Drug also causes false elevations in fluorometric tests for urine catecholamines. Parenteral form may cause false-positive reading of copper sulfate tests (Clinitest).

CONTRAINDICATIONS

Contraindicated in patients with hypersensitivity to drug or other tetracyclines.

SPECIAL CONSIDERATIONS

▶ Use cautiously in patients with impaired renal or hepatic function.
▶ Use of these drugs during last half of pregnancy and in children under age 9 may cause permanent discoloration of teeth, enamel defects, and bone growth retardation.
▶ Renal and liver function test results must be monitored.
▶ A specimen for culture and sensitivity tests should be obtained before first dose. Therapy may begin pending test results.
▶ *Alert:* Expiration date should be checked. Outdated or deteriorated tetracyclines have been associated with reversible nephrotoxicity (Fanconi's syndrome).

▶ Drug should not be exposed to light or heat. Keep cap tightly closed.

▶ With large doses or prolonged therapy, the potential for superinfection exists, especially in high-risk patients.

▶ Patient's tongue should be checked for signs of candidal infection. Stress good oral hygiene.

▶ Drug may cause tooth discoloration in young adults.

▶ Drug is not indicated for the treatment of neurosyphilis.

▶ *Alert:* Don't confuse minocin, niacin, and mithracin.

I.V. administration

▶ 100 mg of powder is reconstituted with 5 ml of sterile water for injection, with further dilution to 500 to 1,000 ml for I.V. infusion. Although reconstituted solution is stable for 24 hours at room temperature, use as soon as possible. Infusions are usually given over 6 hours.

▶ Patient may develop thrombophlebitis with I.V. administration. Extravasation should be avoided. Switch to oral therapy as soon as possible.

Patient teaching

▶ Take entire amount of drug exactly as prescribed, even after feeling better.

▶ Take oral form of drug with a full glass of water. Drug may be taken with food. Don't take within 1 hour of bedtime to avoid esophageal irritation or ulceration.

▶ Avoid driving or other hazardous tasks because of possible adverse CNS effects.

▶ Avoid direct sunlight and ultraviolet light, wear protective clothing, and use sunscreen. Photosensitivity reactions may occur within a few minutes to several hours after exposure. Photosensitivity persists for some time after discontinuation of therapy.

tetracycline hydrochloride

Achromycin V, Apo-Tetra , Novo-Tetra , Nu-Tetra , Panmycin**, Sumycin, Sustamycin§, Tetrachel§

Pregnancy Risk Category D

HOW SUPPLIED
Tablets: 250 mg, 500 mg
Capsules: 100 mg, 250 mg, 500 mg
Oral suspension: 125 mg/5 ml

ACTION
Unknown. Thought to exert bacteriostatic effect by binding to the 30S and possibly 50S ribosomal subunits of microorganisms, thus inhibiting protein synthesis. May also alter the cytoplasmic membrane of susceptible microorganisms.

Route	Onset	Peak	Duration
P.O.	Unknown	1-4 hr	Unknown

INDICATIONS & DOSAGE
Infections due to susceptible gram-negative and gram-positive organisms (including Haemophilus ducreyi, Yersinia pestis, *and* Campylobacter fetus), Rickettsia, Mycoplasma pneumoniae, *and* Chlamydia trachomatis; *psittacosis; granuloma inguinale —*
Adults: 250 to 500 mg P.O. q 6 hours.
Children over age 8: 25 to 50 mg/kg P.O. daily, in divided doses q 6 hours.
Uncomplicated urethral, endocervical, or rectal infections due to C. trachomatis —
Adults: 500 mg P.O. q.i.d. for at least 7 days, 10 days for epididymitis, and 21 days for lymphogranuloma venereum.
Brucellosis —
Adults: 500 mg P.O. q 6 hours for 3 weeks with 1 g of streptomycin I.M. q 12 hours for first week; once daily for second week.

Gonorrhea in patients allergic to penicillin —
Adults: initially, 1.5 g P.O.; then 500 mg q 6 hours for total dose of 9 g; for epididymitis, 500 mg P.O. q 6 hours for 7 days.

Syphilis in patients allergic to penicillin —
Adults: total of 30 to 40 g P.O. in equally divided doses over 10 to 15 days.

Acne —
Adults and adolescents: initially, 250 mg P.O. q 6 hours; then 125 to 500 mg daily or every other day.

Helicobacter pylori *infection —*
Adults: 500 mg P.O. q 6 hours for 10 to 14 days with other agents, such as metronidazole, bismuth subsalicylate, amoxicillin, or omeprazole.

Cholera —
Adults: 500 mg P.O. q 6 hours for 48 to 72 hours.

Malaria due to Plasmodium falciparum —
Adults: 250 to 500 mg P.O. daily for 7 days with quinine sulfate 650 mg P.O. q 8 hours for 3 to 7 days.

ADVERSE REACTIONS
CNS: dizziness, headache, ***intracranial hypertension.***
CV: pericarditis.
EENT: sore throat, glossitis, dysphagia.
GI: anorexia, *epigastric distress, nausea,* vomiting, *diarrhea,* esophagitis, oral candidiasis, stomatitis, enterocolitis, inflammatory lesions in anogenital region.
GU: increased BUN.
Hematologic: ***neutropenia,*** eosinophilia, ***thrombocytopenia.***
Hepatic: elevated liver enzymes.
Musculoskeletal: *bone growth retardation* in children under age 9.
Skin: *candidal superinfection, maculopapular and erythematous rash, urticaria, photosensitivity, increased pigmentation.*
Other: hypersensitivity reactions; *per-*

manent discoloration of teeth, enamel defects.

INTERACTIONS
Drug-drug. *Antacids (including sodium bicarbonate) and laxatives containing aluminum, magnesium, or calcium; antidiarrheals containing kaolin, pectin, or bismuth subsalicylate:* decreased antibiotic absorption. Antibiotic is given 1 hour before or 2 hours after any of these drugs.
Ferrous sulfate and other iron products, zinc: decreased antibiotic absorption. Tetracyclines are given 2 hours before or 3 hours after iron administration.
Lithium carbonate: may alter serum lithium levels. Levels should be monitored.
Methoxyflurane: may cause severe nephrotoxicity with tetracyclines. Monitor carefully.
Oral anticoagulants: potentiated anticoagulant effects. PT and INR must be monitored, and anticoagulant dosage adjusted as needed.
Oral contraceptives: decreased contraceptive effectiveness and increased risk of breakthrough bleeding. A nonhormonal form of birth control should be recommended.
Penicillins: may interfere with bactericidal action of penicillins. Avoid use together.
Drug-food. *Milk, dairy products, other foods:* decreased antibiotic absorption. Antibiotic is given 1 hour before or 2 hours after any of the above.
Drug-lifestyle. *Sun exposure:* photosensitivity reactions may occur. Take precautions.

EFFECTS ON DIAGNOSTIC TESTS
Tetracycline causes false-negative results in urine glucose tests using glucose oxidase reagent (Diastix or Chemstrip uG) and false elevations in fluorometric tests for urine catecholamines.

CONTRAINDICATIONS

Contraindicated in patients with hypersensitivity to drug or other tetracyclines.

SPECIAL CONSIDERATIONS

▶ Use drug with extreme caution in patients with impaired renal or hepatic function. Renal and liver function test results must be monitored.

▶ Also use with extreme caution (if at all) during last half of pregnancy and in children under age 9 because drug may cause permanent discoloration of teeth, enamel defects, and bone growth retardation.

▶ A specimen for culture and sensitivity tests should be obtained before giving first dose. Therapy may begin pending test results.

▶ *Alert:* Expiration date must be checked. Outdated or deteriorated tetracyclines have been associated with reversible nephrotoxicity (Fanconi's syndrome).

▶ Drug exposure to light or heat should be avoided.

▶ With large doses or prolonged therapy, there is the potential for superinfection, especially in high-risk patients.

▶ Patient's tongue should be checked for signs of candidal infection. Stress good oral hygiene.

▶ Drug is not indicated for the treatment of neurosyphilis.

Patient teaching

▶ Take drug exactly as prescribed, even after feeling better; and take the entire amount prescribed.

▶ Effectiveness is reduced when taken with milk or other dairy products, food, antacids, or iron products. Take each dose with a full glass of water on an empty stomach, at least 1 hour before or 2 hours after meals. Also, take it at least 1 hour before bedtime to prevent esophageal irritation or ulceration.

▶ Avoid direct sunlight and ultraviolet light, wear protective clothing, and use sunscreen. Photosensitivity reactions may occur within a few minutes to several hours after sun exposure. Photosensitivity persists after discontinuation of drug.

co-trimoxazole
sulfadiazine
sulfamethoxazole
sulfisoxazole
sulfisoxazole acetyl

COMBINATION PRODUCTS

Azo-Sulfamethoxazole tablets (film-coated): sulfamethoxazole 500 mg and phenazopyridine hydrochloride 100 mg.
Azo-Sulfisoxazole tablets (film-coated): sulfisoxazole 500 mg and phenazopyridine hydrochloride 50 mg.
Eryzole, Pediazole, Sulfimycin suspension: sulfisoxazole 600 mg and erythromycin ethylsuccinate 200 mg/5 ml.

co-trimoxazole (sulfamethoxazole-trimethoprim)

Apo-Sulfatrim , Apo-Sulfatrim DS , Bactrim*, Bactrim DS, Bactrim I.V., Novo-Trimel , Novo-Trimel D.S. , Nu-ᴑotrimox , Resprim‡, Roubac , Septra*, Septra DS, Septra I.V., Septrin‡, SMZ-TMP, Sulfatrim

Pregnancy Risk Category C (contraindicated at term)

HOW SUPPLIED

Tablets (single-strength): trimethoprim 80 mg and sulfamethoxazole 400 mg
Tablets (double-strength): trimethoprim 160 mg and sulfamethoxazole 800 mg
Oral suspension: trimethoprim 40 mg and sulfamethoxazole 200 mg/5 ml
Injection: trimethoprim 16 mg/ml and sulfamethoxazole 80 mg/ml in 5-ml, 10-ml, 20-ml, and 30-ml vials

ACTION

Sulfamethoxazole inhibits formation of dihydrofolic acid from PABA; trimethoprim inhibits dihydrofolate reductase formation. Both decrease bacterial folic acid synthesis; bactericidal.

Route	Onset	Peak	Duration
P.O.	Unknown	1-4 hr	Unknown
I.V.	Immediate	Immediate	Unknown

INDICATIONS & DOSAGE

Shigellosis or urinary tract infections (UTIs) due to susceptible strains of Escherichia coli, Proteus *(indole positive or negative),* Klebsiella, *or* Enterobacter —
Adults: 160 mg trimethoprim/800 mg sulfamethoxazole (double-strength tablet) P.O. q 12 hours for 10 to 14 days in UTIs and for 5 days in shigellosis. If indicated, I.V. infusion is given: 8 to 10 mg/kg/day (based on trimethoprim component) in two to four divided doses q 6, 8, or 12 hours for up to 14 days for severe UTIs. Maximum daily dose is 960 mg trimethoprim.
Children ages 2 months and older: 8 mg/kg/day (based on trimethoprim component) P.O., in two divided doses q 12 hours (10 days for UTIs; 5 days for shigellosis). If indicated, I.V. infusion is given: 8 to 10 mg/kg/day (based on trimethoprim component) in two to four divided doses q 6, 8, or 12 hours. Adult dose shouldn't be exceeded.
Otitis media in patients with penicillin allergy or penicillin-resistant infections —
Children ages 2 months and older: 8 mg/kg/day (based on trimethoprim component) P.O., in two divided doses q 12 hours for 10 to 14 days.
Chronic bronchitis, upper respiratory tract infections —
Adults: 160 mg trimethoprim/800 mg sul-

Reactions may be *common*, uncommon, *life-threatening*, or COMMON AND LIFE-THREATENING.

464

famethoxazole P.O. q 12 hours for 10 to 14 days.

Traveler's diarrhea —

Adults: 160 mg trimethoprim/800 mg sulfamethoxazole P.O. b.i.d. for 3 to 5 days. Some patients may require 2 days or less of therapy.

UTIs in men with prostatitis —

Adults: 160 mg trimethoprim/800 mg sulfamethoxazole P.O. b.i.d. for 3 to 6 months.

Prophylaxis for chronic UTIs —

Adults: 40 mg trimethoprim/200 mg sulfamethoxazole (½ tablet) or 80 mg trimethoprim/400 mg sulfamethoxazole P.O. daily or three times weekly for 3 to 6 months.

Prophylaxis for Pneumocystis carinii *pneumonia —*

Adults: 160 mg of trimethoprim/800 mg sulfamethoxazole P.O. daily.

Children ages 2 months and older: 150 mg/m^2 trimethoprim/750 mg/m^2 sulfamethoxazole P.O daily in two divided doses on 3 consecutive days each week.

P. carinii *pneumonia —*

Adults and children over age 2 months: 15 to 20 mg/kg/day (based on trimethoprim) I.V. or P.O. in three or four divided doses for 14 days.

Dosage adjustment: For patients with renal failure with creatinine clearance of 15 to 30 ml/minute, daily dose should be reduced by 50%. Drug isn't recommended for patients with creatinine clearance below 15 ml/minute.

ADVERSE REACTIONS

CNS: headache, mental depression, aseptic meningitis, tinnitus, apathy, **seizures,** hallucinations, ataxia, nervousness, fatigue, vertigo, insomnia.
CV: thrombophlebitis.
GI: *nausea, vomiting, diarrhea,* abdominal pain, anorexia, stomatitis, pancreatitis, pseudomembranous colitis.
GU: ***toxic nephrosis with oliguria and anuria,*** crystalluria, hematuria, interstitial nephritis, increased BUN and serum creatinine levels.

Hematologic: *agranulocytosis, aplastic anemia,* megaloblastic anemia, ***thrombocytopenia, leukopenia, hemolytic anemia.***

Hepatic: jaundice, ***hepatic necrosis,*** elevated liver function test results.
Musculoskeletal: arthralgia, myalgia, muscle weakness.
Respiratory: pulmonary infiltrates.
Skin: ***erythema multiforme, Stevens-Johnson syndrome,*** *generalized skin eruption,* ***epidermal necrolysis, exfoliative dermatitis,*** photosensitivity, urticaria, pruritus.

Other: ***hypersensitivity reactions, serum sickness, drug fever, anaphylaxis.***

INTERACTIONS

Drug-drug. *Cyclosporine:* may decrease cyclosporine levels and increase nephrotoxicity risk. Avoid concomitant use.
Methotrexate: may increase methotrexate concentrations. Use together cautiously.
Oral anticoagulants: increased anticoagulant effect. Bleeding may occur.
Oral antidiabetics: increased hypoglycemic effect. Blood glucose levels must be monitored.
Oral contraceptives: decreased contraceptive effectiveness and increased risk of breakthrough bleeding. A nonhormonal contraceptive should be recommended.
Phenytoin: may inhibit hepatic metabolism of phenytoin. Monitor closely.
Drug-lifestyle. *Sun exposure:* photosensitivity reactions may occur. Take precautions.

EFFECTS ON DIAGNOSTIC TESTS

Trimethoprim can interfere with serum methotrexate assay as determined by the competitive binding protein technique. No interference occurs if radioimmunoassay is used.

CONTRAINDICATIONS

Contraindicated in patients with severe renal impairment (creatinine clearance below 15 ml/minute), porphyria, megaloblastic anemia due to folate deficiency, or hypersensitivity to trimethoprim or sulfonamides. Also contraindicated in pregnant women at term, in breast-feeding women, and in infants under age 2 months.

SPECIAL CONSIDERATIONS

▶ Use cautiously and in reduced dosages in patients with impaired hepatic or renal function (creatinine clearance 15 to 30 ml/minute), severe allergy or bronchial asthma, G6PD deficiency, and blood dyscrasia.

▶ Renal and liver function test results must be monitored.

▶ A specimen for culture and sensitivity tests should be obtained before first dose. Therapy may begin pending results.

▶ *Alert:* Dosage should be double-checked; dose may be written as trimethoprim component.

▶ *Alert:* Note that the "DS" product means "double strength."

▶ Drug is not to be administered I.M.

▶ Patient must be monitored for complaints of rash, sore throat, fever, cough, mouth sores, or iris lesions — early signs and symptoms of erythema multiforme, which may progress to the sometimes fatal condition, Stevens-Johnson syndrome. These symptoms may also represent early signs of blood dyscrasias.

▶ Superinfection (fever or other signs or symptoms of new infection) is possible.

▶ *Alert:* Adverse reactions, especially hypersensitivity reactions, rash, and fever, occur much more frequently in patients with AIDS.

I.V. administration

▶ Each 5 ml of concentrate for I.V. infusion is diluted in 75 to 125 ml of D_5W before administration. The drug should not be mixed with other drugs or solutions.

The solution is infused slowly over 60 to 90 minutes. The drug is not given by rapid infusion or bolus injection. The drug should not be refrigerated and should be used within 6 hours.

Patient teaching

▶ Take drug as prescribed, even after feeling better.

▶ Take oral medication with 8 oz (240 ml) of water on an empty stomach.

▶ Maintain adequate fluid intake.

▶ Report adverse reactions promptly.

▶ Alert health care provider if discomfort occurs at I.V. insertion site.

▶ Avoid prolonged sun exposure, wear protective clothing, and use sunscreen.

sulfadiazine

Coptin

Pregnancy Risk Category C (contraindicated at term)

HOW SUPPLIED

Tablets: 500 mg

ACTION

Inhibits formation of dihydrofolic acid from PABA, decreasing bacterial folic acid synthesis; bacteriostatic.

Route	Onset	Peak	Duration
P.O.	Unknown	4-6 hr	Unknown

INDICATIONS & DOSAGE

Asymptomatic meningococcal carriers —
Adults: 1 g P.O. q 12 hours for 2 days.
Children ages 1 to 12: 500 mg P.O. q 12 hours for 2 days.
Children ages 2 to 12 months: 500 mg P.O. daily for 2 days.
    Rheumatic fever prophylaxis, as an alternative to penicillin —
Children weighing over 30 kg (66 lb): 1 g P.O. daily.

Children under 30 kg: 500 mg P.O. daily.

Adjunct treatment in toxoplasmosis —
Adults: 2 to 8 g P.O. daily divided q 6 hours for 6 to 8 weeks or until improvement occurs. Usually given with pyrimethamine.
Children: 100 to 200 mg/kg P.O. daily divided q 6 hours (maximum 6 g daily) for 6 to 8 weeks or until improvement occurs. Usually given with pyrimethamine.

Malaria, treatment of chloroquine-resistant Plasmodium falciparum —
Adults: 500 mg P.O. q.i.d. for 5 days with quinine sulfate and pyrimethamine.
Children: 25 to 50 mg/kg P.O. q.i.d. (maximum 2 g daily) for 5 days with quinine sulfate and pyrimethamine.

Nocardiosis —
Adults: 4 to 8 g P.O. daily given in divided doses for a minimum of 6 weeks.

ADVERSE REACTIONS

CNS: headache, mental depression, *seizures,* hallucinations.
GI: *nausea, vomiting, diarrhea,* abdominal pain, anorexia, stomatitis.
GU: *toxic nephrosis with oliguria and anuria,* crystalluria, hematuria, elevated serum creatinine level.
Hematologic: *agranulocytosis, aplastic anemia,* megaloblastic anemia, *thrombocytopenia, leukopenia, hemolytic anemia.*
Hepatic: elevated liver function test results, jaundice.
Skin: *erythema multiforme, Stevens-Johnson syndrome,* generalized skin eruption, *epidermal necrolysis, exfoliative dermatitis,* photosensitivity, urticaria, pruritus.
Other: *hypersensitivity reactions, serum sickness, drug fever, anaphylaxis,* local irritation, extravasation.

INTERACTIONS

Drug-drug. *Methotrexate:* may increase methotrexate levels. Use together cautiously.

Oral anticoagulants: increased anticoagulant effect. Bleeding may occur.
Oral antidiabetics: increased hypoglycemic effect. Blood glucose levels must be monitored.
Oral contraceptives: decreased contraceptive effectiveness and increased risk of breakthrough bleeding. A nonhormonal contraceptive should be recommended.
PABA-containing drugs: inhibited antibacterial action. Don't use together.
Drug-lifestyle. *Sun exposure:* photosensitivity reactions may occur. Take precautions.

EFFECTS ON DIAGNOSTIC TESTS

Drug alters urine glucose tests using cupric sulfate (Benedict's reagent or Clinitest).

CONTRAINDICATIONS

Contraindicated in patients with hypersensitivity to sulfonamides, in those with porphyria, in infants under age 2 months (except in congenital toxoplasmosis), in pregnant women at term, and in breastfeeding women.

SPECIAL CONSIDERATIONS

▶ Use cautiously and in reduced doses in patients with impaired hepatic or renal function, bronchial asthma, history of multiple allergies, G6PD deficiency, and blood dyscrasia.
▶ Drug is administered on a schedule to maintain constant blood level.
▶ Signs of blood dyscrasia include purpura, ecchymoses, sore throat, fever, and pallor.
▶ The patient should be monitored for complaints of rash, sore throat, fever, cough, mouth sores, or iris lesions — early signs and symptoms of erythema multiforme, which may progress to the sometimes fatal Stevens-Johnson syndrome.
▶ Urine cultures, CBCs, and urinalyses should be monitored before and during therapy.

---

*Liquid contains alcohol.   **May contain tartrazine.   †Canada   ‡Australia   §U.K.   ◇OTC

❱ Renal and liver function test results must be monitored.

❱ Superinfection (fever or other signs or symptoms of new infection) may occur.

❱ Folic or folinic acid may be used during rest periods in toxoplasmosis therapy to reverse hematopoietic depression or anemia associated with pyrimethamine and sulfadiazine.

❱ Fluid intake and output is monitored. Intake is maintained between 3,000 and 4,000 ml daily for adults to produce output of 1,500 ml daily. If fluid intake is not adequate to prevent crystalluria, sodium bicarbonate may be administered to alkalinize urine. Urine pH is monitored daily.

❱ *Alert:* Don't confuse sulfadiazine with sulfasalazine. Don't confuse sulfonamide drugs.

Patient teaching

❱ Take drug as prescribed, even after feeling better.

❱ Drink a glass of water with each dose and plenty of water each day to prevent crystalluria.

❱ Report adverse reactions promptly.

❱ Avoid prolonged exposure to sunlight, wear protective clothing, and use sunscreen.

sulfamethoxazole (sulphamethoxazole)

Apo-Sulfamethoxazole, Gantanol

Pregnancy Risk Category C (contraindicated at term)

HOW SUPPLIED

Tablets: 500 mg

ACTION

Inhibits formation of dihydrofolic acid from PABA, decreasing bacterial folic acid synthesis; bacteriostatic.

Route	Onset	Peak	Duration
P.O.	Unknown	2 hr	Unknown

INDICATIONS & DOSAGE

Urinary tract and systemic infections —
Adults: initially, 2 g P.O.; then 1 g P.O. b.i.d. up to t.i.d. for severe infections.

Chlamydia trachomatis *(lymphogranuloma venereum) —*
Adults: 1 g P.O. b.i.d. for 21 days.
Children and infants over age 2 months: initially, 50 to 60 mg/kg P.O.; then 25 to 30 mg/kg b.i.d. Maximum daily dose shouldn't exceed 75 mg/kg.

ADVERSE REACTIONS

CNS: headache, mental depression, *seizures,* hallucinations, aseptic meningitis, tinnitus, apathy.

GI: *nausea, vomiting, diarrhea,* abdominal pain, anorexia, stomatitis, pancreatitis, pseudomembranous colitis.

GU: *toxic nephrosis with oliguria and anuria,* crystalluria, hematuria, interstitial nephritis.

Hematologic: *agranulocytosis, aplastic anemia,* megaloblastic anemia, *thrombocytopenia, leukopenia, hemolytic anemia.*

Hepatic: elevated liver function test results, jaundice.

Skin: *erythema multiforme, Stevens-Johnson syndrome, generalized skin eruption, epidermal necrolysis, exfoliative dermatitis,* photosensitivity, urticaria, pruritus.

Other: *hypersensitivity reactions, serum sickness, drug fever, anaphylaxis.*

INTERACTIONS

Drug-drug. *Methotrexate:* may increase methotrexate levels. Use together cautiously.

Oral anticoagulants: increased anticoagulant effect. Bleeding may occur.

Oral antidiabetics: increased hypoglycemic effect. Blood glucose levels must be monitored.

Oral contraceptives: decreased contraceptive effectiveness and increased risk of

breakthrough bleeding. A nonhormonal contraceptive should be recommended.
Phenytoin: may increase phenytoin effect. Monitor closely.

Drug-lifestyle. *Sun exposure:* may cause photosensitivity reactions. Use precautions.

EFFECTS ON DIAGNOSTIC TESTS

Drug alters results of urine glucose tests using cupric sulfate (Benedict's reagent or Clinitest).

CONTRAINDICATIONS

Contraindicated in patients with hypersensitivity to sulfonamides, in those with porphyria, in infants under age 2 months (except in congenital toxoplasmosis), in pregnant women at term, and in breastfeeding women.

SPECIAL CONSIDERATIONS

▶ Use cautiously and in reduced dosages in patients with impaired hepatic or renal function, severe allergy or bronchial asthma, G6PD deficiency, and blood dyscrasia.

▶ Renal and liver function test results must be monitored.

▶ A specimen for culture and sensitivity tests should be obtained before first dose. Therapy may begin pending results.

▶ Urine cultures, CBCs, and urinalyses before and during therapy must be monitored.

▶ Superinfection (fever or other signs or symptoms of new infection) may occur.

▶ Fluid intake and output is monitored. Intake is maintained between 3,000 and 4,000 ml daily for adults to produce output of 1,500 ml daily. If fluid intake is not adequate to prevent crystalluria, sodium bicarbonate may be administered to alkalinize urine. Urine pH is monitored daily.

▶ *Alert:* Don't confuse sulfamethoxazole with sulfamethizole. Don't confuse the combination products (such as Gantanol) with sulfamethoxazole alone.

Patient teaching

▶ Take drug as prescribed, even after feeling better.

▶ Drink a glass of water with each dose and plenty of water each day to prevent crystalluria.

▶ *Alert:* Notify a health care provider of early signs and symptoms of blood dyscrasia (sore throat, fever, and pallor). Also, be alert for flulike symptoms, cough, and lesions of the iris, skin, and mucous membranes — early signs of erythema multiforme, which can progress to the sometimes fatal Stevens-Johnson syndrome.

▶ Avoid prolonged exposure to sunlight, wear protective clothing, and use sunscreen.

---

sulfisoxazole (sulfafurazole, sulphafurazole)
Novo-Soxazole

sulfisoxazole acetyl
Gantrisin Pediatric
Pregnancy Risk Category C (contraindicated at term)

HOW SUPPLIED
sulfisoxazole
Tablets: 500 mg
sulfisoxazole acetyl
Liquid: 500 mg/5 ml

ACTION
Inhibits formation of dihydrofolic acid from PABA, decreasing bacterial folic acid synthesis; bacteriostatic.

Route	Onset	Peak	Duration
P.O.	Unknown	1-4 hr	Unknown

INDICATIONS & DOSAGE
Urinary tract and systemic infections —

Adults: initially, 2 to 4 g P.O.; then 4 to 8 g daily divided in four to six doses.

Children over age 2 months: initially, 75 mg/kg P.O. daily or 2 g/m² P.O.; then 150 mg/kg or 4 g/m² P.O. daily in divided doses q 6 hours. Total daily dose shouldn't exceed 6 g.

Chlamydia trachomatis *(lymphogranuloma venereum)* —

Adults: 500 mg to 1 g P.O. q.i.d. for 21 days.

Uncomplicated urethral, endocervical, or rectal infections due to C. trachomatis —

Adults: 500 mg P.O. q.i.d. for 10 days.

Dosage adjustment: For patients with renal failure, use normal dose at longer intervals. If creatinine clearance is 10 to 50 ml/minute, give q 8 to12 hours; if clearance is less than 10 ml/minute, give q 12 to 24 hours.

ADVERSE REACTIONS

CNS: headache, mental depression, *seizures,* hallucinations.

CV: tachycardia, palpitations, syncope, cyanosis.

GI: *nausea, vomiting, diarrhea,* abdominal pain, anorexia, stomatitis, pseudomembranous colitis.

GU: *toxic nephrosis with oliguria and anuria,* crystalluria, hematuria, *acute renal failure.*

Hematologic: *agranulocytosis, aplastic anemia,* megaloblastic anemia, *thrombocytopenia, leukopenia, hemolytic anemia.*

Hepatic: jaundice, elevated liver function test results, *hepatitis.*

Skin: *erythema multiforme,* generalized skin eruption, *epidermal necrolysis, exfoliative dermatitis,* photosensitivity, urticaria, pruritus.

Other: *hypersensitivity reactions, serum sickness, drug fever, anaphylaxis.*

INTERACTIONS

Drug-drug. *Methotrexate:* may increase methotrexate levels. Use together cautiously.

Oral anticoagulants: increased anticoagulant effect. Bleeding may occur.

Oral antidiabetics: increased hypoglycemic effect. Blood glucose levels should be monitored.

Oral contraceptives: decreased contraceptive effectiveness, increased risk of breakthrough bleeding. A nonhormonal contraceptive should be recommended.

Drug-lifestyle. *Sun exposure:* photosensitivity reactions may occur. Use precautions.

EFFECTS ON DIAGNOSTIC TESTS

Drug alters results of urine glucose tests using cupric sulfate (Benedict's reagent or Clinitest).

CONTRAINDICATIONS

Contraindicated in patients with hypersensitivity to sulfonamides, in infants under age 2 months (except in congenital toxoplasmosis), in pregnant women at term, and in breast-feeding women.

SPECIAL CONSIDERATIONS

▶ Use cautiously in patients with impaired hepatic or renal function, severe allergy or bronchial asthma, and G6PD deficiency.

▶ Renal and liver function test results must be monitored.

▶ A specimen for culture and sensitivity tests should be obtained before giving first dose. Therapy may begin pending results.

▶ Urine cultures, CBCs, PT, and urinalyses are monitored before and during therapy.

▶ Patient is monitored for moderate to severe diarrhea.

▶ Superinfection (fever or other signs or symptoms of new infection) may occur.

▶ Fluid intake and output is monitored. Intake is maintained between 3,000 and 4,000 ml daily for adults to produce output of 1,500 ml daily. If fluid intake is not adequate to prevent crystalluria, sodium bicarbonate may be administered to alkalinize urine. Urine pH is monitored daily.

▶ *Alert:* Don't confuse sulfisoxazole with sulfasalazine. Don't confuse the combination products (such as Gantrisin) with sulfamethoxazole alone.

Patient teaching

▶ Take drug as prescribed, even after feeling better.

▶ Drink a glass of water with each dose and plenty of water each day to prevent crystalluria.

▶ *Alert:* Notify health care provider if early signs of blood dyscrasia (sore throat, fever, and pallor) and moderate to severe diarrhea occur.

▶ Avoid sunlight, wear protective clothing, and use sunscreen.

alatrofloxacin mesylate
ciprofloxacin
enoxacin
levofloxacin
lomefloxacin hydrochloride
nalidixic acid
norfloxacin
ofloxacin
sparfloxacin
trovafloxacin mesylate

COMBINATION PRODUCTS
None.

---

ciprofloxacin
Cipro, Cipro I.V., Ciproxin‡

Pregnancy Risk Category C

HOW SUPPLIED
Tablets (film-coated): 100 mg, 250 mg, 500 mg, 750 mg
Infusion (premixed): 200 mg in 100 ml D_5W, 400 mg in 200 ml D_5W
Injection: 200 mg, 400 mg

ACTION
Inhibits bacterial DNA synthesis, mainly by blocking DNA gyrase; bactericidal.

Route	Onset	Peak	Duration
P.O.	Unknown	0.5-2.3 hr	Unknown
I.V.	Unknown	Immediate	Unknown

INDICATIONS & DOSAGE
Mild to moderate urinary tract infections (UTIs) due to Escherichia coli, Klebsiella pneumoniae, Enterobacter cloacae, Serratia marcescens, Proteus mirabilis, Providencia rettgeri, Morganella morganii, Citrobacter diversus, C. freundii, Pseudomonas aeruginosa, Staphylococcus epidermidis, *and* Enterococcus faecalis —

Adults: 250 mg P.O. or 200 mg I.V. q 12 hours.
Severe or complicated UTIs; mild to moderate bone and joint infections due to E. cloacae, P. aeruginosa, *and* S. marcescens; *mild to moderate respiratory infections due to* E. coli, K. pneumoniae, E. cloacae, P. mirabilis, P. aeruginosa, Haemophilus influenzae, *and* H. parainfluenzae; *mild to moderate skin and skin-structure infections due to* E. coli, K. pneumoniae, E. cloacae, P. mirabilis, P. vulgaris, Providencia stuartii, M. morganii, C. freundii, Streptococcus pyogenes, P. aeruginosa, Staphylococcus aureus, *and* S. epidermidis; *infectious diarrhea due to* E. coli, Campylobacter jejuni, Shigella flexneri, *and* S. sonnei; *typhoid fever* —
Adults: 500 mg P.O. or 400 mg I.V. q 12 hours.
Severe or complicated bone or joint infections, severe respiratory tract infections, severe skin and skin-structure infections —
Adults: 750 mg P.O. q 12 hours.
Chronic bacterial prostatitis due to E. coli *or* P. mirabilis —
Adults: 500 mg P.O. q 12 hours for 28 days.
Complicated intra-abdominal infections (used with metronidazole) due to E. coli, P. aeruginosa, P. mirabilis, K. pneumoniae, *or* Bacteroides fragilis —
Adults: 500 mg P.O. or 400 mg I.V. q 12 hours for 7 to 14 days.
Acute uncomplicated cystitis —
Adults: 100 mg P.O. q 12 hours for 3 days.
Mild to moderate acute sinusitis —
Adults: 500 mg P.O. q 12 hours for 10 days.
Mild to moderate acute sinusitis due to H. influenzae, Streptococcus pneumoniae, *or* Moraxella catarrhalis; *mild to moderate chronic bacterial prostatitis due to* Escherichia coli *or* P. mirabilis —

Reactions may be *common,* uncommon, *life-threatening*, or COMMON AND LIFE-THREATENING.

472

Adults: 400 mg I.V. infusion given over 60 minutes q 12 hours.

Dosage adjustment: For patients with renal failure, if creatinine clearance is 30 to 50 ml/minute, give 250 to 500 mg P.O. q 12 hours or the usual I.V. dose; if clearance is 5 to 29 ml/minute, give 250 to 500 mg P.O. q 18 hours or 200 to 400 mg I.V. q 18 to 24 hours. If patient is on hemodialysis, give 250 to 500 mg P.O. q 24 hours (after dialysis)

ADVERSE REACTIONS

CNS: headache, restlessness, tremor, dizziness, fatigue, drowsiness, insomnia, depression, light-headedness, confusion, hallucinations, *seizures,* paresthesia.

GI: *nausea, diarrhea,* vomiting, abdominal pain or discomfort, oral candidiasis, pseudomembranous colitis, dyspepsia, flatulence, constipation.

GU: crystalluria, increased serum creatinine and BUN levels, interstitial nephritis.

Hematologic: eosinophilia, *leukopenia, neutropenia, thrombocytopenia.*

Hepatic: elevated liver enzymes.

Musculoskeletal: arthralgia, arthropathy, joint or back pain, joint inflammation, joint stiffness, tendon rupture, aching, neck or chest pain.

Skin: *rash,* photosensitivity, *Stevens-Johnson syndrome, toxic epidermal necrolysis, exfoliative dermatitis.*

Other: hypersensitivity; thrombophlebitis, burning, pruritus, erythema, edema.

INTERACTIONS

Drug-drug. *Antacids containing aluminum hydroxide or magnesium hydroxide, iron supplements, iron- or zinc-containing multivitamins, sucralfate:* decreased ciprofloxacin absorption. Administration times are separated by at least 2 hours.

Probenecid: may elevate serum level of ciprofloxacin. Patient should be monitored for toxicity.

Theophylline: increased plasma theophylline levels and prolonged theophylline half-life. Patient's theophylline blood levels are monitored and patient is observed observe for adverse effects.

Drug-herb. *Yerba maté:* may decrease clearance of yerba maté's methylxanthines and cause toxicity. Use together cautiously.

Drug-food. *Caffeine:* increased effect of caffeine. Monitor closely.

Dairy products, other foods: delayed peak serum levels. Drug is given on an empty stomach.

Drug-lifestyle. *Sun exposure:* photosensitivity reactions may occur. Take precautions.

EFFECTS ON DIAGNOSTIC TESTS

None reported.

CONTRAINDICATIONS

Contraindicated in patients sensitive to fluoroquinolone antibiotics.

SPECIAL CONSIDERATIONS

▶ Use cautiously in patients with CNS disorders, such as severe cerebral arteriosclerosis or seizure disorders, and in those at increased risk for seizures. Drug may cause CNS stimulation.

▶ A specimen for culture and sensitivity tests is obtained before giving first dose. Therapy may begin pending results.

▶ Oral form is administered 2 hours after a meal or 2 hours before or after taking antacids, sucralfate, or products that contain iron (such as vitamins with mineral supplements). Food does not affect absorption but may delay peak serum levels.

▶ Long-term therapy may result in overgrowth of organisms resistant to ciprofloxacin.

▶ Safety in children under age 18 has not been established. Drug may cause cartilage erosion.

▶ Patient's intake and output should be monitored and patient is observed for signs of crystalluria.

▶ Tendon rupture has been reported in patients receiving quinolones. Drug is discontinued if pain, inflammation, or rupture of a tendon occurs.

I.V. administration

▸ Drug is diluted using D_5W or normal saline for injection to a final concentration of 1 to 2 mg/ml before use. The solution is infused slowly (over 1 hour) into a large vein to minimize discomfort and reduce the risk of venous irritation.

▸ If drug is administered through a Y-type set, the other I.V. solution is discontinued during ciprofloxacin infusion.

Patient teaching

▸ Take drug as prescribed, even after feeling better.

▸ Drink plenty of fluids to reduce risk of crystalluria.

▸ Avoid hazardous tasks that require alertness, such as driving, until CNS effects of drug are known.

▸ Avoid caffeine while taking drug because of potential for cumulative caffeine effects.

▸ Hypersensitivity reactions may occur even after first dose. If a rash or other allergic reaction appears, stop drug immediately and notify health care provider.

▸ Avoid excessive sunlight or artificial ultraviolet light during therapy and stop drug and call health care provider if phototoxicity occurs.

▸ Because drug appears in breast milk, discontinue breast-feeding during treatment or ask to be treated with another drug.

▸ Take drug on an empty stomach, 2 hours after a meal.

enoxacin

Penetrex
Pregnancy Risk Category C

HOW SUPPLIED

Tablets (film-coated): 200 mg, 400 mg

ACTION

Inhibits bacterial DNA synthesis, mainly by blocking DNA gyrase; bactericidal.

Route	Onset	Peak	Duration
P.O.	Unknown	1-3 hr	Unknown

INDICATIONS & DOSAGE

Uncomplicated urinary tract infections (UTIs) due to susceptible strains of Escherichia coli, Staphylococcus epidermidis, *and* S. saprophyticus —
Adults ages 18 and older: 200 mg P.O. q 12 hours for 7 days.

Severe or complicated UTIs due to susceptible strains of E. coli, Proteus mirabilis, Pseudomonas aeruginosa, S. epidermidis, *and* Enterobacter cloacae —
Adults ages 18 and older: 400 mg P.O. q 12 hours for 14 days.

Uncomplicated urethral or endocervical gonorrhea —
Adults: 400 mg P.O. as a single dose.

Doxycycline therapy may follow to treat possible coexisting chlamydial infection.
Dosage adjustment: For patients with renal failure, if creatinine clearance is 30 ml/minute or less, therapy is started with usual initial dose. Subsequent doses are decreased by 50%.

ADVERSE REACTIONS

CNS: headache, restlessness, tremor, lightheadedness, confusion, hallucinations, *seizures.*
GI: *nausea, diarrhea,* vomiting, abdominal pain or discomfort, oral candidiasis.
GU: crystalluria.
Hematologic: eosinophilia.

Hepatic: elevated liver enzymes.
Respiratory: dyspnea, cough.
Skin: *rash,* photosensitivity, pruritus.
Other: hypersensitivity.

INTERACTIONS
Drug-drug. *Aminophylline, cyclosporine, theophylline:* increased levels of these drugs because of decreased metabolism. Use together cautiously.
Antacids containing aluminum hydroxide or magnesium hydroxide, oral iron supplements, sucralfate: decreased enoxacin absorption. Administration times are separated by at least 2 hours.
Bismuth subsalicylate: bioavailability of enoxacin is decreased when given within 60 minutes of bismuth subsalicylate. Avoid concomitant use.
Digoxin: may increase digoxin serum levels. Patient is monitored closely for toxicity.
Oral anticoagulants: increased anticoagulant effect. Use together cautiously.
Drug-food. *Any food:* affects absorption. Drug is given on an empty stomach.
Caffeine: increased effect of caffeine. Monitor closely.

EFFECTS ON DIAGNOSTIC TESTS
None reported.

CONTRAINDICATIONS
Contraindicated in patients with hypersensitivity to drug or other fluoroquinolone antibiotics.

SPECIAL CONSIDERATIONS
▶ Use cautiously in patients with CNS disorders, such as severe cerebral arteriosclerosis or seizure disorders, and in those at increased risk for seizures. Drug may cause CNS stimulation.
▶ Use cautiously and with dosage adjustments in patients with impaired renal or hepatic function. Renal function and liver function tests must be monitored.
▶ A specimen for culture and sensitivity tests should be obtained before giving first dose. Therapy may begin pending results.
▶ **Alert:** Before treatment for gonorrhea begins, patient should have an initial serologic test for syphilis. Drug hasn't been effective in treating syphilis and may mask signs and symptoms of infection. Have the serologic test repeated in 1 to 3 months.
▶ Drug is administered 2 hours after a meal or 2 hours before or after antacids containing magnesium hydroxide or aluminum hydroxide, sucralfate, or products that contain iron (such as vitamins with mineral supplements).
▶ Patient is monitored closely for superinfection.
▶ Safety in children under age 18 has not been established. Drug has caused cartilage erosion.
▶ Tendon rupture has been reported in patients receiving quinolones. Drug is discontinued if pain, inflammation, or rupture of a tendon occurs.

Patient teaching
▶ Take drug as prescribed, even after feeling better.
▶ Take drug on an empty stomach.
▶ Drink plenty of fluids to reduce risk of crystalluria.
▶ Don't drink beverages containing caffeine. Enoxacin inhibits the metabolism of caffeine and can result in toxicity.
▶ Avoid hazardous tasks until adverse CNS effects of drug are known.
▶ Avoid overexposure to direct sunlight, use a sunblock, and wear protective clothing while outdoors.
▶ Stop taking drug at first signs of an allergic reaction, and notify health care provider.

---

*Liquid contains alcohol.   **May contain tartrazine.   †Canada   ‡Australia   §U.K.   ◇OTC

levofloxacin

Levaquin
Pregnancy Risk Category C

HOW SUPPLIED

Tablets: 250 mg, 500 mg
Single-use vials: 500 mg
Infusion (premixed): 250 mg in 50 ml
D_5W, 500 mg in 100 ml D_5W

ACTION

Inhibits bacterial DNA gyrase and prevents DNA replication, transcription, repair, and recombination in susceptible bacteria.

Route	Onset	Peak	Duration
P.O., I.V.	Unknown	1-2 hr	Unknown

INDICATIONS & DOSAGE

Note: Indicated for treatment of mild, moderate, and severe infections due to susceptible microorganisms in adults ages 18 and older.

Acute maxillary sinusitis due to susceptible strains of Streptococcus pneumoniae, Moraxella catarrhalis, *or* Haemophilus influenzae —
Adults: 500 mg P.O. or I.V. daily for 10 to 14 days. (See *Dosage adjustment* below.)

Acute bacterial exacerbation of chronic bronchitis due to Staphylococcus aureus, S. pneumoniae, M. catarrhalis, H. influenzae, *or* H. parainfluenzae —
Adults: 500 mg P.O. or I.V. daily for 7 days. (See *Dosage adjustment* below.)

Community-acquired pneumonia due to S. aureus, S. pneumoniae, M. catarrhalis, H. influenzae, H. parainfluenzae, Klebsiella pneumoniae, Chlamydia pneumoniae, Legionella pneumophila, *or* Mycoplasma pneumoniae —
Adults: 500 mg P.O. or I.V. daily for 7 to 14 days. (See *Dosage adjustment* below.)

Mild to moderate skin and skin-structure infections due to S. aureus *or* S. pyogenes —
Adults: 500 mg P.O. or I.V. daily for 7 to 10 days. (See *Dosage adjustment* below.)

Mild to moderate uncomplicated urinary tract infection due to Escherichia coli, K. pneumoniae, *or* S. saprophyticus —
Adults: 250 mg P.O. daily for 3 days.
Dosage adjustment: If creatinine clearance is 20 to 49 ml/minute, subsequent dosages are half the initial dose. If 10 to 19 ml/minute, subsequent dosages are half initial dose and the interval is increased to q 48 hours for above indications.

Urinary tract infections (mild to moderate) due to Enterococcus faecalis, Enterobacter cloacae, E. coli, K. pneumoniae, Proteus mirabilis, *or* Pseudomonas aeruginosa —
Adults: 250 mg P.O. or I.V. daily for 10 days. (See *Dosage adjustment* below.)

Acute pyelonephritis (mild to moderate) due to E. coli —
Adults: 250 mg P.O. or I.V. daily for 10 days. (See *Dosage adjustment* below.)
Dosage adjustment: If creatinine clearance is 10 to 19 ml/minute, dosage interval is increased to q 48 hours.

ADVERSE REACTIONS

CNS: headache, insomnia, dizziness, encephalopathy, paresthesia, *seizures.*
CV: chest pain, palpitations, vasodilation.
GI: nausea, diarrhea, constipation, vomiting, abdominal pain, dyspepsia, flatulence, *pseudomembranous colitis.*
GU: vaginitis.
Hematologic: eosinophilia, hemolytic anemia, lymphopenia.
Metabolic: hypoglycemia.
Musculoskeletal: back pain, tendon rupture.
Respiratory: allergic pneumonitis.
Skin: rash, photosensitivity, pruritus, erythema multiforme, *Stevens-Johnson syndrome.*

Reactions may be *common,* uncommon, *life-threatening,* or COMMON AND LIFE-THREATENING.

Other: pain, hypersensitivity reactions, *anaphylaxis, multisystem organ failure.*

INTERACTIONS

Drug-drug. *Antacids containing aluminum or magnesium, iron salts, products containing zinc, sucralfate:* may interfere with GI absorption of levofloxacin. Drugs are administered at least 2 hours apart.
Antidiabetics: may alter blood glucose levels. Blood glucose levels are monitored closely.
NSAIDs: may increase CNS stimulation. Patient is monitored for seizure activity.
Theophylline: decreased clearance of theophylline with some fluoroquinolones. Theophylline levels must be monitored.
Warfarin and derivatives: increased effect of oral anticoagulant with some fluoroquinolones. PT and INR are monitored.
Drug-lifestyle. *Sun exposure:* photosensitivity reactions may occur. Take precautions.

EFFECTS ON DIAGNOSTIC TESTS

Drug may cause an abnormal ECG.

CONTRAINDICATIONS

Contraindicated in patients with hypersensitivity to drug, its components, or other fluoroquinolones.

SPECIAL CONSIDERATIONS

▸ Safety and efficacy of drug in children under age 18 and in pregnant and breast-feeding women have not been established.
▸ Use cautiously in patients with history of seizure disorders or other CNS diseases, such as cerebral arteriosclerosis. If patient experiences symptoms of excessive CNS stimulation (restlessness, tremor, confusion, hallucinations), the drug is discontinued. Seizure precautions should be instituted.
▸ Use cautiously and with dosage adjustment in patients with renal impairment.
▸ Acute hypersensitivity reactions may require treatment with epinephrine, oxygen,

I.V. fluids, antihistamines, corticosteroids, pressor amines, and airway management.
▸ Most antibacterial drugs can cause pseudomembranous colitis. Drug may be discontinued if diarrhea occurs.
▸ A specimen for culture and sensitivity should be obtained before starting therapy and as needed to determine if bacterial resistance has occurred.
▸ Blood glucose and renal, hepatic, and hematopoietic blood studies must be monitored.

I.V. administration

▸ Levofloxacin injection should be administered only by I.V. infusion. The drug is diluted in single-use vials, according to manufacturer's instructions, with D_5W or normal saline for injection to a final concentration of 5 mg/ml. Reconstituted solution should be clear, slightly yellow, and free of particulate matter. Reconstituted drug is stable for 72 hours at room temperature, for 14 days when refrigerated in plastic containers, and for 6 months when frozen. Thaw at room temperature or in refrigerator only. Drug should not be mixed with other drugs. The solution is infused over 60 minutes.

Patient teaching

▸ Take drug as prescribed, even if symptoms disappear.
▸ Take drug with plenty of fluids and avoid antacids, sucralfate, and products containing iron or zinc for at least 2 hours before and after each dose.
▸ Avoid hazardous tasks until adverse CNS effects of drug are known.
▸ Avoid excessive sunlight, use sunblock, and wear protective clothing when outdoors.
▸ Stop drug and notify health care provider if rash or other signs or symptoms of hypersensitivity develop.
▸ Notify health care provider if experi-

encing pain or inflammation; tendon rupture can occur with drug.
⦁ If diabetic, monitor blood glucose levels and notify health care provider if a hypoglycemic reaction occurs.
⦁ Notify health care provider if loose stool or diarrhea occurs.

lomefloxacin hydrochloride

Maxaquin

Pregnancy Risk Category C

HOW SUPPLIED

Tablets (film-coated): 400 mg

ACTION

Inhibits bacterial DNA gyrase, an enzyme necessary for bacterial replication; bactericidal.

Route	Onset	Peak	Duration
P.O.	Unknown	1.5 hr	Unknown

INDICATIONS & DOSAGE

Acute bacterial exacerbations of chronic bronchitis due to Haemophilus influenzae *or* Moraxella (Branhamella) catarrhalis —
Adults: 400 mg P.O. daily for 10 days.

Uncomplicated urinary tract infections (cystitis) due to Escherichia coli, Klebsiella pneumoniae, Proteus mirabilis, *or* Staphylococcus saprophyticus —
Adults: 400 mg P.O. daily for 10 days.

Complicated urinary tract infections due to E. coli, K. pneumoniae, P. mirabilis, *or* Pseudomonas aeruginosa; *possibly effective against infections due to* Citrobacter diversus *or* Enterobacter cloacae —
Adults: 400 mg P.O. daily for 14 days.
Dosage adjustment: For patients with creatinine clearance of 10 to 40 ml/minute, give loading dose of 400 mg P.O. on first day; then 200 mg daily for duration of therapy.

Hemodialysis removes negligible amounts of drug.
Prophylaxis of infections after transurethral surgical procedures —
Adults: 400 mg P.O. as a single dose 2 to 6 hours before surgery.
Prophylaxis of urinary tract infections after transrectal prostate biopsy —
Adults: 400 mg P.O. as a single dose 1 to 6 hours before procedure.

ADVERSE REACTIONS

CNS: *dizziness, headache,* abnormal dreams, fatigue, malaise, asthenia, agitation, anorexia, anxiety, confusion, depersonalization, depression, insomnia, nervousness, somnolence, *seizures, coma,* hyperkinesis, tremor, vertigo, paresthesia.
CV: flushing, hypotension, hypertension, edema, syncope, arrhythmia, tachycardia, bradycardia, extrasystoles, cyanosis, angina pectoris, *MI, cardiac failure, pulmonary embolism,* cerebrovascular disorder, cardiomyopathy, phlebitis.
EENT: epistaxis, abnormal vision, conjunctivitis, eye pain, earache, tinnitus, tongue discoloration, taste perversion, thirst.
GI: *diarrhea, nausea,* dry mouth, increased appetite, pseudomembranous colitis, abdominal pain, dyspepsia, vomiting, flatulence, constipation, inflammation, dysphagia, bleeding.
GU: dysuria, hematuria, anuria, epididymitis, orchitis, vaginitis, vaginal candidiasis, intermenstrual bleeding, perineal pain.
Hematologic: thrombocythemia, *thrombocytopenia.*
Hepatic: elevated liver enzymes.
Metabolic: hypoglycemia.
Musculoskeletal: leg cramps, arthralgia, myalgia, chest or back pain.
Respiratory: dyspnea, *bronchospasm,* respiratory disorder or infection, increased sputum, stridor.
Skin: pruritus, skin disorder, skin exfoli-

Reactions may be *common,* uncommon, *life-threatening*, or COMMON AND LIFE-THREATENING.

ation, eczema, rash, urticaria, *photosensitivity.*

Other: *anaphylaxis,* increased diaphoresis, lymphadenopathy, chills, allergic reaction, facial edema, flulike syndrome, decreased heat tolerance, gout.

INTERACTIONS

Drug-drug. *Antacids, sucralfate:* impaired absorption after binding with lomefloxacin in GI tract. Drug is given no less than 4 hours before or 2 hours after a dose.

Cimetidine: increased half-life of other fluoroquinolones when administered to patients taking cimetidine; lomefloxacin has not been tested. Patient is monitored for toxicity.

Cyclosporine, warfarin: increased effects on serum levels when combined with other fluoroquinolones; lomefloxacin has not been tested. Patient is monitored for toxicity.

NSAIDs: possibility of increased CNS stimulation and seizures. Use cautiously.

Probenecid: decreased excretion of lomefloxacin. Patient is monitored for toxicity.

Drug-lifestyle. *Sun exposure:* photosensitivity reactions may occur. Take precautions.

EFFECTS ON DIAGNOSTIC TESTS
None reported.

CONTRAINDICATIONS
Contraindicated in patients with hypersensitivity to drug or other fluoroquinolones.

SPECIAL CONSIDERATIONS
▶ Use cautiously in patients with known or suspected CNS disorders, such as seizure disorder or cerebral arteriosclerosis, that may predispose the patient to seizures.
▶ Culture and sensitivity tests should be obtained before giving first dose. Therapy may begin pending results.

▶ Although most fluoroquinolones exhibit photosensitizing effects photosensitization and phototoxicity are more common with lomefloxacin.
▶ Prolonged use may result in overgrowth of organisms resistant to lomefloxacin.
▶ Safety in children under age 18 hasn't been established. Drug has caused cartilage erosion.
▶ Tendon rupture has been reported in patients receiving quinolones. Discontinue if pain, inflammation, or rupture of a tendon occurs.

Patient teaching
▶ Take drug as prescribed, even after feeling better.
▶ Hypersensitivity reactions may occur even after first dose. If rash or other allergic reaction appears, stop taking drug and notify health care provider.
▶ Avoid hazardous tasks until CNS effects of drug are known.
▶ Wear protective clothing, use a sunscreen, and avoid prolonged exposure to sunlight during treatment and for a few days after therapy ends. If sunburn occurs, call health care provider promptly.
▶ Drug may be taken with or without food.
▶ Notify health care provider if loose stool or diarrhea occurs.

---

nalidixic acid
NegGram

Pregnancy Risk Category B (safe use in first trimester unknown)

HOW SUPPLIED
Caplets: 250 mg, 500 mg, 1 g
Oral suspension: 250 mg/5 ml

ACTION
Inhibits microbial DNA synthesis.

Route	Onset	Peak	Duration
P.O.	Unknown	1-2 hr	Unknown

INDICATIONS & DOSAGE

Acute and chronic urinary tract infections due to susceptible gram-negative organisms (Proteus, Klebsiella, Enterobacter, *and* Escherichia coli) —

Adults: 1 g P.O. q.i.d. for 7 to 14 days; 2 g daily for long-term use.

Children over age 3 months: 55 mg/kg P.O. daily divided q.i.d. for 7 to 14 days; 33 mg/kg daily for long-term use.

ADVERSE REACTIONS

CNS: drowsiness, weakness, headache, dizziness, vertigo, *seizures,* malaise, confusion, hallucinations, psychosis, *increased intracranial pressure and bulging fontanelles in infants and children.*

EENT: sensitivity to light, change in color perception, diplopia, blurred vision.

GI: *abdominal pain, nausea, vomiting,* diarrhea.

Hematologic: eosinophilia, *leukopenia, thrombocytopenia,* hemolytic anemia.

Musculoskeletal: arthralgia, joint stiffness.

Skin: pruritus, photosensitivity, urticaria, rash.

Other: *angioedema, anaphylactoid reaction.*

INTERACTIONS

Drug-drug. *Nitrofurantoin:* antagonizes effects of nalidixic acid. Monitor closely. *Oral anticoagulants:* increased anticoagulant effect. Patient is monitored for bleeding.

Drug-lifestyle. *Sun exposure:* photosensitivity reactions may occur. Take precautions.

EFFECTS ON DIAGNOSTIC TESTS

Drug may cause false-positive results in urine glucose tests using cupric sulfate (such as Benedict's reagent, Fehling's solution, and Clinitest). Urine 17-ketosteroid and urine 17-ketogenic steroid levels may be falsely elevated because nalidixic acid interacts with *M*-dinitrobenzene, used to measure these urine metabolites. Urine vanillylmandelic acid levels may also be falsely elevated.

CONTRAINDICATIONS

Contraindicated in patients with hypersensitivity to drug, in those with seizure disorders, and in infants under age 3 months.

SPECIAL CONSIDERATIONS

▶ Use with extreme caution in prepubertal children; drug has caused cartilage erosion.

▶ Use cautiously in patients with impaired hepatic or renal function or with severe cerebral arteriosclerosis. Renal and liver function test results are monitored closely.

▶ A specimen for culture and sensitivity tests should be obtained before starting therapy and repeated as needed. Therapy may begin pending results.

▶ CBC and renal and liver function studies are monitored during long-term therapy.

▶ Resistant bacteria may emerge in the first 48 hours of therapy.

Patient teaching

▶ Take drug as prescribed, even after feeling better.

▶ Take drug with food to prevent GI upset.

▶ Avoid exposure to sunlight, wear protective clothing, and use sunscreen.

▶ Report visual disturbances or CNS symptoms immediately.

norfloxacin

Noroxin, Utinor§

Pregnancy Risk Category C

HOW SUPPLIED

Tablets (film-coated): 400 mg

ACTION

Inhibits bacterial DNA synthesis, mainly by blocking DNA gyrase; bactericidal.

Route	Onset	Peak	Duration
P.O.	Unknown	0.5-2 hr	Unknown

INDICATIONS & DOSAGE

Complicated or uncomplicated urinary tract infections due to susceptible strains of Enterococcus faecalis, Escherichia coli, Klebsiella pneumoniae, Enterobacter aerogenes, E. cloacae, Proteus mirabilis, P. vulgaris, Pseudomonas aeruginosa, Citrobacter freundii, Staphylococcus agalactiae, S. aureus, S. epidermidis, S. saprophyticus, *and* Serratia marcescens —
Adults: for uncomplicated infections, 400 mg P.O. q 12 hours for 7 to 10 days. For complicated infections, 400 mg P.O. q 12 hours for 10 to 21 days. (See *Dosage adjustment* below.)

Cystitis due to E. coli, K. pneumoniae, *or* P. mirabilis —
Adults: 400 mg P.O. q 12 hours for 3 days. (See *Dosage adjustment* below.)

Acute, uncomplicated urethral and cervical gonorrhea —
Adults: 800 mg P.O. as a single dose, followed by doxycycline therapy to treat any coexisting chlamydial infection.

Dosage adjustment: For adult patients with creatinine clearance of 30 ml/minute or less, 400 mg once daily for above indications.

ADVERSE REACTIONS

CNS: fatigue, somnolence, headache, dizziness, *seizures,* depression, insomnia.
GI: nausea, constipation, flatulence, heartburn, dry mouth, abdominal pain, diarrhea, vomiting, anorexia.
GU: increased serum creatinine and BUN levels, crystalluria.
Hematologic: eosinophilia, hematocrit may decrease, *neutropenia.*
Hepatic: ALT, AST, and alkaline phosphatase levels may increase.
Musculoskeletal: back pain.

Skin: rash, photosensitivity.
Other: *hypersensitivity reactions, anaphylaxis,* fever, hyperhidrosis.

INTERACTIONS

Drug-drug. *Antacids, iron products, sucralfate:* may hinder absorption. Administration times are separated by 2 hours.
Cyclosporine: increased serum concentrations of cyclosporine. Serum levels are monitored.
Nitrofurantoin: antagonizes effects of norfloxacin. Monitor closely.
Oral anticoagulants: increased anticoagulant effect. Monitor closely.
Probenecid: may increase serum levels of norfloxacin by decreasing its excretion. Patient is monitored for toxicity.
Theophylline: possibly impaired theophylline metabolism, resulting in increased plasma levels and risk of toxicity. Monitor closely.

EFFECTS ON DIAGNOSTIC TESTS

None reported.

CONTRAINDICATIONS

Contraindicated in patients with hypersensitivity to drug or other fluoroquinolones.

SPECIAL CONSIDERATIONS

▶ Use cautiously in patients with conditions such as cerebral arteriosclerosis that may predispose them to seizure disorders.
▶ Also, use cautiously in those with renal impairment. Renal function must be monitored.
▶ Safety in children under age 18 has not been established. Drug has caused cartilage erosion.
▶ Culture and sensitivity tests should be obtained before starting therapy.
▶ Tendon rupture has been reported in patients receiving quinolones. Discontinue if pain, inflammation, or rupture of a tendon occurs.

Patient teaching

▶ Take drug as prescribed, even after feeling better. Don't exceed recommended dosages.

▶ Take 1 hour before or 2 hours after meals because food, antacids, iron products, and sucralfate may hinder absorption.

▶ Drink several glasses of water throughout the day to maintain hydration and adequate urine output.

▶ Avoid hazardous tasks that require alertness until CNS effects of drug are known.

▶ Avoid exposure to sunlight, wear protective clothing, and use sunscreen while outdoors.

ofloxacin

Floxin, Floxin I.V., Tarivid§

Pregnancy Risk Category C

HOW SUPPLIED

Tablets (film-coated): 200 mg, 300 mg, 400 mg
Injection: 20 mg/ml, 40 mg/ml; 200 mg, 400 mg premixed in D_5W

ACTION

Inhibits bacterial DNA synthesis by blocking DNA gyrase; bactericidal.

Route	Onset	Peak	Duration
P.O.	Unknown	0.5-2 hr	Unknown
I.V.	Unknown	Immediate	Unknown

INDICATIONS & DOSAGE

Lower respiratory tract infections due to susceptible strains of Haemophilus influenzae *or* Streptococcus pneumoniae —
Adults: 400 mg I.V. or P.O. q 12 hours for 10 days.

Cervicitis or urethritis due to Chlamydia trachomatis *or* Neisseria gonorrhoeae —
Adults: 300 mg I.V. or P.O. q 12 hours for 7 days.

Acute, uncomplicated gonorrhea —
Adults: 400 mg I.V. or P.O. as a single dose with doxycycline.

Mild to moderate skin and skin-structure infections due to susceptible strains of Staphylococcus aureus, S. pyogenes, *or* Proteus mirabilis —
Adults: 400 mg I.V. or P.O. q 12 hours for 10 days.

Cystitis due to Escherichia coli *or* Klebsiella pneumoniae —
Adults: 200 mg I.V. or P.O. q 12 hours for 3 days.

Urinary tract infections due to susceptible strains of Citrobacter diversus, Enterobacter aerogenes, E. coli, P. mirabilis, *or* Pseudomonas aeruginosa —
Adults: 200 mg I.V. or P.O. q 12 hours for 7 days. Complicated infections may require therapy for 10 days.

Prostatitis due to E. coli —
Adults: 300 mg I.V. or P.O. q 12 hours for 6 weeks.

Epididymitis —
Adults: 300 mg P.O. q 12 hours for 10 days.

Pelvic inflammatory disease (outpatient) —
Adults: 400 mg P.O. q 12 hours for 14 days with metronidazole.

Dosage adjustment: For renally impaired patients with creatinine clearance of 10 to 50 ml/minute, reduce dosing interval to once q 24 hours. If creatinine clearance is below 20 ml/minute, give half the recommended dose q 24 hours.

ADVERSE REACTIONS

CNS: headache, dizziness, fatigue, lethargy, malaise, drowsiness, sleep disorders, nervousness, insomnia, *seizures.*
CV: chest pain, phlebitis.
EENT: visual disturbances.
GI: *nausea,* anorexia, abdominal pain or discomfort, diarrhea, vomiting, constipation, dry mouth, flatulence, dysgeusia.
GU: vaginitis, vaginal discharge, genital pruritus.

Reactions may be *common,* uncommon, *life-threatening*, or COMMON AND LIFE-THREATENING.

Hepatic: elevated liver enzymes.
Metabolic: hyperglycemia.
Musculoskeletal: trunk pain.
Skin: rash, pruritus, photosensitivity.
Other: *hypersensitivity reactions, anaphylaxis,* fever.

INTERACTIONS

Drug-drug. *Antacids containing magnesium or aluminum hydroxide, iron salts, sucralfate, products containing zinc:* may interfere with GI absorption of ofloxacin. Administration times are separated by at least 2 hours.
Antidiabetics: may cause alterations in blood glucose levels. Levels are monitored closely.
NSAIDs: risk of increased CNS stimulation and seizures. Use cautiously.
Oral anticoagulants: increased effect. The patient is monitored for bleeding and altered PT.
Theophylline: decreased clearance of theophylline with some fluoroquinolones. Theophylline levels are monitored.
Drug-food. *Any food:* decreased absorption. Drug is given on an empty stomach.
Drug-lifestyle. *Sun exposure:* photosensitivity reactions may occur. Take precautions.

EFFECTS ON DIAGNOSTIC TESTS
None reported.

CONTRAINDICATIONS
Contraindicated in patients with hypersensitivity to drug or other fluoroquinolones.

SPECIAL CONSIDERATIONS
▶ Use cautiously in patients with a history of seizure disorders or other CNS diseases such as cerebral arteriosclerosis.
▶ Use cautiously and with dosage adjustment in patients with renal failure because drug is mainly eliminated by renal excretion.

▶ Culture and sensitivity tests are obtained before first dose.
▶ Regular blood studies and hepatic and renal function tests must be monitored during prolonged therapy.
▶ **Alert:** Patients treated for gonorrhea should have a serologic test for syphilis. Drug is not effective against syphilis, and treatment of gonorrhea may mask or delay symptoms of syphilis.
▶ Safety in children under age 18 has not been established. Drug has caused cartilage erosion.
▶ Tendon rupture has been reported in patients receiving quinolones. Discontinue if pain, inflammation, or rupture of a tendon occurs.

I.V. administration
▶ Concentrate for injection is diluted before use. Single-use vials containing 20 or 40 mg/ml must be diluted to a maximum concentration of 4 mg/ml with a compatible I.V. solution, such as D_5W, normal saline for injection, D_5W in normal saline for injection, or sterile water for injection. Solution is infused over at least 60 minutes.
▶ Because compatibility with other drugs is not known, ofloxacin is not mixed with other drugs. If giving infusion at a Y-site, the flow of the other solution should be discontinued.

Patient teaching
▶ Take drug as prescribed, even after feeling better.
▶ Take drug with plenty of fluids, but not with meals, and avoid antacids, sucralfate, and products containing iron or zinc for at least 2 hours before and after each dose.
▶ Avoid hazardous tasks until adverse CNS effects of drug are known.
▶ Use sunscreen and wear protective clothing while outdoors.
▶ Stop drug and notify health care provider if rash or other signs of hypersensitivity develop.

---

sparfloxacin

Zagam
Pregnancy Risk Category C

HOW SUPPLIED
Tablets: 200 mg

ACTION
Inhibits bacterial DNA gyrase and prevents DNA replication, transcription, repair, and deactivation in susceptible bacteria.

Route	Onset	Peak	Duration
P.O.	Unknown	3-6 hr	Unknown

INDICATIONS & DOSAGE
Acute bacterial exacerbation of chronic bronchitis due to Staphylococcus aureus, Streptococcus pneumoniae, Chlamydia pneumoniae, Enterobacter cloacae, Klebsiella pneumoniae, Moraxella catarrhalis, Haemophilus influenzae, *or* H. parainfluenzae —
Adults over age 18: 400 mg P.O. on first day as a loading dose; then 200 mg daily for total of 10 days of therapy.
    Community-acquired pneumonia due to S. pneumoniae, M. catarrhalis, H. influenzae, H. parainfluenzae, C. pneumoniae, *or* Mycoplasma pneumoniae —
Adults over age 18: 400 mg P.O. on first day as a loading dose; then 200 mg daily for total of 10 days of therapy.
Dosage adjustment: For renally impaired patients with creatinine clearance below 50 ml/minute, give a loading dose of 400 mg P.O.; then, 200 mg P.O. q 48 hours for total of 9 days of therapy.

ADVERSE REACTIONS
CNS: headache, dizziness, insomnia, asthenia, somnolence, *seizures.*
CV: prolonged QT interval, vasodilatation.
EENT: dry mouth, taste perversion.
GI: nausea, diarrhea, vomiting, abdominal pain, dyspepsia, flatulence, *pseudomembranous colitis.*
GU: vaginal candidiasis.
Hematologic: elevated WBC counts.
Hepatic: elevated ALT and AST levels.
Musculoskeletal: tendon rupture.
Skin: rash, photosensitivity, pruritus.
Other: hypersensitivity reactions, *anaphylaxis.*

INTERACTIONS
Drug-drug. *Antacids containing aluminum or magnesium, iron salts, sucralfate, zinc:* may interfere with GI absorption of levofloxacin. Drugs are administered at least 4 hours apart.
    Drugs that prolong the QT interval or cause torsades de pointes (including amiodarone, bepridil, cisapride, class IA antiarrhythmics [such as procainamide and quinidine], class III drugs [such as sotalol], disopyramide, erythromycin, pentamidine, phenothiazines, tricyclic antidepressants): may cause torsades de pointes. Sparfloxacin is contraindicated in these patients.
Drug-lifestyle. *Sun exposure:* photosensitivity reactions may occur. Take precautions.

EFFECTS ON DIAGNOSTIC TESTS
Drug may produce false-negative culture results for *Mycobacterium tuberculosis.*

CONTRAINDICATIONS
Contraindicated in patients with a history of hypersensitivity or photosensitivity reactions to drug and in those who cannot avoid the sun. Avoid administration with drugs known to prolong the QT interval or cause torsades de pointes. Drug isn't recommended for patients with heart conditions that predispose them to arrhythmias.

SPECIAL CONSIDERATIONS
▶ Safety and efficacy of levofloxacin in

pregnant and breast-feeding women and in patients under age 18 have not been established.

▶ Use cautiously in patients with history of seizure disorder or other CNS diseases such as cerebral arteriosclerosis. If patient experiences symptoms of excessive CNS stimulation (restlessness, tremor, confusion, hallucinations), discontinue drug. Seizure precautions should be instituted.

▶ Use cautiously and with dosage adjustment in patients with renal impairment. Renal function must be monitored.

▶ Acute hypersensitivity reactions may require treatment with epinephrine, oxygen, I.V. fluids, antihistamines, corticosteroids, and pressor amines, and airway management.

▶ Specimen for culture and sensitivity tests should be obtained before starting therapy and as needed to determine if bacterial resistance has occurred.

Patient teaching

▶ Drug may be taken with food, milk, or products that contain caffeine.

▶ Take drug as prescribed, even if symptoms disappear.

▶ Take drug with plenty of fluids and avoid antacids, sucralfate, and products containing iron or zinc for at least 4 hours after each dose.

▶ Avoid hazardous tasks until adverse CNS effects of drug are known.

▶ *Alert:* Avoid direct, indirect, and artificial ultraviolet light, even with sunscreen on, during treatment and for 5 days after treatment. Stop taking drug and notify health care provider if signs or symptoms of phototoxicity (skin burning, redness, swelling, blisters, rash, itching) occur.

▶ Stop drug and notify health care provider if rash or other signs of hypersensitivity develop.

▶ Stop drug and notify health care provider if experiencing pain or inflammation; tendon rupture can occur with drug use. Rest

and refrain from exercise until diagnosis is made.

▶ Notify health care provider if loose stool or diarrhea occurs.

trovafloxacin mesylate
Trovan Tablets

alatrofloxacin mesylate
Trovan I.V.
Pregnancy Risk Category C

HOW SUPPLIED
Tablets: 100 mg, 200 mg
Injection: 5 mg/ml in 40-ml (200 mg) and 60-ml (300 mg) vials

ACTION
Trovafloxacin is related to the fluoroquinolones with in vitro activity against a wide range of gram-positive and gram-negative aerobic and anaerobic microorganisms. Bactericidal action results from inhibition of DNA gyrase and topoisomerase IV, two enzymes involved in bacterial replication.

Route	Onset	Peak	Duration
P.O., I.V.	Unknown	1 hr	Unknown

INDICATIONS & DOSAGE
Nosocomial pneumonia due to Escherichia coli, Pseudomonas aeruginosa, Haemophilus influenzae, *or* Staphylococcus aureus; *gynecologic and pelvic infections due to* E. coli, Bacteroides fragilis, *viridans group streptococci,* Enterococcus faecalis, Streptococcus agalactiae, Peptostreptococcus *species,* Prevotella *species, or* Gardnerella vaginalis; *complicated intra-abdominal infections including postsurgical infections due to* E. coli, B. fragilis, *viridans group streptococci,* P. aeruginosa, Klebsiella pneumoniae, Pepto-

streptococcus *species, or* Prevotella *species* —
Adults: 300 mg I.V. daily; then, when clinically indicated, 200 mg P.O. daily; total duration of therapy 7 to 14 days (10 to 14 days for pneumonia).

Community-acquired pneumonia due to S. pneumoniae, H. influenzae, K. pneumoniae, S. aureus, Mycoplasma pneumoniae, Moraxella catarrhalis, Legionella pneumophila, *or* Chlamydia pneumoniae; *complicated skin and skin-structure infections including diabetic foot infections due to* S. aureus, S. agalactiae, P. aeruginosa, E. faecalis, E. coli, *or* Proteus mirabilis *(not for treatment of osteomyelitis)* —
Adults: 200 mg P.O. or I.V. daily; then, when clinically indicated, 200 mg P.O. daily; total duration of treatment 7 to 14 days (10 to 14 days for complicated skin and skin-structure infections).

Prophylaxis of infection associated with elective colorectal surgery or vaginal and abdominal hysterectomy —
Adults: 200 mg P.O. or I.V as a single dose 30 minutes to 4 hours before surgery.

Acute sinusitis due to H. influenzae, M. catarrhalis, *or* S. pneumoniae; *chronic prostatitis due to* E. coli, E. faecalis, *or* S. epidermis; *cervicitis due to* C. trachomatis; *and pelvic inflammatory disease (mild to moderate) due to* Neisseria gonorrhoeae *or* C. trachomatis —
Adults: 200 mg P.O. daily for 5 days (cervicitis), 10 days (acute sinusitis), 14 days (pelvic inflammatory disease), or 28 days (chronic prostatitis).

Uncomplicated urinary tract infections due to E. coli; *uncomplicated skin and skin-structure infections due to* S. aureus, S. pyogenes, *or* S. agalactiae; *acute bacterial exacerbation of chronic bronchitis due to* H. influenzae, M. catarrhalis, S. pneumoniae, S. aureus, *or* Haemophilus parainfluenzae; *and uncomplicated gonorrhea due to* N. gonorrhoeae —
Adults: 100 mg P.O. daily for 3 days (urinary tract infections), 7 to 10 days (skin and skin-structure infections, bronchitis) or single dose for treatment of gonorrhea.
Dosage adjustment: For patients with mild to moderate cirrhosis (Child-Pugh Class A and B), reduce 300-mg I.V. dose to 200-mg I.V. and 200-mg I.V. or P.O. dose to 100-mg I.V. or P.O.; no reduction is needed for 100-mg P.O. dose.

ADVERSE REACTIONS

CNS: *dizziness,* light-headedness, headache, ***seizures,*** psychosis.
GI: diarrhea, nausea, vomiting, abdominal pain, pseudomembranous colitis.
GU: vaginitis, increased BUN and creatinine levels.
Hematologic: bone marrow aplasia ***(anemia, thrombocytopenia, leukopenia),*** decreased hemoglobin and hematocrit, increased platelets.
Hepatic: increased ALT and AST.
Musculoskeletal: arthralgia, arthropathy, myalgia.
Skin: pruritus, rash, injection-site reaction, photosensitivity.

INTERACTIONS

Drug-drug. *Antacids containing aluminum, magnesium, or citric acid buffered with sodium citrate (Bicitra), iron-containing preparations, I.V. morphine, sucralfate:* bioavailability of trovafloxacin is significantly reduced following use with these agents. These agents are given 2 hours before or 2 hours after trovafloxacin. Morphine I.V. is avoided for 4 hours if trovafloxacin is taken with food.
Drug-lifestyle. *Sun exposure:* photosensitivity reactions may occur. Take precautions.

EFFECTS ON DIAGNOSTIC TESTS
None reported.

CONTRAINDICATIONS
Contraindicated in patients with hypersensitivity to drug, alatrofloxacin, or oth-

er quinolone antimicrobials or any other components of these products.

SPECIAL CONSIDERATIONS

▶ Use cautiously in patients with CNS disorders (such as cerebral atherosclerosis or epilepsy) and in those at increased risk for seizures. As with other quinolones, drug may cause neurologic complications such as seizures, psychosis, or increased intracranial pressure. Patient with preexisting condition must be monitored closely.

▶ Periodic assessment of liver function is performed because of potential for increases in ALT, AST, and alkaline phosphatase levels.

▶ *Alert:* Using drug for more than 2 weeks greatly increases the risk of serious liver injury. Liver injury has also been reported following reexposure to drug. Therefore, drug should be limited to patients with life- or limb-threatening infections who received their initial treatment as an inpatient in a hospital or a long-term care nursing facility. Drug shouldn't be used if effective and safer alternative antimicrobial therapy is available.

▶ Drug can be given as a single daily dose without regard to food.

▶ Moderate to severe phototoxicity reactions have occurred in patients exposed to direct sunlight.

▶ No dosage adjustment is necessary when switching from I.V. to oral form.

▶ If *P. aeruginosa* is the known or presumed pathogen, treatment with an aminoglycoside or aztreonam may be indicated.

I.V. administration

▶ Alatrofloxacin mesylate is supplied in single-use vials that must be further diluted with an appropriate solution (D_5W, half-normal saline) before administration. Drug is not diluted with normal saline or lactated Ringer's solution. Package insert is referred to for specific instructions regarding preparation of desired dosage.

▶ After dilution, alatrofloxacin mesylate is administered by I.V. infusion over 60 minutes. Rapid bolus or infusion is avoided. Drug and solutions containing multivalent cations (such as magnesium) should not be administered through same I.V. line.

Patient teaching

▶ Drug may be taken without regard to meals; however, products containing iron, aluminum, magnesium (vitamins, minerals, antacids), or sucralfate should be taken at least 2 hours before or 2 hours after trovafloxacin dose.

▶ Take drug with meals or at bedtime if light-headedness or dizziness occurs.

▶ Avoid excessive sunlight or artificial ultraviolet light and use an effective sunscreen to prevent sunburn.

▶ Stop treatment, refrain from exercise, and seek medical advice if pain, inflammation, or rupture of a tendon occurs.

▶ Stop drug at first sign of rash, hives, difficulty swallowing or breathing, or other symptoms suggesting an allergic reaction and to seek medical help immediately.

▶ Notify health care provider if severe diarrhea occurs; this may indicate pseudomembranous colitis.

abacavir sulfate
acyclovir sodium
amantadine hydrochloride
amprenavir
cidofovir
delavirdine mesylate
didanosine
efavirenz
famciclovir
fomivirsen sodium
foscarnet sodium
ganciclovir
indinavir sulfate
lamivudine
lamivudine/zidovudine
nelfinavir mesylate
nevirapine
oseltamivir phosphate
ribavirin
rimantadine hydrochloride
ritonavir
saquinavir
saquinavir mesylate
stavudine
valacyclovir hydrochloride
zalcitabine
zanamivir
zidovudine

COMBINATION PRODUCTS
None.

abacavir sulfate
Ziagen

Pregnancy Risk Category C

HOW SUPPLIED
Tablets: 300 mg
Oral solution: 20 mg/ml

ACTION
Converted intracellularly to the active metabolite carbovir triphosphate, which inhibits the activity of HIV-1 reverse transcriptase, thereby terminating viral DNA growth.

Route	Onset	Peak	Duration
P.O.	Unknown	Unknown	Unknown

INDICATIONS & DOSAGE
HIV-1 infection —
Adults: 300 mg P.O. b.i.d. with other antiretrovirals.
Children ages 3 months to 16 years: 8 mg/kg P.O. b.i.d. (up to maximum of 300 mg P.O. b.i.d.) with other antiretrovirals.

ADVERSE REACTIONS
CNS: insomnia and sleep disorders, headache.
GI: *nausea, vomiting,* diarrhea, loss of appetite, anorexia.
Metabolic: *elevated triglyceride levels.*
Skin: rash.
Other: *hypersensitivity reaction,* fever.

INTERACTIONS
Drug-lifestyle. *Alcohol use:* decreased elimination of abacavir, increasing overall exposure to drug. Alcohol consumption must be monitored. Use together cautiously.

EFFECTS ON DIAGNOSTIC TESTS
None reported.

CONTRAINDICATIONS
Contraindicated in patients with previous hypersensitivity to drug or its components.

SPECIAL CONSIDERATIONS
▶ Use cautiously in patients with known risk factors for liver disease. Lactic acidosis and severe hepatomegaly with steatosis, including fatal cases, have been re-

---

Reactions may be *common,* uncommon, *life-threatening*, or COMMON AND LIFE-THREATENING.

ported with the use of nucleoside analogues alone or in combination, including abacavir and other antiretrovirals.

▶ Women are more likely than men to experience lactic acidosis and severe hepatomegaly with steatosis. Obesity and prolonged nucleoside exposure may be risk factors.

▶ Treatment should be discontinued in patients who develop signs or symptoms of lactic acidosis or pronounced hepatotoxicity, which may include hepatomegaly and steatosis even in absence of elevated transaminase levels.

▶ No adequate studies of the effects of abacavir on pregnancy exist. Use during pregnancy only if the potential benefits outweigh the risk. Register pregnant women taking abacavir with the Antiretroviral Pregnancy Registry at 1-800-258-4263.

▶ *Alert:* Drug therapy must not be restarted after a hypersensitivity reaction because severe signs and symptoms will recur within hours and may include life-threatening hypotension and death. To facilitate reporting of hypersensitivity reactions, register patients with the Abacavir Hypersensitivity Registry at 1-800-270-0425.

▶ *Alert:* Abacavir can cause fatal hypersensitivity reactions; as soon as patient develops signs or symptoms of hypersensitivity (such as fever, rash, fatigue, nausea, vomiting, diarrhea, or abdominal pain), discontinue drug and seek medical attention immediately.

▶ Drug is given with other antiretrovirals, never alone.

▶ Drug may cause mildly elevated blood glucose levels.

Patient teaching

▶ Abacavir can cause a life-threatening hypersensitivity reaction.If signs or symptoms of hypersensitivity (such as fever, rash, severe tiredness, achiness, a generally ill feeling, nausea, vomiting, diarrhea, or stomach pain) develop, stop drug and notify health care provider immediately.

▶ Read drug information leaflet that comes with each new prescription and refill. Carry a warning card summarizing signs and symptoms of abacavir hypersensitivity reaction.

▶ Be aware that this drug isn't a cure for HIV infection. It hasn't been shown to reduce the risk of transmission of HIV to others through sexual contact or blood contamination, and its long-term effects are unknown.

▶ Take drug exactly as prescribed.

▶ Drug can be taken with or without food.

acyclovir sodium

Avirax , Zovirax

Pregnancy Risk Category C

HOW SUPPLIED

Capsules: 200 mg
Tablets: 400 mg, 800 mg
Suspension: 200 mg/5 ml
Injection: 500 mg/vial, 1 g/vial

ACTION

Interferes with DNA synthesis and inhibits viral multiplication.

Route	Onset	Peak	Duration
P.O.	Unknown	2.5 hr	Unknown
I.V.	Immediate	Immediate	Unknown

INDICATIONS & DOSAGE

Initial and recurrent episodes of mucocutaneous herpes simplex virus (HSV-1 and HSV-2) infections in immunocompromised patients; severe initial episodes of genital herpes in patients who are not immunocompromised —

Adults and children ages 12 and older: 5 mg/kg given I.V. at a constant rate over 1 hour q 8 hours for 7 to 14 days (5 to 7 days for severe initial episode of genital herpes).

Children under age 12: 250 mg/m² given I.V. at a constant rate over 1 hour q 8 hours for 7 days.

Initial genital herpes —
Adults: 200 mg P.O. q 4 hours while awake (total of five capsules daily); or 400 mg P.O. q 8 hours. Continue for 7 to 10 days for treatment of initial genital herpes episodes.

Intermittent therapy for recurrent genital herpes —
Adults: 200 mg P.O. q 4 hours while awake (total of five capsules daily). Treatment should continue for 5 days. Initiate therapy at first sign of recurrence.

Long-term suppressive therapy for recurrent genital herpes —
Adults: 400 mg P.O. b.i.d. for up to 12 months. Or, 200 mg P.O. three to five times daily for up to 12 months.

Varicella (chickenpox) infections in immunocompromised patients —
Adults and children ages 12 and older: 10 mg/kg I.V. infused at a constant rate over 1 hour q 8 hours for 7 days. Dosage for obese patients is 10 mg/kg (based on ideal body weight) q 8 hours for 7 days. Don't exceed maximum dosage equivalent of 500 mg/m^2 q 8 hours.
Children under age 12: 500 mg/m^2 I.V. infused at a constant rate over 1 hour q 8 hours for 7 to 10 days.

Varicella infection in immunocompetent patients —
Adults and children ages 2 and older: 20 mg/kg (maximum 800 mg/dose) P.O. q.i.d. for 5 days. Start therapy as soon as symptoms appear to achieve maximum efficacy.

Or, in adults and children weighing over 40 kg (88 lb), 800 mg P.O. q.i.d. for 5 days. In children ages 2 and older weighing 40 kg or less, 20 mg/kg P.O. q.i.d. for 5 days.

Acute herpes zoster infection in immunocompetent patients —
Adults and children ages 12 and older: 800 mg P.O. q 4 hours five times daily for 7 to 10 days.

Herpes simplex encephalitis —
Adults and children over age 6 months: 10 mg/kg I.V. infused at a constant rate over 1 hour q 8 hours for 10 days.

Or, in children ages 6 months to 12 years, 500 mg/m^2 I.V. infused at a constant rate over 1 hour q 8 hours for 10 days.
Dosage adjustment: For patients with renal failure, if creatinine clearance is over 50 ml/minute, I.V. dose is 100% of dose q 8 hours; if clearance is 25 to 50 ml/minute, 100% of dose q 12 hours; if clearance is 10 to 24 ml/minute, 100% of dose q 24 hours; if clearance is below 10 ml/minute, 50% of dose q 24 hours.

P.O. dosage: If normal dose is 200 mg q 4 hours five times daily and creatinine clearance is below 10 ml/minute, 200 mg P.O. q 12 hours. If normal dose is 400 mg q 12 hours and creatinine clearance is below 10 ml/minute, 200 mg q 12 hours. If normal dose is 800 mg q 4 hours five times daily and creatinine clearance is below 10 ml/minute, 800 mg q 12 hours; and if creatinine clearance is 10 to 25 ml/minute, 800 mg q 8 hours.

ADVERSE REACTIONS
CNS: *malaise, headache, **encephalopathic changes,*** including ***lethargy, obtundation, tremor, confusion, hallucinations, agitation, seizures, coma.***
GI: *nausea, vomiting,* diarrhea.
GU: *transient elevations of serum creatinine and BUN levels,* hematuria, ***acute renal failure.***
Hematologic: ***thrombocytopenia, leukopenia,*** thrombocytosis.
Skin: rash, itching, urticaria.
Other: *inflammation, phlebitis at injection site.*

INTERACTIONS
Drug-drug. *Interferon:* may have synergistic effect. Monitor closely.
Probenecid: increased acyclovir blood levels. Patient should be monitored for possible toxicity.

Reactions may be *common*, uncommon, *life-threatening*, or COMMON AND LIFE-THREATENING.

Zidovudine: may cause drowsiness or lethargy. Use together cautiously.

EFFECTS ON DIAGNOSTIC TESTS
None reported.

CONTRAINDICATIONS
Contraindicated in patients with hypersensitivity to drug.

SPECIAL CONSIDERATIONS
▶ Use cautiously in patients with underlying neurologic problems, renal disease, or dehydration and in those receiving other nephrotoxic drugs. Renal function must be monitored.
▶ *Alert:* Drug is not for I.M. or S.C. administration
▶ Encephalopathic changes are more likely to occur in patients with neurologic disorders or in those who have had neurologic reactions to cytotoxic drugs.
▶ No adequate studies in pregnant women exist. Acyclovir should be used during pregnancy only if potential benefits outweigh risks to fetus.

I.V. administration
▶ For I.V. infusion, drug is administered over at least 1 hour to prevent renal tubular damage. Bolus injections are not given. Bolus injection, dehydration (decreased urine output), preexisting renal disease, and concomitant use of other nephrotoxic drugs increase the risk of renal toxicity.
▶ Concentrated solutions (7 mg/ml or more) may be associated with a higher incidence of phlebitis.
▶ Fluid intake should be encouraged because patient must be adequately hydrated during acyclovir infusion. Intake and output must be monitored, especially within the first 2 hours after I.V. administration.

Patient teaching
▶ Take drug as prescribed, even after feeling better.
▶ Drug is effective in managing herpes infection but does not eliminate or cure it. Acyclovir will not prevent spread of infection to others.
▶ Know the early symptoms of herpes infection (such as tingling, itching, or pain); notify health care provider and get a prescription for acyclovir before the infection fully develops. Treatment started early is most effective.

amantadine hydrochloride
Symmetrel

Pregnancy Risk Category C

HOW SUPPLIED
Capsules: 100 mg
Syrup: 50 mg/5 ml
Tablets: 100 mg

ACTION
Unknown. Possibly inhibits the uncoating of the virus.

Route	Onset	Peak	Duration
P.O.	Unknown	1-4 hr	Unknown

INDICATIONS & DOSAGE
Prophylaxis or symptomatic treatment of influenza type A virus, respiratory tract illnesses —
Adults up to age 65 with normal renal function: 200 mg P.O. daily in a single dose.
Children ages 9 to 12: 100 mg P.O. b.i.d.
Children ages 1 to 9 or weighing less than 45 kg (99 lb): 4.4 to 8.8 mg/kg P.O. as a total daily dose given once daily or divided equally b.i.d. Maximum daily dose is 150 mg.
Elderly: 100 mg P.O. once daily in pa-

tients over age 65 with normal renal function.

Begin treatment within 24 to 48 hours after symptoms appear and continue for 24 to 48 hours after symptoms disappear (usually 2 to 7 days of therapy). Start prophylaxis as soon as possible after initial exposure and continue for at least 10 days after exposure. May continue prophylactic treatment up to 90 days for repeated or suspected exposures if influenza vaccine is unavailable. If used with influenza vaccine, continue dose for 2 to 3 weeks until antibody response to vaccine has developed.

Dosage adjustment: For patients with renal failure, if creatinine clearance is 30 to 50 ml/minute, give 200 mg the first day and 100 mg thereafter; if clearance is 15 to 29 ml/minute, give 200 mg the first day, then 100 mg on alternate days; if clearance is below 15 ml/minute, give 200 mg q 7 days.

ADVERSE REACTIONS

CNS: depression, fatigue, confusion, *dizziness,* hallucinations, anxiety, *irritability,* ataxia, *insomnia,* headache, *light-headedness.*
CV: peripheral edema, orthostatic hypotension, *heart failure.*
GI: anorexia, *nausea,* constipation, vomiting, dry mouth.
Skin: *livedo reticularis.*

INTERACTIONS

Drug-drug. *Anticholinergics:* increased anticholinergic effects. Use together cautiously. Dosage of anticholinergic agent may be reduced before initiation of amantadine.
CNS stimulants: additive CNS stimulation. Use together cautiously.
Drug-herb. *Jimsonweed:* may adversely affect CV function. Avoid concomitant use.

EFFECTS ON DIAGNOSTIC TESTS

None reported.

CONTRAINDICATIONS

Contraindicated in patients with hypersensitivity to drug.

SPECIAL CONSIDERATIONS

▶ Use cautiously in patients with seizure disorders, heart failure, peripheral edema, hepatic disease, mental illness, eczematoid rash, renal impairment, orthostatic hypotension, and CV disease and in elderly patients. Renal and liver function tests must be monitored.
▶ *Alert:* Elderly patients are more susceptible to adverse neurologic effects. Mental status changes are signs of these adverse effects.
▶ *Alert:* Don't confuse amantadine with rimantadine.

Patient teaching

▶ If insomnia occurs, take drug several hours before bedtime.
▶ If orthostatic hypotension occurs, don't stand up or change positions too quickly.
▶ Notify health care provider of adverse reactions, especially dizziness, depression, anxiety, nausea, and urine retention.

---

amprenavir

Agenerase

Pregnancy Risk Category C

HOW SUPPLIED

Capsules: 50 mg, 150 mg
Oral solution: 15 mg/ml

ACTION

Inhibits HIV-1 protease by binding to the active site of HIV-1 protease, which causes immature noninfectious viral particles to form.

Route	Onset	Peak	Duration
P.O.	Unknown	1-2 hr	Unknown

INDICATIONS & DOSAGE

HIV-1 infection (with other antiretrovirals) —

Adults and adolescents ages 13 to 16 weighing over 50 kg (110 lb): 1,200 mg (eight 150-mg capsules) P.O. b.i.d. with other antiretrovirals.

Children ages 4 to 12 and adolescents ages 13 to 16 weighing less than 50 kg: *Capsules* — 20 mg/kg P.O. b.i.d. or 15 mg/kg P.O. t.i.d. (to maximum daily dose of 2,400 mg) with other antiretrovirals. *Oral solution* — 22.5 mg/kg (1.5 ml/kg) P.O. b.i.d. or 17 mg/kg (1.1ml/kg) P.O. t.i.d. (to maximum daily dose of 2,800 mg) with other antiretrovirals.

Dosage adjustment: For patients with liver impairment and a Child-Pugh score from 5 to 8, dose for capsules should be reduced to 450 mg P.O. b.i.d. In patients with a Child-Pugh score from 9 to 12, dose for capsules should be reduced to 300 mg P.O. b.i.d.

ADVERSE REACTIONS

CNS: *paresthesia,* depressive or mood disorders.
GI: *nausea, vomiting, diarrhea or loose stools,* taste disorders.
Metabolic: *hyperglycemia, hypertriglyceridemia,* hypercholesterolemia.
Skin: *rash, Stevens-Johnson syndrome.*

INTERACTIONS

Drug-drug. *Amiodarone, lidocaine, quinidine, tricyclic antidepressants:* inhibited metabolism of these drugs. Drug levels must be monitored closely.
Antacids, didanosine: decreased absorption. Administration times should be separated by at least 1 hour.
Anticonvulsants, such as carbamazepine, phenobarbital, and phenytoin: potentially decreased amprenavir levels. Monitor patient closely and adjust dosage as needed.
Bepridil, cisapride, dihydroergotamine, ergotamine, midazolam, triazolam: inhibited metabolism of these drugs, which

may cause serious or life-threatening adverse reactions. Don't use together.
Rifabutin: decreased amprenavir levels and increased rifabutin levels. Rifabutin dosage should be reduced to at least half the recommended dosage. CBC is monitored weekly for neutropenia.
Rifampin: 90% reduced plasma amprenavir levels. Don't use together.
Sildenafil: increased sildenafil levels, which may increase the frequency of sildenafil-associated adverse reactions, such as hypotension, visual changes, and priapism. Use together cautiously.
Warfarin: inhibited metabolism of warfarin, which may cause serious or life-threatening adverse reactions. INR must be monitored closely.
Drug-food. *High-fat foods:* decreased absorption of drug. Avoid taking drug with high-fat foods.

EFFECTS ON DIAGNOSTIC TESTS
None reported.

CONTRAINDICATIONS

Contraindicated in patients with hypersensitivity to drug or its components. Drug can cause severe or life-threatening rash, including Stevens-Johnson syndrome. Therapy should be discontinued if patient develops a severe or life-threatening rash or a moderate rash accompanied by systemic signs and symptoms.

SPECIAL CONSIDERATIONS

▶ Use cautiously in patients with moderate or severe hepatic impairment, diabetes mellitus, a known sulfonamide allergy, or hemophilia A or B.
▶ Use cautiously in pregnant women because no adequate studies exist regarding the effects of amprenavir when administered during pregnancy. Use during pregnancy only if the potential benefits outweigh the risks. Register pregnant woman taking amprenavir with the Antiretroviral

Pregnancy Registry by calling 1-800-258-4263.

▶ *Alert:* Because amprenavir may interact with many drugs, patient's complete drug history should be obtained. Patient must show the drugs he's taking.

▶ High-fat foods may decrease absorption of amprenavir.

▶ Patient must be monitored for adverse reactions. A patient taking a protease inhibitor may experience a redistribution of body fat, including central obesity, dorsocervical fat enlargement (buffalo hump), peripheral wasting, breast enlargement, and cushingoid appearance. The mechanism and long-term consequences of these effects are unknown.

▶ Drug provides high daily doses of vitamin E. Patient taking drug is not to take supplemental vitamin E because high vitamin levels may exacerbate the blood coagulation defect of vitamin K deficiency that anticoagulant therapy or malabsorption causes.

▶ Protease inhibitors have caused spontaneous bleeding in some patients with hemophilia A or B. In some patients, additional factor VIII was required. In many of the reported cases, treatment with protease inhibitors was continued or restarted.

▶ Amprenavir capsules aren't interchangeable with amprenavir oral solution on a milligram-per-milligram basis.

Patient teaching

▶ Drug isn't a cure for HIV infection. Opportunistic infections and other complications from the disease may continue to develop. Also, drug doesn't reduce risk of HIV transmission through sexual contact.

▶ Although drug can be taken without regard to food, don't take it with a high-fat meal because of decreased drug absorption.

▶ Report adverse reactions, especially rash.

▶ Take drug daily, as prescribed, with other antiretrovirals. Don't alter dosage or discontinue drug without health care provider's approval.

▶ Take an antacid or didanosine 1 hour before or after amprenavir to prevent a decrease in amprenavir absorption.

▶ If a dose is missed by more than 4 hours, wait and take the next dose at the regularly scheduled time. If a dose is missed by less than 4 hours, take the dose as soon as possible and then take the next dose at the regularly scheduled time. If a dose is skipped, don't double-dose.

▶ If using hormonal contraception, substitute with another contraceptive measure during drug therapy.

▶ Notify health care provider if pregnancy occurs during therapy.

▶ Don't take supplemental vitamin E because drug contains a significant amount of the vitamin.

cidofovir

Vistide

Pregnancy Risk Category C

HOW SUPPLIED
Injection: 75 mg/ml in 5-ml vial

ACTION
Suppresses CMV replication by selective inhibition of viral DNA synthesis.

Route	Onset	Peak	Duration
I.V.	Unknown	Unknown	Unknown

INDICATIONS & DOSAGE
CMV retinitis in patients with AIDS —
Adults: initially, 5 mg/kg I.V. infused over 1 hour once weekly for 2 consecutive weeks; then maintenance dose of 5 mg/kg I.V. infused over 1 hour once q 2 weeks. Administer probenecid and prehydration with normal saline solution I.V. concomitantly; may reduce potential for nephrotoxicity.

Dosage adjustment: For patients with renal failure, if serum creatinine increases 0.3 to 0.4 mg/dl above baseline, dose is reduced to 3 mg/kg at same rate and frequency. If serum creatinine increases 0.5 mg/dl or more above baseline, drug is discontinued.

ADVERSE REACTIONS

CNS: *asthenia, headache,* amnesia, anxiety, confusion, *seizures,* depression, dizziness, abnormal gait, hallucinations, insomnia, neuropathy, paresthesia, somnolence, malaise.
CV: hypotension, orthostatic hypotension, pallor, syncope, tachycardia, vasodilation.
EENT: amblyopia, conjunctivitis, eye disorders, *ocular hypotony,* iritis, retinal detachment, uveitis, abnormal vision, taste perversion.
GI: *nausea, vomiting, diarrhea, anorexia, abdominal pain,* dry mouth, colitis, constipation, tongue discoloration, dyspepsia, dysphagia, flatulence, gastritis, melena, oral candidiasis, rectal disorders, stomatitis, aphthous stomatitis, mouth ulcerations, weight loss.
GU: *elevated creatinine levels, nephrotoxicity, proteinuria,* decreased creatinine clearance levels, glycosuria, hematuria, urinary incontinence, urinary tract infection.
Hematologic: NEUTROPENIA, *anemia, thrombocytopenia.*
Hepatic: hepatomegaly, abnormal liver function test results, increased alkaline phosphatase levels.
Metabolic: fluid imbalance, hyperglycemia, hyperlipemia, hypocalcemia, hypokalemia, decreased serum bicarbonate level.
Musculoskeletal: arthralgia, myasthenia, myalgia, pain in back, chest, or neck.
Respiratory: asthma, bronchitis, coughing, *dyspnea,* hiccups, increased sputum, lung disorders, pharyngitis, pneumonia, rhinitis, sinusitis.
Skin: *rash, alopecia,* acne, skin discoloration, dry skin, herpes simplex, pruritus, sweating, urticaria.
Other: *fever, infections, chills,* allergic reactions, facial edema, *sarcoma, sepsis.*

INTERACTIONS

Drug-drug. *Nephrotoxic agents (such as aminoglycosides, amphotericin B, foscarnet, I.V. pentamidine):* may increase nephrotoxicity. Avoid concomitant use.
Probenecid: known to interact with the metabolism or renal tubular excretion of many drugs. Monitor closely.

EFFECTS ON DIAGNOSTIC TESTS
None reported.

CONTRAINDICATIONS

Contraindicated in patients with hypersensitivity to drug or history of clinically severe hypersensitivity to probenecid or other sulfur-containing drugs. Also contraindicated in patients receiving agents with nephrotoxic potential and in those with serum creatinine exceeding 1.5 mg/dl, a calculated creatinine clearance of 55 ml/minute or less, or a urine protein of 100 mg/dl or more (equivalent to 2+ proteinuria or more). Don't administer as a direct intraocular injection because it may be associated with significant decreases in intraocular pressure and vision impairment. Don't administer to breast-feeding women.

SPECIAL CONSIDERATIONS

▶ Use cautiously in patients with impaired renal function. Renal function tests and patient's fluid balance must be monitored.
▶ 1 L of normal saline is usually administered over a 1- to 2-hour period immediately before each cidofovir infusion.
▶ Probenecid may be administered with cidofovir.
▶ Renal function (serum creatinine and urine protein) must be monitored before each dose. Dosage may be modified if changes in renal function occur.

▶ Drug shouldn't be used in patients with baseline serum creatinine level exceeding 1.5 mg/dl or calculated creatinine clearance of 55 ml/minute or less unless potential benefits outweigh potential risks.

▶ Fanconi's syndrome and decreased serum bicarbonate levels associated with renal tubular damage have been reported in patients receiving cidofovir. Monitor patient closely.

▶ WBC counts with differential must be monitored before each dose.

▶ Granulocytopenia has been observed with drug treatment. Neutrophil counts should be monitored during therapy.

▶ Intraocular pressure, visual acuity, and ocular symptoms should be monitored periodically.

▶ Cidofovir is indicated only for the treatment of CMV retinitis in patients with AIDS. Safety and efficacy of drug have not been established for treating other CMV infections, congenital or neonatal CMV disease, or CMV disease in patients not infected with HIV.

▶ Cidofovir has been known to be carcinogenic and teratogenic and has caused hypospermia.

▶ Discontinue zidovudine therapy or reduce dosage by 50%, as ordered, on the days cidofovir is administered; probenecid reduces metabolic clearance of zidovudine.

▶ Dosage adjustment may be necessary in elderly patients with renal impairment.

▶ Safety and effectiveness in children have not been established.

▶ It's unknown if cidofovir appears in breast milk.

I.V. administration

▶ Because of the potential for increased nephrotoxicity, recommended dosages or frequency or rate of administration must not be exceeded.

▶ When preparing cidofovir for infusion, extract the appropriate amount of cidofovir from the vial using a syringe and transfer the dose to an infusion bag containing 100 ml of normal saline solution. The entire volume is infused I.V. at a constant rate over a 1-hour period. A standard infusion pump is used for administration.

▶ Because of the mutagenic properties of cidofovir, drug should be prepared in a class II laminar flow biological safety cabinet. Personnel preparing drug should wear surgical gloves and a closed front surgical gown with knit cuffs.

▶ If drug contacts the skin, wash membranes and flush thoroughly with water. Excess drug and all other materials used in the admixture preparation and administration should be placed in a leakproof, puncture-proof container. Recommended method of disposal is high temperature incineration.

▶ Cidofovir infusion admixtures should be administered within 24 hours of preparation; refrigerator or freezer storage shouldn't be used to extend this 24-hour period. If admixtures are not used immediately, they may be refrigerated at 36° to 46° F (2° to 8° C) for no more than 24 hours. Allow cidofovir to reach room temperature before use.

▶ Other drugs or supplements should not be added to admixture for concurrent administration.

▶ Compatibility with Ringer's solution, lactated Ringer's solution, or bacteriostatic infusion fluids has not been evaluated.

Patient teaching

▶ Drug is not a cure for CMV retinitis. Regular ophthalmologic follow-up examinations are necessary.

▶ If also on zidovudine therapy, obtain dosage guidelines on days cidofovir is administered.

▶ Close monitoring of renal function will be needed, and abnormalities may require a change in cidofovir therapy.

▶ Complete a full course of probenecid with each cidofovir dose. Take probenecid after a meal to decrease nausea.

▶ If female and of childbearing age, use effective contraception during and for 1 month following treatment with cidofovir.

▶ If male, practice barrier contraception during and for 3 months after treatment with drug.

▶ If breast-feeding, be aware that it's unknown if cidofovir appears in breast milk.

delavirdine mesylate

Rescriptor

Pregnancy Risk Category C

HOW SUPPLIED

Tablets: 100 mg

ACTION

A nonnucleoside reverse-transcriptase inhibitor of HIV-1. Drug binds directly to reverse transcriptase and blocks RNA- and DNA-dependent DNA polymerase activities.

Route	Onset	Peak	Duration
P.O.	Unknown	1 hr	Unknown

INDICATIONS & DOSAGE

HIV-1 infection when therapy is warranted—

Adults: 400 mg P.O. t.i.d. with other appropriate antiretroviral agents.

ADVERSE REACTIONS

CNS: abnormal coordination, agitation, amnesia, anxiety, change in dreams, cognitive impairment, confusion, depression, disorientation, dizziness, emotional lability, fatigue, hallucinations, headache, hyperesthesia, hyperreflexia, hypoesthesia, impaired concentration, lethargy, malaise, insomnia, manic symptoms, migraine, nervousness, neuropathy, nightmares, pallor, paralysis, paranoid symptoms, paresthesia, restlessness, somnolence, tingling, tremor, vertigo, weakness.

CV: bradycardia, chest pain, edema, orthostatic hypotension, palpitation, syncope, tachycardia, vasodilation.

EENT: blepharitis, conjunctivitis, diplopia, dry eyes, ear pain, epistaxis, nystagmus, pharyngitis, photophobia, rhinitis, sinusitis, taste perversion, tinnitus.

GI: anorexia, aphthous stomatitis, bloody stools, colitis, constipation, decreased appetite, diarrhea, diverticulitis, duodenitis, dry mouth, dyspepsia, dysphagia, enteritis, esophagitis, fecal incontinence, flatulence, gagging, gastritis, gastroesophageal reflux, GI bleeding, gingivitis, gum hemorrhage, increased thirst and appetite, increased saliva, mouth ulcer, *nausea,* nonspecific hepatitis, pancreatitis, rectal disorder, sialadenitis, stomatitis, tongue edema or ulceration, vomiting, abdominal cramps, distention, or pain, weight gain or loss.

GU: epididymitis, hematuria, hemospermia, impotence, renal calculi, renal pain, metrorrhagia, nocturia, polyuria, proteinuria, vaginal candidiasis.

Hematologic: anemia, ecchymosis, eosinophilia, granulocytosis, *neutropenia, pancytopenia,* petechiae, prolonged PTT, purpura, spleen disorder, *thrombocytopenia.*

Hepatic: increased ALT and AST levels.

Metabolic: alcohol intolerance; bilirubinemia; hyperkalemia; hyperuricemia; hypocalcemia; hyponatremia; hypophosphatemia; peripheral edema; increased gamma glutamyl transpeptidase, lipase, serum alkaline phosphatase, serum amylase, serum CK, and serum creatinine levels.

Musculoskeletal: bone disorder, arthralgia or arthritis of single and multiple joints, asthenia, bone pain, back pain, flank pain, leg cramps, muscle cramps, muscular weakness, myalgia, neck rigidity, tendon disorder, tenosynovitis.

Respiratory: chest congestion, bronchitis, dyspnea, laryngismus, cough, upper respiratory tract infection.

Skin: alopecia, angioedema, dermal leuko-cytoblastic vasculitis, dermatitis, desquamation, diaphoresis, dry skin, epidermal cyst, erythema, erythema multiforme, folliculitis, fungal dermatitis, maculopapular rash, nail disorder, petechial rash, pruritus, *rash*, sebaceous cyst, seborrhea, skin nodule, *Stevens-Johnson syndrome,* urticaria, vesiculobullous rash.

Other: allergic reaction, breast enlargement, chills, decreased libido, fever, flu-like syndrome, lip edema, pain, trauma, tetany.

INTERACTIONS

Drug-drug. *Amphetamines, benzodiazepines, calcium channel blockers, cisapride, ergot alkaloid preparations, quinidine:* may result in potentially serious or life-threatening adverse effects. Avoid concomitant use.

Antacids: reduced absorption of delavirdine. Doses should be separated by at least 1 hour.

Carbamazepine, phenobarbital, phenytoin, rifampin: substantially decreased plasma delavirdine levels. Avoid coadministration.

Clarithromycin: increased concentrations of both drugs. Monitor carefully.

Dapsone, warfarin: delavirdine increases plasma concentrations of these drugs. Monitor carefully.

Didanosine: coadministration with delavirdine results in a 20% decrease in absorption of both drugs. Doses should be separated by at least 1 hour.

Fluoxetine, ketoconazole: increased delavirdine trough levels. Monitor patient.

H²-receptor antagonists: may reduce absorption of delavirdine. Chronic use of these drugs with delavirdine isn't recommended.

Indinavir: increased plasma levels of indinavir. A lower dosage of indinavir should be considered.

Rifabutin: decreased delavirdine levels and increased rifabutin levels. Use together cautiously.

Saquinavir: fivefold increase in systemic levels of saquinavir. AST and ALT levels should be monitored frequently when used together.

EFFECTS ON DIAGNOSTIC TESTS

None reported.

CONTRAINDICATIONS

Contraindicated in patients with hypersensitivity to drug's formulation.

SPECIAL CONSIDERATIONS

▶ Use cautiously in patients with impaired hepatic function.

▶ Drug-induced rash is more common in patients with lower CD4+ cell counts and usually occurs within first 3 weeks of treatment. It's typically diffuse, maculopapular, erythematous, and often pruritic. It occurs commonly and its incidence doesn't appear to be significantly reduced by adjusted drug doses.

▶ Rash occurs mainly on the upper body and proximal arms. Using diphenhydramine, hydroxyzine, or topical corticosteroids may relieve symptoms.

▶ Because drug's effects in patients with hepatic or renal impairment have not been studied, renal and liver function test results must be carefully monitored.

▶ Drug has not been shown to reduce risk of transmission of HIV-1.

▶ Because resistance develops rapidly when used as monotherapy, always use drug with appropriate antiretroviral therapy.

▶ Patient's fluid balance and weight must be monitored.

Patient teaching

▶ Discontinue drug and call health care provider if severe rash or such symptoms as fever, blistering, oral lesions, conjunctivitis, swelling, or muscle or joint aches occur.

Reactions may be *common,* uncommon, *life-threatening*, or COMMON AND LIFE-THREATENING.

▶ Drug is not a cure for HIV-1 infection. Illnesses associated with HIV-1 infection, including opportunistic infections, may continue to occur. Therapy has not been shown to reduce the incidence or frequency of such illnesses. Drug has not been shown to reduce transmission of HIV.

▶ Remain under medical supervision when taking drug because the long-term effects are not known.

▶ Take drug as prescribed and don't alter doses without health care provider's approval. If a dose is missed, take next dose as soon as possible; don't double the next dose.

▶ Drug may be dispersed in water before ingestion. Add tablets to at least 5 oz (148 ml) of water, allow to stand for a few minutes, and stir until a uniform dispersion occurs. Drink promptly, rinse glass, and swallow the rinse to ensure that entire dose is consumed.

▶ Drug may be taken without regard to food.

▶ Take drug with an acidic beverage, such as orange or cranberry juice, if you have achlorhydria.

▶ Take drug and antacids at least 1 hour apart.

▶ Report use of other prescription or OTC medications.

didanosine (ddI)

Videx

Pregnancy Risk Category B

HOW SUPPLIED

Tablets (buffered, chewable): 25 mg, 50 mg, 100 mg, 150 mg
Powder for oral solution (buffered): 100 mg/packet, 167 mg/packet, 250 mg/packet,
Powder for oral solution (pediatric): 4-oz, 8-oz glass bottles containing 2 g and 4 g of Videx, respectively

ACTION

Inhibits the enzyme HIV-RNA-dependent DNA polymerase (reverse transcriptase) and terminates DNA chain growth.

Route	Onset	Peak	Duration
P.O.	Unknown	0.5-1 hr	Unknown

INDICATIONS & DOSAGE

HIV infection when antiretroviral therapy is warranted —
Adults weighing 60 kg (132 lb) and over: 200 mg (tablets) P.O. q 12 hours; or 250 mg buffered powder P.O. q 12 hours.
Adults under 60 kg: 125 mg (tablets) P.O. q 12 hours; or 167 mg buffered powder P.O. q 12 hours.
Children: 90 to 150 mg/m^2 P.O. q 12 hours.
Dosage adjustment: Dialysis patients should receive 25% of usual dose.

ADVERSE REACTIONS

CNS: *headache, seizures,* confusion, anxiety, nervousness, abnormal thinking, twitching, depression, *peripheral neuropathy, dizziness,* asthenia, insomnia.
CV: hypertension, edema, ***heart failure.***
EENT: retinal changes, optic neuritis.
GI: *diarrhea, nausea, vomiting, abdominal pain, pancreatitis,* dry mouth, anorexia.
Hematologic: *leukopenia,* granulocytosis, ***thrombocytopenia,*** anemia.
Hepatic: ***hepatic failure,*** elevated liver enzymes.
Respiratory: dyspnea, pneumonia.
Skin: rash, pruritus, alopecia.
Other: pain, infection, sarcoma, allergic reactions, myopathy, increased serum uric acid levels, *chills, fever.*

INTERACTIONS

Drug-drug. *Antacids containing magnesium or aluminum hydroxides:* enhanced adverse effects of the antacid component (including diarrhea or constipation) when administered with didanosine tablets or pediatric suspension. Avoid concomitant use.

Dapsone, drugs that require gastric acid for adequate absorption, ketoconazole: decreased absorption from buffering action. These drugs are administered 2 hours before didanosine.

Fluoroquinolones, tetracyclines: decreased absorption from buffering agents in didanosine tablets or antacids in pediatric suspension. Avoid concomitant use.

Itraconazole: decreased serum levels of itraconazole. Avoid concomitant use.

Drug-food. *Any food:* decreased rate of absorption. Drug is given on an empty stomach at least 30 minutes before a meal.

EFFECTS ON DIAGNOSTIC TESTS
None reported.

CONTRAINDICATIONS
Contraindicated in patients with history of hypersensitivity to any component of the formulation.

SPECIAL CONSIDERATIONS
▶ Use cautiously in patients with history of pancreatitis; fatalities have occurred. Also, it is used cautiously in patients with peripheral neuropathy, renal or hepatic impairment, or hyperuricemia. Liver and renal function tests must be monitored.

▶ Administer didanosine on an empty stomach, regardless of the dosage form used; administering drug with meals can decrease absorption by 50%.

▶ To administer single-dose packets containing buffered powder for oral solution, contents is poured into 4 oz (120 ml) of water. Fruit juice or other beverages that may be acidic should not be used. Then, mixture is stirred for 2 or 3 minutes until the powder dissolves completely. Drug is administered immediately.

▶ The powder for oral solution has been associated with a high incidence of diarrhea. The manufacturer suggests switching to the tablet formulation if diarrhea is a problem.

▶ *Alert:* The pediatric powder for oral solution must be prepared by a pharmacist before dispensing. It must be constituted with purified USP water and then diluted with an antacid (either Mylanta Double Strength Liquid or Maalox TC Suspension) to a final concentration of 10 mg/ml. The admixture is stable for 30 days if refrigerated (at 36° to 46° F [2° to 8° C]). The solution should be shaken well before measuring the dose.

▶ *Alert:* Don't confuse drug with other antivirals that use abbreviations for identification.

Patient teaching
▶ Take drug on an empty stomach.

▶ Because the tablets contain buffers that raise stomach pH to levels that prevent degradation of the active drug, chew tablets thoroughly before swallowing and drink at least 1 oz (30 ml) of water with each dose. Learn how to prepare crushed tablets or buffered powder form for ingestion, if appropriate.

▶ If on a sodium-restricted diet, know that each two-tablet dose of didanosine contains 529 mg of sodium; each single packet of buffered powder for oral solution contains 1.38 g of sodium.

▶ Report symptoms of pancreatitis, such as abdominal pain, nausea, vomiting, diarrhea.

---

efavirenz

Sustiva

Pregnancy Risk Category C

HOW SUPPLIED

Capsules: 50 mg, 100 mg, 200 mg

ACTION

A nonnucleoside, reverse transcriptase inhibitor (NNRTI) that inhibits the transcription of HIV-1 RNA to DNA, a critical step in the viral replication process. Therefore, drug lowers the amount of HIV in the blood (the viral load) and increases CD4 lymphocytes.

Route	Onset	Peak	Duration
P.O.	Unknown	3-5 hr	Unknown

INDICATIONS & DOSAGE

HIV-1 infection —

Adults: 600 mg P.O. once daily.

Children ages 3 and older weighing 40 kg (88 lb) or more: 600 mg P.O. once.

Children ages 3 and older weighing 10 to under 40 kg (22 to under 88 lb):
Children 10 to under 15 kg (22 to under 33 lb): 200 mg P.O. once daily.
Children 15 to under 20 kg (33 to under 44 lb): 250 mg P.O. once daily.
Children 20 to under 25 kg (44 to under 55 lb): 300 mg P.O. once daily.
Children 25 to under 32.5 kg (55 to under 72 lb): 350 mg P.O. once daily.
Children 32.5 to under 40 kg (72 to under 88 lb): 400 mg P.O. once daily.

Note: Give all above doses with a protease inhibitor or nucleoside analogue reverse transcriptase inhibitors.

ADVERSE REACTIONS

CNS: abnormal dreams or thinking, agitation, amnesia, confusion, depersonalization, depression, *dizziness,* euphoria, fatigue, hallucinations, headache, hypoesthesia, impaired concentration, insomnia, somnolence, nervousness.

GI: abdominal pain, anorexia, *diarrhea,* dyspepsia, flatulence, *nausea,* vomiting.

GU: hematuria, kidney stones.

Hepatic: increased AST, ALT, and total cholesterol levels.

Skin: increased sweating, ***erythema multiforme, Stevens-Johnson syndrome, toxic epidermal necrolysis,*** rash, pruritus.

Other: fever.

INTERACTIONS

Drug-drug. *Cisapride, ergot derivatives, midazolam, triazolam:* competition for cytochrome P-450 enzyme system may result in inhibition of the metabolism of these drugs and cause serious or life-threatening adverse effects (such as arrhythmias, prolonged sedation, or respiratory depression). Avoid concomitant use.

Clarithromycin, indinavir: decreased plasma levels. Consider alternative therapy or dosage adjustment.

Drugs that induce the cytochrome P-450 enzyme system (phenobarbital, rifampin, rifabutin): increased clearance of efavirenz resulting in lowered plasma levels. Avoid concomitant use.

Estrogens, ritonavir: increased plasma levels. Monitor patient.

Oral contraceptives: potential interaction of efavirenz with oral contraceptives has not been determined. A reliable method of barrier contraception should be used in addition to oral contraceptives.

Psychoactive drugs: additive CNS effects. Avoid concomitant use.

Saquinavir: plasma levels of saquinavir decreased significantly. Don't use with saquinavir as sole protease inhibitor.

Warfarin: plasma levels and effects potentially increased or decreased. INR should be monitored.

Drug-food. *High-fat meals:* increased absorption of drug. Patient should maintain a proper low-fat diet.

---

*Liquid contains alcohol.   **May contain tartrazine.   †Canada   ‡Australia   §U.K.   ◇OTC

Drug-lifestyle. *Alcohol:* enhanced CNS effects. Avoid concomitant use.

EFFECTS ON DIAGNOSTIC TESTS

Drug therapy may cause false-positive urine cannabinoid test results.

CONTRAINDICATIONS

Contraindicated in patients with hypersensitivity to drug or its components.

SPECIAL CONSIDERATIONS

▶ Use cautiously in patients with hepatic impairment or in those concurrently receiving hepatotoxic drugs. Liver function test results must be monitored in patients with history of hepatitis B or C and in those also taking ritonavir.

▶ Cholesterol levels must be monitored.

▶ *Alert:* Drug should be used with other antiretroviral drugs because resistant viruses emerge rapidly when used alone. Drug shouldn't be used as monotherapy, or added on as a single agent to a failing regimen.

▶ Use with ritonavir is associated with a higher frequency of adverse effects (such as dizziness, nausea, paresthesia) and laboratory abnormalities (elevated liver enzymes).

▶ Drug should be administered at bedtime to decrease noticeable CNS adverse effects.

▶ Pregnancy must be ruled out before starting therapy in women of childbearing age.

▶ Children may be more prone to adverse reactions, especially diarrhea, nausea, vomiting, and rash.

Patient teaching

▶ Take drug with water, juice, milk, or soda. Drug may be taken without regard to meals.

▶ Schedule blood tests to monitor liver function and cholesterol levels.

▶ Use a reliable method of barrier contraception in addition to oral contraceptives and notify health care provider immediately if pregnancy is suspected.

▶ Drug is not a cure for HIV infection and will not affect the development of opportunistic infections and other complications associated with HIV infection or transmission of HIV to others through sexual contact or blood contamination.

▶ Take drug at the same time daily and always with other antiretroviral drugs.

▶ Take drug exactly as prescribed, and don't discontinue it without health care provider's approval.

▶ Report adverse reactions if they occur. Rash is the most common adverse effect; report it immediately because it may be serious (in rare cases).

▶ Report use of other drugs.

▶ Dizziness, difficulty sleeping or concentrating, drowsiness, or unusual dreams may occur the first few days of therapy. These symptoms generally resolve after 2 to 4 weeks and may be less problematic if drug is taken at bedtime.

▶ Avoid alcoholic beverages, driving, or operating machinery until drug's effects are known.

famciclovir

Famvir

Pregnancy Risk Category B

HOW SUPPLIED

Tablets: 125 mg, 250 mg, 500 mg

ACTION

A guanosine nucleoside that's converted to penciclovir, which enters viral cells and inhibits DNA polymerase and viral DNA synthesis.

Route	Onset	Peak	Duration
P.O.	Unknown	1 hr	Unknown

INDICATIONS & DOSAGE

Acute herpes zoster infection (shingles) —

Adults: 500 mg P.O. q 8 hours for 7 days.
Dosage adjustment: For patients with reduced renal function, if creatinine clearance is 60 ml/minute or more, 500 mg P.O. q 8 hours; if clearance is 40 to 59 ml/minute, 500 mg P.O. q 12 hours; if 20 to 39 ml/minute, 500 mg P.O. q 24 hours; and if below 20 ml/minute, 250 mg P.O. q 24 hours.

For hemodialysis patients, 250 mg P.O. after each hemodialysis session.

Recurrent episodes of genital herpes — **Adults:** 125 mg P.O. b.i.d. for 5 days. Therapy begins as soon as symptoms occur.

Dosage adjustment: For patients with reduced renal function, if creatinine clearance is 40 ml/minute or more, 125 mg P.O. q 12 hours; if 20 to 39 ml/minute, 125 mg P.O. q 24 hours; if below 20 ml/minute, 125 mg P.O. q 24 hours.

For hemodialysis patients, 125 mg P.O. after each hemodialysis session.

Recurrent mucocutaneous herpes simplex infections in HIV-infected patients — **Adults:** 500 mg P.O. b.i.d. for 7 days.
Dosage adjustment: For patients with reduced renal function, if creatinine clearance is 40 ml/minute or more, 500 mg P.O. q 12 hours; if 20 to 39 ml/minute, 500 mg P.O. q 24 hours; and if below 20 ml/minute, 250 mg P.O. q 24 hours.

For hemodialysis patients, 250 mg P.O. after each hemodialysis session.

ADVERSE REACTIONS
CNS: *headache,* fatigue, dizziness, paresthesia, somnolence.
EENT: pharyngitis, sinusitis.
GI: diarrhea, *nausea,* vomiting, constipation, anorexia, abdominal pain.
Musculoskeletal: back pain, arthralgia.
Skin: pruritus; zoster-related signs, symptoms, and complications.
Other: fever.

INTERACTIONS
Drug-drug. *Probenecid:* may increase plasma levels of famciclovir. Patient should

be monitored for increased adverse effects.

EFFECTS ON DIAGNOSTIC TESTS
None reported.

CONTRAINDICATIONS
Contraindicated in patients with hypersensitivity to drug.

SPECIAL CONSIDERATIONS
▶ Use cautiously in patients with renal or hepatic impairment. Dosage adjustment may be needed. Renal and liver function tests must be monitored.
▶ Drug may be taken without regard to meals.

Patient teaching
▶ Drug is not a cure for genital herpes, but can decrease the length and severity of symptoms.
▶ Learn how to prevent spread of infection to others.
▶ Early symptoms of herpes infection include tingling, itching, and pain, and should be reported. Treatment is more effective if therapy is started within 48 hours of rash onset.

fomivirsen sodium
Vitravene

Pregnancy Risk Category C

HOW SUPPLIED
Intravitreal injection: preservative-free, 0.25-ml, single-use vials containing 6.6 mg/ml

ACTION
A phosphorothioate oligonucleotide that inhibits human CMV replication by binding to the target mRNA and subsequently inhibiting virus replication.

Route	Onset	Peak	Duration
Intravitreal	Unknown	Unknown	Unknown

INDICATIONS & DOSAGE

Local treatment of CMV retinitis in patients with AIDS, who are intolerant of or have a contraindication to other treatments or who were insufficiently responsive to previous treatment —

Adults: induction dose is 330 mcg (0.05 ml) by intravitreal injection every other week for two doses. Subsequent maintenance dose is 330 mcg (0.05 ml) by intravitreal injection once q 4 weeks after induction.

ADVERSE REACTIONS

CNS: asthenia, headache, abnormal thinking, depression, dizziness, neuropathy, pain.

CV: chest pain.

EENT: abnormal or blurred vision, anterior chamber inflammation, cataract, conjunctival hemorrhage, decreased visual acuity, desaturation of color vision, eye pain, floaters, increased intraocular pressure, photophobia, retinal detachment, retinal edema, retinal hemorrhage, retinal pigment changes, *uveitis, vitreitis,* application site reaction, conjunctival hyperemia, conjunctivitis, corneal edema, decreased peripheral vision, eye irritation, hypotony, keratic precipitates, optic neuritis, photopsia, retinal vascular disease, visual field defect, vitreous hemorrhage, vitreous opacity, sinusitis.

GI: abdominal pain, anorexia, diarrhea, nausea, vomiting, decreased weight, oral candidiasis, *pancreatitis.*

GU: catheter infection, *kidney failure.*

Hematologic: anemia, lymphoma-like reaction, *neutropenia, thrombocytopenia.*

Hepatic: abnormal liver function tests, increased GGT.

Metabolic: dehydration.

Musculoskeletal: back pain.

Respiratory: bronchitis, dyspnea, increased cough, pneumonia.

Skin: rash, sweating.

Other: allergic reactions, cachexia, fever, flulike syndrome, infection, *sepsis,* systemic CMV.

INTERACTIONS

None significant.

EFFECTS ON DIAGNOSTIC TESTS

None reported.

CONTRAINDICATIONS

Contraindicated in patients with hypersensitivity to drug or its components or in those who have recently (within 2 to 4 weeks) been treated with either I.V. or intravitreal cidofovir because of an increased risk of exaggerated ocular inflammation.

SPECIAL CONSIDERATIONS

▸ *Alert:* Drug is for ophthalmic use by intravitreal injection only.

▸ Drug provides localized therapy limited to the treated eye, and does not provide treatment for systemic CMV disease. Patient must be monitored for extraocular CMV disease or disease in the contralateral eye.

▸ Ocular inflammation (uveitis) is more common during induction dosing.

▸ Light perception and optic nerve head perfusion must be monitored postinjection.

▸ Intraocular pressure must be monitored. This is usually transient and returns to normal without treatment or with temporary use of topical medications.

Patient teaching

▸ Drug is not a cure for CMV retinitis. Progression of retinitis may occur during and following treatment.

▸ Drug treats only the eye in which it has been injected, and CMV may also exist in the body. Follow-up visits are important to monitor progress and to check for additional infections.

▸ Patient should have regular ophthalmologic follow-up examinations.
▸ If HIV-infected, continue taking antiretroviral therapy as indicated.

foscarnet sodium (phosphonoformic acid)

Foscavir

Pregnancy Risk Category C

HOW SUPPLIED
Injection: 24 mg/ml in 250- and 500-ml bottles

ACTION
Inhibits all known herpesviruses in vitro by blocking the pyrophosphate binding site on DNA polymerases and reverse transcriptases.

Route	Onset	Peak	Duration
I.V.	Unknown	Immediate	Unknown

INDICATIONS & DOSAGE
CMV retinitis in patients with AIDS —
Adults: Initially, 60 mg/kg I.V. as an induction treatment in patients with normal renal function. Administer q 8 hours for 2 to 3 weeks, depending on clinical response. Follow with a maintenance infusion of 90 to 120 mg/kg daily. Or, 90 mg/kg IV q 12 hours is used for induction.

Acyclovir-resistant HSV infections —
Adults: 40 mg/kg I.V. over 1 hour q 8 to 12 hours for 2 to 3 weeks or until healed.
Dosage adjustment: Refer to package insert for very specific dose adjustments. Dosage must be adjusted when creatinine clearance is below 1.5 ml/minute/kg. If creatinine clearance falls below 0.4 ml/minute/kg, discontinue drug.

ADVERSE REACTIONS
CNS: *headache,* **seizures,** *fatigue, malaise,* *asthenia, paresthesia, dizziness, hypoesthesia, neuropathy,* tremor, ataxia, generalized spasms, dementia, stupor, sensory disturbances, meningitis, aphasia, abnormal coordination, EEG abnormalities, depression, confusion, anxiety, insomnia, somnolence, nervousness, amnesia, agitation, aggressive reaction, hallucinations.
CV: *hypertension, palpitations, ECG abnormalities, sinus tachycardia,* cerebrovascular disorder, *first-degree AV block, hypotension, flushing,* edema.
EENT: visual disturbances, taste perversion, eye pain, conjunctivitis, sinusitis, pharyngitis, rhinitis.
GI: *nausea, diarrhea, vomiting, abdominal pain, anorexia,* constipation, dysphagia, rectal hemorrhage, dry mouth, dyspepsia, melena, flatulence, ulcerative stomatitis, *pancreatitis.*
GU: *abnormal renal function, decreased creatinine clearance and increased serum creatinine levels, albuminuria, dysuria, polyuria, urethral disorder, urine retention, urinary tract infections,* **acute renal failure,** candidiasis.
Hematologic: *anemia, granulocytopenia,* **leukopenia, bone marrow suppression, thrombocytopenia,** platelet abnormalities, thrombocytosis, WBC count abnormalities, lymphadenopathy.
Hepatic: increased liver enzymes; increased serum bilirubin, alkaline phosphatase, ALT, and AST levels; abnormal hepatic function.
Metabolic: hypokalemia, hypomagnesemia, hypophosphatemia or hyperphosphatemia, hypocalcemia, hyponatremia.
Musculoskeletal: leg cramps, arthralgia, myalgia, back or chest pain.
Respiratory: *cough, dyspnea,* pneumonitis, respiratory insufficiency, pulmonary infiltration, stridor, pneumothorax, **bronchospasm,** hemoptysis, flulike symptoms.
Skin: *rash, diaphoresis,* pruritus, skin ulceration, erythematous rash, seborrhea, skin discoloration, facial edema.

Other: *death, fever,* pain, sepsis, rigors, inflammation and pain at infusion site, lymphoma-like disorder, sarcoma, bacterial or fungal infections, abscess.

INTERACTIONS
Drug-drug. *Nephrotoxic drugs (such as aminoglycosides, amphotericin B):* increased risk of nephrotoxicity. Avoid concomitant use.
Pentamidine: increased risk of nephrotoxicity; severe hypocalcemia has also been reported. Avoid concomitant use.
Zidovudine: possible increased incidence or severity of anemia. Blood counts must be monitored.

EFFECTS ON DIAGNOSTIC TESTS
None reported.

CONTRAINDICATIONS
Contraindicated in patients with hypersensitivity to drug.

SPECIAL CONSIDERATIONS
▶ Use cautiously and with reduced dosage in patients with abnormal renal function. Because drug is nephrotoxic, it can worsen renal impairment. Some degree of nephrotoxicity occurs in most patients treated with drug.
▶ Because drug is highly toxic and toxicity is probably dose-related, always use the lowest effective maintenance dose during therapy.
▶ Creatinine clearance is monitored frequently during therapy because of drug's adverse effects on renal function. A baseline 24-hour creatinine clearance is recommended, followed by regular determinations two to three times weekly during induction and at least once every 1 to 2 weeks during maintenance.
▶ Because drug can alter serum electrolytes, levels are monitored using a schedule similar to that established for creatinine clearance. The patient is as-

sessed for tetany and seizures associated with abnormal electrolyte levels.
▶ The patient's hemoglobin and hematocrit levels must be monitored. Anemia is common (in up to 33% of patients treated with drug). It may be severe enough to require transfusions.
▶ Keep in mind that drug administration is associated with a dose-related transient decrease in ionized serum calcium, which may not always be reflected in patient's laboratory values.

I.V. administration
▶ An infusion pump is used to administer foscarnet. To minimize renal toxicity, patient must be adequately hydrated before and during the infusion.
▶ Induction treatment is administered over 1 hour; maintenance infusions over 2 hours.
▶ *Alert:* Don't exceed the recommended dosage, infusion rate, or frequency of administration. All doses must be individualized according to patient's renal function.

Patient teaching
▶ Adequate hydration throughout therapy is important.
▶ Report perioral tingling, numbness in the extremities, and paresthesia.
▶ Alert health care provider if discomfort occurs at I.V. insertion site.

ganciclovir
Cymevene§, Cytovene

Pregnancy Risk Category C

HOW SUPPLIED
Capsules: 250 mg
Injection: 500 mg/vial

ACTION
Inhibits binding of deoxyguanosine tri-

phosphate to DNA polymerase, resulting in inhibition of DNA synthesis.

Route	Onset	Peak	Duration
P.O.	Unknown	1.8-3 hr	Unknown
I.V.	Unknown	Immediate	Unknown

INDICATIONS & DOSAGE

CMV retinitis in immunocompromised individuals, including patients with AIDS and normal renal function —
Adults and children over age 3 months: induction treatment is 5 mg/kg I.V. q 12 hours for 14 to 21 days. Maintenance treatment is 5 mg/kg I.V. daily for 7 days weekly, or 6 mg/kg daily for 5 days weekly. Or, 1,000 mg P.O. t.i.d. with food.
Dosage adjustment: Refer to package insert for very specific dose adjustments. Dosage is adjusted for patients with impaired renal function and is based on creatinine clearance levels.

Dosage adjustment is necessary in patients with creatinine clearance below 70 ml/minute.

Prevention of CMV disease in patients with advanced HIV infection and normal renal function —
Adults: 1,000 mg P.O. t.i.d. with food.

Prevention of CMV disease in transplant recipients with normal renal function —
Adults: 5 mg/kg I.V. (given at a constant rate over 1 hour) q 12 hours for 7 to 14 days; then 5 mg/kg daily for 7 days weekly, or 6 mg/kg daily for 5 days weekly. Duration of therapy depends on degree of immunosuppression.

ADVERSE REACTIONS

CNS: altered dreams, confusion, ataxia, headache, *seizures, coma,* dizziness, somnolence, tremor, abnormal thinking, agitation, amnesia, anxiety, neuropathy, paresthesia, asthenia.
EENT: retinal detachment in CMV retinitis patients.
GI: *nausea, vomiting, diarrhea, anorex-ia, abdominal pain,* flatulence, dyspepsia, dry mouth.
GU: *increased serum creatinine levels.*
Hematologic: *agranulocytosis, thrombocytopenia, leukopenia,* anemia.
Hepatic: abnormal liver function test results.
Respiratory: pneumonia.
Skin: *rash, sweating,* pruritus.
Other: *fever,* infection, chills, sepsis, and inflammation, pain, and phlebitis at injection site.

INTERACTIONS

Drug-drug. *Cytotoxic drugs:* increased toxic effects, especially hematologic effects and stomatitis. Monitor closely.
Didanosine: increased plasma levels of didanosine when used concomitantly. Monitor closely.
Imipenem/cilastatin: heightened seizure activity with concomitant use. Monitor closely.
Immunosuppressants (such as azathioprine, corticosteroids, cyclosporine): enhanced immune and bone marrow suppression. Use together cautiously.
Probenecid: increased ganciclovir blood levels. Monitor closely.
Zidovudine: increased incidence of agranulocytosis with concurrent use. Monitor closely.

EFFECTS ON DIAGNOSTIC TESTS
None reported.

CONTRAINDICATIONS
Contraindicated in patients with hypersensitivity to drug or acyclovir and in those with an absolute neutrophil count below 500 mm³ or a platelet count below 25,000 mm³.

SPECIAL CONSIDERATIONS
▶ Use cautiously and in reduced dosage in patients with renal dysfunction. Renal function tests must be monitored.

▶ Ganciclovir solution is alkaline; use caution.
▶ *Alert:* The drug is not for S.C. or I.M. administration.
▶ Because of the frequency of agranulocytosis and thrombocytopenia, neutrophil and platelet counts are obtained every 2 days during twice-daily ganciclovir dosing and at least weekly thereafter.

I.V. administration
▶ The infusion is administered over at least 1 hour. Too-rapid infusions will result in increased toxicity. An infusion pump must be used. Drug is not to be administered via I.V. bolus.

Patient teaching
▶ Adequate hydration is important during therapy.
▶ Report adverse reactions promptly.
▶ Notify health care provider if discomfort occurs at I.V. insertion site.
▶ The drug causes birth defects. If female, use effective birth control methods during treatment; if male, use barrier contraception during, and for at least 90 days following, treatment with ganciclovir.

indinavir sulfate
Crixivan

Pregnancy Risk Category C

HOW SUPPLIED
Capsules: 200 mg, 400 mg

ACTION
Inhibits HIV protease, enzyme required for the proteolytic cleavage of viral polyprotein precursors into individual functional proteins found in infectious HIV. Indinavir binds to the protease active site and inhibits activity of the enzyme, preventing cleavage of the viral polyproteins and resulting in formation of immature noninfectious viral particles.

Route	Onset	Peak	Duration
P.O.	Unknown	< 1 hr	Unknown

INDICATIONS & DOSAGE
HIV infection when antiretroviral therapy is warranted —
Adults: 800 mg P.O. q 8 hours.
Dosage adjustment: For patients with mild to moderate hepatic insufficiency due to cirrhosis, reduce dosage to 600 mg P.O. q 8 hours.

ADVERSE REACTIONS
CNS: headache, insomnia, dizziness, somnolence, asthenia, malaise, fatigue.
CV: chest pain, palpitations.
EENT: blurred vision, eye pain or swelling.
GI: abdominal pain, *nausea,* diarrhea, vomiting, acid regurgitation, anorexia, dry mouth, taste perversion.
GU: nephrolithiasis, hematuria.
Hematologic: decreased hemoglobin, platelet, or neutrophil count.
Hepatic: elevation in ALT, AST, and serum amylase levels.
Metabolic: *hyperbilirubinemia,* hyperglycemia.
Musculoskeletal: back pain.
Other: flank pain.

INTERACTIONS
Drug-drug. *Cisapride, midazolam, triazolam:* possible inhibition of the metabolism of these drugs because of competition for CYP3A4 by indinavir, creating potential for serious or life-threatening events, such as arrhythmias or prolonged sedation. These drugs should not be administered concurrently.
Clarithromycin: increased serum levels of both drugs. Monitor closely.
Didanosine: possible degradation of didanosine, formulated with buffering agents to increase pH. If administered with indi-

navir, the administration times should be separated by at least 1 hour and be given on an empty stomach. Normal gastric pH (acidic) may be necessary for optimum absorption of indinavir but rapidly degrades didanosine.

Ketoconazole: increased plasma level of indinavir. Consider dosage reduction of indinavir to 600 mg P.O. q 8 hours when coadministered.

Rifabutin: increased plasma levels. Reduce dosage of rifabutin by 50% if administered with indinavir.

Rifampin: markedly diminished plasma levels of indinavir. Avoid concomitant administration of indinavir and rifampin.

Ritonavir: increased indinavir levels. Monitor closely.

Drug-food. *Any food:* substantially decreased absorption of oral indinavir. Don't give together.

EFFECTS ON DIAGNOSTIC TESTS
None reported.

CONTRAINDICATIONS
Contraindicated in patients with hypersensitivity to any component of drug.

SPECIAL CONSIDERATIONS
▶ Use cautiously in patients with hepatic insufficiency due to cirrhosis.
▶ Drug must be taken at 8-hour intervals.
▶ Drug may cause nephrolithiasis. If signs and symptoms of nephrolithiasis occur, drug may be stopped for 1 to 3 days during acute phases.
▶ To prevent nephrolithiasis, patient should maintain adequate hydration (at least 48 oz or 1.5 L of fluids q 24 hours while on indinavir).
▶ Safety and effectiveness in children have not been established.

Patient teaching
▶ Drug is not a cure for HIV infection. Opportunistic infections and other complications associated with HIV infection may continue to occur. Drug has not been shown to reduce the risk of HIV transmission.
▶ Use barrier protection during sexual activity.
▶ Don't adjust dosage or discontinue indinavir therapy without first consulting health care provider.
▶ If a dose of indinavir is missed, take the next dose at the regularly scheduled time and don't double the dose.
▶ Take drug on an empty stomach with water 1 hour before or 2 hours after a meal. Or, take with other liquids (such as skim milk, juice, coffee, or tea) or a light meal. A meal high in fat, calories, and protein reduces absorption of drug.
▶ Store capsules in the original container, and keep desiccant in the bottle; capsules are sensitive to moisture.
▶ Drink at least 48 oz (1.5 L) of fluid daily.
▶ If female, avoid breast-feeding because indinavir may appear in breast milk. If HIV-positive, don't breast-feed, in order to prevent transmitting the virus to the infant

lamivudine
Epivir, Epivir-HBV

Pregnancy Risk Category C

HOW SUPPLIED
Tablets: 100 mg, 150 mg
Oral solution: 5 mg/ml, 10 mg/ml

ACTION
A synthetic nucleoside analogue that inhibits HIV reverse transcription via viral DNA chain termination. RNA- and DNA-dependent DNA polymerase activities are also inhibited.

Route	Onset	Peak	Duration
P.O.	Unknown	1-3 hr	Unknown

INDICATIONS & DOSAGE

HIV infection concomitantly with zidovudine —

Adults weighing 50 kg (110 lb) or more and children ages 12 and older: 150 mg P.O. b.i.d.

Adults under 50 kg: 2 mg/kg P.O. b.i.d.

Children ages 3 months to 12 years: 4 mg/kg P.O. b.i.d. Maximum dose is 150 mg b.i.d.

Dosage adjustment: For patients with renal impairment, if creatinine clearance is 30 to 49 ml/minute, 150 mg P.O. daily. If clearance is 15 to 29 ml/minute, 150 mg P.O. on day 1, then 100 mg daily; if 5 to 14 ml/minute, 150 mg on day 1, then 50 mg daily; if less than 5 ml/minute, 50 mg on day 1, then 25 mg daily.

Chronic hepatitis B associated with evidence of hepatitis B viral replication and active liver inflammation —

Adults: 100 mg P.O. once daily (Epivir-HBV).

Dosage adjustment: For patients with renal impairment, if creatinine clearance is 30 to 49 ml/minute, 100 mg first dose; then 50 mg P.O. once daily. If clearance is 15 to 29 ml/minute, 100 mg first dose; then 25 mg P.O. once daily. If creatinine clearance is 5 to 14 ml/minute, 35 mg first dose; then 15 mg P.O. once daily. If less than 5 ml/minute, 35 mg first dose; then 10 mg P.O. once daily.

ADVERSE REACTIONS

Adverse reactions pertain to the combination therapy of lamivudine and zidovudine.

CNS: *headache, fatigue, neuropathy, malaise, dizziness, insomnia and other sleep disorders,* depressive disorders.

GI: *nausea, diarrhea, vomiting, anorexia,* abdominal pain, abdominal cramps, dyspepsia, pancreatitis.

EENT: *nasal symptoms.*

Hematologic: ***neutropenia,*** anemia, ***thrombocytopenia.***

Hepatic: elevated liver enzymes and bilirubin.

Musculoskeletal: *musculoskeletal pain,* myalgia, arthralgia.

Respiratory: *cough.*

Skin: rash.

Other: *fever, chills.*

INTERACTIONS

Drug-drug. *Trimethoprim/sulfamethoxazole:* may cause increased blood level of lamivudine because of decreased clearance of lamivudine. Monitor patient closely.

Zidovudine: increased serum zidovudine level. Monitor patient closely.

EFFECTS ON DIAGNOSTIC TESTS

None reported.

CONTRAINDICATIONS

Contraindicated in patients with hypersensitivity to drug.

SPECIAL CONSIDERATIONS

▶ ***Alert:*** Use with extreme caution, if at all, in children with history of pancreatitis or other significant risk factors for development of pancreatitis. Lamivudine treatment is stopped immediately and the health care provider must be notified if clinical signs, symptoms, or laboratory abnormalities suggest pancreatitis. Serum amylase level must be monitored.

▶ Use cautiously in patients with renal impairment.

▶ Breast-feeding should be discontinued if lamivudine is prescribed.

▶ Drug is administered with zidovudine. It's not currently indicated for use alone unless for chronic hepatitis B virus infection.

▶ Safety and effectiveness of treatment with Epivir-HBV beyond 1 year have not been established; optimum duration of treatment isn't known. Patients should be tested for HIV before initiating treatment and during therapy because formulation and dosage of lamivudine in Epivir-HBV aren't appropriate for those dually infected with hepatitis B virus and HIV. If lamivudine is administered to patients with hepatitis B virus and HIV, the higher dosage indicated for HIV therapy should be used as part of an appropriate combination regimen.

‣ Patient's CBC, platelet count, renal and liver function studies must be monitored.

‣ An Antiretroviral Pregnancy Registry has been established to monitor maternal-fetal outcomes of pregnant women exposed to lamivudine. To register a pregnant patient, the health care provider can call 1-800-258-4263.

Patient teaching

‣ Long-term effects of lamivudine are unknown.

‣ Take lamivudine exactly as prescribed.

‣ If you're the patient's parent, learn the signs and symptoms of pancreatitis, and report them immediately if they occur in the child.

lamivudine/zidovudine

Combivir

Pregnancy Risk Category C

HOW SUPPLIED

Tablets: 150 mg lamivudine and 300 mg zidovudine

ACTION

Inhibit reverse transcriptase via DNA chain termination. Both drugs are also weak inhibitors of DNA polymerase. Together, they have synergistic antiretroviral activity. Combination therapy with lamivudine and zidovudine is targeted at suppressing or delaying the emergence of resistant strains that can occur with retroviral monotherapy because dual resistance requires multiple mutations.

Route	Onset	Peak	Duration
P.O.	Unknown	Unknown	Unknown

INDICATIONS & DOSAGE

HIV infection —

Adults and children ages 12 and older weighing over 50 kg (110 lb): one tablet P.O. b.i.d.

ADVERSE REACTIONS

CNS: *headache, malaise, fatigue, insomnia, dizziness, neuropathy,* depression.
EENT: *nasal signs and symptoms.*
GI: *nausea, diarrhea, vomiting, anorexia,* abdominal pain, abdominal cramps, dyspepsia.
Hematologic: *neutropenia,* anemia.
Hepatic: increased ALT, AST, amylase.
Musculoskeletal: *musculoskeletal pain,* myalgia, arthralgia.
Respiratory: *cough.*
Skin: rash.
Other: *fever, chills.*

INTERACTIONS

Drug-drug. *Ganciclovir, interferon-alpha, other bone marrow suppressive or cytotoxic agents:* may increase zidovudine's hematologic toxicity. Monitor patient.

EFFECTS ON DIAGNOSTIC TESTS

None reported.

CONTRAINDICATIONS

Contraindicated in patients with known hypersensitivity to drug's components and in those requiring dosage adjustments, such as children under age 12, those weighing under 50 kg, and those with creatinine clearance below 50 ml/minute. Also contraindicated in patients experiencing dose-limiting adverse effects.

SPECIAL CONSIDERATIONS

‣ Use combination cautiously in patients with bone marrow suppression as evidenced by granulocyte count below 1,000 cells/mm³ or hemoglobin level below 9.5 g/dl.

▶ Lactic acidosis and severe hepatomegaly with steatosis have been reported in patients receiving lamivudine and zidovudine alone and in combination. The health care provider is notified if signs of lactic acidosis or hepatotoxicity develop (abdominal pain, jaundice).

▶ Bone marrow toxicity must be monitored by frequent blood counts, particularly in patients with advanced HIV infection. Patients should be monitored for signs and symptoms of lactic acidosis and hepatotoxicity.

▶ A patient's fine motor skills and peripheral sensation should be assessed for evidence of peripheral neuropathies.

▶ An Antiretroviral Pregnancy Registry has been established to monitor maternal-fetal outcomes of pregnant women exposed to Combivir. To register a pregnant patient, health care provider can call 1-800-258-4263.

Patient teaching

▶ The lamivudine/zidovudine combination drug therapy is not a cure for HIV infection; illness, including opportunistic infections, may continue to occur.

▶ HIV transmission can still occur with drug therapy.

▶ Use protection when engaging in sexual activities to prevent disease transmission.

▶ Signs and symptoms of neutropenia and anemia include fever, chills, infection, fatigue; report such occurrences.

▶ Blood counts should be followed closely while on drug, especially if there is advanced disease.

▶ Consult health care provider or a pharmacist before taking other drugs.

▶ Report abdominal pain immediately.

▶ Report signs and symptoms of myopathy or myositis (muscle inflammation, pain, weakness, decrease in muscle size).

▶ Take combination drug therapy exactly as prescribed to reduce the development of resistance.

▶ Combination may be taken with or without food.

▶ Breast-feeding is contraindicated in HIV infection and during drug therapy.

nelfinavir mesylate

Viracept

Pregnancy Risk Category B

HOW SUPPLIED

Tablets: 250 mg
Powder: 50 mg/g powder in 144-g bottle

ACTION

An HIV-1 protease inhibitor, thereby preventing cleavage of the viral polyprotein, resulting in the production of immature, noninfectious virus.

Route	Onset	Peak	Duration
P.O.	Unknown	2-4 hr	Unknown

INDICATIONS & DOSAGE

HIV infection when antiretroviral therapy is warranted —
Adults: 1,250 mg b.i.d. or 750 mg P.O. t.i.d. with meals or light snack.
Children ages 2 to 13: 20 to 30 mg/kg/dose P.O. t.i.d. with meals or light snack; don't exceed 750 mg t.i.d.

Recommended children's dose given t.i.d. is shown below.

Body weight (kg)	Level 1-g scoops	Level teaspoons	Tablets
7 to < 8.5	4	1	–
8.5 to < 10.5	5	1.25	–
10.5 to < 12	6	1.5	–
12 to < 14	7	1.75	–
14 to < 16	8	2	–
16 to < 18	9	2.25	–
18 to < 23	10	2.5	2
23	15	3.75	3

ADVERSE REACTIONS

CNS: anxiety, depression, dizziness, emotional lability, hyperkinesia, insomnia, migraine, headache, paresthesia, *seizures,* sleep disorders, malaise, somnolence, *suicidal ideation.*

EENT: iritis, eye disorder, pharyngitis, rhinitis, sinusitis.

GI: nausea, *diarrhea,* flatulence, anorexia, dyspepsia, epigastric pain, GI bleeding, pancreatitis, mouth ulceration, vomiting.

GU: sexual dysfunction, renal calculus, urine abnormality.

Hematologic: anemia, *leukopenia, thrombocytopenia.*

Hepatic: *hepatitis,* elevated liver function test results, jaundice, bilirubinemia.

Metabolic: dehydration, hyperglycemia, hyperlipidemia, hyperuricemia, hypoglycemia, increased amylase and creatinine phosphokinase levels, metabolic acidosis.

Musculoskeletal: back pain, arthralgia, arthritis, cramps, myalgia, myasthenia, myopathy.

Respiratory: dyspnea.

Skin: rash, dermatitis, folliculitis, fungal dermatitis, pruritus, sweating, urticaria.

Other: allergic reactions, fever, hypersensitivity reactions, including *bronchospasm,* moderate to severe rash, edema.

INTERACTIONS

Drug-drug. *Amiodarone, cisapride, ergot derivatives, midazolam, quinidine, triazolam:* nelfinavir may produce large increases in plasma levels of these drugs, which may increase risk for serious or life-threatening adverse effects. Drugs should not be administered concurrently.

Carbamazepine, phenobarbital, phenytoin: may reduce the effectiveness of nelfinavir by decreasing nelfinavir plasma levels. Monitor closely.

HIV protease inhibitors (indinavir, ritonavir): may increase nelfinavir plasma levels. Use together cautiously.

Oral contraceptives (ethinyl estradiol, norethindrone): nelfinavir may decrease plasma levels. Alternative or additional contraceptive measures should be suggested during nelfinavir therapy.

Rifabutin: nelfinavir dramatically increases rifabutin plasma levels. Therefore, reduce dose of rifabutin to one-half the usual dose.

Rifampin: decreased nelfinavir plasma levels. Don't use together.

EFFECTS ON DIAGNOSTIC TESTS

None reported.

CONTRAINDICATIONS

Contraindicated in patients with hypersensitivity to drug or its components.

SPECIAL CONSIDERATIONS

▸ Use cautiously in patients with hepatic dysfunction or hemophilia types A and B. Liver function test results must be monitored.

▸ Dosage is the same whether drug is used alone or with other antiretroviral drugs.

▸ Twice-daily dosing hasn't been established in pediatric patients.

▸ Oral powder is administered in children unable to take tablets. Oral powder may be mixed with small amount of water, milk, formula, soy formula, soy milk, or dietary supplements. The entire contents must be consumed.

▸ The drug is not to be reconstituted with water in its original container.

▸ Reconstituted powder must be used within 6 hours.

▸ Mixing with acidic foods or juice is not recommended because of bitter taste.

▸ It's not known if drug appears in breast milk. Because safety has not been established, HIV-infected women should be advised not to breast-feed to avoid transmitting the virus to the infant.

▸ *Alert:* Don't confuse nelfinavir with nevirapine.

Patient teaching

▶ Take drug with food.

▶ Drug is not a cure for HIV infection. Drug's long-term effects are currently unknown, and there are no supporting data that nelfinavir reduces risk of transmission of HIV.

▶ Take drug daily as prescribed; don't alter the dose or discontinue drug without health care provider's approval.

▶ If a dose is missed, take the dose as soon as possible and then return to the normal schedule. If a dose is skipped, do not double-dose.

▶ Diarrhea is the most common adverse effect; it can be controlled with loperamide, if necessary.

▶ If taking oral contraceptives, use alternative or additional contraceptive measures while on nelfinavir therapy.

▶ If you have phenylketonuria, be aware that the powder contains 11.2 mg phenylalanine per gram.

▶ Report the use of other prescribed or OTC drugs because of possible drug interactions.

nevirapine

Viramune

Pregnancy Risk Category C

HOW SUPPLIED

Tablets: 200 mg
Oral suspension: 50 mg/5 ml

ACTION

Binds directly to reverse transcriptase and blocks RNA-dependent and DNA-dependent DNA polymerase activities by causing a disruption of the enzyme's catalytic site.

Route	Onset	Peak	Duration
P.O.	Unknown	4 hr	Unknown

INDICATIONS & DOSAGE

Adjunct treatment in patients with HIV-1 infection who have experienced clinical or immunologic deterioration —
Adults: 200 mg P.O. daily for the first 14 days, followed by 200 mg P.O. b.i.d. Used with nucleoside analogue antiretroviral agents.

Adjunct treatment in children infected with HIV-1 —
Children ages 2 months to 8 years: 4 mg/kg P.O. once daily for first 14 days, followed by 7 mg/kg P.O. b.i.d. thereafter. Maximum daily dose is 400 mg.
Children ages 8 and older: 4 mg/kg P.O. once daily for first 14 days; then 4 mg/kg P.O. b.i.d. thereafter. Maximum daily dose is 400 mg.

ADVERSE REACTIONS

CNS: headache, paresthesia.
GI: *nausea,* diarrhea, abdominal pain, ulcerative stomatitis.
Hematologic: *neutropenia,* decreased hemoglobin.
Hepatic: hepatitis, increased ALT, AST, gamma-glutamyl transpeptidase, and total bilirubin levels.
Musculoskeletal: myalgia.
Skin: *rash, blistering,* **Stevens-Johnson syndrome.**
Other: *fever.*

INTERACTIONS

Drug-drug. *Drugs extensively metabolized by P-450 CYP3A:* may lower plasma levels of these drugs, requiring dosage adjustment. Monitor closely.
Protease inhibitors, oral contraceptives, other hormonal contraceptives: may decrease plasma levels of these drugs. These drugs should not be administered concomitantly.
Rifabutin, rifampin: more data needed to assess whether dosage adjustments are necessary. If administering with nevirapine, monitor closely.

Reactions may be *common*, uncommon, *life-threatening*, or COMMON AND LIFE-THREATENING.

EFFECTS ON DIAGNOSTIC TESTS
None reported.

CONTRAINDICATIONS
Contraindicated in patients with hypersensitivity to drug.

SPECIAL CONSIDERATIONS
▶ Use cautiously in patients with impaired renal and hepatic function; pharmacokinetics have not been evaluated in those patients.
▶ Clinical chemistry tests, including renal and liver function tests, should be performed before initiating drug therapy and regularly throughout therapy.
▶ Drug should be used with at least one additional antiretroviral drug.
▶ *Alert:* Patient must be monitored for blistering, oral lesions, conjunctivitis, muscle or joint aches, or general malaise. Be especially alert for a severe rash or rash accompanied by fever. Patients who experience a rash during the initial 14 days of therapy shouldn't have the dosage increased until the rash has resolved. Most rashes occur within the first 6 weeks of therapy.
▶ Moderate and severe liver function test abnormalities may warrant temporary discontinuance of therapy; drug may be restarted at half the previous dose level as ordered.
▶ Patients who have nevirapine therapy interrupted for more than 7 days should restart therapy as if receiving drug for the first time.
▶ Antiretroviral therapy may be changed if disease progresses while patient is receiving nevirapine.
▶ Safety and effectiveness in children have not been established.
▶ Nevirapine appears in breast milk.
▶ *Alert:* Don't confuse nevirapine with nelfinavir.

Patient teaching
▶ Nevirapine is not a cure for HIV; illnesses associated with advanced HIV-1 infection may still occur. The drug does not reduce risk of HIV-1 transmission.
▶ Report rash immediately and discontinue drug until told to resume.
▶ Take drug exactly as prescribed. If a dose is missed, take the next dose as soon as possible. If a dose is skipped, don't double the next dose.
▶ Don't use other drugs unless health care provider approves.
▶ If female and of childbearing age, don't use oral contraceptives and other hormonal methods of birth control during therapy.
▶ Avoid breast-feeding during drug therapy to reduce risk of postnatal HIV transmission.

oseltamivir phosphate
Tamiflu

Pregnancy Risk Category C

HOW SUPPLIED
Capsules: 75 mg

ACTION
Inhibits influenza virus enzyme neuraminidase, which is thought to play a role in viral particle aggregation and release from the host cell. Neuraminidase inhibition, therefore, appears to interfere with viral replication.

Route	Onset	Peak	Duration
P.O.	Unknown	Unknown	Unknown

INDICATIONS & DOSAGE
Uncomplicated, acute illness due to influenza infection in patients who have been symptomatic for 2 days or less —
Adults: 75 mg P.O. b.i.d. for 5 days.
Dosage adjustment: For patients with creatinine clearance less than 30 ml/minute, reduce dose to 75 mg P.O. once daily for 5 days.

ADVERSE REACTIONS
CNS: dizziness, insomnia, headache, vertigo, fatigue.
GI: abdominal pain, diarrhea, nausea, vomiting.
Respiratory: bronchitis, cough.

INTERACTIONS
None significant.

EFFECTS ON DIAGNOSTIC TESTS
None reported.

CONTRAINDICATIONS
Contraindicated in patients with hypersensitivity to drug or its components.

SPECIAL CONSIDERATIONS
▶ Use cautiously in patients with chronic cardiac or respiratory diseases, or any medical condition that may require imminent hospitalization. Also, use cautiously in patients with renal failure, especially those with creatinine clearance less than 10 ml/minute.
▶ There is no evidence supporting drug use in treatment of viral infections other than influenza virus types A and B.
▶ Drug must be given within 2 days of onset of symptoms.
▶ Use to treat flu symptoms, not to prevent influenza.
▶ Drug isn't a replacement for the annual influenza vaccination. Patients for whom vaccine is indicated should continue to receive the vaccine each fall.
▶ Safety and efficacy of repeated treatment courses have not been established.
▶ Drug may be given with meals to decrease GI adverse effects.
▶ It's unknown if drug or its active metabolite appear in breast milk. Use only if potential benefits outweigh potential risks to infant.
▶ Store at controlled room temperature (59° to 86° F [15° to 30° C]).

Patient teaching
▶ Begin treatment as soon as possible after appearance of flu symptoms.
▶ Drug may be taken with or without meals. If nausea or vomiting occurs, take drug with food or milk.
▶ If a dose is missed, take it as soon as possible. Skip a missed dose, however, if next dose is due within 2 hours, and take the next dose on schedule.
▶ Complete the full 5 days of treatment, even if symptoms are resolved.
▶ Drug is not a replacement for the annual influenza vaccination. If vaccine is indicated for you, continue to receive it each fall.

ribavirin
Virazole

Pregnancy Risk Category X

HOW SUPPLIED
Powder to be reconstituted for inhalation: 6 g in 100-ml glass vial

ACTION
Inhibits viral activity by an unknown mechanism, possibly by inhibiting RNA and DNA synthesis by depleting intracellular nucleotide pools.

Route	Onset	Peak	Duration
Inhalation	Unknown	Unknown	Unknown

INDICATIONS & DOSAGE
Hospitalized infants and young children infected by respiratory syncytial virus (RSV) —
Infants and young children: solution in concentration of 20 mg/ml delivered via the Viratek Small Particle Aerosol Generator (SPAG-2) and mechanical ventilator or oxygen hood, face mask, or oxygen tent at a rate of about 12.5 L of mist per minute. Treatment is carried out for 12 to

18 hours/day for at least 3 days, and no more than 7 days.

ADVERSE REACTIONS
CV: *cardiac arrest*, hypotension, ***bradycardia.***
EENT: conjunctivitis.
Hematologic: anemia, reticulocytosis.
Hepatic: elevated bilirubin, AS, and ALT levels.
Respiratory: worsening respiratory state, *apnea*, bacterial pneumonia, pneumothorax.
Other: rash or erythema of eyelids.

INTERACTIONS
None significant.

EFFECTS ON DIAGNOSTIC TESTS
None reported.

CONTRAINDICATIONS
Contraindicated in patients with hypersensitivity to drug. Although drug is used in children, manufacturer states that it's contraindicated in women who are or may become pregnant during treatment.

SPECIAL CONSIDERATIONS
▶ Ribavirin aerosol is administered by the Viratek Small Particle Aerosol Generator (SPAG-2) only. Don't use any other aerosol-generating device.
▶ Sterile USP water for injection is used, not bacteriostatic water. Water used to reconstitute this drug mustn't contain any antimicrobial agent.
▶ Solutions placed in the SPAG-2 unit must be disgarded at least every 24 hours before adding newly reconstituted solution.
▶ The most frequent adverse effects reported in health care personnel exposed to aerosolized ribavirin include eye irritation and headache. Pregnant personnel should be advised of these effects.
▶ **Alert:** Ventilator function must be monitored frequently. Ribavirin may precipitate in ventilator apparatus, causing equipment malfunction with serious consequences.
▶ Reconstituted solutions are stored at room temperature for 24 hours.
▶ Ribavirin aerosol is indicated only for severe lower respiratory tract infection caused by RSV. Although treatment may begin while awaiting diagnostic test results, existence of RSV infection must eventually be documented.
▶ Most infants and children with RSV infection don't require treatment because the disease is commonly mild and self-limiting. Infants with underlying conditions, such as prematurity or cardiopulmonary disease, experience RSV in its severest form and benefit most from treatment with ribavirin aerosol.

Patient teaching
▶ If you're the patient's parent, be aware of need for drug, and report any subtle change in child immediately.

rimantadine hydrochloride
Flumadine

Pregnancy Risk Category C

HOW SUPPLIED
Tablets (film-coated): 100 mg
Syrup: 50 mg/5 ml

ACTION
Unknown. Appears to prevent viral uncoating, an early step in virus reproductive cycle.

Route	Onset	Peak	Duration
P.O.	Unknown	6 hr	Unknown

INDICATIONS & DOSAGE
Prophylaxis of influenza A —
Adults and children over age 10: 100 mg P.O. b.i.d.

Children ages 1 to 9 years: 5 mg/kg (not to exceed 150 mg) P.O. once daily.
Elderly: 100 mg P.O. daily.
Dosage adjustment: For patients with severe hepatic or renal dysfunction or those experiencing adverse effects with normal dosage, 100 mg P.O. daily.

Prophylaxis should begin as soon as possible after initial exposure and should be continued through course of influenza A outbreak. Safety of prolonged therapy over 6 weeks has not been established. Can be used for prophylaxis in children up to 6 weeks after first dose of influenza vaccine or until 2 weeks after second dose of vaccine.

Influenza A —
Adults: 100 mg P.O. b.i.d. initiated within 24 to 48 hours after onset of symptoms and continued for 48 hours after symptoms disappear (usually 7-day total course).

ADVERSE REACTIONS
CNS: insomnia, headache, dizziness, nervousness, fatigue, asthenia.
GI: nausea, vomiting, anorexia, dry mouth, abdominal pain.

INTERACTIONS
Drug-drug. *Acetaminophen, aspirin:* reduced level of rimantadine. Decreased effectiveness of rimantadine is possible.
Cimetidine: may decrease clearance of rimantadine. Monitor for adverse reactions.

EFFECTS ON DIAGNOSTIC TESTS
None reported.

CONTRAINDICATIONS
Contraindicated in patients with hypersensitivity to drug or amantadine.

SPECIAL CONSIDERATIONS
▶ Use cautiously in patients with renal or hepatic impairment and in patients with a history of seizures. Pregnant patients

should consider the risks compared with the benefits before taking drug.
▶ Consider the risk to contacts of treated patients who may be subject to morbidity from influenza A. Influenza A–resistant strains can emerge during therapy. Patients taking drug may still be able to spread the disease.
▶ *Alert:* Don't confuse rimantadine with amantadine.

Patient teaching
▶ Take drug several hours before bedtime to prevent insomnia.
▶ You may still be able to infect others with influenza A; take infection-control precautions.

ritonavir
Norvir

Pregnancy Risk Category B

HOW SUPPLIED
Capsules: 100 mg
Oral solution: 80 mg/ml

ACTION
An HIV protease inhibitor with activity against HIV-1 and HIV-2 proteases. HIV protease is an enzyme required for the proteolytic cleavage of viral polyprotein precursors into the individual functional proteins in infectious HIV. Ritonavir binds to the protease active site and inhibits activity of the enzyme, preventing cleavage of the viral polyproteins and resulting in the formation of immature, noninfectious viral particles.

Route	Onset	Peak	Duration
P.O.	Unknown	2-4 hr	Unknown

INDICATIONS & DOSAGE
HIV infection with nucleoside analogues

or as monotherapy when antiretroviral therapy is warranted —
Adults: 600 mg P.O. b.i.d with meals. If nausea occurs, gradually increasing dose may provide some relief: 300 mg b.i.d. for 1 day, 400 mg b.i.d. for 2 days, 500 mg b.i.d. for 1 day, and then 600 mg b.i.d. thereafter.

ADVERSE REACTIONS
CNS: *asthenia,* headache, malaise, circumoral paresthesia, dizziness, insomnia, paresthesia, peripheral paresthesia, somnolence, thinking abnormality, migraine headache.
CV: vasodilation.
EENT: local throat irritation, blepharitis, diplopia, pharyngitis, photophobia, *taste perversion.*
GI: abdominal pain, anorexia, constipation, *diarrhea, nausea, vomiting,* dyspepsia, flatulence, cramping, jaundice.
GU: dysuria, hematuria, nocturia, polyuria, pyelonephritis, urethritis, hyperuricemia.
Hematologic: decreased hemoglobin and hematocrit levels, ***leukopenia, thrombocytopenia,*** decreased neutrophil and eosinophil levels.
Hepatic: elevated triglycerides, AST, ALT, GGT, alkaline phosphatase, total bilirubin, altered PT and INR.
Metabolic: hyperlipidemia, hyperglycemia, hyperkalemia.
Musculoskeletal: increased CK level, myalgia.
Skin: rash, sweating, urticaria.
Other: fever.

INTERACTIONS
Drug-drug. *Agents that increase CYP3A activity (such as carbamazepine, dexamethasone, phenobarbital, phenytoin, rifabutin, rifampin):* may increase clearance of ritonavir, resulting in decreased ritonavir plasma levels. Monitor patient closely.
Alprazolam, clorazepate, diazepam, dihydroergotamine, ergotamine, estazolam, flurazepam, midazolam, triazolam, zolpidem: significantly increased levels of these drugs. Because of risk of extreme sedation and respiratory depression, don't give these drugs with ritonavir.
Amiodarone, bupropion, cisapride, clozapine, encainide, flecainide, meperidine, piroxicam, propafenone, propoxyphene, quinidine, rifabutin: significantly increased plasma levels of these drugs, which increases patient's risk of arrhythmias, hematologic abnormalities, seizures, or other potentially serious adverse effects. Avoid concomitant use.
Clarithromycin: reduced creatinine clearance. Patients with impaired renal function receiving drug with ritonavir require a 50% reduction in clarithromycin dose if creatinine clearance is 30 to 60 ml/minute and a 75% reduction if it is below 30 ml/minute.
Desipramine: increased overall serum levels of desipramine. Concomitant administration may require a dosage adjustment when administered with ritonavir. Monitor patient.
Directly glucuronidated drugs: ritonavir may increase activity of glucoronosyl transferases with loss of therapeutic effects from these drugs; may signify need for dosage alteration of these drugs. Concomitant use should be accompanied by therapeutic drug level monitoring and increased monitoring of therapeutic and adverse effects, especially for drugs with narrow therapeutic margins, such as oral anticoagulants and immunosuppressants. Dosage reduction greater than 50% may be required for drugs extensively metabolized by CYP3A.
Disulfiram or other drugs that produce disulfiram-like reactions such as metronidazole: increased risk of disulfiram-like reactions. Ritonavir formulations contain alcohol that can produce reactions when co-administered. Monitor patient.
Oral contraceptives containing ethinyl estradiol: decreased overall serum levels

of the contraceptive. Patient should be advised that concomitant therapy may require a dosage increase in the oral contraceptive or use of other contraceptive measures.

Saquinavir: inhibited metabolism of saquinavir, resulting in greatly increased plasma levels. Safety of this combination has not been established.

Theophylline: decreased overall serum levels of theophylline. Increased dosage may be required when coadministered with ritonavir. Theophylline level should be monitored.

Drug-food. *Any food:* increased absorption. Drug is given with food.

Drug-lifestyle. *Smoking:* decreased overall serum levels of ritonavir. Avoid use.

EFFECTS ON DIAGNOSTIC TESTS
None reported.

CONTRAINDICATIONS
Contraindicated in patients with hypersensitivity to drug or its components.

SPECIAL CONSIDERATIONS
▶ Use cautiously in patients with hepatic insufficiency.
▶ Drug may be administered alone or with nucleoside analogues.
▶ Patients beginning combination regimens with ritonavir and nucleosides may improve GI tolerance by starting ritonavir alone and subsequently adding nucleosides before completing 2 weeks of ritonavir.
▶ Safety and effectiveness in children under age 12 have not been established.
▶ It's unknown whether ritonavir appears in breast milk.

Patient teaching
▶ Drug is not a cure for HIV infection. Opportunistic infections and other complications associated with HIV infection may continue to occur. Drug has not been shown to reduce the risk of transmitting HIV to others through sexual contact or blood contamination.
▶ Take drug as prescribed; don't adjust dosage or discontinue therapy without first consulting a health care provider.
▶ The taste of ritonavir oral solution may be improved by mixing it with chocolate milk, Ensure, or Advera within 1 hour of the scheduled dose.
▶ Take drug with a meal to improve absorption.
▶ If a dose is missed, take the next dose as soon as possible. If a dose is skipped, do not double the next dose.
▶ Report use of other drugs, including OTC drugs; ritonavir interacts with some drugs when taken together.
▶ Discontinue breast-feeding to prevent transmission of infection.

---

saquinavir
Fortovase

saquinavir mesylate
Invirase

Pregnancy Risk Category B

HOW SUPPLIED
saquinavir
Capsules (soft gelatin): 200 mg
saquinavir mesylate
Capsules (hard gelatin): 200 mg

ACTION
Inhibits the activity of HIV protease and prevents the cleavage of HIV polyproteins, which are essential for HIV maturation.

Route	Onset	Peak	Duration
P.O.	Unknown	Unknown	Unknown

INDICATIONS & DOSAGE
Adjunct treatment of advanced HIV infection in selected patients —

Adults: 600 mg (Invirase) or 1,200 mg (Fortovase) P.O. t.i.d. taken within 2 hours after a full meal and with a nucleoside analogue such as zalcitabine at a dose of 0.75 mg P.O. t.i.d. or zidovudine at a dose of 200 mg P.O. t.i.d.

ADVERSE REACTIONS

CNS: paresthesia, headache, dizziness, asthenia, numbness.
CV: chest pain.
GI: diarrhea, ulcerated buccal mucosa, abdominal pain, nausea, dyspepsia, pancreatitis.
Hematologic: *pancytopenia, thrombocytopenia.*
Musculoskeletal: musculoskeletal pain.
Respiratory: bronchitis, cough.
Skin: rash.

INTERACTIONS

Drug-drug. *Cisapride:* increased serum level of this drug, increased risk of arrhythmias, and sudden death. Avoid concomitant use.
Ketoconazole, ritonavir: increased serum saquinavir levels. Monitor patient closely.
Phenobarbital, phenytoin, rifabutin, rifampin: reduced steady-state level of saquinavir. Use together cautiously.
Drug-food. *Any food:* increased absorption. Drug is given with food.

EFFECTS ON DIAGNOSTIC TESTS

None reported.

CONTRAINDICATIONS

Contraindicated in patients with hypersensitivity to drug or to any component contained in the capsule.

SPECIAL CONSIDERATIONS

▶ Safety of drug is not established in pregnant or breast-feeding women or in children under age 16.
▶ *Alert:* Don't confuse the two forms of this drug because dosages are different.

▶ CBC, platelets, electrolytes, uric acid, liver enzymes, and bilirubin should be evaluated before therapy begins and at appropriate intervals throughout therapy, as ordered.
▶ If serious toxicity occurs during treatment, drug should be discontinued until cause is identified or the toxicity resolves. Drug may be resumed with no dosage modifications.
▶ Patient's hydration must be monitored if adverse GI reactions occur.
▶ If adverse reactions occur, a physician should be notified. A mild analgesic may be given if drug causes headache, an antiemetic if drug causes nausea, or an antidiarrheal if drug causes diarrhea.
▶ Be alert for adverse reactions associated with adjunct therapy (zidovudine or zalcitabine).

Patient teaching

▶ Take drug within 2 hours after a full meal.
▶ The drug is usually administered with other AIDS-related antivirals.
▶ Take drug around the clock, not missing any doses, to decrease the risk of developing HIV resistance.
▶ A change from Invirase to Fortovase capsules should only be made under health care provider's supervision.
▶ Fortovase capsules are stored in the refrigerator; Invirase capsules can be kept at room temperature.

stavudine (2,3 didehydro-3-deoxythymidine, d4T)

Zerit

Pregnancy Risk Category C

HOW SUPPLIED
Capsules: 15 mg, 20 mg, 30 mg, 40 mg
Oral solution: 1 mg/ml

ACTION
A thymidine nucleoside analogue that prevents replication of retroviruses, including HIV, by inhibiting the enzyme reverse transcriptase and causing termination of DNA chain growth.

Route	Onset	Peak	Duration
P.O.	Unknown	1 hr	Unknown

INDICATIONS & DOSAGE
HIV-infected patients who have received prolonged prior zidovudine therapy —
Adults weighing 60 kg (132 lb) or more: 40 mg P.O. q 12 hours.
Adults under 60 kg: 30 mg P.O. q 12 hours.
Children: 2 mg/kg/day P.O. in divided doses q 12 hours for children under 30 kg (66 lb); adult dose should be used for children 30 kg or more.
Dosage adjustment: For patients with renal impairment, if creatinine clearance is 26 to 50 ml/minute, 20 mg (if weight exceeds 60 kg) or 15 mg (if weight is below 60 kg) P.O. q 12 hours; if creatinine clearance is 10 to 25 ml/minute, 20 mg (if weight exceeds 60 kg) or 15 mg (if weight is below 60 kg) P.O. q 24 hours.

ADVERSE REACTIONS
CNS: peripheral neuropathy, headache, malaise, insomnia, anxiety, *asthenia,* depression, nervousness, dizziness.
CV: chest pain.
EENT: conjunctivitis.
GI: *abdominal pain, diarrhea, nausea, vomiting, anorexia,* dyspepsia, constipation, weight loss, pancreatitis.
Hematologic: *neutropenia, thrombocytopenia,* anemia, increased AST and ALT levels.
Hepatic: *hepatotoxicity.*
Musculoskeletal: *arthralgia, myalgia, back pain.*
Respiratory: *dyspnea.*
Skin: *rash, diaphoresis, pruritus,* maculopapular rash.
Other: *chills, fever*

INTERACTIONS
None significant.

EFFECTS ON DIAGNOSTIC TESTS
None reported.

CONTRAINDICATIONS
Contraindicated in patients with hypersensitivity to drug.

SPECIAL CONSIDERATIONS
▶ Use cautiously in patients with renal impairment or history of peripheral neuropathy. Dosage adjustment is necessary for creatinine clearance below 50 ml/minute; dosage adjustment or discontinuation is necessary in onset of peripheral neuropathy. Also, use cautiously in pregnant women.
▶ *Alert:* Peripheral neuropathy appears to be the major dose-limiting adverse effect of stavudine. It may or may not resolve after drug is discontinued.
▶ CBC and serum levels of creatinine, AST, ALT, and alkaline phosphatase must be monitored.
▶ *Alert:* Don't confuse drug with other antivirals that may use initials for identification.

Patient teaching
▶ Drug may be taken without regard to meals.

» Other drugs for HIV or AIDS should not be taken unless approved.

» Signs and symptoms of peripheral neuropathy include pain, burning, aching, weakness, or pins and needles in the extremities; report them immediately.

» Monitor weight patterns, and report weight loss or gain.

valacyclovir hydrochloride
Valtrex

Pregnancy Risk Category B

HOW SUPPLIED
Tablets: 500 mg, 1 g

ACTION
Rapidly converts to acyclovir, which in turn becomes incorporated into viral DNA, thereby terminating growth of the DNA chain; inhibits viral DNA polymerase, causing inhibition of viral replication.

Route	Onset	Peak	Duration
P.O.	30 min	Unknown	Unknown

INDICATIONS & DOSAGE
Herpes zoster infection (shingles) —
Adults: 1 g P.O. t.i.d. for 7 days.
Dosage adjustment: For renally impaired patients with creatinine clearance of 50 ml/minute or more, use regular dose; if 30 to 49 ml/minute, 1 g P.O. q 12 hours; if 10 to 29 ml/minute, 1 g P.O. q 24 hours; if below 10 ml/minute, 500 mg P.O. q 24 hours.

For hemodialysis patients, 1 g P.O. after hemodialysis.
Initial episode of genital herpes —
Adults: 1 g P.O. b.i.d. for 10 days.
Dosage adjustment:
For renally impaired patients with creatinine clearance of 30 ml/minute or more, dosage is 1 g P.O. q 12 hours; if 10 to 29 ml/minute, 1 g P.O. q 24 hours; if below 10 ml/minute, 500 mg P.O. q 24 hours.

For hemodialysis patients, 1 g P.O. after hemodialysis.
Recurrent genital herpes —
Adults: 500 mg P.O. b.i.d. for 5 days, given at the first sign or symptom of an episode.
Dosage adjustment:
For renally impaired patients with creatinine clearance of 30 ml/minute or more, dosage is 500 mg P.O. q 12 hours; if 29 ml/minute or less, 500 mg P.O. q 24 hours.

For hemodialysis patients, 500 mg P.O. after hemodialysis.

ADVERSE REACTIONS
CNS: *headache,* asthenia, dizziness.
GI: *nausea,* vomiting, diarrhea, constipation, abdominal pain, anorexia.

INTERACTIONS
Drug-drug. *Cimetidine, probenecid:* reduced rate but not extent of conversion of valacyclovir to acyclovir and reduced renal clearance of acyclovir, thus increasing acyclovir blood levels. Monitor for possible toxicity.

EFFECTS ON DIAGNOSTIC TESTS
None reported.

CONTRAINDICATIONS
Contraindicated in patients with hypersensitivity or intolerance to valacyclovir, acyclovir, or components of the formulation.

SPECIAL CONSIDERATIONS
» Valacyclovir isn't recommended for use in patients with HIV infection or in bone marrow or renal transplant recipients due to the occurrence of thrombotic thrombocytopenic purpura and hemolytic uremic syndrome in these patient populations in clinical trials of valacyclovir at doses of 8 g/day.
» Use cautiously in elderly patients, those with renal impairment, and those receiv-

---

ing other nephrotoxic drugs. Renal function test results must be monitored.

▶ Safety and efficacy in children have not been established.

▶ Use during pregnancy should be considered only if the benefits outweigh the risks.

▶ Drug may need to be discontinued in the breastfeeding patient..

▶ Although there have been no reports of overdosage, precipitation of acyclovir in renal tubules may occur when solubility (2.5 mg/ml) is exceeded in the intratubular fluid. With acute renal failure and anuria, the patient may benefit from hemodialysis until renal function is restored.

Patient teaching

▶ Drug may be taken without regard to meals.

▶ Signs and symptoms of herpes infection include rash, tingling, itching, and pain; notify health care provider immediately if they occur. Treatment should be initiated as soon as possible after symptoms appear, preferably within 48 hours of the onset of zoster rash.

▶ Drug is not a cure for herpes but may decrease the length and severity of symptoms.

zalcitabine (dideoxycytidine, ddC)
Hivid
Pregnancy Risk Category C

HOW SUPPLIED
Tablets: 0.375 mg, 0.75 mg

ACTION
Inhibits replication of HIV by blocking viral DNA synthesis.

Route	Onset	Peak	Duration
P.O.	Unknown	1-2 hr	Unknown

INDICATIONS & DOSAGE
Monotherapy for treatment of advanced HIV disease in patients who either can't tolerate zidovudine or who have disease progression while receiving zidovudine —
Adults and children ages 13 and older: 0.75 mg P.O. q 8 hours.

Therapy with zidovudine for treatment of advanced HIV disease (CD4+ cell count 300/mm³ or less) —
Adults and children ages 13 and older: 0.75 mg P.O. q 8 hours given with zidovudine 200 mg P.O. q 8 hours.

Dosage adjustment: For renally impaired patients with creatinine clearance of 10 to 40 ml/minute, dosage is 0.75 mg P.O. q 12 hours; if clearance is below 10 ml/minute, 0.75 mg P.O. q 24 hours.

If patient experiences moderate discomfort with signs and symptoms of peripheral neuropathy, discontinue drug temporarily. If symptoms improve after discontinuation, drug may be reintroduced at 0.375 mg P.O. q 8 hours.

ADVERSE REACTIONS
CNS: *peripheral neuropathy, headache, fatigue,* dizziness, confusion, **seizures,** impaired concentration, amnesia, insomnia, mental depression, tremor, hypertonia, anxiety.
CV: cardiomyopathy, **heart failure,** chest pain.
EENT: pharyngitis, ocular pain, abnormal vision, ototoxicity, nasal discharge.
GI: nausea, vomiting, diarrhea, abdominal pain, anorexia, constipation, stomatitis, esophageal ulcer, glossitis, pancreatitis.
Hematologic: anemia, *neutropenia, leukopenia, thrombocytopenia.*
Hepatic: increased AST, ALT and alkaline phosphatase.
Metabolic: hypoglycemia.
Musculoskeletal: myalgia, arthralgia.
Respiratory: cough.
Skin: pruritus; night sweats; *erythema-*

---

tous, maculopapular, or follicular rash; urticaria.

Other: *fever.*

INTERACTIONS

Drug-drug. *Aminoglycosides, amphotericin B, foscarnet, other drugs that may impair renal function:* increased risk of nephrotoxicity. Avoid concomitant use when possible.

Antacids containing aluminum or magnesium: decreased bioavailability of zalcitabine. Don't use together.

Chloramphenicol, cisplatin, dapsone, didanosine, disulfiram, ethionamide, glutethimide, gold salts, hydralazine, iodoquinol, isoniazid, metronidazole, nitrofurantoin, other drugs that can cause peripheral neuropathy, phenytoin, ribavirin, stavudine, vincristine: increased risk of peripheral neuropathy. Avoid concomitant use.

Cimetidine, probenecid: increased serum zalcitabine levels. Monitor patient carefully.

Pentamidine: increased risk of pancreatitis. Avoid concomitant use when possible.

Drug-food. *Any food:* decreased rate of absorption. Drug is given on an empty stomach.

EFFECTS ON DIAGNOSTIC TESTS

None reported.

CONTRAINDICATIONS

Contraindicated in patients with hypersensitivity to drug or its components.

SPECIAL CONSIDERATIONS

▶ Use with extreme caution in patients with preexisting peripheral neuropathy.
▶ Use cautiously in patients with hepatic failure, history of pancreatitis or heart failure, or baseline cardiomyopathy. Liver function test results and pancreatic enzymes must be monitored.
▶ Toxic effects of drug may cause abnormalities in several laboratory tests, including CBC, hemoglobin, leukocyte, reticulocyte, granulocyte, and platelet counts; and AST, ALT, and alkaline phosphatase levels.
▶ Drug is not to be administered with food because it decreases the rate and extent of absorption.
▶ Signs and symptoms of peripheral neuropathy characterized by numbness and burning in the extremities are the drug's major toxic effects. If drug isn't withdrawn, peripheral neuropathy can progress to sharp shooting pain or severe continuous burning pain requiring opioid analgesics. The pain may or may not be reversible.
▶ **Alert:** Don't confuse drug with other antivirals that may use initials for identification.

Patient teaching

▶ Take drug on an empty stomach.
▶ Drug doesn't cure HIV infection; opportunistic infections may still occur despite continued use. Know and observe safe sex practices.
▶ If you're of childbearing age, use an effective contraceptive while taking drug.
▶ Peripheral neuropathy is the major toxic condition associated with drug and pancreatitis is the major life-threatening toxic reaction. The signs and symptoms of these adverse reactions should be reviewed, and the patient should alert the health care provider promptly if any appear.

zanamivir

Relenza

Pregnancy Risk Category B

HOW SUPPLIED

Powder for inhalation: 5 mg/blister

ACTION

Likely exerts its antiviral action by inhibiting neuraminidase on the surface of the influenza virus, potentially altering virus particle aggregation and release.

Route	Onset	Peak	Duration
Inhalation	Unknown	1-2 hr	Unknown

INDICATIONS & DOSAGE

Uncomplicated acute illness due to influenza virus in patients who have been symptomatic for no more than 2 days —
Adults and adolescents ages 12 and older: 2 oral inhalations (one 5-mg blister per inhalation for total dose of 10 mg) b.i.d. using the Diskhaler inhalation device for 5 days. Two doses should be taken on first day of treatment provided there is at least 2 hours between doses. Subsequent doses should be about 12 hours apart (in the morning and evening) at about the same time each day.

ADVERSE REACTIONS

CNS: headache, dizziness.
EENT: nasal signs and symptoms; sinusitis; ear, nose, and throat infections.
GI: diarrhea, nausea, vomiting.
Respiratory: bronchitis, cough.

INTERACTIONS

None significant.

EFFECTS ON DIAGNOSTIC TESTS

None reported.

CONTRAINDICATIONS

Contraindicated in patients with known hypersensitivity to drug or its components.

SPECIAL CONSIDERATIONS

▶ Use cautiously in patients with severe or decompensated chronic obstructive pulmonary disease, asthma, or other underlying respiratory disease.
▶ Patients with underlying respiratory disease should have a fast-acting bronchodilator available in case of wheezing while taking zanamivir. Patients scheduled to use an inhaled bronchodilator for asthma should use their bronchodilator before taking zanamivir.
▶ No data are available to support safety and efficacy of zanamivir in patients who begin treatment after 48 hours of symptoms.
▶ Safety and efficacy of drug haven't been established for influenza prophylaxis. Use of drug shouldn't affect evaluation of patient for annual influenza vaccination.
▶ Lymphopenia, neutropenia, and a rise in liver enzyme and CK levels have been reported during zanamivir treatment.
▶ Patient should be monitored for bronchospasm and decline in lung function. Stop drug in such situations.

Patient teaching

▶ Carefully read instructions for proper use of the Diskhaler inhalation device to administer drug.
▶ Keep Diskhaler level when loading and inhaling zanamivir. Always check inside the mouthpiece of the Diskhaler before each use to make sure it's free of foreign objects.
▶ Exhale fully before putting the mouthpiece in the mouth; then, keeping the Diskhaler level, close lips around the mouthpiece and breathe in steadily and deeply. Hold your breath for a few seconds after inhaling to help drug stay in the lungs.
▶ If you have underlying respiratory disease and are scheduled to use an inhaled bronchodilator, do so before taking zanamivir. Have a fast-acting bronchodilator available in case of wheezing while taking zanamivir.
▶ Finish the entire 5-day course of treatment even if you start to feel better and symptoms improve before the fifth day.
▶ Use of zanamivir has not been shown to reduce the risk of transmission of influenza virus to others.

Reactions may be *common*, uncommon, *life-threatening*, or COMMON AND LIFE-THREATENING.

zidovudine (azidothymidine, AZT)
Apo-Zidovudine , Novo-AZT , Retrovir

Pregnancy Risk Category C

HOW SUPPLIED
Capsules: 100 mg
Tablets: 300 mg
Syrup: 50 mg/5 ml
Injection: 10 mg/ml

ACTION
Inhibits replication of HIV by blocking DNA synthesis.

Route	Onset	Peak	Duration
P.O., I.V.	Unknown	0.5-1.5 hr	Unknown

INDICATIONS & DOSAGE
Symptomatic HIV infection, including AIDS —
Adults and children ages 12 and older: 100 mg P.O. q 4 hours around the clock, 300 mg (1 tablet) P.O. q 12 hours, 200 mg P.O. q 8 hours, or 1 mg/kg I.V. q 4 hours six times daily.
Children ages 3 months to 12 years: 180 mg/m^2 P.O. q 6 hours (720 mg/m^2/day), not to exceed 200 mg q 6 hours.
Asymptomatic HIV infection —
Adults and children ages 12 and older: 100 mg P.O. q 4 hours while awake (500 mg daily). Or, 1 mg/kg I.V. q 4 hours while awake (5 mg/kg/day).
Children ages 3 months to 12 years: 180 mg/m^2 P.O. q 6 hours (720 mg/m^2/day), not to exceed 200 mg q 6 hours.
To reduce risk of transmission of HIV from infected mother with a baseline CD4+ lymphocyte count exceeding 200 cells/mm^3 to the newborn —
Adults: 100 mg P.O. five times daily given initially between 14 and 34 weeks' gestation and continued throughout pregnancy. During labor, administer loading dose of 2 mg/kg I.V. over 1 hour followed by continuous I.V. infusion of 1 mg/kg/hour until umbilical cord is clamped.
Neonates: 2 mg/kg P.O. (syrup) q 6 hours for 6 weeks, beginning within 12 hours after birth. Or, 1.5 mg/kg I.V. q 6 hours.
Therapy with zalcitabine or other antiretroviral agents for treatment of advanced HIV disease —
Adults and children ages 13 and older: 200 mg P.O. q 8 hours or 300 mg (1 tablet) P.O. q 12 hours given with zalcitabine 0.75 mg P.O. q 8 hours or other antiretroviral agents.
Dosage adjustment: For patient with end-stage renal disease or patient receiving hemodialysis or peritoneal dialysis, 100 mg P.O. or 1 mg/kg I.V. q 6 to 8 hours.

ADVERSE REACTIONS
CNS: *headache, seizures,* paresthesia, *malaise,* insomnia, *asthenia, dizziness,* somnolence.
GI: nausea, anorexia, abdominal pain, vomiting, constipation, diarrhea, taste perversion, dyspepsia, pancreatitis.
Hematologic: *severe bone marrow suppression, anemia, agranulocytosis, thrombocytopenia.*
Hepatic: increased liver enzyme levels.
Musculoskeletal: myalgia.
Skin: *rash.*
Other: diaphoresis, *fever,* lactic acidosis.

INTERACTIONS
Drug-drug: *Acetaminophen, aspirin, indomethacin:* may impair hepatic metabolism of zidovudine, increasing drug's toxicity. Monitor closely.
Acyclovir: possible seizures, lethargy, and fatigue. Use together cautiously.
Amphotericin B, dapsone, flucytosine, pentamidine: increased risk of nephrotoxicity and bone marrow suppression. Monitor closely.
Fluconazole, methadone, valproic acid:

increased zidovudine level. Monitor for toxicity.

Ganciclovir, interferon-alpha: increased risk of hematologic toxicity. Monitor closely.

Other cytotoxic drugs: additive adverse effects on the bone marrow. Avoid concomitant use.

Probenecid: may decrease the renal clearance of zidovudine. Avoid concomitant use.

Ribavirin: antagonized antiviral activity of zidovudine against HIV. Avoid concomitant use.

EFFECTS ON DIAGNOSTIC TESTS

Drug may cause depression of formed elements (erythrocytes, leukocytes, and platelets) in peripheral blood.

CONTRAINDICATIONS

Contraindicated in patients with hypersensitivity to drug.

SPECIAL CONSIDERATIONS

▶ Use cautiously and with close monitoring in patients with advanced symptomatic HIV infection and in patients with severe bone marrow depression.

▶ Use with caution in patients with hepatomegaly, hepatitis, or other known risk factors for liver disease and in those with renal insufficiency. Renal and liver function tests must be monitored.

▶ Blood studies should be monitored every 2 weeks to detect anemia or agranulocytosis. Patients may require dosage reduction or temporary discontinuation of drug.

▶ Drug may temporarily decrease morbidity and mortality in certain patients with AIDS.

I.V. administration

▶ The drug is diluted before administration. The calculated dose is removed from the vial; the dose is added to D_5W to achieve a concentration that doesn't exceed 4 mg/ml. The drug is infused over 1 hour at a constant rate. Rapid infusion or bolus injection must be avoided. Adding mixture to biological or colloidal fluids (for example, blood products, protein solutions) isn't recommended. Protect undiluted vials from light.

Patient teaching

▶ Take drug exactly as directed, and do not share it with others.

▶ Take drug on an empty stomach. To avoid esophageal irritation, take drug while sitting upright and with adequate amount of fluids.

▶ Carefully follow the dosage schedule. Explore ways to avoid missing doses, perhaps by using an alarm clock.

▶ Blood transfusions may be needed during treatment. Zidovudine frequently causes a low RBC count.

▶ Other drugs for AIDS should not be taken unless approved.

▶ If you're pregnant and HIV-infected, be aware that drug therapy only reduces the risk of HIV transmission to the newborn. Long-term risks to infants are unknown.

▶ Be aware that monotherapy is no longer recommended.

▶ If you're a health care worker considering zidovudine prophylaxis after occupational exposure (following needle-stick injury, for example), know that the drug's safety and efficacy have not yet been proved.

azithromycin
clarithromycin
dirithromycin
erythromycin base
erythromycin estolate
erythromycin ethylsuccinate
erythromycin lactobionate
erythromycin stearate

COMBINATION PRODUCTS

Eryzole, Pediazole, Sulfimycin: ery-thromycin (200 mg) and sulfisoxazole (600 mg)/5 ml.

azithromycin

Zithromax

Pregnancy Risk Category B

HOW SUPPLIED

Capsules: 250 mg; Z-pak (contains 5 days of therapy)
Injection: 500 mg
Oral suspension: 100 mg/5 ml, 200 mg/5 ml
Single-dose powder for oral suspension: 1 g
Tablets: 250 mg, 600 mg

ACTION

Binds to the 50S subunit of bacterial ri-bosomes, blocking protein synthesis; bac-teriostatic or bactericidal, depending on concentration.

Route	Onset	Peak	Duration
P.O.	Unknown	2.5-4.4 hr	Unknown
I.V.	Unknown	Unknown	Unknown

INDICATIONS & DOSAGE

Acute bacterial exacerbations of COPD due to Haemophilus influenzae, Moraxel-la (Branhamella) catarrhalis, *or* Strepto-coccus pneumoniae; *uncomplicated skin and skin-structure infections due to* Staphylococcus aureus, Streptococcus pyogenes, *or* S. agalactiae; *second-line therapy of pharyngitis or tonsillitis due to* S. pyogenes —
Adults and adolescents ages 16 and old-er: 500 mg P.O. as a single dose on day 1; then 250 mg daily on days 2 through 5. Total dose is 1.5 g.

Community-acquired pneumonia due to Chlamydia pneumoniae, H. influenzae, Mycoplasma pneumoniae, S. pneumoni-ae; *I.V. form can also be used for* Legion-ella pneumophila, M. catarrhalis, *and* S. aureus —
Adults and adolescents ages 16 and older: 500 mg P.O. as a single dose on day 1; then 250 mg P.O. daily on days 2 through 5. Total dose is 1.5 g. For patients requiring initial I.V. therapy, 500 mg I.V. as a single daily dose for 2 days; then 500 mg P.O. as a single daily dose to com-plete a 7-to 10-day course of therapy. Switch from I.V. to P.O. therapy should be done at the health care provider's dis-cretion and based on patient's clinical re-sponse.

Nongonococcal urethritis or cervicitis due to C. trachomatis —
Adults and adolescents ages 16 and older: 1 g P.O. as a single dose.

Prevention of disseminated Mycobac-terium avium *complex disease in patients with advanced HIV infection* —
Adults: 1,200 mg P.O. once weekly, as indicated.

Urethritis and cervicitis due to Neis-seria gonorrhoeae —
Adults: 2 g P.O. as a single dose.

Pelvic inflammatory disease due to C. trachomatis, N. gonorrhoeae, *or* M. ho-minis *in patients who require initial I.V. therapy* —
Adults: 500 mg I.V. as a single daily dose

for 1 to 2 days; then 250 mg P.O. daily to complete a 7-day course of therapy. Switch from I.V. to P.O. therapy should be at health care provider's discretion and based on patient's clinical response.

Genital ulcer disease in men caused by H. ducreyi *(chancroid)* —
Adults: 1 g P.O. as a single dose.

Otitis media —
Children over age 6 months: 10 mg/kg (maximum 500 mg) P.O. on day 1; 5 mg/kg (maximum 250 mg) on days 2 to 5.

Pharyngitis, tonsillitis —
Children over age 2: 12 mg/kg (maximum 500 mg) P.O. daily for 5 days.

Dental prophylaxis in patients allergic to penicillin —
Adults: 500 mg P.O. 1 hour before procedure.
Children: 15 mg/kg P.O. 1 hour before procedure.

ADVERSE REACTIONS
CNS: dizziness, vertigo, headache, fatigue, somnolence.
CV: palpitations, chest pain.
GI: *nausea, vomiting, diarrhea, abdominal pain,* dyspepsia, flatulence, melena, cholestatic jaundice, pseudomembranous colitis.
GU: candidiasis, vaginitis, nephritis.
Skin: rash, photosensitivity.
Other: *angioedema.*

INTERACTIONS
Drug-drug. *Aluminum- and magnesium-containing antacids:* lowered peak plasma levels of azithromycin. Administration times should be separated by at least 2 hours.
Carbamazepine, cyclosporine, phenytoin: may increase levels of these drugs. Monitor closely.
Digoxin: may cause elevated digoxin levels. Monitor closely.
Ergotamine: acute ergotamine toxicity has occurred. Monitor closely.
Pimozide: prolongation of QT interval and

ventricular tachycardia have been associated with other macrolide anti-infectives. Monitor patient closely.
Theophylline: may increase plasma theophylline levels with other macrolides; effect of azithromycin is unknown. Theophylline levels should be monitored carefully.
Triazolam: may decrease clearance of triazolam. Monitor closely.
Warfarin: may increase INR with other macrolides; effect of azithromycin is unknown. INR must be monitored carefully.
Drug-food. *Any food:* decreased absorption of capsules and multidose oral suspension formulation. The preparations should be taken on an empty stomach.
Drug-lifestyle. *Sun exposure:* photosensitivity reactions may occur. Take precautions.

EFFECTS ON DIAGNOSTIC TESTS
None reported.

CONTRAINDICATIONS
Contraindicated in patients with hypersensitivity to erythromycin or other macrolides.

SPECIAL CONSIDERATIONS
▶ Use cautiously cautiously in patients with impaired hepatic function.
▶ A specimen for culture and sensitivity tests should be obtained before first dose is given. Therapy may begin pending results.
▶ Capsules and multidose oral suspension are administered 1 hour before or 2 hours after meals; the drug should not be administered with antacids. Tablets and single-dose packets for oral suspension can be taken with or without food.
▶ Superinfection may occur. The drug may cause overgrowth of nonsusceptible bacteria or fungi.
▶ Single-dose, 1-g packets for suspension should be reconstituted with 2 oz (60 ml)

---

of water, mixed, and administered to patient. Patient should rinse glass with additional 2 oz of water and drink to ensure he has consumed entire dose. Packets are not for pediatric use.

I.V. administration
▶ The drug is reconstitute in a 500-mg vial with 4.8 ml of sterile water for injection and shaken well until all the drug is dissolved (yields a concentration of 100 mg/ml). The solution is further diluted in at least 250 ml of normal saline, half-normal saline, D_5W, or lactated Ringer's solution to yield a concentration range of 1 to 2 mg/ml.
▶ *Alert:* A 500-mg dose of azithromycin is infused I.V. over 1 hour or more. A bolus or I.M. injection is never given.

Patient teaching
▶ Take drug as prescribed, even after feeling better.

clarithromycin
Biaxin, Klaricid§

Pregnancy Risk Category C

HOW SUPPLIED
Tablets (film-coated): 250 mg, 500 mg
Suspension: 125 mg/5 ml, 250 mg/5 ml

ACTION
Binds to the 50S subunit of bacterial ribosomes, blocking protein synthesis; bacteriostatic or bactericidal, depending on concentration.

Route	Onset	Peak	Duration
P.O.	Unknown	2-4 hr	Unknown

INDICATIONS & DOSAGE
Pharyngitis or tonsillitis due to Streptococcus pyogenes —

Adults: 250 mg P.O. q 12 hours for 10 days.
Children: 15 mg/kg/day P.O. in divided doses q 12 hours for 10 days.
Acute maxillary sinusitis due to S. pneumoniae, Haemophilus influenzae, *or* Moraxella (Branhamella) catarrhalis —
Adults: 500 mg P.O. q 12 hours for 14 days.
Children: 15 mg/kg/day P.O. in divided doses q 12 hours for 10 days.
Acute exacerbations of chronic bronchitis due to M. catarrhalis *or* S. pneumoniae; *pneumonia due to* S. pneumoniae, Chlamydia pneumoniae, *or* Mycoplasma pneumoniae —
Adults: 250 mg P.O. q 12 hours for 7 to 14 days.
Acute exacerbations of chronic bronchitis due to H. influenzae —
Adults: 500 mg P.O. q 12 hours for 7 to 14 days.
Uncomplicated skin and skin-structure infections due to Staphylococcus aureus *or* S. pyogenes —
Adults: 250 mg P.O. q 12 hours for 7 to 14 days.
Children: 15 mg/kg/day P.O. in divided doses q 12 hours for 10 days.
Acute otitis media caused by H. influenzae, M. catarrhalis, *or* S. pneumoniae —
Children: 7.5 mg/kg P.O. q 12 hours for 10 days.
Mycobacterium avium *complex (MAC) disease in patients with HIV infection* —
Adults: 500 mg P.O. q 12 hours, with other antimycobacterial drugs, for life.
Children: 7.5 mg/kg P.O. (maximum of 500 mg) q 12 hours, with other antimycobacterial drugs, for life.
Prophylaxis against MAC disease in patients with advanced HIV infection —
Adults: 500 mg P.O. q 12 hours.
Children: 7.5 mg/kg P.O. (maximum of 500 mg) q 12 hours.
Active duodenal ulcer associated with Helicobacter pylori *infection* —

Adults: 500 mg P.O. t.i.d. for 14 days with omeprazole 40 mg P.O. each morning. Omeprazole therapy should continue at a dose of 20 mg P.O. each morning for days 15 to 28. Or, 500 mg P.O. t.i.d. for 14 days with ranitidine bismuth citrate 400 mg P.O. b.i.d. Ranitidine bismuth citrate therapy continues for days 15 to 28. Or, 500 mg P.O. b.i.d. plus lansoprazole 30 mg P.O. b.i.d. and amoxicillin 1 g P.O. b.i.d. for 14 days.

Dental prophylaxis in patients allergic to penicillin —
Adults: 500 mg P.O. 1 hour before procedure.
Children: 15 mg/kg P.O. 1 hour before procedure.

ADVERSE REACTIONS
CNS: headache.
CV: *ventricular arrhythmias.*
GI: *diarrhea, nausea, abnormal taste,* dyspepsia, abdominal pain or discomfort, pseudomembranous colitis.
GU: *increased BUN.*
Hematologic: *increased INR,* **leukopenia, thrombocytopenia.**
Hepatic: elevated liver studies.
Skin: rash, ***Stevens-Johnson syndrome,*** urticaria.

INTERACTIONS
Drug-drug. *Cisapride, pimozide:* altered metabolism of these drugs, with prolongation of QT interval and ventricular tachycardia. Don't use these drugs with clarithromycin.
Carbamazepine: may increase serum levels of carbamazepine. Blood levels must be monitored.
Digoxin: may increase serum digoxin levels. Digitalis toxicity may occur.
Fluconazole: increased clarithromycin levels. Monitor closely.
Theophylline: increased plasma theophylline levels possible with other macrolides; effect of clarithromycin is unknown.

Theophylline levels must be monitored carefully.
Warfarin: increased INR possible with other macrolides; effect of clarithromycin is unknown. INR must be monitored carefully.
Zidovudine: decreased zidovudine levels. Effectiveness of zidovudine must be monitored closely.

EFFECTS ON DIAGNOSTIC TESTS
None reported.

CONTRAINDICATIONS
Contraindicated in patients with hypersensitivity to erythromycin or other macrolides and in those receiving cisapride, and pimozide.

SPECIAL CONSIDERATIONS
▶ Use cautiously in patients with hepatic or renal impairment.
▶ A specimen for culture and sensitivity tests must be obtained before giving first dose. Therapy may begin pending results.
▶ Patient must be monitored for superinfection. Drug may cause overgrowth of nonsusceptible bacteria or fungi.

Patient teaching
▶ Take drug as prescribed, even after feeling better.
▶ Report persistent adverse reactions.
▶ Drug may be taken with or without food. The suspension form should not be refrigerated. Discard unused portion after 10 days.

---

dirithromycin
Dynabac
Pregnancy Risk Category C

HOW SUPPLIED
Tablets (enteric-coated): 250 mg

ACTION
Inhibits bacterial RNA-dependent protein synthesis by binding to the 50S subunit of the ribosome.

Route	Onset	Peak	Duration
P.O.	Unknown	4 hr	Unknown

INDICATIONS & DOSAGE
Acute bacterial exacerbations of chronic bronchitis due to Moraxella (Branhamella) catarrhalis, Streptococcus pneumoniae, *or* Haemophilus influenzae; *secondary bacterial infection of acute bronchitis due to* M. catarrhalis *or* S. pneumoniae; *uncomplicated skin and skin-structure infections due to* Staphylococcus aureus *(methicillin-susceptible strains) or* S. pyogenes —
Adults and children ages 12 and older: 500 mg P.O. daily with food (or within 1 hour after eating) for 5 to 7 days.

Community-acquired pneumonia due to Legionella pneumophila, Mycoplasma pneumoniae, *or* S. pneumoniae —
Adults and children ages 12 and older: 500 mg P.O. daily with food (or within 1 hour after eating) for 14 days.

Pharyngitis or tonsillitis due to S. pyogenes —
Adults and children ages 12 and older: 500 mg P.O. daily with food (or within 1 hour after eating) for 10 days.

ADVERSE REACTIONS
CNS: headache, dizziness, vertigo, asthenia, insomnia.
GI: abdominal pain, nausea, diarrhea, vomiting, dyspepsia, flatulence.

Hepatic: increased liver enzyme levels.
Hematologic: increased platelet, eosinophil, and neutrophil counts.
Metabolic: hyperkalemia.
Respiratory: increased cough, dyspnea.
Skin: rash, pruritus, urticaria.
Other: pain, decreased bicarbonate levels, increased CK level.

INTERACTIONS
Drug-drug. *Antacids, H2-antagonists:* may slightly increase the absorption of dirithromycin when it is administered immediately after these drugs. Do not give together.
Theophylline: may alter steady-state plasma levels of theophylline. Theophylline plasma levels must be monitored. Dosage adjustments may be needed.
 Note: Alfentanil, oral anticoagulants, bromocriptine, carbamazepine, cyclosporine, digoxin, disopyramide, ergotamine, hexobarbital, lovastatin, phenytoin, triazolam, and valproate have been reported to interact with erythromycin products. It's unknown whether these same drugs interact with dirithromycin. Until further data are available, use caution during coadministration.
Drug-food. *Any food:* increased absorption. Drug should be administered with food.

EFFECTS ON DIAGNOSTIC TESTS
None reported.

CONTRAINDICATIONS
Contraindicated in patients with hypersensitivity to drug, erythromycin, or other macrolide antibiotics.

SPECIAL CONSIDERATIONS
▶ Use cautiously in patients with hepatic insufficiency and in breast-feeding women. Liver function test results must be monitored.
▶ Safety of drug in children under age 12 hasn't been established.

---

*Liquid contains alcohol.   **May contain tartrazine.   †Canada   ‡Australia   §U.K.   ◇OTC

▶ Culture and sensitivity results must be obtained to ensure organism is sensitive to dirithromycin. Drug isn't recommended for empiric use.

▶ Drug shouldn't be used in patients with known, suspected, or potential bacteremias because serum levels are inadequate to provide antibacterial coverage of organisms within the bloodstream.

▶ Drug should be administered with food or within 1 hour of food intake.

▶ Patient should be monitored for superinfection. Drug may cause overgrowth of nonsusceptible bacteria or fungi.

Patient teaching
▶ Take drug as prescribed, even after feeling better.
▶ Take drug with food or within 1 hour after eating and do not cut, chew, or crush the tablet.

erythromycin base

Apo-Erythro Base , EMU-V Tablets‡, E-Base, E-Mycin, Erybid , Eryc, Ery-Tab, Erythromid , Erythromycin Base Filmtab, Erythromycin Delayed-Release, Novo-Rythro Encap, PCE Dispertab

erythromycin estolate

Ilosone, Ilosone Pulvules, Novo-Rythro

erythromycin ethylsuccinate

Apo-Erythro-ES , E.E.S., EES-400‡, EES granules‡, Erymin§, EryPed, EryPed 200, EryPed 400, Erythroped§, Erythroped A§, Novo-Rythro

erythromycin lactobionate

Erythrocin, Erythromycin Lactobionate

erythromycin stearate

Apo-Erythro-S , Erythrocin Stearate, Novo-Rythro

Pregnancy Risk Category B

HOW SUPPLIED
erythromycin base
Tablets (enteric-coated): 250 mg, 333 mg, 500 mg
Tablets (filmtabs): 250 mg, 500 mg
Capsules (delayed-release): 250 mg
erythromycin estolate
Tablets: 500 mg
Capsules: 250 mg
Oral suspension: 125 mg/5 ml, 250 mg/5 ml
erythromycin ethylsuccinate
Tablets (film-coated): 400 mg
Tablets (chewable): 200 mg
Oral suspension: 200 mg/5 ml, 400 mg/5 ml, 100 mg/2.5 ml
erythromycin lactobionate
Injection: 500-mg, 1-g vials
erythromycin stearate
Tablets (film-coated): 250 mg, 500 mg

ACTION
Inhibits bacterial protein synthesis by binding to the 50S subunit of the ribosome. Bacteriostatic or bactericidal, depending on concentration.

Route	Onset	Peak	Duration
P.O.	Unknown	1-4 hr	Unknown
I.V.	Unknown	Immediate	Unknown

INDICATIONS & DOSAGE
Acute pelvic inflammatory disease due to Neisseria gonorrhoeae —

Adults: 500 mg I.V. (lactobionate) q 6 hours for 3 days; then 250 mg (base, estolate, stearate) or 400 mg (ethylsuccinate) P.O. q 6 hours for 7 days.
Children: initially, 20 mg/kg (base, ethylsuccinate, stearate) P.O. 1½ to 2 hours before procedure; then half the initial dose 6 hours later.

Intestinal amebiasis due to Entamoeba histolytica —
Adults: 400 mg P.O. (ethylsuccinate) q.i.d. for 10 to 14 days. I.V. therapy not effective.
Children: 30 to 50 mg/kg (ethylsuccinate) P.O. daily, in divided doses, for 10 to 14 days. I.V. therapy not effective.

Erythrasma —
Adults: 250 mg P.O. (base, estolate, stearate) t.i.d. for 21 days.

Rheumatic fever prophylaxis —
Adults: 250 mg (base, estolate, stearate) P.O. q 12 hours.

Mild to moderately severe respiratory tract, skin, and soft-tissue infections due to sensitive group A beta-hemolytic streptococci, Streptococcus pneumoniae, Mycoplasma pneumoniae, Corynebacterium diphtheriae, *or* Bordetella pertussis —
Adults: 250 to 500 mg (base, estolate, stearate) P.O. q 6 hours; or 400 to 800 mg (ethylsuccinate) P.O. q 6 hours; or 15 to 20 mg/kg I.V. daily, as continuous infusion or in divided doses q 6 hours for 10 days (3 weeks for Mycoplasma infection).
Children: 30 to 50 mg/kg (oral erythromycin salts) P.O. daily, in divided doses q 6 hours; or 15 to 20 mg/kg I.V. daily, in divided doses q 4 to 6 hours for 10 days (3 weeks for Mycoplasma infection).

Listeria monocytogenes infection —
Adults: 250 mg (base, estolate, stearate) P.O. q 6 hours or 500 mg P.O. q 12 hours.

Nongonococcal urethritis due to Ureaplasma urealyticum —
Adults: 500 mg (base, estolate, stearate) P.O. q 6 hours for at least 7 days.

Syphilis in patients allergic to penicillin —
Adults: 500 mg (base, estolate, stearate) P.O. q.i.d. for 2 weeks.

Legionnaires' disease —
Adults: 500 mg to 1 g I.V. or P.O. (base, estolate, stearate) or 800 to 1,600 mg (ethylsuccinate) q 6 hours for 10 to 14 days.

Uncomplicated urethral, endocervical, or rectal infections due to Chlamydia trachomatis *when tetracyclines are contraindicated* —
Adults: 500 mg (base, estolate, stearate) or 800 mg (ethylsuccinate) P.O. q.i.d. for 14 days.

Urogenital C. trachomatis *infections during pregnancy* —
Adults: 500 mg (base, estolate, stearate) P.O. q.i.d. for at least 7 days or 250 mg (base, estolate, stearate) or 400 mg (ethylsuccinate) P.O. q.i.d. for at least 14 days.

Conjunctivitis due to C. trachomatis *in neonates* —
Neonates: 50 mg/kg (base, estolate, stearate) P.O. daily in four divided doses for 14 days.

Pneumonia in infants caused by C. trachomatis —
Infants: 50 mg/kg/day (base, estolate, stearate) P.O. in four divided doses for 21 days or 15 to 20 mg/kg/day (lactobionate) I.V. as a continuous infusion or in four divided doses.

ADVERSE REACTIONS
CV: *ventricular arrhythmias.*
EENT: hearing loss (with high I.V. doses).
GI: *abdominal pain and cramping, nausea, vomiting, diarrhea.*
Hepatic: cholestatic jaundice (with erythromycin estolate).
Skin: urticaria, rash, eczema.
Other: overgrowth of nonsusceptible bacteria or fungi; *anaphylaxis;* fever; *vein irritation, thrombophlebitis after I.V. injection.*

INTERACTIONS

Drug-drug. *Carbamazepine:* increased carbamazepine blood levels and increased risk of toxicity. Monitor closely.

Cisapride: may increase cisapride levels, leading to toxicity including arrhythmias.

Clindamycin, lincomycin: may be antagonistic. Don't use together.

Cyclosporine: increased levels of cyclosporine. Monitor closely.

Digoxin: increased serum digoxin levels. Digoxin toxicity is possible.

Disopyramide: increased disopyramide plasma levels resulting, in some cases, in arrhythmias and prolonged QT intervals. ECG must be monitored.

Midazolam, triazolam: increased effects of these drugs. Monitor closely.

Oral anticoagulants: increased anticoagulant effect. PT and INR must be monitored closely.

Theophylline: decreased erythromycin blood level and increased theophylline toxicity. Use together cautiously.

Drug-herb. *Pill-bearing spurge:* may inhibit CYP3A enzymes, affecting drug metabolism. Use together cautiously.

EFFECTS ON DIAGNOSTIC TESTS

Erythromycin may interfere with fluorometric determination of urine catecholamines. AST and ALT may become falsely elevated during erythromycin therapy (rare).

CONTRAINDICATIONS

Contraindicated in patients with hypersensitivity to drug or other macrolides. Erythromycin estolate is contraindicated in patients with hepatic disease.

SPECIAL CONSIDERATIONS

‣ Use erythromycin salts cautiously in patients with impaired hepatic function. Liver function test results must be monitored.

‣ Erythromycin estolate isn't recommended during pregnancy because of the potential adverse effects on the mother and fetus.

‣ A urine specimen should be obtain for culture and sensitivity tests before first dose is given. Therapy may begin pending results.

‣ When administering suspension, the concentration should be noted.

‣ Patient should be monitored for superinfection. Drug may cause overgrowth of nonsusceptible bacteria or fungi.

‣ Hepatic function (increased serum levels of alkaline phosphatase, ALT, AST, and bilirubin may occur) must be monitored. Erythromycin estolate may cause serious hepatotoxicity in adults (reversible cholestatic jaundice). Other erythromycin salts cause hepatotoxicity to a lesser degree.

‣ Drug may falsely elevate levels of urinary 17-hydroxycorticosteroids and 17-ketosteroids.

‣ Drug may interfere with colorimetric assays, resulting in falsely elevated AST and ALT levels.

‣ Keep in mind that coated tablets or encapsulated pellets have caused fewer instances of GI upset; they may be better tolerated by patients who cannot tolerate erythromycin.

‣ Drug isn't indicated for the treatment of neurosyphilis.

I.V. administration

‣ Drug is reconstituted according to manufacturer's directions; each 250 mg is diluted in at least 100 ml of normal saline solution. Dosage is infused over 1 hour.

‣ *Alert:* Erythromycin lactobionate should not be administered with other drugs.

Patient teaching

‣ Take drug as prescribed, even after feeling better.

‣ Take oral form of drug with full glass of water 1 hour before or 2 hours after meals for best absorption. Drug may be taken with food if GI upset occurs. Coated tablets may be taken with meals. Don't drink fruit juice with drug. Chewable erythromycin tablets shouldn't be swallowed whole.

▶ Report adverse reactions, especially nausea, abdominal pain, and fever.

aztreonam
bacitracin
chloramphenicol sodium
   succinate
clindamycin hydrochloride
clindamycin palmitate
   hydrochloride
clindamycin phosphate
imipenem and cilastatin
   sodium
meropenem
nitrofurantoin macrocrystals
nitrofurantoin microcrystals
quinupristin/dalfopristin
spectinomycin hydrochloride
trimethoprim
vancomycin hydrochloride

COMBINATION PRODUCTS
Macrobid: nitrofurantoin macrocrystals
25 mg and nitrofurantoin monohydrate 75
mg.

---

aztreonam

Azactam

Pregnancy Risk Category B

HOW SUPPLIED
Injection: 500-mg vials, 1-g vials, 2-g vials

ACTION
Inhibits bacterial cell-wall synthesis, ultimately causing cell-wall destruction; bactericidal.

Route	Onset	Peak	Duration
I.V.	Unknown	Immediate	Unknown
I.M.	Unknown	< 1 hr	Unknown

INDICATIONS & DOSAGE
*Urinary tract infections, lower respirato-
ry tract infections, septicemia, skin and
skin-structure infections, intra-abdominal
infections, surgical infections, and gynecologic infections due to susceptible strains
of the following gram-negative aerobic
organisms:* Escherichia coli, Klebsiella
pneumoniae, Proteus mirabilis, Pseudomonas aeruginosa, Enterobacter cloacae,
Klebsiella oxytoca, *and* Citrobacter
species, Serratia marcescens; *respiratory
infections due to* Haemophilus influenzae —
Adults: 500 mg to 2 g I.V. or I.M. q 8 to
12 hours. For severe systemic or life-threatening infections, 2 g q 6 to 8 hours may
be given. Maximum dose is 8 g daily.
Children ages 9 months to 15 years:
30 mg/kg q 6 to 8 hours I.V. Maximum
dose is 120 mg/kg/day.
Dosage adjustment:
For adults with renal impairment, if creatinine clearance is 10 to 30 ml/minute,
dose is 1 to 2 g; then 50% usual dose at
the usual interval. If clearance is less than
10 ml/minute, 500 mg to 2 g; then 25%
usual dose at usual interval. For adults
with alcoholic cirrhosis, decrease dose by
20% to 25%.

ADVERSE REACTIONS
CNS: *seizures,* headache, insomnia, con-
fusion.
CV: hypotension.
GI: diarrhea, nausea, vomiting,
pseudomembranous colitis.
GU: increased BUN and serum creatinine
levels.
Hematologic: *neutropenia,* anemia, *pan-
cytopenia, thrombocytopenia,* leukocy-
tosis, thrombocytosis, prolonged PT, INR,
and PTT.
Hepatic: transient elevation of ALT and
AST.
Other: *hypersensitivity reactions (rash,
anaphylaxis),* thrombophlebitis, discom-

Reactions may be *common*, uncommon, *life-threatening*, or COMMON AND LIFE-THREATENING.

fort and swelling at I.M. injection site, increased LD.

INTERACTIONS

Drug-drug. *Aminoglycosides, beta-lactam antibiotics, other anti-infectives:* synergistic effectiveness. Avoid concomitant use.

Cefoxitin, imipenem: possible antagonistic effect. Avoid concomitant use.

Probenecid: increased serum aztreonam levels. Avoid concomitant use.

EFFECTS ON DIAGNOSTIC TESTS

Drug therapy alters urine glucose determinations using cupric sulfate (Clinitest or Benedict's reagent). Coombs' test results may become positive during therapy.

CONTRAINDICATIONS

Contraindicated in patients with hypersensitivity to drug.

SPECIAL CONSIDERATIONS

▶ Use cautiously in elderly patients and in those with impaired renal function. Dosage adjustment may be necessary. Renal function tests must be monitored.

▶ Culture and sensitivity tests must be obtained before giving first dose. Therapy may begin pending results.

▶ I.M. injections must be administered deep into a large muscle mass, such as the upper outer quadrant of the gluteus maximus or the lateral aspect of the thigh. Doses exceeding 1 g should be given I.V.

▶ I.M. injections are not given to children.

▶ Patient should be obseved for signs of superinfection.

▶ Because drug is ineffective against gram-positive and anaerobic organisms, anticipate using it with other antibiotics for immediate treatment of life-threatening illnesses. Aztreonam is a narrow-spectrum antibiotic, effective only against gram-negative organisms.

▶ Patients who are allergic to penicillins

or cephalosporins may not be allergic to aztreonam. However, close monitoring of those who have had an immediate hypersensitivity reaction to these antibiotics is recommended.

I.V. administration

▶ To administer a bolus of aztreonam, drug is injected slowly (over 3 to 5 minutes) directly into a vein or I.V. tubing. Infusions are given over 20 minutes to 1 hour.

Patient teaching

▶ I.M. drug injection may cause pain and swelling at injection site.

▶ Alert health care provider if discomfort occurs at I.V. insertion site.

▶ Report adverse reactions and signs of superinfection promptly.

bacitracin

BACI-IM, Bacitin

Pregnancy Risk Category C

HOW SUPPLIED

Injection: 50,000-U vials

ACTION

Hinders bacterial cell-wall synthesis, damaging the bacterial plasma membrane and making the cell more vulnerable to osmotic pressure.

Route	Onset	Peak	Duration
I.M.	Unknown	1-2 hr	Unknown

INDICATIONS & DOSAGE

Pneumonia or empyema due to susceptible staphylococci —

Infants weighing over 2.5 kg (5.5 lb): 1,000 U/kg I.M. daily, divided q 8 to 12 hours for up to 12 days.

Infants under 2.5 kg: 900 U/kg I.M. daily, divided q 8 to 12 hours for up to 12 days.

ADVERSE REACTIONS

EENT: ototoxicity.
GI: nausea, vomiting.
GU: *nephrotoxicity (albuminuria, cylindruria, oliguria, anuria, tubular and glomerular necrosis),* increased BUN and serum creatinine.
Skin: urticaria, rash.
Other: injection site pain.

INTERACTIONS

Drug-drug. *Inhalation anesthetics, neuromuscular blockers:* prolonged muscle weakness. Patient should be monitored for excessive muscle weakness or respiratory distress.
Nephrotoxic drugs (such as aminoglycosides): increased nephrotoxicity. Use together cautiously.

EFFECTS ON DIAGNOSTIC TESTS

Urinary sediment tests may show increased protein and cast excretion.

CONTRAINDICATIONS

Contraindicated in patients with impaired renal function or hypersensitivity to drug. Because of significant risk of neurotoxicity, limit I.M. use to infants with staphylococcal pneumonia.

SPECIAL CONSIDERATIONS

▶ Use cautiously in patients with myasthenia gravis and neuromuscular disease.
▶ Culture and sensitivity tests should be obtained before giving first dose.
▶ Baseline renal function studies must be assessed before and during therapy.
▶ Drug is administered by deep I.M. injection only.
▶ Concentration of bacitracin should be between 5,000 and 10,000 U/ml. A 50,000-U vial is reconstituted with 9.8 ml of diluent. Reconstituted vials are stored in a refrigerator. Drug is inactivated if stored at room temperature.
▶ Adequate fluid intake must be maintained and urine output monitored closely.
▶ Keep urine pH above 6 to reduce risk of nephrotoxicity.
▶ Prolonged therapy may result in overgrowth of nonsusceptible organisms, especially *Candida albicans.*

Patient teaching

▶ Injection may be painful.
▶ Report adverse reactions promptly.

---

chloramphenicol sodium succinate

Chloromycetin Sodium Succinate, Kemicetine§, Pentamycetin
Pregnancy Risk Category C

HOW SUPPLIED

Injection: 1-g vial; 1 g, 2 g premixed (frozen)

ACTION

Inhibits bacterial protein synthesis by binding to the 50S subunit of the ribosome; bacteriostatic.

Route	Onset	Peak	Duration
I.V.	Unknown	1-3 hr	Unknown

INDICATIONS & DOSAGE

Haemophilus influenzae *meningitis, acute* Salmonella typhi *infection, and meningitis, bacteremia, or other severe infections due to sensitive* Salmonella *species,* Rickettsia, *lymphogranuloma, psittacosis, or various sensitive gram-negative organisms —*
Adults: 50 to 100 mg/kg I.V. daily, divided q 6 hours. Maximum dose is 100 mg/kg daily.
Full-term infants over age 2 weeks with normal metabolic processes: up to 50 mg/kg I.V. daily, divided q 6 hours.
Premature infants, neonates ages 2

weeks or less, and children and infants with immature metabolic processes: 25 mg/kg I.V. once daily. I.V. route must be used to treat meningitis.

ADVERSE REACTIONS

CNS: headache, mild depression, confusion, delirium, peripheral neuropathy with prolonged therapy.
EENT: optic neuritis (in patients with cystic fibrosis), decreased visual acuity.
GI: nausea, vomiting, stomatitis, diarrhea, enterocolitis, glossitis.
Hepatic: jaundice.
Hematologic: *aplastic anemia, hypoplastic anemia, granulocytopenia, thrombocytopenia.*
Other: *hypersensitivity reactions, anaphylaxis, gray syndrome in neonates.*

INTERACTIONS

Drug-drug. *Anticoagulants, barbiturates, hydantoins, iron salts, sulfonylureas:* increased blood levels of these drugs possible. Patient should be monitored for toxicity.
Penicillins: synergistic effects may develop in the treatment of certain microorganisms, but antagonism may also occur. Patient should be monitored for effectiveness closely.
Rifampin: may reduce chloramphenicol levels. Patient should be monitored for changes in effectiveness.
Vitamin B$_{12}$: may decrease response of vitamin B in patients with pernicious anemia. Monitor closely.

EFFECTS ON DIAGNOSTIC TESTS

False elevation of urine PABA levels result if chloramphenicol is administered during a bentiromide test for pancreatic function. Treatment with chloramphenicol causes false-positive results on tests for urine glucose using cupric sulfate (Clinitest).

CONTRAINDICATIONS

Contraindicated in patients with hypersensitivity to drug.

SPECIAL CONSIDERATIONS

▶ Use cautiously in patients with impaired hepatic or renal function, acute intermittent porphyria, and G6PD deficiency and with other drugs that cause bone marrow suppression or blood disorders.
▶ *Alert:* Use with caution in premature infants and newborns because potentially fatal gray syndrome may occur. Symptoms include abdominal distention, gray cyanosis, vasomotor collapse, respiratory distress, and death within a few hours of symptom onset.
▶ A specimen for culture and sensitivity tests should be obtained before giving first dose. Therapy may begin pending results.
▶ Plasma levels must be monitored. Therapeutic plasma levels are as follows: peak, 10 to 20 mcg/ml; trough, 5 to 10 mcg/ml.
▶ CBC, platelets, serum iron, and reticulocytes should be monitored before and every 2 days during therapy, as ordered. Drug must be stopped immediately if anemia, reticulocytopenia, leukopenia, or thrombocytopenia develops.
▶ The patient should be monitored for evidence of superinfection.

I.V. administration

▶ The drug is given I.V. slowly over at least 1 minute. Injection site is checked daily for phlebitis and irritation.
▶ A 1-g vial of powder for injection is reconstituted with 10 ml of sterile water for injection. Concentration will be 100 mg/ml. Stable for 30 days at room temperature, but refrigeration recommended. Cloudy solutions should not be used.

Patient teaching

▶ Notify health care provider if adverse reactions occur, especially nausea, vomiting, diarrhea, fever, confusion, sore throat, or mouth sores.
▶ If receiving drug I.V., alert health care

provider if discomfort occurs at I.V. insertion site.

▶ Report symptoms of superinfection.

clindamycin hydrochloride
Cleocin HCl, Dalacin C ‡

clindamycin palmitate hydrochloride
Cleocin Pediatric, Dalacin C
Flavored Granules

clindamycin phosphate
Cleocin Phosphate, Dalacin C ‡,
Dalacin C Phosphate ‡

Pregnancy Risk Category B

HOW SUPPLIED
clindamycin hydrochloride
Capsules: 75 mg, 150 mg, 300 mg
clindamycin palmitate hydrochloride
Granules for oral solution: 75 mg/5 ml
clindamycin phosphate
Injection: 150-mg base/ml, 300-mg base/
2 ml, 600-mg base/4 ml, 900-mg base/
6 ml, 9,000-mg base/60 ml
Injectable infusion (in 5% dextrose):
300 mg (50 ml), 600 mg (50 ml), 900 mg
(50 ml)

ACTION
Inhibits bacterial protein synthesis by binding to the 50S subunit of the ribosome.

Route	Onset	Peak	Duration
P.O.	Unknown	45-60 min	Unknown
I.V.	Unknown	Immediate	Unknown
I.M.	Unknown	3 hr	Unknown

INDICATIONS & DOSAGE
Infections due to sensitive staphylococci, streptococci, pneumococci, Bacteroides,
Fusobacterium, Clostridium perfringens, *and other sensitive aerobic and anaerobic organisms —*
Adults: 150 to 450 mg P.O. q 6 hours; or 300 to 600 mg I.M. or I.V. q 6, 8, or 12 hours.
Children over age 1 month: 8 to 20 mg/kg P.O. daily, in divided doses q 6 to 8 hours; or 15 to 40 mg/kg I.M. or I.V. daily, in divided doses q 6 or 8 hours.
Pelvic inflammatory disease —
Adults: 900 mg I.V. q 8 hours with gentamicin. Continue at least 48 hours after improvement in symptoms; then switch to oral clindamycin 450 mg 4 times daily for a total course of 10 to 14 days or doxycycline 100 mg P.O. q 12 hours for total of 10 to 14 days.
Pneumocystis carinii pneumonia —
Adults: 600 mg I.V. q 6 hours (or, 900 mg IV q 8 hours) or 300 to 450 mg P.O. q 6 hours with primaquine.

ADVERSE REACTIONS
CV: thrombophlebitis.
GI: *nausea,* vomiting, abdominal pain, *diarrhea, pseudomembranous colitis.*
Hematologic: *transient leukopenia,* eosinophilia, *thrombocytopenia.*
Hepatic: jaundice; transient increases in serum bilirubin, alkaline phosphatase, and AST.
Skin: maculopapular rash, urticaria.
Other: *anaphylaxis.*

INTERACTIONS
Drug-drug. *Erythromycin:* may block access of clindamycin to its site of action. Avoid concomitant use.
Kaolin: decreased absorption of oral clindamycin. Administration times must be separated.
Neuromuscular blockers: potentiated neuromuscular blockade possible. Monitor closely.
Drug-food. *Diet foods with sodium cyclamate:* decreased serum level of drug. Don't use together.

EFFECTS ON DIAGNOSTIC TESTS
None reported.

CONTRAINDICATIONS
Contraindicated in patients with hypersensitivity to drug or lincomycin.

SPECIAL CONSIDERATIONS
▶ Use cautiously in neonates and patients with renal or hepatic disease, asthma, history of GI disease, or significant allergies.
▶ Drug does not penetrate blood-brain barrier.
▶ Culture and sensitivity tests should be obtained before giving first dose. Therapy may begin pending results.
▶ For I.M. administration, inject deeply. Rotate sites. Doses over 600 mg per injection are not recommended.
▶ I.M. injection may raise CK in response to muscle irritation.
▶ Reconstituted oral solution should not be refrigerated because it will thicken. Drug is stable for 2 weeks at room temperature.
▶ Renal, hepatic, and hematopoietic functions must be monitored during prolonged therapy.
▶ The patient must be observed for signs of superinfection.
▶ *Alert:* Opioid antidiarrheals should not be given to treat drug-induced diarrhea; they may prolong and worsen diarrhea.

I.V. administration
▶ When giving I.V., the site should be checked daily for phlebitis and irritation. For I.V. infusion, each 300 mg is diluted in 50-ml solution, and given no faster than 30 mg/minute (over 10 to 60 minutes). Drug is never given undiluted as a bolus.

Patient teaching
▶ If taking capsules, take them with a full glass of water to prevent esophageal irritation.
▶ I.M. injection may be painful.

▶ Alert health care provider if discomfort occurs at I.V. insertion site.
▶ Notify health care provider if adverse reactions, especially diarrhea, occur. Do not self-treat such diarrhea.

imipenem and cilastatin sodium
Primaxin IM, Primaxin IV
Pregnancy Risk Category C

HOW SUPPLIED
Powder for injection: 250 mg, 500 mg, 750 mg

ACTION
Imipenem is bactericidal and inhibits bacterial cell-wall synthesis. Cilastatin inhibits the enzymatic breakdown of imipenem in the kidneys, thereby achieving adequate antibacterial levels of imipenem in the urine.

Route	Onset	Peak	Duration
I.V.	Unknown	Immediate	Unknown
I.M.	Unknown	1-2 hr	Unknown

INDICATIONS & DOSAGE
Serious infections of the lower respiratory and urinary tracts, intra-abdominal and gynecologic infections, bacterial septicemia, bone and joint infections, skin and soft-tissue infections, and endocarditis. Most known microorganisms are susceptible: Acinetobacter, Enterococcus, Staphylococcus, Streptococcus, Escherichia coli, Haemophilus, Klebsiella, Morganella, Proteus, Enterobacter, Pseudomonas aeruginosa, *and* Bacteroides, *including* B. fragilis —
Adults weighing over 70 kg (154 lb): 250 mg to 1 g by I.V. infusion q 6 to 8 hours. Maximum daily dose is 50 mg/kg/day or 4 g/day, whichever is less. Or,

500 to 750 mg I.M. q 12 hours. Maximum daily dose is 1,500 mg.

Dosage adjustment:
For children over age 12, patients under 70 kg, and those who are renally impaired, refer to package insert for dosage adjustments based on weight, creatinine clearance, and severity of infection.

ADVERSE REACTIONS
CNS: *seizures,* dizziness, somnolence.
CV: hypotension.
GI: nausea, vomiting, diarrhea, *pseudomembranous colitis.*
GU: increased BUN or serum creatinine levels.
Hematologic: eosinophilia, *thrombocytopenia, leukopenia.*
Hepatic: transient increases in AST, ALT, alkaline phosphatase, and bilirubin.
Skin: rash, urticaria, pruritus.
Other: *hypersensitivity reactions, anaphylaxis,* fever; increased LD; thrombophlebitis, injection site pain.

INTERACTIONS
Drug-drug. *Aminoglycosides:* synergistic effect. Monitor closely.
Beta-lactam antibiotics: possible in vitro antagonism. Avoid concomitant use.
Ganciclovir: may cause seizures. Avoid concomitant use.
Probenecid: increased serum levels of cilastatin. Avoid concomitant use.

EFFECTS ON DIAGNOSTIC TESTS
Drug may interfere with glucose determination by Benedict's solution or Clinitest.

CONTRAINDICATIONS
Contraindicated in patients with hypersensitivity to drug.

SPECIAL CONSIDERATIONS
▶ Use cautiously in patients allergic to penicillins or cephalosporins because drug has similar properties.

▶ Also, use cautiously in patients with history of seizure disorders, especially if they also have compromised renal function.
▶ Use with caution in children under age 3 months.
▶ Culture and sensitivity tests should be obtained before giving first dose. Therapy may begin pending results.
▶ Dosage adjustment is necessary for patients with a creatinine clearance below 70 ml/minute. Renal function tests must be monitored.
▶ *Alert:* Drug should be discontinued if seizures develop and persist despite anticonvulsant therapy.
▶ Patient should be monitored for bacterial or fungal superinfections and resistant infections during and after therapy.

I.V. administration
▶ The drug must not be administered by direct I.V. bolus injection. Each 250- or 500-mg dose should be given by I.V. infusion over 20 to 30 minutes. Each 1-g dose should be infused over 40 to 60 minutes. If nausea occurs, the infusion may be slowed.
▶ When reconstituting powder, shake until the solution is clear. Solutions may range from colorless to yellow; variations of color within this range don't affect drug's potency. After reconstitution, solution is stable for 10 hours at room temperature and for 48 hours when refrigerated.

Patient teaching
▶ Report adverse reactions promptly.
▶ Alert health care provider if discomfort occurs at I.V. insertion site.
▶ Notify health care provider if loose stool or diarrhea occurs.

---

meropenem

Meronem§, Merrem I.V.

Pregnancy Risk Category B

HOW SUPPLIED

Powder for injection: 500 mg, 1 g

ACTION

Inhibits cell-wall synthesis in bacteria. It readily penetrates cell wall of most gram-positive and gram-negative bacteria to reach penicillin-binding-protein targets.

Route	Onset	Peak	Duration
I.V.	Unknown	1 hr	Unknown

INDICATIONS & DOSAGE

Complicated appendicitis and peritonitis due to viridans group streptococci, Escherichia coli, Klebsiella pneumoniae, Pseudomonas aeruginosa, Bacteroides fragilis, Bacteroides thetaiotaomicron, *and* Peptostreptococcus *species; bacterial meningitis (pediatric patients only) due to* Streptococcus pneumoniae, Haemophilus influenzae, *and* Neisseria meningitidis —

Adults: 1 g I.V. q 8 hours over 15 to 30 minutes as I.V. infusion or over 3 to 5 minutes as I.V. bolus injection (5 to 20 ml).

Children ages 3 months and older weighing below 50 kg (110 lb): 20 mg/kg (intra-abdominal infection) or 40 mg/kg (bacterial meningitis) q 8 hours over 15 to 30 minutes as I.V. infusion or over 3 to 5 minutes as I.V. bolus injection (5 to 20 ml). Maximum dosage is 2 g I.V. q 8 hours.

Children 50 kg and over: 1 g I.V. q 8 hours for intra-abdominal infections and 2 g I.V. q 8 hours for meningitis.

Dosage adjustment:

For patients with renal insufficiency or renal failure and creatinine clearance of 26 to 50 ml/minute, usual dose q 12 hours; if clearance is 10 to 25 ml/minute, half the usual dose q 12 hours; and if it is below 10 ml/minute, half the usual dose q 24 hours.

ADVERSE REACTIONS

CNS: *seizures,* headache.

GI: diarrhea, nausea, vomiting, constipation, pseudomembranous colitis, oral candidiasis, glossitis.

GU: increased creatinine or BUN levels, presence of RBCs in urine.

Hematologic: increased or decreased platelet count, increased eosinophil count, positive direct or indirect Coombs' test, decreased hemoglobin level or hematocrit, decreased WBC count, prolonged or shortened PT, INR, or PTT.

Hepatic: increased levels of ALT, AST, alkaline phosphatase, LD, and bilirubin.

Respiratory: *apnea,* dyspnea.

Skin: rash, pruritus.

Other: *hypersensitivity, anaphylactic reaction;* inflammation, phlebitis, thrombophlebitis (at injection site).

INTERACTIONS

Drug-drug. *Probenecid:* inhibited renal excretion of meropenem. Drug competes with meropenem for active tubular secretion, which significantly increases elimination half-life of drug and the extent of systemic exposure. Administration of probenecid with meropenem is not recommended.

EFFECTS ON DIAGNOSTIC TESTS

Drug may cause a positive direct or indirect Coombs' test.

CONTRAINDICATIONS

Contraindicated in patients with hypersensitivity to components of drug or other drugs in same class and in those who have demonstrated anaphylactic reactions to beta-lactams.

SPECIAL CONSIDERATIONS

▶ Use cautiously in elderly patients and in

those with a history of seizure disorders or impaired renal function.

▶ Safety and effectiveness of drug have not been established for patients under age 3 months.

▶ It's unknown whether meropenem appears in breast milk. Use drug cautiously in breast-feeding women.

▶ Drug is not used to treat methicillin-resistant staphylococci.

▶ A specimen for culture and sensitivity test should be obtained before giving first dose. Therapy may begin pending test results.

▶ *Alert:* Serious and occasionally fatal hypersensitivity reactions have been reported in patients receiving therapy with beta-lactams. Before therapy is initiated, determine whether previous hypersensitivity reactions to penicillins, cephalosporins, other beta-lactams, or other allergens have occurred.

▶ Discontinue drug if an allergic reaction occurs. Serious anaphylactic reactions require immediate emergency treatment.

▶ Seizures and other CNS adverse reactions associated with meropenem therapy can occur in patients with CNS disorders, bacterial meningitis, and compromised renal function.

▶ If seizures occur during drug therapy, discontinue infusion. Dosage adjustment may be necessary.

▶ Patient should be monitored for signs and symptoms of superinfection. Drug may cause overgrowth of nonsusceptible bacteria or fungi.

▶ Periodic assessment of organ system functions, including renal, hepatic, and hematopoietic function, is recommended during prolonged therapy.

▶ Patient's fluid balance and weight must be monitored carefully.

I.V. administration

▶ For I.V. bolus administration, 10 ml of sterile water for injection is added to 500 mg/20-ml vial or 20 ml to 1 g/30-ml vial. The vial is shaken to dissolve, and let standing until clear.

▶ For I.V. infusion, infusion vials (500 mg/100 ml and 1 g/100 ml) may be directly reconstituted with a compatible infusion fluid. Or, an injection vial may be reconstituted, then the resulting solution added to an I.V. container and further diluted with an appropriate infusion fluid. Don't use ADD-Vantage vials for this purpose. For ADD-Vantage vials, constitute only with half-normal saline injection, normal saline injection, or 5% dextrose injection in 50-, 100-, or 250-ml Abbott ADD-Vantage flexible diluent containers. The manufacturer's guidelines must be followed closely when using ADD-Vantage vials.

▶ Meropenem should not be added or mixed with solutions containing other drugs.

▶ Freshly prepared solutions of drug should be used immediately whenever possible. Stability of drug varies with type of drug used (injection vial, infusion vial, or ADD-Vantage container). Consult manufacturer's literature for details.

Patient teaching

▶ If breast-feeding, be aware of the risk of transmitting drug to infant through breast milk.

▶ Report adverse reactions or signs and symptoms of superinfection.

---

nitrofurantoin macrocrystals
Macrobid, Macrodantin

nitrofurantoin microcrystals
Apo-Nitrofurantoin , Furadantin, Furalan, Macrodantin, Novo-Furantoin

Pregnancy Risk Category B

HOW SUPPLIED
nitrofurantoin macrocrystals
Capsules: 25 mg, 50 mg, 100 mg
nitrofurantoin microcrystals
Oral suspension: 25 mg/5 ml

ACTION
Unknown. Appears to interfere with bacterial enzyme systems and possibly with bacterial cell-wall formation.

Route	Onset	Peak	Duration
P.O.	Unknown	Unknown	Unknown

INDICATIONS & DOSAGE
Urinary tract infections due to susceptible Escherichia coli, Staphylococcus aureus, *enterococci; or certain strains of* Klebsiella *and* Enterobacter —
Adults and children over age 12: 50 to 100 mg P.O. q.i.d. with meals and h.s.
Children ages 1 month to 12 years: 5 to 7 mg/kg P.O. daily, divided q.i.d.
Long-term suppression therapy —
Adults: 50 to 100 mg P.O. daily h.s.
Children: 1 mg/kg P.O. daily in a single dose h.s. or divided into two doses given q 12 hours.

ADVERSE REACTIONS
CNS: *peripheral neuropathy,* headache, dizziness, drowsiness, *ascending polyneu-*

ropathy with high doses or renal impairment.
GI: *anorexia, nausea, vomiting,* abdominal pain, *diarrhea.*
Hematologic: *hemolysis in patients with G6PD deficiency, agranulocytosis, thrombocytopenia.*
Hepatic: *hepatitis, hepatic necrosis,* elevated bilirubin and alkaline phosphatase.
Metabolic: hypoglycemia.
Respiratory: *pulmonary sensitivity reactions, asthmatic attacks.*
Skin: maculopapular, erythematous, or eczematous eruption; transient alopecia; pruritus; urticaria; *exfoliative dermatitis; Stevens-Johnson syndrome.*
Other: *hypersensitivity reactions, anaphylaxis,* drug fever, overgrowth of nonsusceptible organisms in urinary tract.

INTERACTIONS
Drug-drug. *Magnesium-containing antacids:* decreased nitrofurantoin absorption. Administration times should be separated by 1 hour.
Probenecid, sulfinpyrazone: increased blood levels and decreased urine levels. May result in increased toxicity and lack of therapeutic effect. Don't use together.
Drug-food. *Any food:* increased absorption. Drug is given with food.

EFFECTS ON DIAGNOSTIC TESTS
Nitrofurantoin may cause false-positive results in urine glucose tests using cupric sulfate (such as Benedict's reagent, Fehling's solution, or Clinitest) because it reacts with these agents.

CONTRAINDICATIONS
Contraindicated in infants ages 1 month and under and in patients with moderate to severe renal impairment, anuria, oliguria, or creatinine clearance under 60 ml/minute. Contraindicated in pregnancy at term (38 to 42 weeks) and during labor and delivery.

---

*Liquid contains alcohol.   **May contain tartrazine.   †Canada   ‡Australia   §U.K.   ◇OTC

SPECIAL CONSIDERATIONS

▶ Use cautiously in patients with renal impairment, anemia, diabetes mellitus, electrolyte abnormalities, vitamin B deficiency, debilitating disease, and G6PD deficiency. Drug may precipitate an asthma attack in patients with a history of asthma.

▶ Urine specimen for culture and sensitivity tests should be obtained before starting therapy and repeat as needed. Therapy may begin pending results.

▶ Drug is given with food or milk to minimize GI distress and improve absorption.

▶ Fluid intake and output is monitored carefully. May turn urine brown or darker.

▶ CBC and pulmonary status is monitored regularly.

▶ The patient should be monitored for signs of superinfection. Use of nitrofurantoin may result in growth of nonsusceptible organisms, especially Pseudomonas.

▶ The patient should be monitored for pulmonary sensitivity reactions including cough, chest pain, fever, chills, dyspnea, pulmonary infiltration with consolidation or effusions.

▶ *Alert:* Hypersensitivity may develop when used for long-term therapy.

▶ Some patients may experience fewer adverse GI effects with nitrofurantoin macrocrystals.

▶ Dual-release capsules (25 mg nitrofurantoin macrocrystals combined with 75 mg nitrofurantoin monohydrate) enable patients to take drug only twice daily.

▶ Continue treatment for 3 days after sterile urine specimens have been obtained.

▶ Store drug in amber container. Keep away from metals other than stainless steel or aluminum to avoid precipitate formation.

Patient teaching

▶ Take drug for as long as prescribed, exactly as directed, even after feeling better.

▶ Take drug with food or milk to minimize stomach upset.

▶ Report adverse reactions.

▶ Drug may turn urine a harmless dark yellow or brown color.

▶ Do not store drug in container made of metal other than stainless steel or aluminum.

quinupristin/dalfopristin
Synercid

Pregnancy Risk Category B

HOW SUPPLIED
Injection: 500 mg/10 ml (150 mg quinupristin and 350 mg dalfopristin)

ACTION
The two antibiotics work synergistically to inhibit or destroy susceptible bacteria through combined inhibition on protein synthesis in bacterial cells. Without the ability to manufacture new proteins, the bacterial cells are inactivated or die.

Route	Onset	Peak	Duration
I.V.	Unknown	Unknown	Unknown

INDICATIONS & DOSAGE
Serious or life-threatening infections associated with vancomycin-resistant Enterococcus faecium *(VREF) bacteremia —*
Adults and adolescents ages 16 and older: 7.5 mg/kg I.V. infusion over 1 hour every 8 hours. Treatment duration should be determined by site and severity of infection.

Complicated skin and skin structure infections due to Staphylococcus aureus *(methicillin susceptible) or* Streptococcus pyogenes —
Adults and adolescents ages 16 and older: 7.5 mg/kg by I.V. infusion over 1 hour every 12 hours for at least 7 days.

ADVERSE REACTIONS

CNS: headache, pain.
CV: thrombophlebitis.
GI: nausea, diarrhea, vomiting.
Hepatic: *elevated total and conjugated bilirubin levels,* altered liver function studies.
Musculoskeletal: arthralgia, myalgia.
Skin: rash, pruritus.
Other: *inflammation, pain, edema at infusion site; infusion site reaction.*

INTERACTIONS

Drug-drug. *Cyclosporine:* metabolism is reduced and levels may be increased. Cyclosporine levels must be monitored.
Drugs metabolized by cytochrome P-450 3A4 (carbamazepine, delavirdine, diazepam, diltiazem, disopyramide, docetaxel, indinavir, lidocaine, lovastatin, methylprednisolone, midazolam, nevirapine, nifedipine, paclitaxel, ritonavir, tacrolimus, verapamil, vinblastine, and others): increased plasma levels of these drugs that could increase their therapeutic effects and adverse reactions. Use together cautiously.
Drugs metabolized by cytochrome P-450 3A4 that may prolong the QT^c interval (such as cisapride, quinidine): decreased metabolism of these drugs, resulting in prolongation of QT^c interval. Avoid concomitant use.

EFFECTS ON DIAGNOSTIC TESTS

None reported.

CONTRAINDICATIONS

Contraindicated in patients with hypersensitivity to drug or other streptogramin antibiotics.

SPECIAL CONSIDERATIONS

▶ Quinupristin/dalfopristin isn't active against *Enterococcus faecalis.* Appropriate blood cultures are needed to avoid misidentifying *E. faecalis* as *E. faecium.*
▶ Because mild to life-threatening pseudomembranous colitis has been reported with use of quinupristin/dalfopristin, consider this diagnosis in patients who develop diarrhea during or following therapy with drug.
▶ Adverse reactions, such as arthralgia and myalgia, may be reduced by decreasing dosage interval to every 12 hours.
▶ Because overgrowth of nonsusceptible organisms may occur, the patient is monitored closely for signs and symptoms of superinfection.
▶ Liver function tests should be monitored during therapy.

I.V. administration

▶ The powder for injection is reconstituted by adding 5 ml of either sterile water for injection or D$_5$W and gently swirling the vial by manual rotation to ensure dissolution; avoid shaking to limit foaming. Reconstituted solutions must be further diluted within 30 minutes.
▶ The appropriate dose, according to patient's weight, of reconstituted solution should be added to 250 ml of D$_5$W to make a final concentration of no more than 2 mg/ml. This diluted solution is stable for 5 hours at room temperature or 54 hours if refrigerated.
▶ Fluid restricted patients with a central venous catheter may receive dose in 100 ml of D$_5$W. This concentration isn't recommended for peripheral venous administration.
▶ If moderate to severe peripheral venous irritation occurs, consider increasing infusion volume to 500 or 750 ml, changing injection site, or infusing by a central venous catheter.
▶ All doses are administered by I.V. infusion over 1 hour. An infusion pump or device may be used to control rate of infusion.
▶ *Alert:* Quinupristin/dalfopristin is incompatible with saline and heparin solutions. The drug must not be diluted with solutions containing saline or infuse into lines that con-

tain saline or heparin. The line should be flushed with D_5W before and after each dose.

Patient teaching
▶ Immediately report irritation at I.V. site, pain in joints or muscles, and diarrhea.
▶ Report persistent or worsening signs and symptoms of infection, such as pain or erythema.

spectinomycin hydrochloride
Trobicin

Pregnancy Risk Category B

HOW SUPPLIED
Powder for injection: 2 g

ACTION
Inhibits protein synthesis by binding to the 30S subunit of the ribosome.

Route	Onset	Peak	Duration
I.M.	Unknown	1-2 hr	Unknown

INDICATIONS & DOSAGE
Acute gonococcal urethritis and proctitis in men and cervicitis and proctitis in women; alternative therapy for patient allergic to beta-lactam antibiotics —
Adults: 2 g I.M. single dose injected deeply into the upper outer quadrant of the buttock.
  Disseminated gonococcal infection —
Adults: 2 g I.M. q 12 hours for 24 to 48 hours; then switch to cefixime, ciprofloxacin, or ofloxacin.

ADVERSE REACTIONS
CNS: insomnia, dizziness.
GI: nausea.
GU: decreased urine output and creatinine clearance, increased BUN.
Hematologic: decreased hemoglobin levels and hematocrit.

Hepatic: increased AST, serum alkaline phosphatase.
Skin: urticaria.
Other: *anaphylaxis,* fever, chills, injection site pain.

INTERACTIONS
None significant.

EFFECTS ON DIAGNOSTIC TESTS
None reported.

CONTRAINDICATIONS
Contraindicated in patients with hypersensitivity to drug.

SPECIAL CONSIDERATIONS
▶ Spectinomycin isn't effective for pharyngeal gonorrhea.
▶ Know that fever and chills may mask or delay the symptoms of incubating syphilis.
▶ The vial is shaken vigorously after reconstitution and before withdrawing dose. The drug is stored at room temperature after reconstitution and use within 24 hours.
▶ A 20G needle is used to administer drug.

Patient teaching
▶ Drug is not effective in the treatment of syphilis. Serologic test for syphilis should be performed before therapy begins and for 3 months afterward.
▶ Report adverse reactions promptly.
▶ All infection sites should be cultured 7 days after treatment to confirm eradication of organism.

trimethoprim
Ipral§, Monotrim§, Proloprim, Trimopan§, Trimpex, Triprim‡

Pregnancy Risk Category C

HOW SUPPLIED
Tablets: 100 mg, 200 mg

ACTION

Interferes with the action of dihydrofolate reductase, inhibiting bacterial synthesis of folic acid.

Route	Onset	Peak	Duration
P.O.	Unknown	1-4 hr	Unknown

INDICATIONS & DOSAGE

Uncomplicated urinary tract infections due to susceptible strains of Escherichia coli, Proteus mirabilis, Klebsiella pneumoniae, Enterobacter *species, and coagulase-negative* Staphylococcus, *including* S. saprophyticus —

Adults: 200 mg P.O. daily as a single dose or in divided doses q 12 hours for 10 days.

Note: Drug is not recommended for children under age 12.

Dosage adjustment:

For patients with creatinine clearance of 15 to 30 ml/minute, 50 mg P.O. q 12 hours; if clearance is below 15 ml/minute, don't use drug.

ADVERSE REACTIONS

GI: *epigastric distress, nausea, vomiting,* glossitis.

GU: increased BUN and serum creatinine.

Hematologic: *thrombocytopenia, leukopenia,* megaloblastic anemia, methemoglobinemia.

Hepatic: elevated liver function test results.

Skin: *rash, pruritus, exfoliative dermatitis.*

Other: fever.

INTERACTIONS

Drug-drug. *Phenytoin:* may decrease phenytoin metabolism and increase its serum levels. The patient must be monitored for toxicity.

EFFECTS ON DIAGNOSTIC TESTS

Drug interferes with serum methotrexate assays.

CONTRAINDICATIONS

Contraindicated in patients with hypersensitivity to drug and in those with documented megaloblastic anemia due to folate deficiency.

SPECIAL CONSIDERATIONS

▶ Use cautiously in patients with impaired hepatic or renal function. Dosage should be decreased in patients with severely impaired renal function. Also, use cautiously in patients with possible folate deficiency. Renal and liver function test results must be monitored.

▶ Urine specimen for culture and sensitivity tests should be obtained before giving first dose. Therapy may begin pending results.

▶ CBC is monitored routinely. Clinical signs and symptoms, such as sore throat, fever, pallor, or purpura, may be early indications of serious blood disorders.

▶ The patient's fluid balance should be monitored.

▶ *Alert:* Prolonged use of trimethoprim at high doses may cause bone marrow suppression.

▶ Because resistance to trimethoprim develops rapidly when administered alone, it's usually given with other drugs.

▶ *Alert:* Trimethoprim is also used with sulfamethoxazole; don't confuse the two products.

Patient teaching

▶ Take entire amount of drug as prescribed, even after feeling better.

▶ Report adverse reactions promptly, especially signs of infection or unusual bruising.

▶ Adequate hydration is necessary during therapy.

---

vancomycin hydrochloride

Vancocin, Vancoled

Pregnancy Risk Category C

HOW SUPPLIED

Capsules: 125 mg, 250 mg
Powder for oral solution: 1-g bottles, 10-g bottles
Powder for injection: 500-mg vials, 1-g vials, 5 g, 10 g

ACTION

Hinders bacterial cell-wall synthesis, damaging the bacterial plasma membrane and making the cell more vulnerable to osmotic pressure. Also interferes with RNA synthesis.

Route	Onset	Peak	Duration
P.O.	Unknown	Unknown	Unknown
I.V.	Unknown	Immediate	Unknown

INDICATIONS & DOSAGE

Serious or severe infections when other antibiotics are ineffective or contraindicated, including those caused by methicillin-resistant Staphylococcus aureus, Staphylococcus epidermidis, *or diphtheroid organisms —*
Adults: 1 to 1.5 g I.V. q 12 hours (dose based on weight and renal function; longer dosing intervals necessary in renal dysfunction).
Children: 10 mg/kg I.V. q 6 hours.
Neonates and young infants: 15 mg/kg I.V. loading dose, followed by 10 mg/kg I.V. q 12 hours if child is under age 1 week or 10 mg/kg I.V. q 8 hours if age is over 1 week but under 1 month.
Antibiotic-associated pseudomembranous (Clostridium difficile) *and* staphylococcal enterocolitis —
Adults: 125 to 500 mg P.O. q 6 hours for 7 to 10 days.
Children: 40 mg/kg P.O. daily, in divided doses q 6 hours for 7 to 10 days. Maximum daily dose is 2 g.
Endocarditis prophylaxis for dental procedures —
Adults: 1 g I.V. slowly over 1 hour, starting 1 hour before procedure.
Children: 20 mg/kg I.V. over 1 hour, starting 1 hour before procedure.

ADVERSE REACTIONS

CV: hypotension.
EENT: tinnitus, ototoxicity.
GI: nausea, pseudomembranous colitis.
GU: *nephrotoxicity,* increased BUN and serum creatinine levels.
Hematologic: *neutropenia, leukopenia,* eosinophilia.
Respiratory: wheezing, dyspnea.
Skin: "red-neck" syndrome with rapid I.V. infusion.
Other: chills, fever, *anaphylaxis,* superinfection, pain, thrombophlebitis at injection site.

INTERACTIONS

Drug-drug. *Aminoglycosides, amphotericin B, cisplatin, pentamidine:* increased risk of nephrotoxicity and ototoxicity. Monitor closely.

EFFECTS ON DIAGNOSTIC TESTS

None reported.

CONTRAINDICATIONS

Contraindicated in patients with hypersensitivity to drug.

SPECIAL CONSIDERATIONS

‣ Use cautiously in patients receiving other neurotoxic, nephrotoxic, or ototoxic drugs; in patients over age 60; and in those with impaired hepatic or renal function, preexisting hearing loss, or allergies to other antibiotics. Patients with renal dysfunction require dosage adjustment. Serum levels should be monitored to adjust I.V. dosage. Normal therapeutic levels of vancomycin are as follows: peak, 30 to

40 mg/L (drawn 1 hour after infusion ends); trough, 5 to 10 mg/L (drawn just before next dose is given).

▶ Patient's fluid balance is monitored and patient is observed for oliguria and cloudy urine.

▶ Culture and sensitivity tests should be obtained before giving first dose. Therapy may begin pending results.

▶ Hearing evaluation and renal function studies must be obtained before therapy.

▶ Patient is carefully monitored for "red-neck" syndrome, which can occur if drug is infused too rapidly. Signs and symptoms include maculopapular rash on face, neck, trunk, and extremities, pruritis and hypotension associated with histamine release. If this reaction occurs, the infusion is stopped.

▶ Drug is not for I.M. use.

▶ *Alert:* Oral administration is ineffective for systemic infections, and I.V. administration is ineffective for pseudomembranous (*C. difficile*) diarrhea.

▶ Keep in mind that the oral preparation is stable for 2 weeks if refrigerated.

▶ Renal function (BUN, serum creatinine, urinalysis, creatinine clearance, and urine output) is monitored during therapy. Also, the patient should be monitored for signs and symptoms of superinfection.

▶ The patient's hearing should be evaluated during prolonged therapy.

▶ When drug is used to treat staphylococcal endocarditis, it will be given for at least 4 weeks.

I.V. administration

▶ For I.V. infusion, the drug is diluted in 200 ml normal saline for injection or D₅W, and infused over 60 minutes; if dose is greater than 1 g, it is infused over 90 minutes. The site must be checked daily for phlebitis and irritation. Report pain at infusion site. Avoid extravasation; severe irritation and necrosis can result.

▶ I.V. solution must be refrigerated after reconstitution and use within 14 days.

Patient teaching

▶ Take entire amount of drug exactly as directed, even after feeling better.

▶ If receiving drug I.V., alert health care provider if discomfort occurs at I.V. insertion site.

Pregnancy Risk Categories

Each systemically absorbed drug has been assigned a pregnancy risk category based upon available clinical and preclinical information. The Pregnancy Risk Category parallels the five Pregnancy Categories (A, B, C, D, and X) assigned by the Food and Drug Administration (FDA) to reflect a drug's potential to cause birth defects. Although drugs are best avoided during pregnancy, this rating system permits rapid assessment of the risk-benefit ratio should drug administration to a pregnant woman become necessary.

Drugs in category A are generally considered safe to use in pregnancy; drugs in category X are generally contraindicated.

▶ A: Adequate studies in pregnant women have failed to show a risk to the fetus.

▶ B: Animal studies have not shown a risk to the fetus, but controlled studies have not been conducted in pregnant women; or animal studies have shown an adverse effect on the fetus, but adequate studies in pregnant women have not shown a risk to the fetus.

▶ C: Animal studies have shown an adverse effect on the fetus, but adequate studies have not been conducted in humans. The benefits from use in pregnant women may be acceptable despite potential risks.

▶ D: The drug may cause risk to the human fetus, but the potential benefits of use in pregnant women may be acceptable despite the risks (such as a life-threatening situation or a serious disease for which safer drugs can't be used or are ineffective).

▶ X: Studies in animals or humans show fetal abnormalities, or adverse reaction reports indicate evidence of fetal risk. The risks involved clearly outweigh potential benefits.

▶ NR: Not rated.

APPENDICES
SELECTED REFERENCES
INDEX

APPENDIX A:
RARE INFECTIOUS DISEASES

RARE DISEASE	CAUSE AND DESCRIPTION	TREATMENT
African trypanosomiasis: sleeping sickness	*Trypanosoma* transmitted by tsetse fly bite. Febrile illness followed months or years later by progressive neurologic impairment and death; occurs in two forms: Gambian — typically found in west and central Africa — and Rhodesian — a more virulent type found in East Africa.	For Gambian form, stage 1 (normal cerebrospinal fluid [CSF]), pentamidine; stage 2 (abnormal CSF), eflornithine or melarsoprol. For Rhodesian form, stage 1, use suramin; stage 2, melarsoprol.
American trypanosomiasis: Chagas' disease	*Trypanosoma cruzi* transmitted by the infected species of triatomine bugs; can also be transmitted through transfusion of blood donated by an infected person. Febrile illness prevalent in Mexico, Central America, South America, Texas, and southwestern United States; often benign in adults, although cardiomyopathy may develop; can be severe in children.	Nifurtimox or benznidazole
Anthrax: woolsorters' disease	Acute bacterial infection caused by *Bacillus anthracis;* affects people who have contact with contaminated animals or their hides, bones, fur, hair, or wool. Three forms in humans: cutaneous, inhalational, and GI.	High-dose penicillin; isolation

RARE DISEASE	CAUSE AND DESCRIPTION	TREATMENT
Armstrong's disease: lymphocytic choriomeningitis	Form of meningitis caused by an arenavirus infection that follows exposure to food or dust contaminated by rodents; virus found to occur naturally in guinea pigs, monkeys, dogs, and swine. Occurs in adults ages 20 to 40 during fall and winter; usually asymptomatic or mild, although severe meningoencephalitis may occur.	Supportive and symptomatic treatment. Infection can be prevented by careful hand washing (although mode of transmission may be airborne).
Babesiosis	*Babesia microti* transmitted by infected ticks. Disease occurs in coastal areas of northeastern United States; rarely fatal. Attacks RBCs; initial symptoms include fatigue, loss of appetite, and general malaise; then fever, drenching sweats, muscle aches, and headache. Symptoms may last several days to months; may be severe if immune system is already compromised.	Quinine and clindamycin
Barometer-maker's disease: chronic mercury poisoning	Mercury poisoning resulting from chronic exposure to mercury or its vapors or to contaminated fish or fungicides used on seeds. Soreness of gums, loosening of teeth, salivation, fetid breath, abdominal cramping and diarrhea, weakness, ataxia, intention tremors, irritability and depression, birth defects, and death.	Evacuate stomach, lavage with milk or sodium bicarbonate, and administer activated charcoal, but treat with dimercaprol promptly to prevent fatal progression. Neurologic toxicity is not considered reversible, although some recommend trial dose of penicillamine.
Basal cell carcinoma of the eye	Cause unknown; predisposing factors include exposure to sunlight, radiation, chemicals, and other carcinogens. Common extraorbital cancer affects the eyelids, conjunctivae, and cornea.	Surgery; possibly radiation therapy

RARE DISEASE	CAUSE AND DESCRIPTION	TREATMENT
Bouillaud's disease: rheumatic endocarditis	Delayed sequel to pharyngeal infection by group B streptococci. Manifests as a heart murmur of either mitral or aortic insufficiency; in severe cases, pericarditis and heart failure may occur.	No specific cure; supportive therapy to reduce mortality and morbidity
Bovine spongiform encephalopathy: mad cow disease	Proteinaceous infectious particle (prion) causes degenerative brain disorder in cattle. Loss of coordination, abandonment of routine habits, and unpredictable behavior may occur; may be transferred to humans through infected milk or beef products.	No specific cure; supportive therapy
Brainerd diarrhea	Infectious agent, possibly a chemical toxin in unpasteurized milk and untreated well water. Self-limited, noncontagious illness; 10 to 20 episodes per day of explosive, watery diarrhea is characterized by urgency and fecal incontinence. Accompanying symptoms include gas, mild abdominal cramping, and fatigue.	Supportive therapy includes high doses of opioid antimotility drugs, such as loperamide, diphenoxylate, and paregoric
Brill-Zinsser disease	*Rickettsia prowazekii;* relapse of typhus, which can occur years after the primary attack.	Tetracycline, chloramphenicol, analgesics, antipyretics
Brown-Symmers disease	Viral pathogens (rabies, measles, mumps, rubella, influenza) cause acute serous encephalitis in children.	Supportive therapy; control of intracranial pressure; correction of metabolic problems, disseminated intravascular coagulation, bleeding, renal failure, pulmonary emboli, and pneumonia; invariably fatal

RARE DISEASE	CAUSE AND DESCRIPTION	TREATMENT
Burkitt's tumor: Burkitt's lymphoma	Unknown, but Epstein-Barr virus suspected in some cases. Undifferentiated malignant lymphoma that usually begins as a large mass in the jaw (African's Burkitt) or an an abdominal mass (American Burkitt's)	Chemotherapy; radiation therapy; surgical resection in extensive local disease; in patients with a relapse, autologous bone marrow transplantation
Cat-scratch fever: cat-scratch disease	Subacute self-limiting disease due to *Bartonella henoelae* that is characterized by a primary local lesion and regional lymphadenopathy; more common in children and young adults in contact with cats and dogs; disseminated form — bacillary angiomatosis — found in immunocompromised persons such as those infected with human immunodeficiency virus.	Symptomatic management; if patient is ill, can use trimethoprim-sulfamethoxazole, ciprofloxacin, gentamicin, or rifampin
Charrin's disease	Pyogenic infections due to *Pseudomonas aeruginosa* that results in formation of blue pus; may cause urinary tract infections or otitis externa.	Fluoroquinolone, gentamicin, or imipenem; increased fluid intake to flush urinary tract
Chromomycosis: chromoblastomycosis	Slowly spreading fungal infection of the skin and subcutaneous tissues due to *Phialophora verrucosa*, *Fonsecaea pedrosoi*, and *Cladosporium carrioni*. Cauliflower-like lesions on the legs or arms may spread to the brain, causing an abscess.	Lesion removal with liquid nitrogen, electrocoagulation, or surgery; flucytosine alone or with ketoconazole. Itraconazole may also be effective.
Concato's disease	Causative organism is *Mycobacterium tuberculosis*. Progressive malignant polyserositis with large effusions into the pericardium, pleura, and peritoneum; associated with tuberculosis.	Thoracentesis and parenteral or oral antitubercular antibiotics, such as para-aminosalicylate and ethionamide

RARE DISEASE	CAUSE AND DESCRIPTION	TREATMENT
Dengue: breakbone or dandy fever	Group B arboviruses transmitted by female *Aedes* mosquito cause acute febrile disease that's endemic during warmer months in tropics and subtropics. Rarely fatal, unless it progresses to hemorrhagic shock syndrome.	Symptomatic management, nonaspirin analgesics, and I.V. fluid replacement
Diamond-skin disease: swine erysipelas	Acute febrile vascular disease due to *Streptococcus pyogenes;* capillary congestion follows dilation of superficial capillaries resulting from stress, inflammation, or external heat stimulation. Localized swelling and inflammation of the skin and subcutaneous tissue results.	Penicillin or erythromycin, application of cool magnesium sulfate compresses, aspirin for pain, and fluid replacement as needed
Dracunculiasis	Nonfatal infection due to *Drarunculus medinensis* (guinea worm) occurring in southern Africa and India. Worm migrates through the body causing severe pain, especially in joints. When it emerges (from the feet in 90% of cases), it causes an intensely painful edema, blister and, finally, an ulcer. After perforation, intolerable pain is followed by fever, nausea, and vomiting.	Supportive therapy
Dubois' disease: congenital syphilis	*Treponema pallidum,* a spirochete transmitted by venereal contact, causes multiple thymic abscesses in congenital syphilis.	Penicillin or, in allergic patients, oxytetracycline, chlortetracycline, or erythromycin
Dukes' disease: fourth disease	Likely caused by a viral exanthema of the coxsackievirus or echovirus group. Disease marked by myalgia, headache, fever, pharyngitis, conjunctivitis, generalized adenopathy, and desquamation following confluent raised erythema.	Symptomatic and supportive management

RARE DISEASE	CAUSE AND DESCRIPTION	TREATMENT
Durand's disease	Causative organism is *Chlamydia trachomatis*. Transient vesicles on penis or vagina frequently inflame inguinal lymph nodes.	Incision and drainage of infected lymph nodes; tetracycline
Economo's disease: lethargic encephalitis	Possibly neurotropic virus, but may be arthropod-borne virus or sequela of influenza, rubella, varicella, or vaccinia. Epidemic encephalitis marked by increasing languor, apathy, and drowsiness, progressing to lethargy; usually occurs in winter.	Symptomatic management, including appropriate antibiotics for secondary infection
Elephantiasis	Filaria, a parasitic worm, is transmitted from person-to-person by mosquitoes; endemic disease of Africa, Asia, the Western Pacific, and Latin America. Invades lymphatic system, causing dramatic swelling of limbs (usually the leg) and genitals (usually the scrotum).	Mectizan and albendazole; compression bandages to affected limbs
Engman's disease	Infectious eczematoid dermatitis caused by Staphylococci.	Topical application of corticosteroids, bath oils, lubricants, and topical antibiotics for secondary infections
Epstein-Barr disease: pseudodiphtheria, mononucleosis	Epstein-Barr virus causes classic heterophil-positive infectious mononucleosis, occasionally complicated by neurologic diseases such as encephalitis or transverse myelitis.	Symptomatic management; generally benign course
Erysipeloid	*Erysipelothrix insidiosa* transmitted by contact with infected meat, fish, poultry, animal hides, bones, or manure. Acute, self-limiting skin infection occurring in butchers, fishermen, and others who handle infected material; may progress to infective endocarditis if primary lesions untreated.	Penicillin G or erythromycin; cloxacillin or cephalexin for persistent cases

RARE DISEASE	CAUSE AND DESCRIPTION	TREATMENT
Erythrasma	Superficial, bacterial skin infection due to *Corynebacterium minutissimum* that usually affects the skin folds, especially in the groin, axillae, and toe webs.	Keratolytics or topical antibiotics
Fifth disease: erythema infectiosum	Human parvovirus, probably transmitted by respiratory tract. Contagious disease characterized by rose-colored eruptions diffused over the skin, usually starting on the cheeks; mainly affects children ages 4 to 10.	Symptomatic treatment. Screening of donated blood, which might prevent transfusion-related transmission, is under investigation.
Fish-slime disease	Septic substances introduced into blood through puncture wound. Rapidly progressive septicemia following a puncture wound by the spine of a fish.	Supportive and symptomatic management of septicemia and secondary infections
Filariasis	Tropical infection of round, thread-like parasitic worms of *Wuchereria bancrofti, Brugia malayi,* or *B. timori* transmitted by mosquitoes; rarely fatal. Tissue damage caused by the worms restricts the normal flow of lymph fluid and results in swelling, scarring, and infections, mostly in the legs and groin. Severe disfigurement, decreased mobility, and long-term disability results.	Albendazole with diethylcarbamazine or ivermectin; prevention of opportunistic bacterial and fungal "superinfection"; hygiene and compression to affected limbs
Friedländer's disease: endarteritis obliterans	Trauma, pyogenic bacterial infection, infective thrombi, or syphilis. Chronic progressive thickening of the intima, leading to stenosis or obstruction of the lumen.	Endarterectomy
Geotrichosis	Fungal infection due to *Geotrichum candidum* that affects the mouth, throat, lungs, or intestines.	Gentian violet for oral, throat, or intestinal infections; oral potassium iodide for pulmonary infections

RARE DISEASE	CAUSE AND DESCRIPTION	TREATMENT
Habermann's disease	Unknown, possibly viral. Sudden onset of a polymorphous skin eruption of macules, papules and, occasionally, vesicles, with hemorrhage.	Supportive therapy; topical steroids, light therapy, antibiotics, and antihistamines
Heavy-chain disease	Possibly caused by microorganisms and immune deficiency syndrome due to malnutrition or genetic predisposition. Neoplasms of the lymphoplasmacytes, in which abnormal proliferation occurs among cells that produce immunoglobulins, causes incomplete heavy chains and no light chains in their molecular structure.	Supportive and palliative therapy with chemotherapy, radiation therapy, antibiotics, and steroids
Heubner's disease	*Treponema pallidum* causes a syphilitic inflammation of tunica intima of cerebral arteries.	Supportive therapy, including antibiotic therapy
Hutinel's disease	*Mycobacterium tuberculosis* causes tuberculous pericarditis, with cirrhosis of the liver in children.	Tuberculostatic agents
Hydatid disease, alveolar	*Echinococcus multilocularis* (larvae) infection is characterized by invasion and destruction of tissue by cysts, which undergo endogenous budding and form an aggregate of innumerable small cysts that honeycomb the affected organ — usually the liver — and may metastasize.	Symptomatic management and surgery; usually fatal
Hydatid disease, unilocular	Infestation by *Echinococcus granulosus* (larvae); hydatid tapeworm in dogs and cats causes marked formation of single or multiple unilocular cysts	Surgery, drug therapy with albendazole or mebendazole

RARE DISEASE	CAUSE AND DESCRIPTION	TREATMENT
Iceland disease: epidemic neuromyasthenia, benign myalgic encephalomyelitis	Probably infection but possibly psychosocial phenomenon. Marked by headaches, muscle pain, low-grade fever, lymphadenopathy, fatigue, and paresthesia; outbreaks occur in summert, usually in young women.	Symptomatic management
Isambert's disease	Acute miliary tuberculosis of the larynx and pharynx, probably caused by infection but possibly psychosocial phenomenon.	Tuberculostatic agents
Jaksch's disease: anemia pseudoleukemica infantum	Malnutrition, chronic infection, malabsorption, hemoglobinopathies. Syndrome of anisocytosis, peripheral red blood cell immaturity, leukocytosis, and hepatosplenomegaly that usually occurs in children under age 3	Treatment of underlying causes
Kawasaki disease: Mucocutaneous lymph node syndrome	Viral or bacterial cause unknown; rarely fatal. Illness in children characterized by fever, rash, swollen hands and feet, irritation and redness of the sclera, swollen lymph glands in the neck, and irritation and inflammation of the mouth, lips and throat.	Aspirin to reduce fever, rash, joint inflammation, and pain, and to help prevent formation of blood clots. Early treatment with gamma globulin may decrease risk of developing coronary artery abnormalities.
Kuru	Slow virus or possibly prion associated with cannibalism causes a chronic, progressive, and fatal neurologic disease found only in New Guinea.	No effective treatment; invariably fatal
Lewandowsky-Lutz disease: epidermodysplasia verruciformis	Opportunistic virus associated with an autosomal recessive disorder causes widespread red or red-violet lesions resembling verruca plana; lesions have tendency to become malignant.	Ablative techniques, topical retinoids, or 5-FU

RARE DISEASE	CAUSE AND DESCRIPTION	TREATMENT
Loiasis: Loa loa (African eyeworm)	*Loa loa,* a filarial nematode that occurs in the rain forest and swamp forest areas of West Africa, is transmitted to humans by biting *Chrysops* flies where larvae mature to adults. Adult worm may migrate to the eye and may be seen moving slowly across surface of conjunctiva and cornea of the eye or bridge of the nose. Immune reactions to the migrating worms may cause calabar swellings in the arms and legs. Recurrent swelling can lead to painful cystlike enlargements of the connective tissues around the tendon sheaths. Dying worms may cause chronic abscesses followed by granulomatous reactions and fibrosis. Infection is only fatal if worms migrate to the brain and cause encephalitis.	Diethylcarbamazine or ivermectin
Ludwig's angina	Abscesses of the second and third mandibular molars usually cause infection of the sublingual and submandibular spaces that is characterized by brawny induration of the submaxillary region, edema of the sublingual floor of the mouth, and elevation of the tongue.	Significant airway obstruction may require tracheotomy. Antibiotics such as nafcillin are effective against streptococci and staphylococci.
Lung fluke disease: Paragonimus westermani, Paragonimus heterotrema	Infestation by trematodes or flukes cause parasitic hemoptysis, or oriental hemoptysis from pulmonary cysts.	Parasitotropic agents, symptomatic and supportive management of hemoptysis
Magitot's disease	Osteoperiostitis of the alveoli of the teeth occurs, usually secondary to gingivitis	Steroid therapy for extreme inflammation, antibiotics for secondary infection

RARE DISEASE	CAUSE AND DESCRIPTION	TREATMENT
Marburg disease: Marburg virus disease	Exposure to African green monkeys may result in severe viral disease that is characterized by skin lesions, conjunctivitis, enteritis, hepatitis, encephalitis, and renal failure.	Symptomatic and supportive management; usually fatal
Mushroom picker's disease	Airborne irritant, usually mold: *Micropolyspora faeni* or *Thermoactinomycoces vulgaris*. Allergic respiratory disease of persons working with moldy compost prepared for growing mushrooms.	Supportive and symptomatic management
Mycetoma: maduromycosis, Madura foot	*Allescheria boydii* or *Actinomycetales* bacteria or fungi causes chronic infection of the skin, subcutaneous tissues, and bone, usually affecting the foot.	Sulfonamides, streptomycin, itraconazole, or ketoconazole
Neurocycticercosis	*Parastrongylus cantonensis* is transmitted by ingestion of raw or improperly cooked mollusks; disease is endemic in Hawaii, Pacific islands, Vietnam, Thailand, China, and Indonesia. Invasion of the meninges causes severe headache, stiffness of neck and back, and paresthesias; rarely fatal.	No specific treatment
Onchocerciasis: blinding filarial disease, river blindness, Robles' disease	*Onchocerca volvulus* infects the skin and subcutaneous tissue; transmission is by bite of female black fly, which in Africa belongs to the *Simulium damnosum* species complex; less frequently found in the Americas and Yemen. Initial symptoms include fatigue and headache, then progresses to wrinkled, itchy skin and, finally, blindness.	Annual doses of ivermectin

RARE DISEASE	CAUSE AND DESCRIPTION	TREATMENT
Paracoccidioido-mycosis: South American blastomycosis	Fungal infection of the skin, lungs, mucous membranes, lymphatics, and viscera, due to *Paracoccidioides brasiliensis;* occurrs primarily in the tropical forests of South America and Mexico.	Ketoconazole, itraconazole, or fluconazole
Q fever	Acute systemic disease due to *Coxiella burnetii* that strikes people exposed to infected cattle, sheep, or goats.	Tetracycline (doxycycline, co-trimoxazole, or rifampin) for endocarditis; possible valve replacement
Rat-bite fever: sodoku	Gram-negative bacterial infection due to *Streptobacillus moniliformis* or *Spirillum minor* that occurs 1 to 3 weeks after bite from an infected rat or mouse.	Penicillin G procaine, tetracycline, or streptomycin
Rhinosporidiosis	Fungal infection due to *Rhinosporidium seeberi* that produces painless, vascularized, friable, and often large tumor-like lesions; most common in Ceylon and India.	Electrocauterization or surgical excision, followed by dapsone
Rickettsialpox	*Rickettsia akari,* transmitted by bites of mites carried by infected mice, causes a mild, self-limiting disease characterized by lesions and fever.	Tetracycline or chloramphenicol, antipyretics, analgesics, and increased fluid intake
Saint Louis encephalitis	A group B arbovirus, transmitted by *Culex* mosquitoes; disease occurs in late summer and early fall. Severity varies in range and occurrence is strongly age-dependent; people over age 60 are at most risk. Severe cases suffer long-term residual neurologic sequelae; may include paralysis, memory loss, or deterioration of fine motor skills.	Supportive therapy

RARE DISEASE	CAUSE AND DESCRIPTION	TREATMENT
Sponge-diver's disease: sponge dermatitis	Irritation by toxins of sea anemones of the *Sagartia* and *Actinia* genera causes burning, itching, erythema, necrosis, and ulceration of skin; common in Mediterranean divers.	Symptomatic management, including local application of calamine lotion and administration of antihistamines for hives and itching
Toxocariasis: visceral larva migrans	Ingestion of *Toxocara* larvae, usually from dirt, results in chronic, frequently mild syndrome common in children, involving roundworm migration from the intestine to various organs and tissues; characterized by hepatosplenomegaly and eosinophilia.	Diethylcarbamazine, mebendazole, albendazole, or ivermectin
Trench fever: Wolhynia fever, shin bone fever, His-Werner disease, quintana fever	*Rochalimaea quintana* transmitted by body lice causes a self-limiting illness occurring sporadically in Eastern Europe, Asia, North Africa, and Mexico, and produces multiple symptoms.	Analgesics, antipyretics, and delousing with lindane or other pediculicide
Trichuriasis: whipworm disease	Ingestion of food contaminated with *Trichuris* causes nematode infection of the cecum and the anterior parts of the large intestine, producing various GI effects.	Mebendazole or albendazole
Tropical sprue	GI disorder that causes atrophy of the small intestine, resulting in malabsorption, malnutrition, and folic acid deficiency; characterized by bulky, pale, frothy stools with increased fecal fat and macrocytic anemia. Occurs mainly in Puerto Rico, Cuba, Haiti, Hong Kong, and India; cause unknown.	Tetracycline or oxytetracycline, phthalylsulfathiazole, diphenoxylate with atropine sulfate, folic acid

RARE DISEASE	CAUSE AND DESCRIPTION	TREATMENT
Tularemia: deer fly fever, rabbit fever, Ohara's disease (in Japan)	*Francisella tularensis* is transmitted by contact with secretions of an infected animal; by the bite of a tick, deer fly, or flea that feeds on these animals; or by ingestion of contaminated water or meat. Acute, gram-negative infection that has five forms — ulceroglandular, oculoglandular, typhoidal (enteric), oropharyngeal (pneumonic), and glandular — each with varying symptoms.	Streptomycin with tetracycline or chloramphenicol
Typhus, endemic: murine, rat, or flea typhus	*Rickettsia typhi* transmitted by bites of infected fleas or lice or by inhalation of contaminated flea feces causes a mild form of typhus; systemic illness characterized by fever, headache, rash, and myalgia.	Tetracycline, doxycycline, or chloramphenicol; analgesics; antipyretics
Typhus, epidemic: European, classic, or louse-borne typhus	*Rickettsia prowazekii* transmitted by *Pediculus humanus trichiura* causes an acute systemic illness that may be fatal.	Tetracycline, doxycycline, or chloramphenicol; analgesics; antipyretics; delousing with lindane or other pediculicide
Typhus, scrub: Japanese river or flood fever, tsutsugamushi fever	*Rickettsia tsutsugamushi* transmitted by mite larvae causes an acute systemic disease that occurs almost exclusively in the western Pacific, Japan, and Southeast Asia.	Chloramphenicol or tetracycline
Tyzzer's disease	*Bacillus piliformis* transmitted through contact with rodents or dogs causes necrotic lesions of liver and intestine.	Symptomatic management and appropriate antibiotics

RARE DISEASE	CAUSE AND DESCRIPTION	TREATMENT
Venezuelan equine encephalomyelitis	Mosquito-borne Togaviridae, alphavirus from infected horses in South and Central America, Mexico, Florida, and Texas caues healthy adults to experience flulike symptoms, such as high fever, headache, loss of appetite, weakness, and eventually CNS disorders. Severe illness or death may occur in the young, the elderly, or patients with weakened immune systems.	Supportive therapy
Verneuil's disease	Syphilitic disease of the bursae due to *Treponema pallidum*.	Early treatment of syphilis
***Vibrio vulnificus* septicemia**	*Vibrio vulnificans* causes an overwhelming sepsis in a cirrhotic patient who has ingested oysters; typically affects men over age 40 in coastal states between May and October.	Tetracycline, chloramphenicol, or penicillin
Wegner's disease	Osteochondritic separation of the epiphyses due to congenital syphilis.	Effective treatment of syphilis during pregnancy
Whipple's disease: intestinal lipodystrophy, lipophagia granulomatosis	GI malabsorption disorder due to *Trophenyma whippelii*; characterized by chronic diarrhea and progressive wasting.	Co-trimoxazole, penicillin G procaine with streptomycin
Yaws: frambesia tropica	Chronic relapsing infection due to *Treponema pertenue*; characterized by lesions and systemic signs and symptoms.	Penicillin in aluminum monostearate 2%, oxytetracycline, or chlortetracycline
Yellow fever	Flavivirus transmitted by the *Aedes* mosquito. Infection causes sudden illness accompanied by fever, slow pulse rate, and headache; endemic in tropical Africa and Central and South America.	High-protein, high-carbohydrate liquid diet; analgesics; sedatives; antipyretics; bed rest; fluids to maintain adequate blood volume

RARE DISEASE	CAUSE AND DESCRIPTION	TREATMENT
Zygomycosis: phycomycosis, mucormycosis	Fungal infection due to Zygomycetes that commonly occurs in immunocompromised patients; several forms, including rhinocerebral, GI, pulmonary, and disseminated mucormycosis.	Amphotericin B, surgical removal of necrotic tissue

APPENDIX B:
REPORTABLE INFECTIOUS DISEASES

Disease reporting laws vary from state to state. Local agencies report certain diseases to state health departments, which determine which diseases are reported to the Centers for Disease Control and Prevention. Reportable infectious diseases include:

- acquired immunodeficiency syndrome
- amebiases
- animal bites
- anthrax (cutaneous or pulmonary)
- arbovirus
- aseptic meningitis
- botulism
- brucellosis
- campylobacteriosis
- chancroid
- chlamydial infections
- cholera
- diarrhea of the newborn (epidemic)
- diptheria (cutaneous or pharyngeal)
- encephalitis (postinfectious or primary)
- food poisoning
- gastroenteritis (hospital outbreak)
- giardiasis
- gonococcal infections
- gonorrhea
- group A beta-hemolytic streptococcal infections (including scarlet fever)
- Guillain-Barre syndrome
- hepatitis (types A, B, C and unspecified)
- histoplasmosis
- influenza
- Kawasaki disease
- lead poisoning
- *Legionella* infections (Legionnaires' disease)
- leprosy
- leptospirosis
- listeriosis
- Lyme disease
- lymphogranuloma venereum
- malaria
- measles
- meningitis
- meningococcal disease
- mumps
- neonatal hypothyroidism
- pertussis
- phenylketonuria
- plague
- poliomyelitis
- psittacosis
- rabies
- Reye's syndrome
- rheumatic fever
- rickettsial diseases (including Rocky Mountain spotted fever)
- rubella and congenital rubella syndrome
- salmonellosis (excluding typhoid fever)
- shigellosis
- staphylococcal infections (neonatal)
- syphilis (congenital)
- syphilis (primary or secondary)
- tetanus
- toxic shock syndrome
- toxoplasmosis
- trichinosis
- tuberculosis
- tularemia, typhoid, and paratyphoid fever
- typhus
- varicella
- yellow fever

ALTERNATIVE THERAPIES FOR SELECTED INFECTIONS

HERBAL AGENT	REPORTED USE	DOSE
Chaparral Creosote bush, greasewood, *Hediondilla*	Tea derived from plant leaves; widely used by Native Americans for treatment of bronchitis, colds, skin disorders, and pain. Human clinical trials confirming anticancer properties are lacking.	No consensus exists. Daily consumption of tea recommended.
Cloves Caryophyllum, *Eugenia aromatica*, oil of cloves, oleum caryophylli	Oil used topically for treatment of toothache; also added to mouth washes as an antiseptic. Some in vitro data have confirmed its anti-inflammatory and antimicrobial activity.	Dose varies depending on product. *Fluid extract:* 5 to 30 drops. *Oil extract:* 1 to 5 drops. *Oral mouth rinse containing clove oil:* ¼ to 1 oz.
Cranberry Bog cranberry, isokarpalo (Finland), marsh apple, mountain cranberry, pikkukarpalo (Finland), small cranberry	Proposed as a nonantibiotic, preventive treatment for urinary tract infections (UTIs), cranberry has a 100-year history of being used to prevent recurrent UTI. In animals, cranberry juice significantly inhibited bacterial adherence in urine. Human clinical trials are promising. Although anticancer properties have been proposed by Europeans, well-designed trials are lacking. Cranberry is thought to help urostomy patients with skin irritations from urine, and has also been used in patients with drug overdoses to help urinary excretion of phencyclidine.	Most studies used 10 to 16 oz juice P.O. daily or 1 to 2 capsules of concentrate P.O. daily.

HERBAL AGENT	REPORTED USE	DOSE
Juniperus communis A'ra'r a'di, ardic, baccal juniper, common juniper, dwarf, gemener, genievre, ground juniper, hackmatack, harvest, horse savin, juniper mistletoe, *Juniperi fructus*, yoshu-nezu, zimbro	Used traditionally for treatment of kidney infections, a decoction of *J. communis* branch with berries is still used in some parts of the world. Plant was considered an adjuvant to diuretics in the relief of dropsy due to tubular kidney obstruction. Diluted fresh berry juice is believed to be an effective diuretic for children. Although *Juniper* is considered a diuretic, there are no confirming studies. Native Americans used bruised inner bark of plant to relieve the odor of putrid-smelling wounds. Because of its antiflatulent properties, oil has been used for flatulence and colic.	Dosage varies. *For hypoglycemic activity,* in vivo doses ranged between 250 to 500 mg/kg every 24 hours. *For anti-inflammatory activity,* in vitro studies used 0.2 mg/ml. *For antimicrobial activity,* in vitro studies used 20 mg/ml. *For flatulence and colic,* 0.05 to 0.2 ml of juniper oil.
Marjoram Common marjoram, knotted marjoram, oleum majoranae (oil), oregano, sweet marjoram, wild marjoram	Dried leaves and flowering tops of marjoram plant used mainly in cooking. Although labeled as oregano, it has a milder flavor. Medicinally, it has been used as an antidote for snakebite and for treatment of muscle and joint pain, bruises, nausea, infant colic, cough, headache, insomnia, motion sickness, menstrual cramps, amenorrhea, conjunctivitis, and certain cancers. *O. majorana* and *O. vulgare* have been used to stimulate digestion and prevent flatulence.	*Tea:* steep 1 to 2 teaspoons of dried leaves and flower tops for 10 minutes in 1 cup of boiling water; no more than 3 cups should be taken P.O. daily. Alternatively, three doses of ¼ to 1 teaspoon of tincture P.O. daily.

HERBAL AGENT	REPORTED USE	DOSE
Oregano Mountain mint, origanum, wild marjoram	Used as a mild tonic, diaphoretic, and menstrual stimulant and as flavoring agent and preservative in the kitchen. Oregano's antibacterial and antioxidant properties have led to its recommended use in superficial and systemic infections.	*As a dietary supplement,* 2 capsules P.O. once or twice daily, preferably with meals; or add few drops of oil of oregano to milk or juice. *For topical use,* apply oil of oregano directly to affected region once or twice daily. As a shampoo, add small amount of oil of oregano to commercial shampoo. After shampooing, allow it to remain for a few minutes, then rinse hair. Add to pump soaps and use during showering and hand washing as an antiseptic cleanser.
Pill-bearing spurge Asthma weed, catshair, euphorbia, garden spurge, milkweed, queensland asthmaweed, snake weed	Therapeutic claims include treatment of asthma, hay fever, coughs, bronchitis, diarrhea, dysentery, intestinal amebiasis, gonorrhea, thrush, snakebites, and ophthalmic disorders.	*Dried plant:* 120 to 300 mg P.O. or by infusion P.O. t.i.d. *Liquid extract (1:1 in 45% alcohol):* 0.12 to 0.3 ml P.O. t.i.d. *Tincture (1:5 in 60% alcohol):* 0.6 to 2 ml P.O t.i.d.
Pomegranate Granatum	Claimed to be useful as an anthelmintic; also used as an antidiarrheal in Asia and South America. Although in vitro studies appear to support these uses, human clinical trials are lacking.	No consensus exists. Infusions (tea) or extracts of plant parts are often the source of pomegranate studied during in vitro studies.

HERBAL AGENT	REPORTED USE	DOSE
Sage Dalmatian, garden sage, meadow sage, scarlet sage, tree sage	Used as an astringent, antioxidant, and antispasmodic; also claimed to be therapeutic for dysmenorrhea, diarrhea, gastritis, sore throats, gingivitis, and galactorrhea. However, supporting clinical trial data are lacking. Sage has been used for many years as a food flavoring and fragrance for soaps and perfumes. It is listed by the Council of Europe as a natural source of food flavoring.	*For sore throat,* 1 to 4 g leaf as a gargle P.O. t.i.d. *For menstrual disorders,* 1 to 4 ml leaf extract (1:1 in 45% alcohol) P.O. t.i.d.
Tea tree Australian tea tree oil, *Melaleuca alternifolia,* melaleuca oil, tea tree oil	Oil has long been used as a local antiseptic; Australian aborigines used it for burns, cuts, insect bites, and athlete's foot, among other disorders. Some studies indicate that oil is promising as a treatment for skin problems, including acne, eczema, lice infestation, furuncles, psoriasis, wound infections, vaginal candidiasis, chronic cystitis, and bacterial and fungal infections of the skin and oral mucosa. Melaleuca oil has been compared with tolnaftate and clotrimazole solution for various skin conditions with some effect. It has also been studied against 5% benzoyl peroxide for the treatment of acne vulgaris. More research is needed to prove its value in the treatment of skin infections, acne, and vaginal infections.	*For topical use,* oil applied locally in concentrations from 0.4% to 100%, depending on type of product and nature and location of skin disorder.

HERBAL AGENT	REPORTED USE	DOSE
Turmeric *Curcuma*, curcumin, Indian saffron, Indian valerian, jiang huang, radix, red valerian, tumeric	Used in cancer prevention and as a treatment adjunct. According to the American Institute for Cancer Research, curcumin prevents stomach, colon, oral, esophageal, breast, and skin cancers; it also is used in the treatment of inflammatory conditions (injuries, osteoarthritis, and rheumatoid arthritis), irritable bowel syndrome, atherosclerosis, liver disorders, cholelithiasis, GI diseases (ulcerations, gastritis, and flatulence), and in infections due to viruses, GI bacterial overgrowth, and parasitic infestation. Traditional Chinese and Indian (Ayurvedic) philosophies of medicine involve the use of turmeric for flatulence, jaundice, menstrual problems, bloody urine, hemorrhage, toothache, bruises, chest pain, and colic. Poultices of turmeric have been used to relieve local pain and inflammation.	*Curcumin:* 400 to 600 mg P.O. t.i.d. *Turmeric:* equivalent dose is 8 to 60 g P.O. t.i.d., taken on an empty stomach.

APPENDIX D:
REVISED C.D.C. ISOLATION PRECAUTIONS

To help hospitals maintain up-to-date isolation practices, the Centers for Disease Control and Prevention (CDC) and the Hospital Infection Control Practices Advisory Committee recently revised the CDC's Guideline for Isolation Precautions in Hospitals.

Standard precautions

The revised guidelines contain two tiers of precautions. The first — called standard precautions — are those designated for the care of all hospital patients regardless of their diagnosis or presumed infection. Standard precautions are the primary strategy for reducing the risk of and control-

PRECAUTIONS	INDICATIONS
Standard precautions	All patients regardless of diagnosis or presumed infection
Airborne precautions (used in addition to standard precautions)	Patients known to have or suspected of having a serious illness transmitted by airborne droplet nuclei, such as: ▶ measles ▶ varicella ▶ tuberculosis
Droplet precautions (used in addition to standard precautions)	Patients known to have or suspected of having a serious illness transmitted by large-particle droplets, such as: ▶ invasive Haemophilus influenzae type B disease, including meningitis, pneumonia, epiglottitis, and sepsis ▶ invasive Neisseria meningitidis disease, including meningitis, pneumonia, and sepsis ▶ other serious viral infections spread by droplets, including: – diphtheria – mycoplasma pneumonia – pertussis – pneumonic plaque – streptococcal pharyngitis, pneumonia, or scarlet fever in infants and young children ▶ other serious viral infections spread by droplets, including: – adenovirus – influenza – mumps – rubella – parvovirus B19

ling nosocomial infections. They have replaced universal precautions as the standard of care. These precautions apply to:
- blood
- all body fluids, secretions, and excretions, except sweat, regardless of whether or not they contain visible blood
- skin that is not intact
- mucous membranes.

Transmission-based precautions

The second tier of precautions are known as transmission-based precautions. These precautions are instituted for patients who are known to be or suspected of being infected with a highly transmissible infection — one that needs precautions beyond those set forth in the standard precautions. There are three types of transmission-based precautions: airborne precautions, droplet precautions, and contact precautions.

Airborne precautions

Airborne precautions are designed to reduce the risk of airborne transmission of infectious agents. Microorganisms carried through the air can be dispersed widely by air currents, making them available for inhalation or deposit on a susceptible host in the same room or a longer distance away from the infected patient. Airborne pre-

PRECAUTIONS	INDICATIONS
Contact precautions (used in addition to standard precautions)	Patients known to have or suspected of having a serious illness easily transmitted by direct patient contact or by contact with items in the patient's environment. Examples of such illnesses include:
	- GI, respiratory, skin or wound infections or colonization with multidrug-resistant bacteria judged by the infection control program (based on current state, regional, or national recommendations) to be of special clinical and epidemiologic significance
	- enteric infections with a low infectious dose or prolonged environmental survival, including Clostridium difficile for diapered or incontinent patients; enterohemorrhagic Escherichia coli 0157: H7, Shigella, hepatitis A, or rotavirus•respiratory syncytial virus, parainfluenza virus, or enteroviral infections in infants and young children
	- skin infections that are highly contagious or that may occur on dry skin, including diphtheria (cutaneous), herpes simplex virus (neonatal or mucocutaneous), impetigo, major (noncontained) abscesses, cellulitis, or decubiti, pediculosis, scabies, staphylococcal furunculosis in infants and young children, and zoster (disseminated or in the immunocompromised host)
	- viral or hemorrhagic conjunctivitis
	- viral hemorrhagic infections (Ebola, Lassa, or Marburg)

cautions include special air handling and ventilation procedures to prevent the spread of infection. They require the use of respiratory protection such as a particulate respirator — in addition to standard precautions — when entering an infected patient's room.

Droplet precautions

Droplet precautions are designed to reduce the risk of transmitting infectious agents through large-particle (exceeding 5 micrometers) droplets. Such transmission involves the contact of infectious agents to the conjunctivae or to the nasal or oral mucous membranes of a susceptible person. Large-particle droplets do not remain in the air and generally travel short distances of 3 feet or less. They require the use of a mask – in addition to standard precautions — to protect the mucous membranes.

Contact precautions

Contact precautions are designed to reduce the risk of transmitting infectious agents by direct or indirect contact. Direct-contact transmission can occur through patient care activities that require physical contact. Indirect-contact transmission involves a susceptible host coming in contact with a contaminated object, usually inanimate, in the patient's environment. Contact precautions require the use of gloves, a mask, a gown, and dedicated patient care equipment (thermometer, stethoscope, and blood pressure cuff) — in addition to standard precautions— to avoid contact with the infectious agent. Stringent hand washing is also necessary after removal of the protective items. The following chart sets forth the different types of precautions and provides examples of infections for which specific precautions would be used.

Standard precautions

The CDC recommends that the following standard precautions be used for all patients. This is especially important in emergency care settings, where the risk of blood exposure is increased and the patient's infection status is usually unknown. Implementing standard precautions doesn't eliminate the need for other transmission-based precautions, such as airborne, droplet, and contact precautions.

Sources of potential exposure

Standard precautions apply to blood, semen, vaginal secretions, cerebrospinal fluid, synovial fluid, pleural fluid, peritoneal fluid, pericardial fluid, and amniotic fluid. These fluids are most likely to transmit human immunodeficiency virus (HIV). Standard precautions also apply to other body fluids — including feces, nasal secretions, saliva, sputum, tears, vomitus, urine, and breast milk.

Barrier precautions

▶ Wear gloves when touching blood and body fluids, mucous membranes, or broken skin of all patients; when handling items or touching surfaces soiled with blood or body fluids; and when performing venipuncture and other vascular access procedures.

▶ Change gloves and wash hands after contact with each patient.

▶ Wear a mask and protective eyewear or a face shield to protect mucous membranes of the mouth, nose, and eyes during procedures that may generate drops of blood or other body fluids.

▶ In addition to a mask and protective eyewear or a face shield, wear a gown or an apron during procedures that are likely to generate splashing of blood or other body fluids.

Precautions for invasive procedures

▶ Wear gloves during all invasive procedures. Also wear a surgical mask and goggles or a face shield.

▶ During procedures that commonly generate droplets or splashes of blood or other body fluids, or that generate bone chips, wear protective eyewear and a mask, or a face shield.

▶ During invasive procedures that are likely to cause splashing or splattering of blood or other body fluids, wear a gown or an impervious apron.

▶ If you perform or assist in vaginal or cesarean deliveries, wear gloves and a gown when handling the placenta or the infant and during umbilical cord care.

Work practice precautions

Prevent injuries caused by needles, scalpels, and other sharp instruments or devices when cleaning used instruments, when disposing of used needles, and when handling sharp instruments after procedures.

▶ To prevent needle-stick injuries, do not recap used needles, bend or break needles, remove them from disposable syringes or manipulate them.

▶ Place disposable syringes and needles, scalpel blades, and other sharp items in puncture-resistant containers for disposal, making sure these containers are located near the area of use.

▶ Place large-bore reusable needles in a puncture-resistant container for transport to the reprocessing area.

▶ If a glove tears or a needle-stick or other injury occurs, remove the gloves, wash your hands, and wash the site of the needle-stick thoroughly; then put on new gloves as quickly as patient safety permits. Remove the needle or instrument involved in the incident from the sterile field. Promptly report injuries and mucous-membrane exposure to the appropriate infection-control officer.

Additional precautions

▶ Use available safety devices, such as safety syringes, safety angiocatheters, and needleless I.V. systems, to reduce the risk of injury from sharp objects.

▶ Make sure mouthpieces, one-way valve masks, resuscitation bags, or other ventilation devices are available in areas where the need for resuscitation is likely.

Note: Saliva has not been implicated in HIV transmission.

▶ If you have exudative lesions or weeping dermatitis, refrain from direct patient care and handling patient care equipment until the condition resolves.

APPENDIX E: IMMUNIZATION SCHEDULE

Before an immunization, obtain the child's medication, illness, and allergy history. Instruct the parents to report a severe reaction to the vaccine to the doctor. Childhood immunizations are usually given on a fixed schedule, as follows:

AGE	IMMUNIZATION
Birth to 2 months	First dose: Hepatitis B vaccine (HBV)
1 to 4 months	Second dose: HBV[1] First dose: diphtheria-tetanus acellular-pertussis (DTaP) vaccine, inactivated polio vaccine (IPV), Haemophilus influenzae type b conjugate (Hib) vaccine
2 months	Second dose: DTaP, IPV, and Hib
4 months	Third dose: DTaP and Hib
6 months	Third dose: HBV and IPV
6 to 18 months	First dose: Measles-mumps-rubella (MMR) vaccine.
12 to 15 months	Fourth dose: Hib
12 to 18 months	Fourth dose: DTaP[2]. First dose: varicella zoster virus vaccine
4 to 6 years	Fifth dose: DTaP. Fourth dose: IPV. Second dose: MMR
11 to 12 years	MMR (if not given at age 4 to 6); varicella zoster (catchup vaccination[3])
11 to 16 years	Tetanus (booster every 10 years)

[1] The second dose of HBV is given at least 1 month after the first dose. The third dose is given at least 6 months after the second dose.
[2] A fourth dose of DTaP may be given as early as age 12 months through 18 months provided that 6 months have elapsed since the third dose. The acellular form of the vaccine can now be used for all doses in the vaccination series, even for children who started the series with standard whole-cell D vaccine.
[3] Unvaccinated children with no history of chickenpox should be vaccinated at ages 11 to 12 years.

SELECTED REFERENCES

Armstrong, D., et al. *Infectious Diseases.* Philadelphia: Mosby-Year book, 1999.

Ball, P., and Gray, J.A. *Infectious Diseases.* Philadelphia: W.B. Saunders Co., 1999.

Diseases, 3rd ed. Springhouse, Pa.: Springhouse Corp., 2000.

Fauci, A.S., et al., eds. *Harrison's Principles of Internal Medicine,* 14th ed. New York: McGraw-Hill Book Co., 1998.

Gorbach, S.L., et al. *Infectious Diseases,* 2nd ed. Philadelphia: W.B. Saunders Co., 1998.

Handbook of Diseases, 2nd ed. Springhouse, Pa.: Springhouse Corp., 1999.

Isada, C., et al. *Infectious Diseases Handbook,* 3rd ed. Hudson, Ohio: Lexi-Comp Inc., 1999.

McQuiston, J.H., et al. "The Human Ehrlichioses in the United States," *Emerging Infectious Diseases* 5(5):635-42, 1999.

Muirhead, G., et al. "Targeting Therapy for Infective Endocarditis," *Patient Care* 33(16):127-30, 133-4, 136+, Oct 15, 1999.

Nilsson, I.M., et al. "Protection Against *Staphylococcus aureus* Sepsis by Vaccination with Recombinant Staphylococcal Enterotoxin A Devoid of Superantigenicity," *Journal of Infectious Disease* 180(4):130-3, April 1999.

Professional Guide to Diseases, 6th ed. Springhouse, Pa.: Springhouse Corp., 1998.

Safety and Infection Control. Springhouse, Pa.: Springhouse Corp., 1998.

Schlossberg, D., and Shulman, J. *Differential Diagnosis of Infectious Diseases.* Philadelphia: Williams and Wilkins, 1996.

Shulman, S., et al. *The Biologic and Clinical Basis of Infectious Diseases,* 5th ed. Philadelphia: W.B. Saunders Co., 1997.

Websites

Centers for Disease Control and Prevention (2000, March). Available: http://www.cdc.gov/

Medscape, Infectious Diseases (2000, February). Available: http://id.medscape.com

National Institutes of Health (2000, February). Available: http://www.nih.gov/

National Institutes of Health (2000, March). Available: http://clinicaltrials.gov/ct/gui/c/b

SUBJECT INDEX

A

B

Note: i indicates illustration; t indicates table; c indicates color page.

Note: i indicates illustration; t indicates table; c indicates color page.

Note: i indicates illustration; t indicates table; c indicates color page.

Note: i indicates illustration; t indicates table; c indicates color page.

Note: i indicates illustration; t indicates table; c indicates color page.

Note: i indicates illustration; t indicates table; c indicates color page.

Note: i indicates illustration; t indicates table; c indicates color page.

Note: i indicates illustration; t indicates table; c indicates color page.

Note: i indicates illustration; t indicates table; c indicates color page.

DRUG INDEX